Adventures in Medical Research

ADVENTURES
IN MEDICAL RESEARCH

A Century
of Discovery at
Johns Hopkins

A. McGehee Harvey

THE JOHNS HOPKINS
UNIVERSITY PRESS
BALTIMORE AND
LONDON

SUPPLEMENT TO THE JOHNS HOPKINS MEDICAL JOURNAL

Manufactured in the United States of America

The Johns Hopkins University Press, Baltimore, Maryland 21218
The Johns Hopkins University Press Ltd., London

Portions of this book have previously appeared in the *Johns Hopkins Medical Journal*.

Library of Congress Catalog Card Number 75-36955
ISBN 0-8018-1785-4

Contents

Preface   xi

Acknowledgments   xv

1. A Century of Clinical Science at Johns Hopkins: Contributions to Medicine by Students, House Officers, and Faculty   1
2. Pioneers in Urology: James R. Brown and Howard A. Kelly   8
3. Medical Students on the March: Brown, MacCallum, and Opie   18
4. Two Mycoses First Described at Johns Hopkins   32
5. Teacher and Distinguished Pupil: William Henry Welch and George Hoyt Whipple   39
6. Pharmacology's Giant: John Jacob Abel   49
7. Neurosurgical Genius: Walter Edward Dandy   60
8. Early Contributions to the Surgery of Cancer: William S. Halsted, Hugh H. Young, and John G. Clark   69
9. Fountainhead of American Physiology: H. Newell Martin and His Pupil William Henry Howell   84
10. A New School of Anatomy: The Story of Franklin P. Mall, Florence R. Sabin, and John B. MacCallum   97
11. Johns Hopkins—The Birthplace of Tissue Culture: The Story of Ross G. Harrison, Warren H. Lewis, and George O. Gey   114
12. Creators of Clinical Medicine's Scientific Base: Franklin Paine Mall, Lewellys Franklin Barker, and Rufus Cole   124
13. Compleat Clinician and Renaissance Pathologist: Louis Hamman and Arnold R. Rich   139
14. Classical Descriptions of Disease   152
15. The Second Professor of Gynecology and the Department of Art as Applied to Medicine   173
16. John Whitridge Williams—His Contributions to Obstetrics   188
17. The First Full-time Academic Department of Pediatrics: The Story of the Harriet Lane Home   195
18. Johns Hopkins—Its Role in Medical Education for Women   225
19. Contributions of the Part-time Staff of The Johns Hopkins Hospital: Moore, King, and Gay   248
20. Cardiovascular Research at Johns Hopkins   261
21. Hematological Firsts at Hopkins   288
22. Research at Johns Hopkins on the Thyroid Gland and Its Diseases   314
23. More Bright Stars in the Johns Hopkins Galaxy   333
24. Johns Hopkins and Biomedical Communication   364

25. The Story of Chemotherapy at Johns Hopkins: Perrin H. Long,
    Eleanor A. Bliss, and E. Kennerly Marshall, Jr.   390
26. Discoveries at Johns Hopkins Related to the Nervous System and
    Its Diseases   401
    References   425
    Name Index   451
    Subject Index   456
    About the Author— A. McGehee Harvey and Scientific Clinical
    Medicine, by Richard J. Johns, M.D.   461

Illustrations

Thomas Henry Huxley   3
John Shaw Billings   3
Howard A. Kelly   13
James R. Brown   13
Eugene L. Opie   25
William George MacCallum   25
Pithotomy Club founders   25
Thomas Caspar Gilchrist   34
Benjamin Robinson Schenck   34
William Henry Welch in 1884   44
"The Welch and Nuttall Gas Plant"   44
The Pathological Building   44
A laboratory in the Pathological Building   44
"Some Welch Rabbits"   45
Staff of the Department of Pathology, 1908–1909   45
John Timothy Geraghty   55
Leonard George Rowntree   55
John Jacob Abel   55
Walter Edward Dandy   63
Walter Edward Dandy at play   63
Hugh Hampton Young   77
John Goodrich Clark   77
William Stewart Halsted in 1922   77
First surgical operation for which the operator
    wore gloves, 1893   77
H. Newell Martin   88
William Henry Howell   88
Biological Laboratory   89
Jay McLean   89
Florence Rena Sabin   105
John Bruce MacCallum   105
Franklin Paine Mall   105
George Otto Gey   117
Ross Granville Harrison   117
Warren Harmon Lewis   117
Arthur D. Hirschfelder   131
Lewellys F. Barker   131

Carl Voegtlin   131
Rufus Cole   131
George S. Bond   131
Louis Hamman   145
Arnold R. Rich and Louis Hamman   145
Arnold R. Rich at work in his laboratory   145
Augustus Roi Felty   162
Frank Alexander Evans   162
Chester Scott Keefer   162
William Osler, W. W. Francis, William S.
    Thayer, and H. A. LaFleur   163
Thomas Peck Sprunt   163
Warfield Theobald Longcope   163
Max Broedel   177
Thomas S. Cullen   177
William Wood Russell   185
Richard W. TeLinde   185
An operation by W. W. Russell   185
J. Whitridge Williams   191
The nursery in the Department of Obstetrics, 1903   191
John F. Howland   201
William David Booker   201
Kenneth D. Blackfan   201
William McKim Marriott   201
James Lawder Gamble   218
Benjamin Kramer   218
Lawson Wilkins and the "Boys," 1963   218
Paul G. Shipley   219
Edwards Albert Park   219
Lawson Wilkins   219
Patients with Hodgkin's disease studied by
    Dorothy Reed   234
House officers of the Johns Hopkins Hospital,
    1901   234
Helen Brooke Taussig   235
Philip S. Hench and Caroline Bedell Thomas   235
Mary Ellen Avery   235
Joseph Earle Moore   253
Leslie N. Gay   253
John Theodore King, Jr.   253
Joseph Erlanger   267
Theodore C. Janeway   267
Edward Perkins Carter   267
William Sydney Thayer   267
E. Cowles Andrus and Richard S. Ross   278
William Hofmeyr Craib   278

William B. Kouwenhoven   279
Vivian Thomas   279
Richard J. Bing   279
Alfred Blalock   279
William Lorenzo Moss   300
Mildred C. Clough   300
John Auer   301
Irving J. Sherman   301
Verne Rheem Mason   301
Charles A. Janeway and A. McGehee Harvey   307
Maxwell M. Wintrobe   307
Regina Weistock   307
Julia B. Mackenzie   321
Bruce Peck Webster   321
Alan Mason Chesney   321
Cosmo G. Mackenzie   321
William F. Rienhoff, Jr.   321
Jonas Friedenwald   348
John Eager Howard   348
W. Barry Wood, Jr.   348
George W. Thorn   349
Curt P. Richter   349
Henry E. Sigerist   381
Henry Mills Hurd   381
The original library and the residents' reading
    room, Johns Hopkins Hospital, 1903   381
Eleanor A. Bliss   393
Perrin H. Long   393
E. Kennerly Marshall, Jr.   393
Howard A. Howe and David Bodian   412
Philip Bard   412
Frank Rodolph Ford   412
Joseph L. Lilienthal, Jr., and Richard Riley   412
Isabel Morgan   413
Stephen W. Kuffler   413
Poliomyelitis research group   413

Figures

Dr. Brown's modification of the cystoscope, 1893   13

The double-contoured spore   34

The fungus *Sporotrichum Schenckii*   35

Apparatus of "vividiffusion"   55

Blood supply of the pituitary body   63

New method of studying the mammalian heart,
   1895   88

Two views of the same nerve fiber   117

The heart station, 1909   130

Electrocardiogram, complete heart block, 1909   130

Phonocardiogram, systolic murmur, 1909   130

The "blue navel," 1919   176

The operation for exophthalmic or hyperplastic
   goiter, 1917   176

Drawing of the ear by Max Broedel   177

A drawing of the skull by Dr. Harvey Cushing   181

Aberrant portions of the Müllerian duct found in
   an ovary, 1899   184

Reed-Sternberg cell   234

Electrocardiogram taken by Einthoven, 1902   267

The doublet concept in heart function   278

Demonstration of the cold auto-agglutinin   301

Preface

RESEARCH IS DEFINED by Webster as "investigation or experimentation aimed at the discovery and interpretation of facts, revision of accepted theories or laws in the light of new facts, or practical application of such new or revised theories or laws." At the time of the industrial revolution, and more clearly during the twentieth century, research achieved firm status as a major contributor to social and economic welfare.

Research as a principal concern of medical schools and their associated hospitals received an important supporter with the opening of the Johns Hopkins Hospital. At that time John Shaw Billings commented on the widespread hope and expectation that the new Johns Hopkins Institutions would endeavor "to produce investigators as well as practitioners, to give to the world men who can not only sail by the old charts, but who can make new and better ones for the use of others."

The Johns Hopkins Hospital opened its doors in 1889, and the Johns Hopkins School of Medicine began the instruction of its first class a little over four years later, in October 1893. Thus the history of these two great institutions has paralleled that of the century in which the greatest progress has been made in the advance of medical science and the treatment and prevention of the diseases affecting man. Early members of the hospital staff and the medical school faculty played a major role in bringing the new scientific approaches and the new era of experimental medical science to this country from Germany. What took place in Baltimore from 1889 onward was a revolutionary change in medical education, important contributions to the medical sciences, and the evolution of a new member of the medical team who has come to occupy a position interposed between the basic scientist and the practicing physician—the clinical scientist or clinical investigator.

Welch, Mall, and others on the original faculty stressed the importance to medicine of science, of scientific methods, of scientific thinking and techniques of expression. They recognized the need for laboratories and strove to provide career opportunities for talented young men motivated to become full-time medical scientists. It has been said that Welch's greatest contribution to medical education was his insistence on the importance of the medical sciences.

Members of the Johns Hopkins medical community, as we shall see, made vital contributions to many of the outstanding medical research accomplishments of the past century, including the development of chemotherapy in the treatment of infectious diseases, the development of an effective vaccine against poliomyelitis, the emergence of cardiac surgery, and the evolution of cell culture as an important technique for medical research.

Great research contributions do not come about overnight as the brainchild
of a single individual. The process is one of steps, with a series of discoveries by
different individuals, often as the result of research done merely for the sake of
seeking out the truth rather than specifically related to the area of concern represented by the ultimate practical triumph. Finally, one scientist supplies the last
research result, which represents the breakthrough to a practical, clinically applicable discovery. Much had to be done over many years, for example, before Salk
and Sabin brought their poliomyelitis vaccine research to the long-sought stage
of practicality, and dozens of pieces of information had to be accumulated before
open heart surgery became a reality.

A superficial survey of the evidence indicates that basic undirected research
is the foundation on which the discoveries relating to the prevention, diagnosis,
and treatment of disease are based, but a more careful evaluation of the way in
which discoveries come about is important to provide confirmatory evidence of
this conclusion. Dr. Julius H. Comroe, Jr., and Dr. Robert D. Dripps have been
conducting "research on research" in an effort to demonstrate how clinical advances of practical importance evolve. Their first step was to consult a group of
physicians and surgeons as to the most important clinical advances made in the
past thirty years. The following achievements related to advances in the cardio-
vascular-pulmonary area were given the highest priority: open heart surgery;
cardiac resuscitation, defibrillation, cardioversion, pacing; intensive cardiovascular
and respiratory care; chemotherapy and antibiotics; vascular surgery; medical
treatment of coronary insufficiency; oral diuretics; new diagnostic methods; drug
treatment of hypertension; and prevention of poliomyelitis. Many of the discoveries relevant to these major research accomplishments were made at Johns Hopkins. Thse various achievements, among many others, will be described in these
essays, and although a systematic study of the type now under way by Comroe
and Dripps is not possible, the way in which the discovery came about will be
indicated.

The contributions to our basic and clinical knowledge of medicine and
surgery that have been made at Johns Hopkins serve well to emphasize what
must be the major concern of a true university—creative scholarship. Alan Gregg
gave the unique spirit of creative scholarship at Johns Hopkins a special and
meaningful name in 1950, when he made the following statement:

I suggest that something extraordinarily precious comes out of the close but entirely
free association of really superior people. To this emergent quality I give the name—
the heritage of excellence, mostly because it lasts so long and because it never comes
from, nor appeals to, mediocrities.
. . . What more do men of superior character and capacity require for their association than freedom, responsibility and expectation? The wisdom of the university is
to provide those three—freedom, responsibility and expectation. It is the interaction of
such men that attracts great young men, leads to great living and itself lives on long
afterwards as a heritage of excellence ready at any time to burst into bloom again.

These essays will demonstrate that a true heritage of excellence exists when
every member of the medical environment has this keen sense of inquiry—the
drive to develop new knowledge and to advance in every way our resources for

alleviating and preventing illness in man. The discoveries presented were not made by professors alone, but by residents, interns, students, and technicians as well—all a vital part of what Gregg labeled "the heritage of excellence." Moreover, these discoveries are only samples chosen from a total number of contributions far too numerous to be included in a single volume; many important ones have not been mentioned. The author hopes that others will ultimately make the recording of all these research accomplishments complete. For the most part, research done after 1947 has not been included. Significant research accomplishments at Hopkins during the past twenty-five years will be presented in the next volume of the history of the Johns Hopkins Medical Institutions.

Acknowledgments

MY DEEP APPRECIATION goes to Ms. Carol Bocchini for her expert help in editing most of these essays.

Information and materials useful in the writing of this book were kindly given to me by the following: Richard W. TeLinde, the late Houston S. Everett, Mrs. Harry F. Klinefelter, Francis C. Wood, Frederick Bang, John Hanks, Kenneth Kohlstaedt, Benjamin M. Baker, Charles W. Wainwright, Dr. Katherine Sprunt, Dr. Jean Felty Kenny, Mrs. Stewart Lindsay, Mrs. Ranice Crosby, Claude Migeon, Hugh Josephs, John Whitridge, Jr., Leslie N. Gay, and Arnall Patz.

I wish to thank Ms. Susan L. Boone for permission to quote unpublished material from the biography of Dorothy Reed in the Sophia Smith Collection at Smith College.

I would also like to express my appreciation to the following for their help in reviewing parts of the manuscript: R. Carmichael Tilghman, Thomas B. Turner, Richard W. TeLinde, Owsei Temkin, Richard S. Ross, E. Cowles Andrus, John E. Howard, Mary Betty Stevens, Carol Johns, Harold Harrison, Claude Migeon, C. Lockard Conley, Frank Walsh, A. E. Maumenee, Patrick Murphy, William R. Bell, R. Robinson Baker, Hugh J. Jewett, David Bodian, Philip Bard, Stephen Kuffler, and Irwin Pollack.

1 ❧ A Century of Clinical Science at Johns Hopkins: Contributions to Medicine by Students, House Officers, and Faculty

To give to the world men who can not only sail by the old charts, but who can make new and better ones for the use of others.—John Shaw Billings

ONE OF THE IMPORTANT events associated with the opening of the Johns Hopkins University was the address delivered on September 12, 1876, by Thomas H. Huxley. The address was given under rather difficult circumstances. The day prior to his talk Huxley returned from a trip to Washington very tired, only to be told that he was to attend a formal dinner and reception the same evening. He attempted to finish preparing his address before going out since it had to be ready for simultaneous publication in the New York papers. Since the lecture was to be given from notes only, the reporter took it down in shorthand, promising to provide a longhand copy before the lecture the following morning. The copy, which arrived at the last moment, was written upon such flimsy paper that Huxley was unable to read it. He quickly made up his mind to deliver the lecture as best he could from memory.

There was an audience of two thousand people, and when Huxley began to talk about dangers of overpopulation and poverty in future America one could have heard a pin drop. At the end of the lecture amid the enthusiastic applause of the crowd he made his way to the box in which his hosts and their party were seated and received their warm congratulations. These were the prophetic words with which Huxley so impressed that audience in Baltimore almost one hundred years ago:

I cannot say that I am in the slightest degree impressed by your bigness or your material resources as such. Size is not grandeur and territory does not make a nation. The great issue about which hangs a true sublimity and the terror of overhanging fate is what are you going to do with all these things. What is to be the end to which these are to be the means. You are making a novel experiment in politics on the greatest scale which the world has yet seen. Forty million at your first centenary, it is reasonably to be expected that at the second, these States will be occupied by two hundred million of English speaking people spread over an area as large as that of Europe, and with climates and interests as diverse as those of Spain and Scandinavia, England and Russia. You and your descendants have to ascertain whether this great mass will hold together under the form of a Republic and the despotic reality of universal suffrage; whether state rights will hold out against centralization without separation; whether centralization will get the better, without actual or disguised monarchy; whether shifting corruption is better than a permanent bureaucracy; and as population thickens in your great cities and the pressure of want is felt, the gaunt spector of pauperism will stalk among you, and communism and socialism will claim to be heard. Truly America has a great future before her; great in toil and care and in responsibility; great in true glory if she be guided in wisdom and righteousness; great in shame if she fails. I cannot understand why other Nations should envy you or be blind to the fact that it is for the highest interest of mankind that you should succeed. But the one condition of success, your sole safeguard, is the moral worth and intellectual clearness of the individual citizen. Education cannot give these but it may cherish them and bring them to the front in whatever station of society they are to be found *and the Universities ought to be and may be the fortresses of the higher life of the Nation.*

How well Huxley foresaw what was ahead for America in the century just about to end. Certainly the accomplishments to be portrayed in these essays give ample evidence that the Johns Hopkins Medical Institutions have represented during this past century one of the "fortresses of the higher life of the Nation."

It is worthy of note that not all of the responses to the plans for The Johns Hopkins University were favorable. In general the South was apathetic, and in Baltimore many were quite hostile. Those citizens of Baltimore who disapproved apparently did so for two main reasons. The first was a feeling that local rights were being disregarded. The second reason for disapproval, perhaps less articulate but just as deeply rooted, was the obvious leaning of the university toward natural science and the fear that its influence would be hostile to religion. Strange as it may seem now, Thomas Huxley was looked upon as a dangerous person whose writings were subversive to religious faith. French points out that it was a very disquieting event when Huxley's disciple, Newell Martin, was recruited as professor of biology at the Johns Hopkins. When Huxley himself was invited to lecture on "University Education," apprehensions were increased. Huxley was openly assailed in an editorial in the Baltimore *Bulletin* as an adherent of the doctrine of evolution, than which, declared the writer, "There is no more frightful heresy extant." The fact that there was no public prayer preceding the lecture was seized upon as specific evidence of the irreligious character of the new university. It is interesting that there is no reason why there should have been a prayer, for the occasion was not a formal university function. In addition, all of the main representatives of the university, or most of them, were Quakers not accustomed to opening meetings with a prayer.

This gives some idea of the public reaction to science at the time the medical school and hospital were about to open. Times have changed and the catalogue of original contributions by members of the community of the Johns Hopkins Medical Institutions played a significant role in changing the public attitude toward science.

Some thirteen years after Huxley's lecture, at the formal opening of the

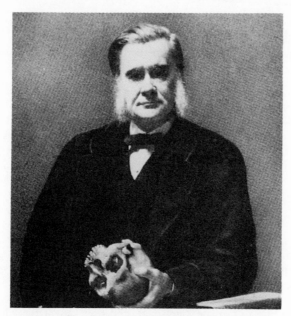

Thomas Henry Huxley

From the National Portrait Gallery, London. Reproduced with permission.

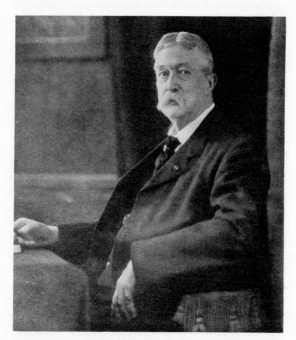

John Shaw Billings

From F. H. Garrison, *John Shaw Billings, a Memoir* (New York: G. P. Putnam's Sons, 1915). Reproduced with permission.

Johns Hopkins Hospital on May 7, 1889, the principal address was given by John Shaw Billings, entitled "The Plans and Purposes of the Johns Hopkins Hospital." The following comments on the principles to be kept in mind in such a hospital are taken from this address:

The third principle to be kept in view in such a hospital as this is, that it should provide the means of giving medical instruction, for the sake of the sick in the institution as well as those out of it.... The very act of teaching clarifies and crystallizes his own knowledge; in attempting to explain, the dark places become more prominent and demand investigation, and hence it is that those cases which are lectured on receive the best treatment.... Johns Hopkins understood all this and specially directed that "in all your arrangements in relation to this hospital you will bear constantly in mind that it is my wish and purpose that the institution shall ultimately form a part of the Medical School of The University."... As the majority of the trustees were also trustees of the university, they knew well the principles which underlie the organization of that institution, and that the same principles would govern the organization of the medical department when that came to be taken in hand. One of these principles is the thorough teaching of that which is known, another is to increase that which is known, and furnish the men and means for doing this. So also the hospital should not only teach the best methods of caring for the sick now known, but aim to increase knowledge, and thus benefit the whole world by its diffusion.

Later Dr. Billings goes on to say:

The probable length of life of the new-born infant today is not much more than half what it ought to be; the practical productive period of the life of our men and women is shortened and interrupted by unnecessary disease and suffering; but remember, that if these things are due to be amended, it is not merely by teaching old doctrines; we must open fresh windows and let in more light so that we can see what these obstacles really are. It is in this work of discovery that it is hoped that this hospital will join hands with the university, and it is in this hope that some of the structures around you have been planned and provided.... *It is because it is believed that this will be the case that there is a widespread hope and expectation that these combined institutions will endeavor to produce investigators as well as practitioners, to give to the world men who can not only sail by the old charts, but who can make new and better ones for the use of others.** This can only be done where the professors and teachers are themselves seeking to increase knowledge, and doing this for the sake of knowledge itself;—and hence it is supposed that from this hospital will issue papers and reports giving accounts of advances in, and of new methods of acquiring knowledge, obtained in its wards and laboratories, and that thus all scientific men and all physicians shall share in the benefits of the work actually done within these walls. *But, however interesting and valuable this work may be in itself, it is of secondary importance to the future of science and medicine, and to the world at large, in comparison with the production of trained investigators, full of enthusiasm, and imbued with the spirit of scientific research, who will spread the influence of such training far and wide.** It is to young men thus fitted for the work that we look for the solution of some of the myriad problems which now confront the biologist and the physician.

* The italics are those of the author (AMH).

It is now a matter of history how Welch, Halsted, Osler, Kelly, and the other excellent men who assembled here in the early days of the hospital carried out these principles laid down by Dr. Billings.

In commenting on the early days Dr. Osler said twenty-five years later:

It was not the men, though success could not have come without them, so much as the method, the organization and a collective new outlook on old problems. They were gathered here from all parts to do one thing, to show the primary function of a university was to contribute to the general sum of human knowledge. . . . Individuals here and there for generations had had in this country these ideals but never before a *studium generale,* a whole body of men gathered in one place to form a university. That part of the university with which the hospital forms the medical school has only had 25 years of existence, not a generation, a mere fraction of time in the long history of the growth of science so that it seems presumptuous to claim any powerful influence on the profession at large. The feeling, however, is strong, too strong to be passed over, that the year 1889 did mean something in the history of medicine in this country. One thing certainly it meant as originally designed by that great leader, Daniel Coit Gilman, that the ideals of the men [in the medical school] were to be the same as those of the men in the laboratories [of the university], that a type of medical school was to be created new to this country in which teacher and student alike should be in the fighting line. That is lesson number one of our first quarter-century. . . . Lesson number two was the demonstration that the student of medicine has his place in the hospital as part of its machinery just as much as he has in the anatomical laboratory and that to combine successfully in his education practice with science, the academic freedom of the university must be transplanted to the hospital . . . And binding us all together there came as a sweet influence the spirit of the place; whence we know not, but teacher and taught alike felt the presence and subtle domination. Comradeship, sympathy one with another, devotion to work and its fruits and its guidance drove from each heart hatred and malice and all uncharitable-ness. Looking back these are my impressions of the work of the Johns Hopkins Hospital.

What this meant was clearly stated many years later in an address by Alan Gregg on Dr. Welch's influence on medical education. At the celebration of Dr. Welch's hundredth birthday, he spoke as follows:

Let me begin the final section of this paper with a rather stark question. Can you think of some part of the world where there is a college or university but where the establishment of a six-thousand-dollar fellowship without closely defined objective but tenable for six successive years would almost certainly be an inexcusable waste of money? If you can think of such a university, you will agree that there are, on the other hand, universities where such a fellowship would be magnificently used. What is the probable principal difference between a university that could not safely be given such a fellowship and another university that would be able to use so much money to the greatest advantage? I think it is that the first university lacks what I would call the *heritage of excellence** and the second has it. I must admit that in the phrase *"heritage of excellence"** I am inventing a name for what I've sensed but never seen. I am sure it has been recognized but has it ever been described. Though I

* The italics are those of the author (AMH).

believe it is a psychological reality I shall introduce it as an hypothesis—as befits this audience.

I suggest that something extraordinarily precious comes out of the close but entirely free association of really superior people. To this emergent quality I give the name—the *heritage of excellence*,* mostly because it lasts so long and because it never comes from, nor appeals to, mediocrities. I doubt if a human being can maintain really close relationships with more than six or seven people. Therefore large numbers of excellent persons are not necessary to create it. By really superior people I mean persons so spirited and yet so balanced, so gifted and yet so incomplete, so mature and yet so eager that they can remain in close contact with but a few of their kind and yet experience no surfeit, boredom or friction.

The exact nature of the contacts between a few absolutely first-rate people is completely unpredictable except in point of its astonishing quality. All you can know about it in advance is that it will be memorable and that it will spread outward and afterward. This almost unearthly and certainly intangible product of the interchange between superior persons cannot be seen but it can be felt and truly like an atmosphere it can be breathed. Indeed, it is an inspiration. . . .

What Welch and his colleagues did and believed and wrote is not as important now—nor anywhere near as important—as the *heritage of excellence* their contacts with each other have left us. We are met today to talk about Dr. Welch and his influence. What we are talking about is not Dr. Welch alone but the quality of interchange among a relatively small number of first-rate human beings—an atmosphere in which Dr. Welch was Popsy—a relationship whose larval form was eager work and whose imago I have tried to name as the *heritage of excellence*. It does not depend on numbers; it depends on the quality of the participants in the life of the university. . . .

In this sense Johns Hopkins is enviably rich. The legend, the *heritage of excellence* that came from the unflagging interchange between Welch and Osler and Halsted and Abel and Howell and Mall and a few others—in this you have what makes a generous fellowship a safe investment here at Hopkins, safer than in a university that has never witnessed the contagious companionship of excellence. What more do men of superior character and capacity require for their association than freedom, responsibility and expectation? The wisdom of the university is to provide those three—freedom, responsibility and expectation. It is the interaction of such men that attracts great young men, leads to great living and itself lives on long afterwards as a *heritage of excellence* ready at any time to burst into bloom again.

This marvelous *heritage of excellence*, this atmosphere of creative scholarship that has been the traditional atmosphere at Hopkins, still persists as we approach our hundredth year of being.

The chapters which follow will try to recapture some of the men and their contributions to medicine that have stemmed from their being in the Johns Hopkins Medical Institutions where such an atmosphere of excellence prevails. Perhaps these fine scientific contributions will act as a further stimulus to students, house officers, and faculty alike in the second century of Johns Hopkins.

There is a documented tale of a Danish church where well into the nineteenth century parishioners maintained a long-standing custom of kneeling

* The italics are those of the author (AMH).

when they passed by an area of the church wall. The reason was only made known when removal of the white wash in this spot uncovered the likeness of the Madonna. These worshipers had bowed down for centuries before the place where this Madonna was once visible. Physicians have traditionally had a reverence for those who by their lives and accomplishments have added, even in some small way, to the body of knowledge useful in medical practice. Our *heritage of excellence* can be enhanced by a knowledge of the creative scholarship of those who have done their work in these institutions. These essays will not represent a complete catalogue of all the contributions made from Johns Hopkins. The author has exercised the right of personal choice in the hope that the reader will be stimulated to seek for himself knowledge of other new additions to medical knowledge by our colleagues past and present.

2 ❦ Pioneers in Urology:
James R. Brown and Howard A. Kelly

IN THE EARLY DAYS after the opening of the Johns Hopkins Hospital, there were many exciting activities in motion which clearly indicated that the intended goal of developing new knowledge for the benefit of patient care would be achieved in full measure. Among the most fruitful accomplishments were two which changed dramatically the field of urology. The first was the successful catheterization of the male ureters by Dr. James R. Brown and the second was the development of the technique of air cystoscopy with catheterization of the female ureters by Dr. Howard A. Kelly. Which achievement came first is difficult to determine, and in a letter written in 1918 in response to a query by Dr. Henry Hurd in regard to the question, Dr. W. S. Halsted side-stepped the issue. In any event Dr. Brown's preliminary report was published in the *Johns Hopkins Hospital Bulletin* a few months before Dr. Kelly's first paper appeared in print.

The First Successful Catheterization
of the Male Ureter by Dr. James Brown

The scene: the outpatient clinic for genito-urinary diseases at the Johns Hopkins Hospital. The witnesses: ten medical gentlemen connected with that institution. The event: the first catheterization of the male ureter, performed on the ninth of June 1893 by Dr. James Brown. Dr. Brown, a modest man, gave the principal credit to Dr. Brenner of Vienna. In December 1888 Dr. Brenner had Leiter, the well-known instrument maker of Vienna, construct for him a modification of the Nitze-Leiter cystoscope, whereby the fluid in the bladder could be changed without removing the cystoscope. The modification consisted of a small tube incorporated with the shaft of the instrument at its lower part. Subsequently, by passing a fine catheter through this cannula, Dr. Brenner attempted to catheterize the ureters. He apparently succeeded in one female case, but failed in the male subject.

The instrument which Dr. Brown used was similar to that of Dr. Brenner. The only modification which proved to be of importance consisted of a stylet terminating in a slight spring, which being introduced into the catheter gave it a slight curve for a distance of about 3 centimeters at its tip (Fig. 1). Dr. Brown's method of procedure was as follows: The cystoscope having been passed into the bladder, which contained about 200 cubic centimeters of fluid, the stylet was withdrawn from the cannula and replaced by the catheter armed with its stylet. This was passed as far as the inner opening of the cannula. The ureteral orifice of the supposed sound side could now be searched for and when found the catheter directed into it, the stylet having been withdrawn before it passed beyond the inner opening of the cannula. The curve given by the spring stylet to the catheter enabled the operator, by rotating the part projecting outside between the thumb and index finger, to direct its point when free in the cavity of the bladder upward, downward, or to either side. The posture of the patient was important. The pelvis and thighs were raised on an incline of about 35 degrees, with the shoulders and head low. This threw the abdominal viscera toward the thorax and thus prevented the respiratory movements from being communicated to the bladder. The ureteral orifices were also presented better in this than in the horizontal position.

The first case was a man suffering from partial anesthesia of the bladder and urethra, as well as the lower extremities, due to the effects of an injury to the spinal cord received some six years previously. No anesthetic was necessary, while in the second case the only anesthetic employed was 2 cubic centimeters of a 3 percent solution of cocaine injected into the deep urethra.

All of the ten gentlemen stated that they had seen clearly the catheter entering the ureteral orifice, and the ridge formed by the catheter passing obliquely through the vesical wall also was plainly visible, the catheter being passed 8 to 9 centimeters into the ureter. The manner in which the urine issued from the catheter was noted. Five, six, or seven drops would come and then there would be a pause of several seconds' duration when several drops would come again in quick succession to be followed by a pause as before. It seemed as if a certain amount of urine would collect in the ureter above the catheter. Then by stimulating the muscular walls of this tube to contraction, it would be forced out through the eye of the catheter. The catheter, being laterally placed about 1.5 centimeters from its tip, would be naturally occluded by the walls of the tube during the intervals of contraction.

Dr. Brown pointed out that, in considering the advisability of an operation upon one of the kidneys and the kind of operation which had best be performed, if any, one would be largely influenced in his decision by the conclusion he arrived at respecting the second kidney. "It has been generally recognized," he said, "that the best possible way to determine the condition of the second kidney would be to collect its secretions unmixed with that of its diseased companion."

One of the early patients studied by this method was a nineteen-year-old boy under the care of Dr. Osler. The specimen from the right side obtained by ureteral catheterization was cloudy and contained numerous polymorphonuclear leukocytes. Urine from the other side was found to be essentially normal. On the following day the right kidney was removed by Dr. Halsted and a stone was found occupying one of the infundibula. After the operation, the urine was found to be perfectly normal.

The way in which Dr. Brown began work with ureteral catheterization adds interest to his accomplishment. In a letter written to Dr. Henry Hurd on May 10, 1918, Dr. W. S. Halsted commented:

I recall quite distinctly that Brown began work on the problem not later than the summer of 1890 and possibly in 1889. I had taken lessons in catheterization of the female ureter with Pawlik in Vienna in 1879 or 1880 and urged Brown to try to catheterize the male ureter. We had many conferences on the subject in the course of his endeavors; indeed, it was for several years prior to his success our usual conversational piece. Kelly's procedure is a great improvement on Pawlik's, but Pawlik had become very skillful in the practice of his own method.

James Brown was born in Baltimore, November 12, 1854, the son of Thomas R. Brown and Mary Elizabeth Hynson. He attended what is now the University of Maryland for his medical degree, which he received in 1875. He was a resident physician at Bayview Hospital, Baltimore, and assumed charge of the genito-urinary dispensary in the Johns Hopkins Hospital at its opening in 1889. From 1893 to 1894 he was a lecturer and from 1894 to 1895 associate in genito-urinary surgery at the Johns Hopkins University. He was married first to Amanda Bechtel and later to Imogene Bechtel. He had two children. A granddaughter, Mrs. Harry Klinefelter, resides in Baltimore.

Dr. Brown had been in delicate health for several years prior to his death on June 16, 1895, while enroute to Boston on a steamer. During the spring of 1895 he became infected from an accidental wound received in performing a surgical operation and for many weeks was in critical condition. While convalescing, symptoms of pulmonary disease developed which were thought to be caused by tuberculosis and which led him to seek a change of climate. He died on this journey in his forty-first year.

Dr. James Brown was the uncle of Dr. Thomas R. Brown, a graduate of the first class of the Johns Hopkins medical school in 1897.

After Dr. Brown's death the post of head of genito-urinary disease was held for a short period by Dr. Bradley Gaither. Dr. Gaither was born in Baltimore in 1863, received his A.B. from Princeton in 1885 and his M.A. from Princeton in 1888. He graduated from what is now the medical school of the University of Maryland in 1887 and became resident physician at the Bayview Asylum. From 1890 to 1897 he was assistant in the Genito-Urinary Division of the Johns Hopkins Hospital dispensary. He was succeeded in 1897 by Dr. Hugh Hampton Young, who held the position of surgeon-in-charge of the Genito-Urinary Division for many years and became internationally famous.

The "Kensington Colt" and the
Development of Female Urology

In 1893, several months after James Brown's epoch-making catheterization of the male ureter, Kelly succeeded in catheterizing female ureters under direct vision through an open tubular endoscope, the bladder having been filled with air and lighted by a head mirror from an electric lamp without.

Dr. Kelly was born in Camden, New Jersey, on February 20, 1858. His father, Henry Kuhl Kelly, a successful man of affairs and a public-minded citizen of Philadelphia, later served in the Union Army during the Civil War. His mother, Louisa Warner Hard Kelly, was the daughter of an Episcopal minister. Thomas Kelly, Dr. Kelly's great-grandfather, migrated from Port Au Doun, Ireland, to Philadelphia, late in the eighteenth century. The Kuhls and Hillegases migrated to Philadelphia from Germany very early in the eighteenth century. These ancestors were active in the business, public, and religious enterprises of Philadelphia during their lives. The most outstanding, perhaps, was Dr. Kelly's great-great-grandfather, Michael Hillegas, who was born in Philadelphia in 1729. He was the first treasurer of the United States (1776–1789). His business interests were manifold and included merchandising, banking, sugar refining, iron manufacturing, and coal prospecting, among others. From his earliest days he served in one public capacity after another. Exceptionally well educated, he loved music and wrote a pamphlet entitled "An Easy Method for the Flute." He was also greatly interested in historical research. In his mental equipment, vast energy, multiple interests, and physical appearance, he was very much like the subject of this chapter. It is of interest that there were no doctors of medicine or scientists among Dr. Howard Kelly's ancestors. Even when Dr. Kelly was scarcely able to comprehend, his mother, "who gave him his real start in life" and "who had convictions and tastes which he inherited," began teaching him the Bible and fostering an interest in natural sciences and books.

In 1867 at the age of nine, Dr. Kelly was entered as a pupil in Fiare's Classical Institute, where he remained as a day student for six years. He received an excellent grounding in English, Latin and Greek, penmanship and drawing but stated that mathematics was a bugbear. His ability to sketch was striking and served him in good stead later in life. His training in the classics probably accounts for his ability to write, read and speak German, French, and Spanish fluently. He read the testaments in the Bible in the original Greek and Hebrew.

On entering as an undergraduate student at the University of Pennsylvania in 1873, he was awarded the Matriculate Latin Prize and received his B.A. four years later. He entered the medical school at Pennsylvania in 1877 and graduated in 1882. During the year 1880–1881, he had to interrupt his medical course on account of insomnia. This period was spent in Colorado on the O.Z. Ranch, where he acted as cowboy, postman, and doctor. As a medical student he was apparently much more impressed by teachers of the scientific branches than by clinicians and especially by Joseph Leidy, Edward Cope, and Harrison Allen. All of these men were scientists and personages of unusual abilities. His viewpoint as to the relative importance of vocations was changed by a year's internship in the Episcopal Hospital of Kensington. Contact with patients and guidance by sympathetic and skillful chiefs brought the conviction that his "real education began in the wards and dispensary of the hospital and that richer rewards followed caring for the sick than even the greatest of the sciences could bestow." Entering clinical medicine had not been Dr. Kelly's first choice but seemed a way of earning a living and continuing his explorations in natural history. However, to one who knew Dr. Kelly this change in attitude was inevitable. He was an extremely human individual who loved people, reveled in trust and affection, and rejoiced in aiding those in trouble.

Between the ages of twenty-five and thirty-one, the period of life now usually spent in a surgical residency, our budding gynecologist was furiously engaged in many activities. In his own words, "After my residency it seemed better to locate in Kensington where work was waiting than to settle down assisting the older doctors." A two-room hospital was started on the second floor of a residence; a year later it was moved into a larger building, and a third move was made into Kensington Hospital, which was incorporated in 1887. Along with hospital organization, he was building up a large practice and developing new methods of abdominal and particularly gynecological surgery. It was here that Kelly started his work on the diagnosis and treatment of urological conditions, then a *terra incognita*. His skill as an operator drew visitors to his modest clinic from far and wide. Indeed, Dr. Kelly's facility with his hands, a facility he maintained until the end of his life, was extraordinary, and this combined with an ability to think and improvise on a moment's notice marked the great surgeon. To this was added a thorough knowledge of gross anatomy and a willingness to go back to dissections time and again.

It was during this Kensington period that he first became acquainted with Dr. Osler and others at the University of Pennsylvania. Osler is responsible for labeling him the "Kensington Colt." With his excellent judgment of men, Osler picked Dr. Kelly as a man of exceptional promise, and when an important post became vacant in the University of Pennsylvania and several were being considered for the position, the following course of events took place. As described by Osler:

Goodell had resigned and there was no end of discussion as to who should take his place. On several occasions I had gone to Kensington to see Kelly operate and I happened to mention to Pepper that I'd never seen anybody do abdominal work with the same skill. He knew of Kelly but had not, I believe, seen him operate which he immediately arranged to do. Then one evening at the Biological Club, Horatio Wood and Mitchell were discussing Goodell's successor and I said that Pepper and I were backing a dark horse—a "Kensington Colt." With that Leidy chipped in with a remark that if it was young Howard Kelly, his former prosector, he would back him heartily. This is how I remember the story.

During this period Dr. Kelly managed three trips to Europe, which broadened his vision and created many new friends. The first trip was in 1886, the second in 1888, and the third in the summer of 1889. On the twenty-seventh of June of that year he was married in Marienkirche in Danzig to Fraulein Laetitia Bredow, daughter of Dr. Justus Bredow of Berlin.

The rudimentary condition of surgery in the late portion of the nineteenth century is now difficult to believe. Anesthesia was still in its infancy. Many of the leaders in obstetrics and gynecology still opposed the ideas of asepsis, and those who did not were dominated by the necessity for antiseptic procedures rather than asepsis. Bacteriology and cellular pathology were just beginning to take hold of the minds of the clinicians and were being translated into effectual application in the wards and operating rooms. During the 1888 trip in the company of Hunter Robb and Constantine Goodell, Dr. Kelly visited Berlin, where he met Virchow and worked on cadavers in an attempt to determine a

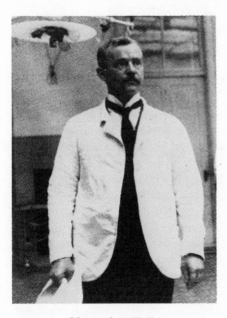

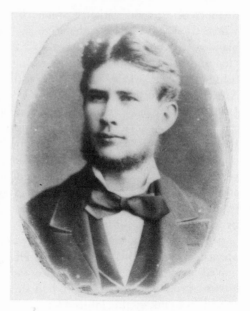

Howard A. Kelly

From A. M. Chesney, *The Johns Hopkins Hospital and the Johns Hopkins University School of Medicine: A Chronicle*, vol. 2, *1893–1905* (Baltimore: The Johns Hopkins University Press, 1958), p. 322

James R. Brown

Courtesy of Mrs. Harry F. Klinefelter

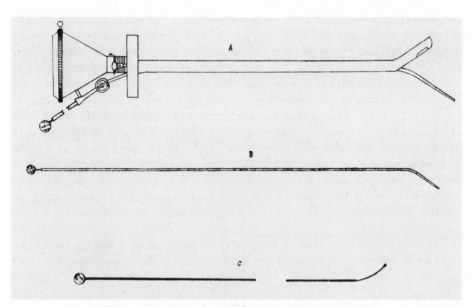

Fig. 1. Dr. Brown's modification of the cystoscope

From *Johns Hopkins Hosp. Bull.* 4 (1893): 74

method of ureteral catheterization. From Berlin the party went to Prague, where they saw Pawlik catheterize the ureters blindly through the water-filled bladder. After this visit to Pawlik's clinic in 1888, Kelly returned to Philadelphia and began to practice catheterizing ureters blindly by Pawlik's method, by fishing for the orifices in the water-filled bladder. He described this to the American profession as Pawlik's method in 1893. It was during this period (1888) that he was appointed associate professor of obstetrics at the University of Pennsylvania. Then in the fall of 1889 there was a preliminary visit to Baltimore, which permitted a view of the Johns Hopkins Hospital and an opportunity to meet the men with whom he was to be associated for so many years. He had an interview with President Gilman, who outlined the high aims and ideals of the new institution in a way that "fired his imagination." He returned that same fall, having accepted the professorship of obstetrics and gynecology in the Johns Hopkins University and the directorship of these departments in the hospital. First he lived on Broadway near the hospital, later he opened an office on Charles Street, where he practiced until 1892. In 1892 he moved his residence to Eutaw Place and acquired some houses nearby in which his first resident, Hunter Robb, had started a private hospital. The facilities for private patients at the Johns Hopkins Hospital at that time were limited and available only to the heads of departments. Dr. Robb had received a call too, and had accepted the chair of gynecology and obstetrics in Western Reserve University in Cleveland. Almost certainly it was to help Dr. Robb that he started the "Sanitorium." This name was changed to the "Howard A. Kelly Hospital," and it was incorporated in 1913. After Dr. Kelly's retirement in 1940 it continued as the Kelly Clinic. But now let us return to our story.

In 1892 Dr. Kelly began viewing the water-distended bladder through a cystoscope of his own invention, with the patient in the knee-chest posture. The instrument which was made for him had a glass partition to prevent the water from running out of the bladder. He inspected the bladder by direct vision, using a head mirror. One day the cystoscope was dropped by an assistant, and the mirror was shattered. Shortly after this accident, Kelly happened to notice that with a patient in the knee-chest posture, air spontaneously rushed into the vagina. It occurred to him that the bladder might similarly be distended with air. To quote his resident of that year, John Clark, "The idea suddenly struck Dr. Kelly that the same effect would be produced on the bladder if air was allowed to enter it and he called for the short speculum from which the glass had fallen out and inserted it into the urethra. The bladder at once ballooned out, its walls could be inspected and after some search the ureteral orifice on one side was located and the ureter catheterized under direct inspection for the first time."

In November 1893, several months after James Brown had published his paper on catheterization of the ureter in the male, Dr. Kelly published his paper on catheterization of the ureter in the female, in the *Johns Hopkins Hospital Bulletin*, entitled "The Examination of the Female Bladder and Catheterization of the Ureters under Direct Inspection." In the same year he had delivered an address describing his method, perhaps for the first time, before the Washington,

D.C., Obstetrical and Gynecological Society entitled "The Direct Examination of the Female Bladder with Elevated Pelvis—The Catheterization of the Ureters Under Direct Inspection With and Without Elevation of the Pelvis."

As an outgrowth of this pioneer work of Dr. Kelly, examination of the urinary tract and treatment of its diseases became an integral part of the work in his gynecological department at the Johns Hopkins Hospital. Gradually a female cystoscopic clinic for examination and treatment of both hospitalized and outpatients was established as a definite unit of the gynecological service. Dr. Guy L. Hunner, who early in his career became especially interested in this phase of gynecological practice, was for many years the guiding influence of this clinic, and he was followed by Dr. Houston S. Everett. As a result of the examples and teachings first of Kelly, later of Hunner and then of Everett, there have been trained and spread about this country a group of gynecologists who have come to look upon their specialty as one dealing with the genital and urinary tracts in the female.

This discovery, however, plunged Dr. Kelly into the greatest controversy of his career. In 1896 there appeared in the *American Journal of Obstetrics* an article by Dr. W. Rubeska, an assistant of Dr. Pawlik, entitled "A Criticism of Professor Howard Kelly and his Discoveries in the Domain of Urinary Diseases." He stated that Kelly had observed a demonstration of ureteral catheterization in Pawlik's clinic in Prague and that Pawlik told him of his yet unpublished method of cystoscopy by distending the bladder with air with the patient in the knee-chest posture. Rubeska concluded by stating: "One, a Kelly ureteral catheter does not exist. Two, the so-called cystoscope of Kelly is entirely the discovery and intellectual property of Professor Pawlik." Kelly had always had a keen interest in medical history, and in many of his scientific articles he prefaced the report of his contributions by a short chronological review of the discoveries up to that time, being careful to give credit where credit belonged. He had no intention of letting Rubeska's claims go unchallenged. Fortunately, in Prague Kelly had had with him a traveling companion, Dr. W. C. Goodell, who later wrote Kelly verifying the latter's statement that only the blind method of ureteral catheterization by "fishing" had been demonstrated by Pawlik to him and Dr. Kelly.

When Dr. Kelly appeared at Hopkins at the age of thirty-one, he had a very youthful appearance, which was the occasion of many practical jokes, especially by Osler, who took pleasure in portraying Kelly to his patients as a man of mature age and dignity. Then he would usher in the boyish, smooth-shaven Kelly and delight in watching the patients' reaction. On one occasion Osler asked Kelly to cystoscope one of his patients, which he did by the air method. As Dr. Kelly put his eye to the cystoscope, the patient suddenly sneezed, allowing a blast of urine to hit him in the face. Kelly immediately picked up the patient's history and wrote: "Dear Osler: All I know about your patient is that her urine is salty."

Immediately on the opening of the Johns Hopkins Hospital, Kelly established, as Osler had in medicine, a long-term residency training program in gynecology, with Hunter Robb as the first resident. Judging by the quality of his many residents, one may wonder whether this was not his greatest contribution to his specialty. Kelly's postgraduate discipline by means of this long-term residency was an entirely new concept in surgical training at that time. Each year the assistant residents were given increasing responsibilities in the care of patients and in procedures in the operating room. Surgery upon the ward patients was done almost exclusively by the resident and his assistants, subject to consultation and help when necessary by the senior staff. When asked on one occasion why he did so much for his house staff, he replied, "When I was resident in a Philadelphia hospital the head of the surgical department wanted to do everything himself. When I amputated a finger on one occasion, the surgeon reported me to the trustees for overstepping my authority. I made up my mind right then and there that if I ever were head of a surgical department, my men would be given every opportunity."

Dr. Kelly's primary efforts in surgery were directed at techniques of hysterectomy, myomectomy, vesicovaginal fistula, rectovaginal fistula, ureteral and kidney surgery and uterine suspensions, while Drs. Clark and Sampson, his residents, worked on the radical operation with lymph node dissection for cervical cancer. By temperament, he was too impatient to be suited to obstetrics, and in 1899 he delegated the Department of Obstetrics to the able direction of Dr. J. Whitridge Williams. Kelly was also not the man to spend hours at the microscope and he placed Dr. Thomas S. Cullen in charge of the pathological laboratory. Dr. Kelly all of his life was open-minded and inclined promptly to adopt methods and means which promised simplification and improvement in the clinic. Undoubtedly Dr. Halsted's fundamental researches on the way to obtaining aseptic conditions influenced greatly the operating room technique. However, as far as the Johns Hopkins Hospital is concerned, the preparation and use of absorbable sutures were attributable to the gynecological department. The introduction into the operating room of nitrous oxide as a convenient anesthetic has also been ascribed to Dr. Kelly. Cullen's frozen section method of tissue diagnosis at the operating table is another brainchild of the department. In the employment of radium and Roentgen radiation and of electrical coagulation and fulguration methods, notable advances were made in gynecological therapy, which likewise exercised profound influence in all the surgical and medical specialties.

Dr. Kelly was a facile sketcher. The early gynecological histories at the Johns Hopkins Hospital as well as those at his private hospital are filled with his drawings. He began taking photographs through the aid of Mr. Anthony S. Murray, an enthusiastic amateur photographer and friend, almost at the beginning of his work in Baltimore. Also, he was a pioneer in the use of lantern slides for teaching, slides which were made and used to illustrate his lectures. In 1908 he produced the first of a series of stereo-photographs of operations. Mr. Max Broedel joined Dr. Kelly in 1893 and remained with him until he became the director of his Department of Art as Applied to Medicine of the Johns Hopkins University in 1911. Broedel was not only a magnificent artist but became an anatomist of the highest order. Through him a number of artists, notably Hermann Becker, 1895, and August Horn, 1898, joined the gynecological staff. All of them were subsidized by Dr. Kelly. Where Broedel thought necessary, he was encouraged to and would work for weeks at a time at anatomical studies in order to draw a single picture clearly and accurately. Dr. Kelly's rough sketches helped the artists complete their sketches made at the operating table. Broedel's anatomical studies and drawings added greatly to the value of some of Dr. Kelly's publications, but without the freedom and help given him in his formative years, Broedel might never have become the marvelous illustrator into which he developed. Together the pair constituted a great team.

After thirty years as active head of the gynecology department of the John Hopkins University, Kelly resigned as professor of gynecology in 1919 at the age of sixty. The circumstances leading to his resignation are recorded in the files of Dr. Edward H. Richardson in the form of a sheaf of personal letters of Howard Kelly to Sir William Osler, covering the period from 1911 to 1913. They were presented to Dr. Richardson in March 1950 by Dr. W. W. Francis, nephew of Dr. Osler and librarian and literary executor of the Osler Library at McGill University. They clearly indicate that Dr. Kelly thought injustices were perpetrated against him by the formulation of plans by certain faculty members for a transition to the full-time system at Hopkins. These plans were circulated among the trustees and served the purpose of making Kelly believe that his services were no longer acceptable as professor of gynecology. His own feelings were expressed in a letter to Sir William Osler, written in May 1911, from which the following is an excerpt:

Dear Osler: We confabulated last night from 8-11 o'c. All were for the change putting the men on salary and cutting off all private work except Meyer and myself. Meyer's objection to the change was that he was unwilling to yield his liberty but he did not expect to do any practice. Finding I stood alone and that my minority report was looked upon rather as an attempt at personal vindication than any criticism of the real matters at issue, I told them to go ahead and do whatever they conscientiously felt to be right without reference to me. I shall be very sorry but it will mean my retirement wholly into my private work. Williams will also be able to realize the great ambition of his life, the control of both Gyn. and Ob. This, I think, is a bad arrangement but it may work well for a term of years especially under his able management.

On January 12, 1943, Dr. Kelly died of pneumonia, his wife following him a few hours later. Thus was terminated, at the age of eighty-five, the life of one of the most dynamic men of medical history, a man who did more to establish American gynecology as a surgical specialty than anyone before or since his generation. How true his prediction in 1912 has become: "Accordingly as we remember others so those yet to come will remember us." Probably the man best able to evaluate the life of Dr. Kelly was Dr. Welch. On the occasion of Dr. Kelly's seventy-fifth birthday, Welch sent the following letter: "I have always felt as did Osler that you did more than any of us to extend the fame of the Johns Hopkins University to distant parts and the hospital offered no greater attraction than the opportunity to see you and your work and the new methods that you were so rapidly developing."

3 ❧ Medical Students on the March: Brown, MacCallum, and Opie

THE FIRST CLASS of the Johns Hopkins University School of Medicine entered in 1893 and graduated in 1897. There were fifteen members of the class, many of whom were eminently successful in their subsequent careers. Theirs was the good fortune to study medicine in a new and very exciting educational environment. Like all great teachers, Welch, Osler, Halsted, Kelly, and the others "possessed the ability to make students independent in their thought and action, seeking not to make them mere imitators of themselves, but rather to have them develop that which was distinctive in themselves, inspiring them through their own aspirations and striving to obtain new heights of knowledge and power."

In such a stimulating and inspiring atmosphere it is not surprising that one finds a high level of creative endeavor among the students in this first class *during* their undergraduate years. This chapter will describe the contributions of three members of the class of 1897, each of whom had notable research achievements during this period at Johns Hopkins.

Thomas R. Brown

On March 3, 1896, Mr. Robert T., a twenty-three-year-old white male, English by birth, was admitted to the hospital complaining of generalized pain and assigned to one of the medical students, acting as clinical clerk. Mr. Robert T. was a real hobo, a rider of the rails, a true wanderer. He had been complaining of generalized pains, particularly in the joints, bones, and muscles, for about six weeks. For the past fortnight his complaints had been so severe that he was scarcely able to move about.

The young medical student assigned to this patient was a member of the first class to enter the Johns Hopkins medical school. He had taken a course in clinical microscopy given by Dr. William S. Thayer. Dr. Thayer, while studying in Europe, had learned the techniques developed by Ehrlich for staining the blood cells with aniline dyes. When he came to Baltimore, Thayer stimulated with his youthful enthusiasm, the interest of students and colleagues in this new technique of blood examination. The examination of Mr. Robert T.'s blood by the medical student, Mr. Thomas R. Brown, revealed that there were 17,000 leukocytes present, but the most interesting observation was that 68 percent of them were eosinophiles. The absence of rose spots and of any palpable enlargement of the spleen, as well as the presence of a leukocytosis and the extraordinary increase of eosinophilic cells, rendered unlikely the diagnosis of typhoid fever, which was at first considered probable. The extreme muscular tenderness on pressure and on voluntary or passive motion and the irregular temperature suggested rather a myositis, and a diagnosis of trichinosis was made.

Further questioning of the patient revealed that six or seven weeks previously he remembered repeatedly having eaten raw or incompletely cooked pork. To confirm the diagnosis, a small piece of muscle was removed under cocaine from the right biceps where the pain was greatest. A teased specimen of this showed on microscopic examination trichinae, the majority being actively motile. None was encapsulated. The patient's symptoms gradually abated, and by the time of his discharge on May 13 he felt quite well.

Mr. Brown presented his case before the Johns Hopkins Hospital Medical Society, and an abstract of the remarks and the discussion which took place at that meeting were published in the *Johns Hopkins Hospital Bulletin* in April 1897. Thus, one can see that the spirit of creative scholarship which had become the trademark of the Johns Hopkins Hospital and Medical School in those early days involved the students as well as the members of the faculty.

Dr. Brown later studied similar cases and published a comprehensive article entitled "Studies on Trichinosis With the Special Reference to the Increase of the Eosinophilic Cells in the Blood and Muscle, the Origin of these Cells and Their Diagnostic Importance." In other papers reviewing the various situations associated with eosinophilia, he was among the first, if not the first, to note the eosinophilia seen in adrenal insufficiency, and he pointed out that the marked increase in the percentage of eosinophilic cells in the blood in trichinosis is a useful diagnostic sign, being accompanied by a leukocytosis in contrast to the eosinophilia in other situations.

Thomas Richardson Brown was born in Baltimore on September 11, 1872. After a year of graduate work in chemistry, he entered the first class of the Johns Hopkins Medical School. After an internship at the Johns Hopkins Hospital, Dr. Brown began the practice of internal medicine in Baltimore and in 1899 was appointed to the teaching staff of the Johns Hopkins Medical School. In 1912 Dr. Brown was asked to develop the work in gastroenterology as a separate division in the Department of Medicine at the Johns Hopkins Hospital. In order to do this he felt the need of a year of study abroad, so he started almost at once in the biochemical laboratory in the University of Berlin under Bickel and Wohlgemuth. He also spent time with Ewald, a pioneer in the field of digestive diseases. Dr. Ewald was an old friend of Sir William Osler. Later Brown spent time in the laboratory of Hans Eppinger in Vienna. After a short visit to Innsbruck he then went on to Munich, which in those days meant the clinic of Friedrich Müller, that brilliant diagnostician who spoke four languages fluently, and whose medical clinics were a constant delight. The one which he gave every Saturday afternoon was singularly intriguing because student attendance was not obligatory, and he regarded it as a test of his drawing qualities. It must have been quite a struggle for the students those Saturday afternoons, to decide between the clinical charms of Friederich Müller and the lovely lakes and steep slopes of the nearby Bavarian Alps. But usually Müller won out. After this impressive experience in Munich, Brown went to London, where he spent the major portion of his time with Arthur Hurst at Guy's Hospital but managed to maintain contacts with the great physiologists Bayliss and Starling, whose work on various digestive problems was epoch-making.

In developing the gastroenterology clinic, which began in 1913 in two small rooms and later became one of the largest and most active in the Outpatient Department, Dr. Brown had two principles from which he never deviated. First, that gastroenterology could never be a narrow specialty and was only safe in the hands of those fundamentally trained in internal medicine and that a complete general history and medical examination should always precede the intensive studies of the digestive tract itself. Second, that the Outpatient Department was a fertile field for research. That this is true is shown by the fact that from two hundred to three hundred papers were published by the members of the staff of the gastrointestinal clinic while Dr. Brown was in charge. These publications were based not only on clinical but on laboratory studies. Included in this work are the observations on ulcerative colitis by Dr. Moses Paulson, on digestive ferments by Dr. Lay Martin, and in the field of gastroscopy by Dr. John Tilden Howard. Weekly surgical-digestive conferences and monthly meetings at the home of Dr. Brown were held regularly, and talks were given by many, including Dr. Howell, Dr. MacCallum, Dr. Hurst of London, and many others. The last talk Dr. John J. Abel ever gave, one on tetanus, was at one of these meetings.

In 1943 Dr. Brown was awarded the Julius Friedenwald Medal by the American Gastroenterological Association. The previous recipients of this medal were Max Einhorn and Walter B. Cannon. Thus, one can see that he was highly respected by his colleagues.

In 1919, at the request of his former classmate, Dr. Richard P. Strong, Dr. Brown assumed the post of director of the medical section of the newly formed League of Red Cross Societies at Geneva, which was soon to become part of the League of Nations. He spent a year in this post and rendered conspicuous service. Dr. Brown served as a trustee of the university for a number of years. In 1937 he became the first chairman of the advisory board of the newly endowed orthopedic hospital in Wilmington, Delaware, having been invited by Mrs. Alfred I. DuPont to plan and organize the hospital provided for in the will of her husband. The July 1950 issue of *Gastroenterology* was dedicated to Dr. Brown in recognition of his accomplishments as a teacher, clinician, and contributor to *Gastroenterology*.

There are numerous interesting sidelights of the discovery of the eosinophilia in trichinosis and of Dr. Brown's student days. In commenting on the patient with eosinophilia, he noted that when he first saw the high figure of 68 percent of the blood cells being eosinophiles, he wondered if this had any relationship to the young man's muscular pain. He excised bits of muscle and found large numbers of trichinae and made daily blood counts, always with the same results. Dr. Brown recalled that he was very eager to continue his studies after the patient left the hospital. He taught the patient to make very creditable blood smears and furnished him with needles and coverslips, even giving him what seemed a large sum from his meager purse on the promise that he would send specimens back at weekly intervals for follow-up examination. Although, as pointed out, the man was a real hobo, he kept his promise for several months.

One of the interesting by-products of Dr. Brown's discovery is chronicled in Colonel Bailey Ashford's book entitled *A Soldier of Science*. Not long after Dr. Brown's report appeared, Dr. Ashford was struggling to discover the cause of what appeared to be an epidemic of fatal anemia in an area of Puerto Rico. He tried feeding his patients an ample diet, but in his own words, "But I feed them by order ... and the ungrateful things keep on dying." This in reply to his wife, who had tried to comfort him by saying, "This is the anemia of the country. They all die of it eventually. They say it is due to lack of food." But Dr. Ashford did not believe that he was doing the best he could. He began with the most obvious thing and proceeded to examine the blood. The results were shocking to him. The picture was that of true pernicious anemia and profound at that. But who ever heard of a whole agricultural class dying of an epidemic of pernicious anemia? It was unthinkable. "Hold on," he admonished himself, "look at those eosinophiles. What were they doing so numerous in pernicious anemia?" He goes on to say:

And now I had to explain to my patient wife that the white corpuscles of the blood are normally five in variety, the polys, the lymphocytes, the monocytes, the basophiles and the eosinophiles, and that the latter should not exceed 4%, yet here they are impudently running up to forty. What on earth—? Oh yes, now I remember something I read out of a journal not long ago, I murmured to myself. A man by the name of Brown found these prominent, strawberry-looking eosinophiles to be increased in an infection by the worm causing "pork measles." Maybe these anemics have worms. And I began to laugh ... by myself ... at myself. I sent my tired wife to bed, but I sat up far into the night until the chilly morning land breeze began to blow.

And I went to bed still intrigued with eosinophiles shooting like comets before my eyes. The idea that a frightful epidemic anemia with a high death rate might be caused by anything so commonplace as worms! There were charlatans who made a living by treating worms in dogs and man and they were known as worm doctors, too. I remember that lots of patients in the Children's Hospital back in Washington had had worms but those cases were all rosy enough save the black ones. The next day I would go again at this blood and then I would examine the feces—a tremendous jolt to my pride if not actually unscientific. The next day came and what happened is told at the beginning of this chronicle. The veil had lifted from the face of the anemia of Puerto Rico. Now to remove the cause, watch those people get well and publish the results. It never occurred to me at any time that anybody would have the temerity to doubt that cause or to be indifferent in applying that knowledge. I had visions of everybody falling over each other in their eagerness to cure all these wretched people overnight. But it was to be more than four years before I could attract the slightest attention to the meaning even of my find. [The finding was that the anemia was due to hookworm infestation.]

In later years Colonel Ashford and Dr. Brown met many times and had friendly arguments as to the cause of tropical sprue in which both were interested and had done some investigation, Dr. Ashford on a large scale, Dr. Brown on a comparatively small one.

As has been mentioned, Dr. Brown was a member of that fortunate band of pioneers in the first class of the Johns Hopkins Medical School, a group unhampered by precedent, unfettered by tradition. Among his closest friends in that group were Charles Bardeen, who became professor of anatomy at the University of Wisconsin; Dr. William G. MacCallum, who returned to become professor of pathology; and Dr. Richard P. Strong, who later became a dynamic figure in the field of tropical medicine, first in the Philippines and later at Harvard.

Because of his training in chemistry, Dr. John J. Abel, the professor of pharmacology, took Dr. Brown into his private laboratory as his first research assistant. Among the problems that Dr. Brown helped him with in his investigations was the cause of light in lightning bugs. What a surprise to those who saw a great professor and his young assistant chasing those elusive insects as they faded into darkness!

It is interesting to note, as pointed out by Dr. Chesney, that the name of Dr. Thomas R. Brown does not appear on the original list of those whom Dr. Welch interviewed on the opening day of the medical school. This omission was due to the fact that Dr. Brown did not make up his mind to study medicine until after the school had opened and was under way. Although both his father and his father's brother, Dr. James R. Brown, were physicians, the latter being a member of Dr. Halsted's staff and assigned as the surgeon-in-charge of the genito-urinary dispensary, Dr. Brown had not up to that time directed his thoughts to medicine but had decided upon a career in chemistry. He had seriously considered one in journalism and even professional baseball. While an undergraduate student in the Johns Hopkins University, he elected the physical-chemical group of studies and upon graduation in 1892 enrolled as a candidate for the Ph.D. degree in chemistry. He had actually begun his second year of work in that subject under Remsen when he suddenly made up his mind to study medicine—"overnight," according to his own words. There was, however, one thing that stood in his way. He had not studied biology while an undergraduate student. Unable to dissuade him from giving up chemistry. Dr. Remsen sent Brown to President Gilman, who arranged to have him study biology with the undergraduate students while he was taking his first year of work as a student of medicine.

MacCallum and Opie

On August 24, 1897, the British Association for the Advancement of Science met in Toronto with Lord Lister, the father of antiseptic surgery, in the chair. A shy, sensitive young man with moist palms stepped to the rostrum and presented a paper on the haematozoan infections of birds—work done while a student of medicine in the first class of the new Johns Hopkins School of Medicine. The youthful speaker was none other than William G. MacCallum.

Dr. William S. Thayer, prior to his appointment to the resident staff at the

Johns Hopkins Hospital, had studied in Europe and learned the new techniques that Ehrlich had developed for staining the cells in smears of the peripheral blood. In 1895 Dr. Thayer, then resident physician, was appointed an associate in medicine as part of an effort to provide additional personnel to conduct the third year instruction in the School of Medicine. It was the result of his enthusiasm that two of the young medical students, William G. MacCallum, who presented the paper referred to above, and Eugene L. Opie, received their stimulus to study the haematozoan infections of birds. Baltimore was the scene of much malarial infection in those days, and it was the subject of intensive study by Dr. Osler, Dr. Thayer and others on the hospital staff. It was believed that there was sufficient similarity between the infection in birds and that in man to warrant further investigation.

In the adult examples of the Halteridium of Labbe, which occurs abundantly in crows in Ontario, Opie in 1896–1897 had pointed out a distinction between two forms—a hyaline, nonstaining form and a form which was granular and took on a comparatively dark stain with methylene blue—and suggested that the hyaline form alone might become flagellated. This distinction was readily confirmed by MacCallum, and he noted clearly that only the hyaline forms became flagellated, the granular forms being extruded, and lying quietly as spheres beside the free nuclei of the red corpuscles which lately contained them. By carefully watching the two adult forms on extrusion from the corpuscle, MacCallum noted that the flagella from the flagellated forms, tearing themselves free, constituted themselves fertilizing agents or spermatozoa, and proceeding directly to the granular sphere, wriggled about it. He noted that only one of these gained admission, and plunged itself into the sphere, which after some agitation of the pigment became quiet for a period of fifteen or twenty-five minutes. After this it put out a conical process, which grew and drew the protoplasm into itself until there was finally a fusiform body with a small pigmented appendage and a refractive, nucleus-like body such as described by Danilewsky as a "vermiculus." He recognized that this was a sexual process, with a resulting motile form occurring under favorable circumstances and comparable with analogous processes observed in lower plants and animals. A few weeks later MacCallum examined the blood of a woman suffering from an infection with aestivo-autumnal malaria in which a great number of crescent forms were to be seen in a freshly made slide of blood. With few exceptions these retained their crescent shape for only a few minutes. They soon drew themselves up, straightening out the curve of the crescent, while shortening themselves into the now well-known ovoid form. After a lapse of ten to twelve minutes, most of them were quite round and extracorpuscular. After twenty to twenty-five minutes certain ones of these spherical forms became flagellated; others, and especially those in which the pigment formed a definite ring and was not diffused throughout the organism, remained quiet and did not become flagellated. In a field where an example of each form could be watched, the flagella broke from the flagellated form and struggled about among the corpuscles, finally approaching the quiet spherical form; one of them entered, agitating the pigment greatly, sometimes spinning the ring about. The rest were refused admission, but swarmed about, beating their heads against the wall of the organism. MacCallum recognized that this was the same event in the human form of malaria, which he had predicted from his studies on the organisms of the bird. Some years later Sir Ronald Ross said about this discovery by the young medical student: "I have ever since felt disgraced as a man of science!"; for Ross had erroneously interpreted the sperm cell wriggling into the penetrated female cell as being a flagellated spore trying to escape from it.

Medical students Opie and MacCallum presented some of their earlier studies on the pathology of haematozoan infections of birds before a meeting of the Johns Hopkins Medical Society held on November 16, 1896. It was pointed out in the discussion that Dr. Osler and his staff had become deeply interested in the study of the malarial parasite which Laveran had discovered in 1880, the life history of which was being actively investigated in Italy and elsewhere at the time. The observation was made in 1885 in Europe that birds harbored a similar parasite, a haematozoan, which stimulated the studies at Johns Hopkins. In Opie's studies, which were done in the clinical laboratory of the hospital during the months of June, July, August, and September, over 125 birds were examined. Of these the greater number, 100, were from the neighborhood of Baltimore, including 80 English sparrows, 9 of which were infected with intracorpuscular parasites; 12 red-winged black birds, 6 of whom were infected; 2 swamp sparrows and 1 song sparrow, whose blood contained organisms. Of 25 birds, including a variety of species of the neighborhood of Dunnville, the MacCallum home near Toronto, Ontario, 5 birds were similarly infected, namely 1 great horned owl and 4 crows. It was on the crows that MacCallum did his classic work on the pathology of the infection.

Osler, in his discussion, pointed out that in 1886, when he was busily engaged for the first time in the study of the malarial parasite, Mr. William G. MacCallum's father, Dr. MacCallum of Dunnville, Ontario, sent to the biological laboratory in Toronto a goose which was supposed to have malaria. Osler noted that he was extremely skeptical about it, as he knew nothing at that time about the parasites in birds. To his astonishment there were large numbers of pigmented intracellular organisms entirely similar to those that he had just seen demonstrated by Mr. Opie.

We shall hear more later about Opie. Let us now find out more about the background and career of this brilliant young medical student, William G. MacCallum. He was born in Dunnville, Ontario, on the eighteenth of April, 1874, the second of four children. His younger brother was John Bruce MacCallum, whose brilliant career in medical research was cut short by his death from tuberculosis at the age of thirty. MacCallum's mother was Florence Octavia Eakins, an accomplished pianist and singer, and it was from her that he acquired his deep and life-long love of music. His father, Dr. George Alexander MacCallum, was a general practitioner with an active practice in the countryside surrounding Dunnville. As a youth, "our" MacCallum often rode with his father on visits to patients, helping him at times during operations by administering ether, and by "purifying the air of the room" with the Lister

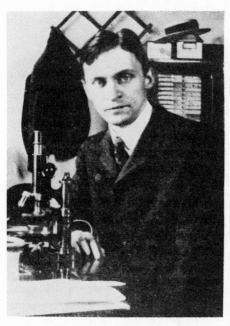

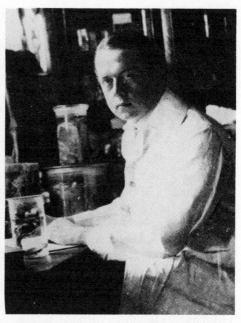

Eugene L. Opie

From Chesney's *Chronicle*, vol. 2

William George MacCallum

From A. M. Chesney, *The Johns Hopkins Hospital and the Johns Hopkins University School of Medicine: A Chronicle*, vol. 2, *1893–1905* (Baltimore: The Johns Hopkins University Press, 1958)

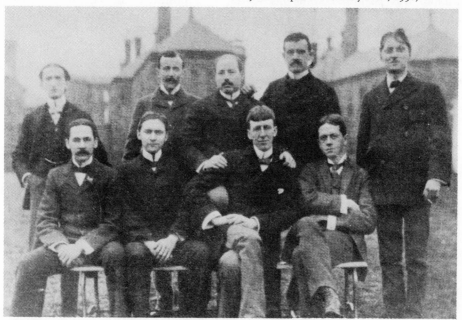

Pithotomy Club founders

Bottom row, second from left, is Eugene Opie, next is Thomas Brown, and on the right is William G. MacCallum

From J. A. Brown, *Dr. Tom Brown, Memories* (New York: Richard R. Smith, 1949)

carbolic spray, the originator of which he was later to encounter, as we have already seen.

His father had a consuming interest in natural history, and the home was filled with stuffed wildcats, foxes, snakes, birds, and other animals. MacCallum was taught at home until he was nine years of age. Then he attended public school, and at the early age of fifteen passed the entrance examinations to the University of Toronto, where he completed in four years the requirements for a B.A. degree and in addition a sufficient number of medical courses to enable him to enter the second-year class of the Johns Hopkins Medical School in the company of the small group who the preceding year had been the first students to be admitted to the newly opened school. At the suggestion of Dr. Archibald E. Malloch, a friend of Dr. Osler and of the MacCallums, he wrote to Osler asking if he could be admitted to the second-year class. Osler replied that admission with advanced standing could not be permitted as no such precedent existed in the school. Since the school itself had not been in existence long enough to have had a precedent of that sort, young MacCallum then directed his correspondence to Dr. William H. Welch, the dean, and was accepted.

In 1897, at the age of twenty-three, MacCallum was graduated at the head of the class. After a year spent in a rotating internship at the Johns Hopkins Hospital, he applied without success for a place on Dr. Osler's staff. The competition in medicine must have been great at that time! Fortunately, Dr. Welch offered him an assistantship in pathology, which he accepted. This turned out to be a most perceptive appointment on Dr. Welch's part, as Mac-Callum was later to become his successor as professor and chairman of the Department of Pathology. In 1908 Dr. MacCallum was made professor of pathological physiology and lecturer in forensic medicine. This was probably the first new chair created after the opening of the university. The following year he accepted the position as professor of pathology at Columbia University, where he remained until 1917, when he returned to Johns Hopkins to succeed Dr. Welch as Baxley Professor of Pathology.

At the University of Toronto, MacCallum came under the tutelage of Ramsey Wright, an Edinburgh graduate, zoologist and professor of biology, whose particular field was comparative anatomy. At an early age, therefore, MacCallum was the beneficiary of another source of stimulation toward work in the biological sciences.

MacCallum's interest in the parathyroid glands, a subject on which he did his most outstanding work, began in 1902 while he was a member of the staff in Pathology. In March 1902, Gont Scharukov, of Kiev, published a short paper in the *Zentralblatt fur Allgemeine Pathologie,* on the production of a specific antithyroid serum, in which article he stated that after the injection of emulsions of dogs' thyroids into sheep, he was able to produce in other dogs by the injection of the serum of the sheep, certain tetanic symptoms which he thought indicated the existence of a specific antithyroid toxin. MacCallum, knowing the literature on the physiological properties of the parathyroid glands as contrasted to those of the thyroid, decided to repeat these experiments with better controlled observations. He knew at this point that destruction of the thyroid gland alone produced a disturbance of metabolism which appeared slowly and led to myxedema; and that destruction of the parathyroid alone, on the other hand, produced the acute, rapidly fatal nervous phenomenon which had for many years been thought due to the extirpation of the thyroid. He set out in an attempt to produce a specific cytotoxin for the thyroid alone and similarly a specific cytotoxin for the parathyroid alone. The results of his experiments completely disproved Gont Scharukov's conclusions. In the course of these experiments, MacCallum's interest became so strongly attached to the problem of the nature of the parathyroid glands and their function in the body and role in disease that he for the next several years worked intensively in this area. He pointed out that the objective of his preliminary investigations was mainly concerned with determining the role of the parathyroid glands under normal conditions. In extirpating these organs from dogs and observing under various conditions the results, he confirmed the fact that under these circumstances the dogs developed tetany. However, several important problems in connection with this phenomenon presented themselves to him. The first question, Was one dealing with a condition in which there was a lack of some necessary secretion of the parathyroid? Two, Was there, on the other hand, a poison produced somewhere in the body which was circulating in the blood and which produced these phenomena but which in the normal animal was neutralized either by the parathyroid cells themselves or by their secretion? Three, Was this poison produced by the metabolism of any particular group of cells or, in other words, were there specific relationships between the parathyroid and any other particular organ?

MacCallum and his co-workers decided to study experimental tetany and the influence of various factors, such as diet. They showed, as did others, that the symptoms of tetany could be made to disappear by the subcutaneous or intravenous injection of an extract of the parathyroid gland. He described a very interesting patient who developed tetany after subtotal thyroidectomy. An emulsion of four or five parathyroid glands of the cow was prepared aseptically and injected beneath the breast. Several hours later the tetany disappeared. Four days later the tetany was combatted again in the same way. He and Carl Voegtlin then studied the chemical nature of the processes which result from parathyroidectomy. They showed that tetany was due to nervous system rather than muscle aberration, and as a result of the experiments of Forster and Voigt on the effects of deprivation of calcium in the diet on muscular or nervous hyperexcitability, their interest returned in this direction. They noted also that Jacques Loeb, in studies on the production of the muscular twitchings by electrolytes, found that the injection into the animal body of any salt liable to precipitate calcium produced twitching of the muscles and that the administration of calcium salts might cure the disease. Similarly, his brother, J. B. MacCallum, had pointed out that the peristaltic activity in the intestine and secretory activity in certain organs may be stirred up by certain salts which have an action antagonistic to that of calcium, and that such activity was suppressed by the addition of soluble calcium salts.

The experiments of MacCallum and Voegtlin fell into two groups. In one they endeavored to ascertain, in cases of outspoken tetany produced by para-thyroidectomy, the effect of the administration of various substances, chiefly mineral salts, and especially calcium, which might occur normally or under pathological conditions in the animal body. The second group of experiments related to the changes in metabolism in tetany and in the chemical composition of the tissue of animals dying in that condition. They had previously shown that the transfusion of blood from a normal dog would suppress the symptoms of tetany when a sufficiently large amount was introduced. Their experiments were conclusive in demonstrating the immediate and specific curative effect of the administration of a soluble calcium salt upon the tetany of parathyroidectomy. Shortly thereafter, Dr. John J. Musser of Philadelphia allowed them to see a case of postoperative tetany, which had followed surgical extirpation of an extensively invading malignant growth of the thyroid. In this patient, calcium lactate was administered in frequent and quite large doses, resulting in the disappearance of the tetany in the course of one day. In their conclusions they stated that calcium salts have a moderating effect upon the nerve cells.

The parathyroid secretion in some way controls the calcium exchange in the body. It may be possible that in the absence of the parathyroid secretion substances arise which can combine with calcium extracted from the tissues and cause its excretion and that the parathyroid secretion prevents the appearance of such bodies. The mechanism of the parathyroid action is not determined, but the result, the impover-ishment of the tissues with respect to calcium and the consequent development of hyperexcitability of the nerve cells and tetany, is proven. Only the restoration of calcium to the tissues can prevent this.

These results were reported on May 18, 1908, at a meeting of the Johns Hopkins Medical Society. A report of these studies appeared in preliminary form in the *Johns Hopkins Hospital Bulletin* in March 1908, and a full paper on the "Relation of Tetany to the Parathyroid Glands and to Calcium Metabo-lism" was published in the *Journal of Experimental Medicine*.

No discussion of MacCallum's contributions should fail to mention that work which has had so wide an influence throughout the English-speaking world, namely, his *Textbook of Pathology*. This book, which appeared in 1916, was written in a lucid and engaging style and with an inquiring critical attitude made sound by rich personal experience with the subject matter. It was a landmark in the history of textbooks of pathology, for it represented the first effort to treat the entire subject from the standpoint of etiology. In this book the attempt was made to present the effects that each form of injury, each cause of disease, produced in the whole body, instead of following the traditional method of cataloguing all of the heterogeneous and unrelated injuries that can affect each separate organ. The extraordinary success of the book in this coun-try and abroad for almost three decades, during which it passed through seven editions, attest plainly enough to the approval aroused by his treatment of the subject. As a student who had the good fortune to be assigned to Dr. Mac-Callum's "group" in pathology, I can recall that the clarity, informality, and effectiveness of his teaching was superb.

Dr. MacCallum shrank from the familiarity that most men find agreeable, and would actually wince on rare occasions when some venturesome colleague would call him "Bill." It is, therefore, somewhat anomalous that through his association with J. L. Nichols, he became one of the founders of the Society of Pithotomists, a medical students' club which is still very much in active existence. In his last year as a medical student (1896) he and Nichols, a classmate, rented a house at 1200 Guilford Avenue. As a housewarming, they invited Dr. Welch, Dr. Osler, other members of the faculty and a few friends, and entertained them with a small keg of beer. Everyone had such a good time that the performance was repeated, and shortly thereafter seven classmates joined with MacCallum and Nichols to perpetuate the idea, some of them taking rooms in the house. A club was thus formed, and MacCallum coined from the Greek the word "pithotomy" for the periodic operation of opening the keg. If he had no other claim to fame, the organization of the Pithotomy Club would suffice, since it has provided a most effective and entertaining relationship between students and faculty over the many years of its existence and has been a very important part of the Johns Hopkins Medical Institutions.

Let us now turn to the research career of Dr. MacCallum's classmate, Dr. Opie, and his work on diabetes. Here we shall see that again they had common interests, and we shall hear of Dr. MacCallum's further work on the relation of the islets of Langerhans to glycosuria.

Dr. Eugene L. Opie, also a member of the first class of the Johns Hopkins Medical School, grew up in a house at the corner of Howard and Little Ross Streets in the heart of the Johns Hopkins University. His father, a general practitioner, was for thirty years dean of the College of Physicians and Surgeons of Baltimore. Opie attended this school for one year and then transferred to Johns Hopkins, joining the first class to be graduated from this new medical school. After graduation, perhaps on account of his excellent work as a student, but particularly his demonstrated potential for research, vouched for by his work on bird malaria, two of the giants at Johns Hopkins, Osler and Welch, each tried to recruit Opie to their departments. Osler lost again, as Opie chose pathology, presumably because of the greater appeal to him of the German school, stressing basic science and pathogenesis, in contrast to the English school, emphasizing anatomy and definition of disease. Although as previously described, Opie's first paper, published in the *Journal of Experimental Medicine* in 1898, reported work that he did between his third and fourth years of medical school on a malaria-like parasite in Baltimore birds, his first interest in research appeared even earlier, as he describes in his own words: "During the laboratory course in Pathology I found in a section of the pancreas a strange body which I showed to Dr. Welch when he made his unhurried rounds of the class. He told me it was a structure described by Langerhans in 1869. Find out all you can about the islets of Langerhans, Welch said to me." It is recorded of Opie's father that on his way South to fight for the Confederacy he stopped over in Washington to attend Lincoln's Inaugural Ball. One can see, in this action, the same intellectual curiosity tempered with humor which had proved so effective in his son. As pointed out by Peyton Rous, it is plain from Opie's early papers that he started to discover by asking himself urgently what each and everything meant that came under his eye. "When examining post-mortem material, he was no recorder of final states. The changes met in the dead had for him the livest of implications. He was an inquirer into riddles who sought after the meaning of diseased organs much as one might seek for the answers to charades." It was with this approach to the unknown, and remembering what Dr. Welch had told him, that he observed in post-mortem sections from the pancreas of a diabetic person the nearly complete destruction by hyaline changes of the islets of Langerhans. The hint was enough. He had proved to himself while yet a medical student that the islets were not modified or unde-veloped acinar cells, as was currently thought, and had discriminated the inter-lobular and interstitital types of chronic inflammatory pancreatitis. Now he went on to demonstrate by the perceptive collection of cases that severe injury to Langerhans' islets is followed by diabetes. Another autopsy provided him with the clue to the cause of some other pancreatic disorders. This time the patient had died of hemorrhagic pancreatitis with fat necrosis and Opie found a stone blocking the ampulla of Vater. By recourse to animal experiment and diligent post-mortem search, he demonstrated that the diversion of bile to the pancreas will cause hemorrhagic pancreatitis, and that fat necrosis is secondary to digestion by a ferment liberated from the gland tissue. Studying the pancreas further, reconstructing natural processes with the aid of thought and test, he dispelled much of the mystery that hung about the disorders of the organ and in less than five years had become by right of achievement the authority on pancreatic disease; all this done within the first five years of his graduation from medical school.

MacCallum in the meanwhile followed with interest the paper of Opie on the relations of the islets of Langerhans to the development of glycosuria, and was aware that in certain cases of diabetes with intense glycosuria the lesion may apparently consist in their being destroyed while the rest of the pancreas is intact. However, he noted that it was still far from proven that the islets of Langerhans had any such special function and that diabetes was rather the result of injury to the whole tissue of the pancreas. Dr. MacCallum knew that if the ducts of the pancreas were ligated so that the secretion of that gland is obstructed from passing into the intestine, there followed certain digestive dis-turbances and injuries to the gland but no glycosuria. He knew that this was generally ascribed to the fact that, although such obstruction causes atrophy of the secreting acini, the islets of Langerhans not being connected with the ducts, do not suffer. He was also aware of the experiments of Mering and Minkowski that total extirpation of the pancreas in dogs resulted in a severe and total diabetes, which they attributed to the lack of some substance which the pan-creas secreted into the blood stream. At this point, MacCallum concluded that a satisfactory solution to the question could be arrived at if the secreting tissue of the pancreas could be made to atrophy completely. Then if the islets of Langerhans remained intact, they might finally be secured in a pure state so that their specific function could be studied. The difficulty of previous experi-ments was that after ligation of the duct and separation from the intestines the dog had to be kept alive for a considerable period of time to allow atrophy of the acini to occur. This was very difficult to do. What MacCallum did was to separate a portion of the pancreas from the rest and to ligate its duct. After it had undergone extensive atrophy the remaining tissue was removed. The atrophied remnant was shown to be capable of warding off glycosuria, even when considerable amounts of dextrose were ingested. When the remnant itself was removed, glycosuria appeared at once, spontaneously. This clearly proved the specific control of carbohydrate metabolism by the islets of Langherhans.

The procedure (duct ligation) employed by Dr. MacCallum in order to destroy the acinar tissue while leaving the islets intact was later adopted by Banting and Best in their successful attempt to extract from the islets the antidiabetic hormone (insulin), which Dr. MacCallum's experiments had shown to be secreted by these cells. Thus, the paths of these two classmates, Opie and MacCallum, crossed as far as their research interests were concerned, in two important areas.

After six years in the Department of Pathology at Johns Hopkins, Dr. Opie, at the age of thirty-one, was appointed one of the first group of members of the Rockefeller Institute for Medical Research. In 1910, while in the midst of his studies on tuberculosis, he was asked to go to St. Louis to help reorganize the medical school of Washington University and to become professor of pathology. Soon after arriving there he discovered how diet can prevent the hepatic and renal effects of alcohol, phosphorus, and chloroform, knowledge which has proved applicable in practice.

In 1923 he was invited to be professor of pathology at the University of Pennsylvania and director of the Laboratories of the Henry Phipps Institute for the Study, Treatment, and Prevention of Tuberculosis. He had fashioned his abilities to precisely such purposes. Opie had a long-standing interest in tuberculosis, and the opportunity to study this disease under ideal circumstances was apparently a major factor that led him to accept the call to Philadelphia in 1923. His work there provided convincing evidence for the communicability of tuberculosis within households and for the high susceptibility to this disease of young adults of rural background on moving to crowded city environments.

In 1932 Opie moved to New York to head the pathology department at Cornell, a post he held for the next decade. He trained a large number of men who later assumed positions of prominence in experimental medicine and pathology. The single largest block of Opie's life at one institution was the nearly thirty years of his retirement spent as a "guest investigator" at the Rockefeller Institute.

In spite of his excellent work in the field of inflammation and allergy, including that on tuberculosis, he is best known for his description of the hyaline degeneration of the islets of Langerhans in cases of diabetes mellitus. This finding attracted attention to the islets as the probable source of an internal secretion lacking in diabetes mellitus. Opie's discovery led Sir Edward Sharpey-Schafer to postulate, in 1916, the theory that diabetes is caused by the lack of a hypothetical internal secretion. MacCallum's additional work served as a firm foundation for this hypothesis.

4 ❧ Two Mycoses First Described
at Johns Hopkins

ACCORDING TO Garrison, the latter part of the nineteenth century marked the scientific or parasitic period of dermatology, in which many cutaneous diseases were directly traced to microscopic organisms, especially under the leadership of Sabouraud and Unna. Earlier David Gruby described a contagious tinea sycosis due to a fungus (1841–1843), and Carl Eichstedt established a relationship between pityriasis versicolor and microsporon furfur (1846). Gruby's work received little attention until the bacteriological and parasitological period, when it was taken up by Raymond Sabouraud of Paris, who made extensive studies of the different varieties of trichophyton (1894). Americans made two important contributions to this field, both emanating from the Johns Hopkins Hospital in the period between 1894 and 1898. The first case of blastomycosis of the skin was reported in 1894 by T. Caspar Gilchrist and the first recognized case of sporotrichosis was studied by Benjamin R. Schenck in 1898.

T. Caspar Gilchrist

In June 1894 Gilchrist discussed blastomycetic dermatitis before the American Dermatological Association at Washington, D.C., and exhibited microscopical sections from a patient who had been under the care of Dr. Louis A. Duhring of Philadelphia. Dr. Duhring described the case as a typical chronic scrofuloderma of the back of the man's hand. A portion was excised and sent to Dr. Gilchrist. In this tissue Gilchrist found large numbers of bodies which were round, doubly contoured, and refractive. After the unstained sections were treated with liquor potassae, these bodies appeared very distinct compared to the blurred appearance of the tissue. The tissue consisted of hypertrophied epidermis, throughout which were scattered numerous miliary abscesses, each one of which contained from one to nine of these bodies. Numerous budding forms were observed, and the mode of reproduction was found to be by gemmation. No opportunity was afforded for making cultures or for inoculation experiments, as the patient was operated on before the tissues had been examined. The opinion was expressed by Gilchrist that these organisms belonged more to plant than to animal life and should be so classified.

It was in the rete mucosum of Gilchrist's case that the chief pathological changes were to be observed. The epithelium was enormously hypertrophied and consisted of irregular prolongations of various shapes and sizes extending downward into the corium. The most noticeable feature in the rete was the presence of numerous well-defined miliary abscesses of different sizes. The smallest of these were about equal in area to that of three adjoining epithelial cells, while the largest were just visible to the naked eye. The contents consisted of polymorphonuclear leukocytes, nuclear detritus, a few detached epithelial cells, now and then a giant cell, a number of peculiar nuclear cells, and the organisms which characterized the disease. The organisms were almost always present in the miliary abscesses and scattered through the corium, but none was found on the surface of the skin. The number present varied, as many as fifteen having been found in one abscess, though the average was only four, five, or six.

Gilchrist made a careful search of the literature dealing with protozoa, sporozoa, and coccidia and concluded that the present case was a unique one at the time it was exhibited at Washington in June 1894. "The main characteristics of the organism were its mode of reproduction by gemmation and its comparatively small size pointing unmistakably to a classification among the yeast or blastomycetes. The subsequent finding by Busse and other observers of similar bodies which had produced pathological changes in man or animals is strong corraborative evidence in support of this view." Thus, Gilchrist is given the credit for having described the first case of cutaneous blastomycosis. The definitive article was published in the *Johns Hopkins Hospital Reports* under the title of "A Case of Blastomycetic Dermatitis in Man."

When the Johns Hopkins Hospital opened in 1889 there was no chair or designated department of dermatology. There was a Dispensary Department of Dermatology, which in 1889 was under the supervision of Robert Brown Morison, who with Atkinson and Rohe were the real stalwarts of Baltimore dermatology and who since 1885 had been members of the American Dermatological Association. Morison was active in the general journal club and frequently reviewed papers on skin diseases and allied subjects. His lectures on skin diseases were as follows: on May 22, he lectured on the anatomy of the skin, hyperemias, erythemas, and eczema; on May 29, his subject was parasitic diseases of the skin; on June 5, the application of remedies for the common forms of skin diseases.

At this time dermatology was under the domain of surgery, just as it was at the University of Maryland. Assisting Morison were Jere Williams Lord and T. Caspar Gilchrist. Gilchrist also lectured on skin diseases to the nurses of the Johns Hopkins Hospital. Morison continued as dermatologist until 1893, when he became ill. He died in 1897. One year after Morison's death, Gilchrist was made clinical professor of dermatology, and since until this time Jere Williams Lord had shared equal rank, he also was made clinical professor of dermatology, a post which both held until their deaths. Gilchrist simultaneously held the position of clinical professor of dermatology at the School of Medicine of the University of Maryland. In 1917 he became professor of dermatology at the University of Maryland, a rank which he held until his death in 1927.

Dr. Gilchrist was born on June 15, 1862 at Crewe, Cheshire, England, the son of Robert and Emma Gilchrist. His early education was received at Fair-

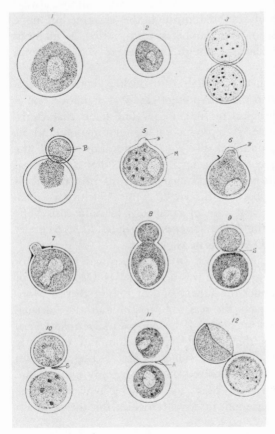

Fig. 1. The double-contoured spore

Plate 46 from "A Case of Blastomycosis Dermatitis in Man," Johns Hopkins Hospital Reports, vol. 1 (1896)

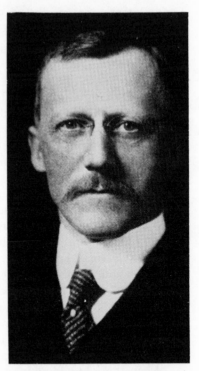

Thomas Caspar Gilchrist

From A. M. Chesney, *The Johns Hopkins Hospital and the Johns Hopkins University School of Medicine: A Chronicle,* vol. 2, *1893–1905* (Baltimore: The Johns Hopkins University Press, 1958)

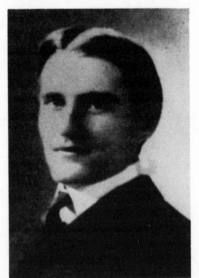

Benjamin Robinson Schenck

From Chesney's *Chronicle,* vol. 2

34

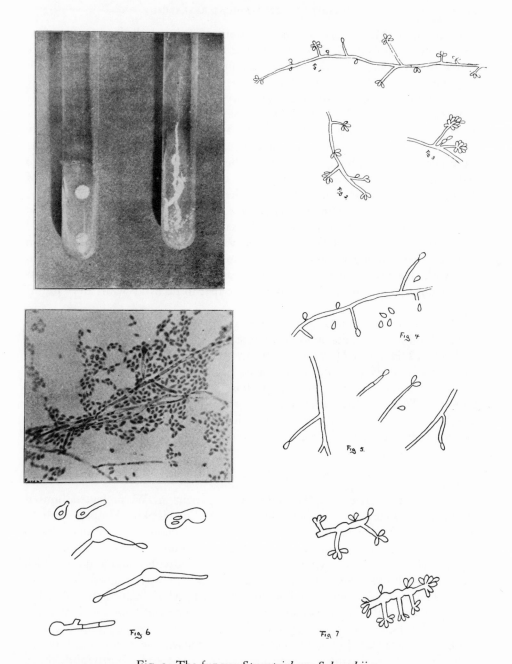

Fig. 2. The fungus *Sporotrichum Schenckii*

Plate 1 from "On Refractory Subcutaneous Abscesses Caused by a Fungus Possibly Related to the Sporotricha," *Johns Hopkins Hosp. Bull.*, vol. 9 (1898)

field Academy, Manchester. From 1882 until 1888 he studied at Owens College, Victoria University, Manchester. He graduated and received his M.B. degree in London, and came to America in October 1889. After a time spent with Duhring in Philadelphia, he elected to settle in Baltimore to practice medicine. In 1907 he was given the honorary title of Doctor of Medicine by the University of Maryland. At the Johns Hopkins Hospital he was made assistant dermatologist in 1892, associate in 1896, and clinical professor in 1898. He worked in Dr. Welch's laboratory and made many scientific contributions of the highest value. Although he cultured the acne bacillus and was the first to make an acne vaccine, his most important contribution was the description of the disease blastomycetic dermatitis and the isolation and proof of its cause—the double-contoured spore, the *blastomyces dermatitidis* (Fig. 1). Being a gifted artist, he drew the organisms as he saw them under the microscope, and these drawings are still of great value today. Gilchrist was a pioneer in radium and Roentgen-ray therapy, and sustained injuries to his hands while carrying on this work. He was probably the first to teach undergraduate medical students morphological methods of diagnosis and the first to do away with "dry" lecturing.

Dr. Gilchrist was president of the American Dermatological Association in 1909, and an enormous amount of research work in dermatology was done at the Johns Hopkins Hospital under his direction. Besides Blastomycosis the most important were studies of the acne bacillus, pemphigus, mast cells, and urticaria factitia. He was also the author of a volume entitled *Outlines of Common Skin Diseases Including Eruptive Fevers* (1927). Dr. Gilchrist's daughter, who lives in Baltimore, is married to Dr. Monte Edwards, a surgeon who has been a member of the University of Maryland staff for many years.

Benjamin Robinson Schenck

On the thirtieth day of November 1896, patient A. W. presented himself at Dr. Finney's surgical outpatient clinic at the Johns Hopkins Hospital with an infection of the right hand and arm of an unusual nature. The primary lesion was on the index finger, whence it extended up the outside of the arm following the lymph channels and giving rise to several circumscribed indurations, which were in part broken down and ulcerated. The patient was assigned to a senior medical student, Mr. Benjamin Robinson Schenck, who obtained the following history: During the latter part of August 1896, some three months before the visit to the Johns Hopkins Hospital dispensary, while working at the iron worker's trade in St. Louis, the patient had scratched the index finger of the right hand on a nail while reaching into a keg of red lead. Shortly after this a small abscess formed which had been opened with a pin. A slight amount of watery fluid escaped. Three weeks later an ulcer appeared between the second and third metacarpophalangeal joints. The inflammation traveled up the arm, and seven weeks after the infection several similar abscesses had formed. Being unable to work, the patient returned to his home in Baltimore late in November. By this time a "waxen kernel" about the size of a walnut had appeared in the axilla. One of the indurated areas was incised, and deep in the tissues a thimbleful of gelatinous puriform material was found. A culture from this fluid was made on agar, and an abundant growth of an organism not resembling bacteria but evidently in pure culture was seen. On December 7 Dr. Finney, under aseptic precautions, removed an indurated area just above the elbow and in three days a growth in pure culture, of the peculiar organism previously seen, was isolated. Dr. Finney thereafter removed a second, larger piece of tissue for microscopic examination.

The young medical student pursued the study of this case, and after extensive bacteriological studies, in which he had the cooperation of Dr. Erwin F. Smith of the United States Department of Agriculture in Washington, the identity of the organism was established. The description from Dr. Smith's report is as follows: "When a little of the bouillon containing the colorless elliptical or cylindrical conidia was inoculated into hanging drops of alkaline beef broth and set away under a moist bell jar for 48 hours, there was an abundant growth of the fungus. The spore-bearing branches of which being undisturbed, retained their spores in the normal condition and the appearance of the fungus under such conditions is shown in the sketches" (Fig. 2).

The life history of the organism was studied from bouillon cultures and from hanging drops. The conidia germinated by sending out one or more straight unbranched germ tubes, sometimes from the end, again from the side. These germ tubes gave off spores of the same character, the attachment being either terminal or lateral by means of short pedicle sterigmata. Although the classification of fungi existing at that time was a purely artificial one and incomplete in many details, the young medical student, with the help of Dr. Smith, correctly identified it as a *sporotrichum*. It was subsequently named *Sporotrichum Schenckii* in honor of the budding physician who first recognized it as a cause of disease in man. He further did experiments upon dogs and mice, proving the pathogenicity of the organism and indicating that under different circumstances it may remain local in its development or it may invade the internal organs and produce a pyemia. Dr. Schenck expressed indebtedness to Dr. Simon Flexner for his advice and assistance in the course of these studies, which were published in the *Johns Hopkins Bulletin* in December 1898.

Benjamin Robinson Schenck was born in Syracuse, New York on August 19, 1872, the son of Adrian A. and Harriet Robinson Schenck. His ancestry dates back to the Holland Schencks in unbroken line to 1346. His first American ancestor, Roelof Martense Schenck (1619–1704), who was born in Amsterdam, came to New Amsterdam and settled in Flatlands, Long Island. Benjamin Baird Schenck VII (1809–1883), the grandfather of our Dr. Benjamin Schenck, was a physician, a graduate of the Geneva Medical College in 1835. Dissatisfied with the often vague and always heroic methods of the "old school," he turned to homeopathy, where he became a bright light. Also, he was an ordained minister of the gospel from 1846. Benjamin's father held a number of important political positions and built up a flourishing manufacturing business. He collected a massive amount of geneological data, which his son assembled with characteristic care and thoroughness. The outcome was a volume of 160 pages entitled *The Descendants and Ancestors of Rulef Schenck, a Geneology of the Onandaga County Branch of the Schenck Family,* by Benjamin Robinson Schenck, from records and notes compiled by Adrian Adelbert Schenck, Detroit, Michigan, 1911.

Benjamin took his A.B. degree in 1894 from Williams College and graduated from the Johns Hopkins School of Medicine in 1898. After graduation Schenck became a resident on the gynecological staff under Dr. Howard A. Kelly (1898–1903) and also instructor in gynecology (1901–1902). Schenck succeeded Dr. Guy L. Hunner as resident gynecologist in the hospital when Hunner resigned that post in April 1902 in order to enter private practice in Baltimore. Since the custom had by that time been firmly established that those attaining the rank of resident on any of the services of the hospital should be given an appointment on the medical faculty because of the teaching duties which they were called upon to perform, Schenck's appointment in the school followed as a matter of course, although he remained on the medical faculty for less than a year, resigning in April 1903 to enter private practice in Detroit, Michigan, where he became associated with the Detroit College of Medicine and Surgery as associate professor in gynecology.

In addition to the description of sporotrichosis, he wrote a number of other papers, including: "Four Cases of Calculi Impacted in the Ureter with Nephroureterectomy"; "Abdominal Ureterolithotomy"; "Vaginal Ureterolithotomy," 1901; in conjunction with W. W. Russell, "An Ovarian Sarcoma Developing from the Theca Externa of the Graafian Follicle," 1902; "A Resume of 48 Cases of Postoperative Crural Thrombosis," 1902. No more model clinical study can be found in the early literature than his "Symptoms, Diagnosis, and Treatment of Ureteral Calculi" (1902), written at a date when the method of discovering calculi by passing a waxed-tipped catheter up the ureter and recognizing the pathognomonic scratch marks was still comparatively new.

Schenck became secretary of the Michigan State Medical Society and editor of the journal of that society from 1905 to 1910. It also fell to his lot to organize the state society meetings. The medical library at Detroit owes its excellent status to his brooding care.

In 1916 he was forced to move to Colorado with his family in search of health. Here he died on June 30, 1920, after several years of a brave fight against pulmonary tuberculosis.

5 ❧ Teacher and Distinguished Pupil: William Henry Welch and George Hoyt Whipple

WILLIAM HENRY WELCH became the first full-time professor of pathology at the new Johns Hopkins University in 1884. He immediately departed for Europe to familiarize himself with the latest methods in bacteriology and for the purpose of purchasing apparatus and books for his future laboratory in Baltimore. The trustees of the university voted a sum of $2,000 for this purpose, but when Welch returned in the autumn of 1885 he informed the trustees that he had exceeded the appropriation by $500. They promptly approved his request for this additional sum. However, Welch found that the laboratory was not ready for him when he returned.

The original plans for the "Pathological Building" of the hospital provided for a two-story building containing an "autopsy theater" with an elaborate autopsy table. The proposed arrangement was not entirely satisfactory to Welch, and he persuaded the hospital authorities to make certain alterations. When the original plans were drawn it had been assumed that most of the instruction of the medical students in pathology would be conducted in buildings to be erected on the medical school grounds. Dr. Welch, however, thought that the activities of the Department of Pathology had such an important bearing upon the work in the hospital that they should be conducted in close proximity to the wards. This view was accepted, and while Welch was awaiting the completion of his hospital laboratory, he worked in the new biology laboratory of the university. In January 1886 the rooms in the upper story of the pathology building were ready for his occupancy. It was in the winter of 1886, while the construction of the laboratory was still under way, that he delivered his first lectures in the university on "Microorganisms and Disease" to an audience of physicians and students in biology. The following autumn he organized systematic courses in pathology and bacteriology in "the Pathological," and there Welch and Councilman, with Franklin P. Mall as fellow in pathology to assist them, began the first formal instruction in these subjects.

The students for that first course were nearly all young physicians from Baltimore but there were others as well. The official list of sixteen is impressive indeed, and includes Alexander C. Abbott, B. Meade Bolton, William D. Booker, Harry Friedenwald, Frank D. Gavin, William S. Halsted, Christian A. Herter, Robert W. Johnson, George M. Sternberg, and Henry M. Thomas among others. Some of these students were engaged in special work, while others took the formal course. At least five of the group later became members of the medical faculty. The time was right, and the courses offered by Welch appealed to recent medical graduates eager to gain new knowledge of pathology and the newer science of bacteriology. The pathological laboratory under Welch's direction soon became a mecca for young men from various parts of the country. To it came Walter Reed and James Carroll of yellow fever fame; Simon Flexner, who was later to organize and direct so successfully the Rockefeller Institute for Medical Research; J. H. Wright, who subsequently developed the reticulocyte count, which was of such help to George Minot in his work on liver therapy in pernicious anemia; Reid Hunt, who became professor of pharmacology at Harvard; and J. Whitridge Williams, the first professor of obstetrics at Johns Hopkins.

When the hospital opened in 1889, many of the younger members of the staff took advantage of the opportunity to attend the courses in the pathological laboratory or to participate in the work going on there. On this list appear the names of such distinguished individuals as Lewellys F. Barker, William S. Thayer, John M. T. Finney, T. S. Cullen, and Hunter Robb. As Chesney notes, the chief source of pathological material for the laboratory was that obtained from the autopsies done at Bayview (later Baltimore City Hospitals) by Councilman, who brought back the specimens in pails suspended from the handlebars of his bicycle. Some of these students were encouraged to remain in the laboratory and undertake the study of special problems. As a result, more than one received a stimulus toward important investigative work which would influence them greatly for the rest of their lives. This was Welch's most active period in the laboratory, during which time he discovered the bacillus of gas gangrene. One of his most distinguished pupils was George Hoyt Whipple, who later shared the Nobel Prize with Minot and Murphy.

Welch and the Gas Bacillus

On October 25, 1891, there came to autopsy in the Johns Hopkins Hospital a mulatto from Osler's ward with an aneurysm of the aorta. The large aneurysmal sac had pressed on the bony structures of the chest, eroding them away, and on the skin, resulting in ulcerations from which several hemorrhages had occurred.

During the autopsy, Welch noted a peculiar swelling of the skin over the neck, arms and chest which on pressure gave forth a crackling sound. The veins of the skin were easily visible and contained gas. The examination was made soon after death, so that decomposition could not explain these unusual changes. Welch nicked one of the exposed veins, to which he then held a lighted match. The escaping gas ignited with a slight explosion and was noted to burn with a pale bluish flame, demonstrating that it was not air. Examination of blood from the heart and great vessels showed numerous short bacilli, and similar organisms were found in the laminated clot lining the aneurysm, as well as in the liver, spleen, and kidneys. These bacilli were present in pure culture, stained with aniline dyes and were surrounded by a capsule. They grew readily in culture under anaerobic conditions.

The bacilli were not pathogenic for animals. However, when animals injected intravenously with the organisms later were killed, the bacilli quickly multiplied in the blood vessels of various organs, simulating the appearances observed at the autopsy. Dr. Welch concluded that the organisms developed in the thick clots of the sac, entered the blood stream, and were thus distributed throughout the body before death. He believed that the entrance of gas and of bacilli into the circulation were related to the sudden death of the patient.

Welch and his associate, Dr. George H. F. Nuttall, studied the characteristics of the organism and reported the case in the *Johns Hopkins Hospital Bulletin* under the title "A Gas Producing Bacillus (Bacillus Aerogenes Capsulatus, nov. spec.) Capable of Rapid Development in the Blood Vessels After Death." The opening paragraph reads as follows: "There are to be found in medical literature many cases in which the blood-vessels after death contained air or gas which did not seem attributable to post-mortem decomposition. Various explanations of this occurrence have been offered. The observation to be here reported is calculated to shed light upon some of these mysterious cases."

The first issue of the *Journal of Experimental Medicine*, of which Welch was the editor, appeared in January 1896. The first article was a description of the gas bacillus and the report of additional instances in which the bacillus had been isolated from patients in the Johns Hopkins Hospital suffering from gas gangrene, intestinal perforation with peritonitis, morbid conditions of the urinary tract, hemorrhagic infarction of the lung, gas cysts of the intestine, and biliary tract infection.

Two years after the original report of Welch and Nuttall, E. Frankel of Germany published a monograph on gas phlegmons in which he described a bacillus isolated from four cases of gas gangrene. Welch recognized that this bacillus was identical with the one which he and Nuttall had described. He later proved this by studying cultures sent him by Frankel and by the effects of the two microorganisms in animals. The bacillus has subsequently been known as the "Welch bacillus." As pointed out by Flexner, the common occurrence of gas-producing bacilli in contaminated wounds had a profound significance during World War I, when there was a high incidence of gas gangrene. Antitoxin was developed, and subsequently chemotherapy proved beneficial in the treatment of these infections.

This discovery was perhaps Welch's most significant scientific contribution. It was an important discovery in a period when bacteriology was expanding rapidly and the specific causes of many of the infectious diseases were being unearthed. Welch brought the excitement of this whole era to the United States, and he, more than any other scientist, was the generator of the magnificent period of fruitful scientific discovery, which allowed America to pay back her long-standing debt to Europe.

On his eightieth birthday Welch sat at the side of President Hoover in Washington. Simultaneous dinners were being held in his honor in London, Paris, Geneva, Tokyo, and Peking. His friends all over the world listened with keen attention to the radio, which transmitted the words of the President and the comments of many distinguished friends and admirers. They recalled Welch's achievements as a scientist and his contributions to medical education and public health. In reply Welch spoke as follows:

Did I accept merely as a personal tribute these words of praise and this manifestation of appreciation and good will marked by this large and distinguished gathering and by meetings elsewhere, I should be overpowered with a sense of unreality depriving me of utterance, but I shall assume, as I feel that I am justified in doing, that by virtue of certain pioneering work and through over a half-century of service I stand here to represent an army of teachers, investigators, pupils, associates, and colleagues, whose work and contributions during this period have advanced the science and art of medicine and public health to the eminent position which they now hold in this country.... If I have handed on any intellectual heritage to pupils, assistants, and associates, whose work and achievements have been the greatest satisfaction and joy of my life it is derived from that which I received from my own masters.

Who were these masters and what was the itinerary that led Welch to the Hopkins, the discovery of the gas bacillus, and all of the tremendous contributions which followed? When it came time for him to choose his life's work, he was eager to become a teacher of Greek. As there was no opportunity to secure an attractive post, he reluctantly turned to medicine and selected the College of Physicians and Surgeons in New York City. The school, like all other medical schools at that time in the United States, was a poor one, but the teachers were fine gentlemen. Welch was much impressed by the course given in nervous diseases by Dr. Edward C. Seguin. He thought for a time that he would devote his life to the study of neurology. However, he made such an admirable report on Dr. Seguin's lectures that he received a microscope as a prize. This instrument transformed for him the study of anatomy, and he soon became enthusiastic about pathological anatomy. Six months after graduation he received an appointment at Bellevue, where he made the acquaintance of Dr. Abraham Jacobi, who was greatly impressed with Welch and occasionally asked him to dine at his home. During the after-dinner conversations there, Jacobi introduced Welch to the great achievements of the German scientists in medicine and public health. In March 1875 Welch wrote to his father that he wished to spend a year in Germany. On April 19, 1876 he sailed on a voyage of exploration which was in its ultimate results perhaps the most important ever taken by an American doctor, at least in the eyes of his biographers, Simon and James Thomas Flexner. By a fortunate series of events, Welch entered the physiological laboratory of Karl Ludwig—a period which determined his whole subsequent career. On February 25, 1877, Welch wrote as follows:

My work with Prof. Ludwig has been very profitable, especially in giving me an insight into the apparatus and methods of modern physiology, which is by far the most exact of any of the branches of medicine, this position of exactness having been obtained more through the efforts of Prof. Ludwig than of any living man.... I hope I have learned from Prof. Ludwig's precept and practice that most important lesson for a microscopist, as well as for every man of science, not to be satisfied with loose thinking and half proofs, not to speculate and theorize but to observe closely and carefully facts.

Later, when he was working in Wagner's laboratory, he was introduced to John Shaw Billings, who had been appointed to organize the Johns Hopkins Hospital and medical department of the Johns Hopkins University and who was spending a short time in Germany for the purpose of studying the laboratories and methods. That night Billings and Welch drank beer at Aurbach's Keller, in the room where Faust was reputed to have met the devil. Under sixteenth-century murals depicting this classic rendezvous, these two men had a long conversation, which marked a turning point in Welch's career. Welch learned that the medical department of the Hopkins would not be organized for four years, which gave him some time to prove himself. Billings drew Welch out not only about his studies in Germany but also about his attitude toward science and many other things. At the end he took Welch's name and address and said that he would have to look to such men as he, who were pursuing their studies abroad, when the time came to organize Johns Hopkins.

Welch expected to study with Virchow in Berlin, but Ludwig advised him to go to Breslau to Julius Cohnheim, whose brilliant pioneering in the application of physiological methods to pathology was making him world famous. Welch recognized that Wagner, with whom he had been working, was usually satisfied with the possession of a bare fact, but he soon learned that Cohnheim's interest did not stop there but demanded an explanation of the fact. Cohnheim had taken for his special study such important subjects as inflammation, dropsy, and embolism. Through his work these had become the subjects in pathology in which knowledge approached in exactness what was known concerning physical or chemical processes. During this trip, Welch also became intimate with Karl Weigert, the pathologist who first stained bacteria, and also with the youthful Paul Ehrlich.

Welch returned to New York, where he was successful in setting up a small pathology laboratory and in beginning some experimental work, which soon brought him into prominence with students and physicians in that city. But his great opportunity was just around the corner. He received another visit from Dr. Billings, who asked if he might see Welch do an autopsy the following day. They again had a long conversation and Welch was very enthusiastic as he described to Billings what he had seen in Germany and what he considered the opportunities to be for original research in the United States.

On March 1, 1884, Billings wrote a very laudatory letter to President Gilman about this young thirty-three-year-old pathologist, whom he had heard lecture and had seen working in the laboratory. He characterized him as modest and quiet, a gentleman in every sense and a good teacher. Cohnheim wrote to Gilman as follows: "The person best fitted for the chair of general pathology is Mr. Welch of New York." On March 31 Welch accepted the offer of Gilman to come to Hopkins, effective September 1, 1884. Welch was given the opportunity to return to Germany while the laboratories in Baltimore were being organized, and he sailed on September 16, 1884. From Leipzig, he wrote to Gilman: "I am convinced that for some years the relations of microorganisms to the causation of disease is to be the most important subject in pathology. I have therefore endeavored to make myself thoroughly familiar with the present

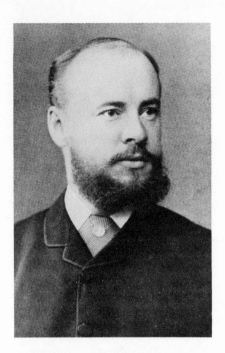

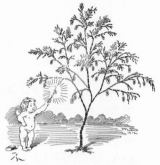

"The Welch and Nuttall Gas Plant"

Drawing by Max Broedel in the program of a dinner honoring Dr. George H. F. Nuttall on the occasion of his Herter Foundation Lectures in 1912 From the Archives Office, The Johns Hopkins Medical Institutions

William Henry Welch in 1884

Welch returned to Germany in that year to work with Robert Koch after his appointment to Johns Hopkins.
From *Bull. Johns Hopkins Hosp.*, vol. 87, August suppl., 1950

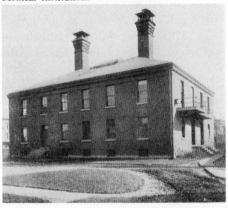

The Pathological Building

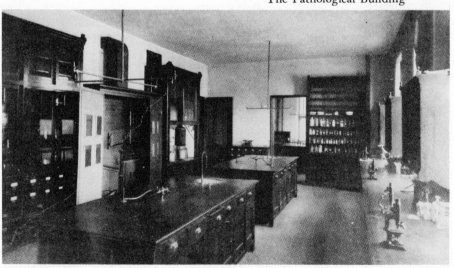

A laboratory in the Pathological Building

Photos from A. M. Chesney, *The Johns Hopkins Hospital and the Johns Hopkins University School of Medicine: A Chronicle*, vol. 1, *1867–1893* (Baltimore: The Johns Hopkins University Press, 1943)

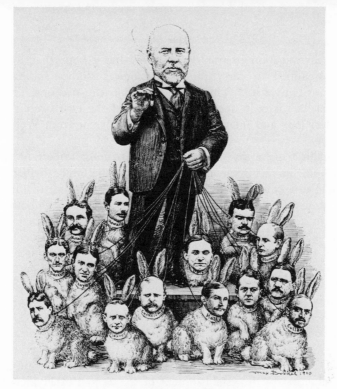

"Some Welch Rabbits"
Cartoon by Max Broedel

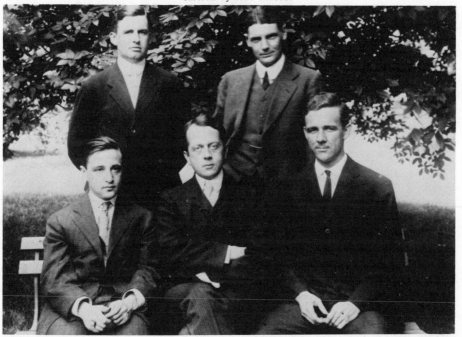

Staff of the Department of Pathology, 1908–1909
Standing: Dr. John T. King (*left*), Dr. Stewart; seated (*left to right*): Dr. Milton C. Winternitz,
Dr. William G. MacCallum, Dr. George Whipple
From the Archives Office, The Johns Hopkins Medical Institutions

methods of investigation in this department, and I hope that we shall be in every way qualified to carry on bacteriological studies successfully at the Johns Hopkins University." This is the way that it turned out. The description of the gas bacillus is only one finite evidence of the far-reaching work in the field of bacteriology and infectious diseases which came from Welch's pathological laboratory.

During this trip he saw things which were most important in the subsequent developments in his career. He worked in the famed hygienic laboratory of Max von Pettenkofer, where he discovered how methods of sanitary reform and purification of soil and water had almost abolished typhoid fever, once very prevalent in Munich. In the hospital there he saw Dr. Hugo Wilhelm von Ziemssen in a laboratory for the investigation of disease in the living patient that equaled the laboratory designed to study autopsies and other dead materials. He worked in Leipzig again with Ludwig and with Weigert, Cohnheim's brilliant assistant, who lectured on pathology after Cohnheim's death. The following July he spent in Robert Koch's new laboratory and returned to begin his appointment in Baltimore on October 1, 1885.

Welch had an extraordinary capacity to recognize the importance of events and ideas as he came in contact with them. The experience with Pettenkofer became very important years later and led to his interest in hygiene and public health, culminating in the establishment of the School of Hygiene and Public Health. He recognized, long before Osler, the tremendous significance of the work of Koch, Pasteur, and others; and he foresaw the golden era of medicine that was heralded by the advent of bacteriology and the demonstration of the cause of most of the infectious diseases.

Whipple's Disease

On April 12, 1907, a thirty-seven-year-old medical missionary was admitted to the Johns Hopkins Hospital with a disease "characterized clinically by gradual loss of weight and strength, stools consisting chiefly of neutral fat and fatty acids, indefinite abdominal signs, and a peculiar multiple arthritis." Some five years before, while working in Turkey, this physician had noted interrupted episodes of migratory polyarthritis. Six months prior to his death he returned to the United States (September 1906) because he thought that he had tuberculosis. He spent a month in the Adirondacks and later went to Mexico. During this time no evidence of tuberculosis could be obtained. He gradually developed swelling of the abdomen and was admitted to the hospital because of low-grade fever, steatorrhea, and an abdominal mass. Clinical and laboratory investigations narrowed the differential diagnosis to: (1) pulmonary and mesenteric tuberculosis, (2) erythema multiforme exudativum with arthritis, and/or (3) sarcoma or Hodgkin's disease of the mesenteric glands. These diagnoses are still among the commonly considered ones in the patient with this disease. An exploratory laparotomy was done which was thought to have demonstrated Hodgkin's disease, and he died shortly thereafter.

The case was reported by Dr. George Hoyt Whipple in the *Johns Hopkins*

Hospital Bulletin under the title, "A Hitherto Undescribed Disease Characterized Anatomically by Deposits of Fats and Fatty Acids in the Intestinal and
Mesenteric Lymphatic Tissues." Pathologically the lesions of interest were
found in the intestines and the lymphatic tissue draining this region. The intestinal mucosa showed enlarged villi, due to deposits of large masses of neutral
fats and fatty acids in the lymph spaces and an infiltration of the interglandular
tissue by large mononuclear and polynuclear giant cells. Examination of the
submucosa in many places revealed similar deposits in the enlarged lymph
spaces and invasion by large mononuclear cells. Grossly the mesenteric nodes
were the site of the most striking changes, but under the microscope the picture
closely resembled that seen in the intestine. The nodes showed the same deposits in even greater amounts, a chronic inflammatory reaction with replacement of much of the node by fibrous scar tissue and masses of large
mononuclear cells or polynuclear giant cells of the foreign body type.

Of the greatest interest was the observation that microscopically there
were many rod-shaped organisms. These Whipple described as about the diameter of the spirochete of syphilis, but not of spiral shape, and rarely exceeding two microns in length. The majority closely resembled in form the
tubercle bacillus. He did not claim that these bacillus-like bodies represented
the etiological factor in this disease, but their presence in the nodes was suggestive. He concluded that no suitable name could be applied to this condition
until the etiological factor was determined, but he suggested that the term
"intestinal lipodystrophy" had more in its favor than any other designation.

Little has been added to Dr. Whipple's lucid description of this entity
except the reaction of material in the foamy macrophages to periodic-acid-
Schiff reagent. Many years later (1961) sections of the intestine, lymph node,
heart, and pancreas from Whipple's original case were made and stained by
techniques not available to Whipple. The characteristic PAS-positive material
was found in the macrophages.

Whipple's disease is a rare disorder, and only about two hundred cases
have been reported. There are more articles in the literature on Whipple's
disease than patients reported. It is now clear that this disease is a systemic
rather than primarily an intestinal disorder. There has been increasing interest
in the disease in recent years as the methods of studying intestinal abnormalities have grown in effectiveness. In the later stages all of these patients show
malabsorption of some degree. Pathological studies have now demonstrated
that essentially any organ may contain infiltrates of Whipple cells or PAS-
positive macrophages and the degree of involvement varies from patient to
patient. The diagnosis can be made in most instances by biopsy of lymph nodes
or of the jejunum with demonstration of the characteristic PAS-positive cells.
The use of electron microscopy has brought about not only the "re-discovery"
of the organisms first pointed out by Dr. Whipple, but has also increased the
knowledge of the character, location, and relationship of these organisms to the
PAS-positive material within macrophages. These findings, of course, strongly
suggest that bacteria play a role in the etiology of Whipple's disease. Whipple
himself cultivated a "bacillus of the colon group" from a mesenteric lymph

node of his case. In a recent study of a patient with Whipple's disease, Charache and her colleagues isolated an atypical beta-hemolytic streptococcus (Type D). This finding has not been confirmed, as the opportunity to study cases of Whipple's disease in patients who have not received antibiotic therapy is unusual. When corticosteroids were first introduced into clinical medicine, encouraging results were obtained in the treatment of Whipple's disease. Later there were isolated reports of the efficacy of antibiotics in controlling the symptoms of Whipple's disease, but their importance was firmly established by the large series of cases reported from Duke University Medical Center by Davis and his colleagues and later by Ruffin et al. A successful outcome has followed the administration of penicillin and streptomycin in combination, followed by tetracycline, and also in certain instances with chloramphenicol. The etiology of Whipple's disease still remains an enigma, and it is not certain whether it is primarily a bacterial infection or whether other factors are also concerned with its causation.

George Hoyt Whipple was born in Ashland, New Hampshire, on August 28, 1878. He was educated at Andover Academy and Yale University, receiving his M.D. degree from Johns Hopkins in 1905. With the exception of one year, 1907–1908, as pathologist at the Ancon Hospital in Panama, Dr. Whipple was at the Johns Hopkins Medical School from 1905 to 1914 as assistant, instructor, and associate professor in pathology. From 1914 to 1921 he was professor of research medicine at the University of California Medical School and director of the Hooper Foundation for Medical Research, University of California. During the year 1920–1921 he was dean of the University of California Medical School. In 1921 Dr. Whipple became professor of pathology and dean of the School of Medicine and Dentistry at the University of Rochester.

In 1920 he began to study the influence of food on blood regeneration. The transformation of hematology into the dynamic and exciting field it is today began with these systematic studies of George Whipple and his associates. The method adopted in these experiments was to withdraw from dogs a certain quantity of blood, feeding them afterwards with foods of various kinds. By that method he discovered that certain foods were superior to others inasmuch as they stimulated the bone marrow to a more vigorous manufacture of red blood corpuscles. Most effective was liver, then kidney, then meat, and next certain vegetable articles of food.

These investigations of Whipple's gave George Minot and William Murphy the idea of feeding patients with pernicious anemia foods that Whipple had found to yield favorable results in his experiments. Their work, of course, led to the discovery of liver therapy of pernicious anemia, and subsequently to the isolation of vitamin B_{12}, the specific factor which cures this type of anemia. In 1934, along with Drs. Minot and Murphy, Dr. Whipple shared the Nobel Prize in Medicine.

6 ❦ Pharmacology's Giant: John Jacob Abel

PHARMACOLOGY, the study of the action of drugs, like medicine in general, had an empirical beginning hampered by superstition, metaphysical speculation, and rationalization. Its scientific base had to await that of physiology and biochemistry, since most of the effects of drugs are functional. The first scientific investigations of pharmacology began when drugs were used as tools by physiologists. One of the earliest studies was that of Claude Bernard on curare, made almost 120 years ago. It was conducted as a project of "experimental medicine," without any thought of its ultimate practical therapeutic application.

In the mid-nineteenth century the German academic community perceived that pharmacology was a field worth cultivating for itself, and in 1856 the first university department of pharmacology for the scientific study of drug action was established in Dorpat under Buchheim. It was quite successful, and other German universities soon followed the example. When the German university of Strasbourg was founded after the Franco-German War, its "Pharmakologische Institute," headed by Oswald Schmiedeberg, soon became the heart of pharmacology. News of this stimulating new scientific focus spread over the world, including, of course, the United States. Progressive universities were beginning to establish full-time chairs in various important medical subjects. Victor Vaughan, dean of the medical school of the State of Michigan, had gathered a notable group of medical scientists and this school was the first to put pharmacology on a full-time basis, although still under the title of Materia Medica and Therapeutics. Being a perceptive dean, he turned for advice to Schmiedeberg at Strasbourg, who recommended John Jacob Abel as the first professor of pharmacology in the United States. Subsequently, Abel came to Baltimore and established a department which has continued to be unsurpassed in its contributions to research and teaching. This is the story of Abel and his multitude of important research adventures.

John Jacob Abel

John Jacob Abel was one of the pioneers who helped develop American scientific medicine to the high place it now occupies. He was the first professor of pharmacology in the United States, and his important influence extended over a quarter of a century. The story of his training and subsequent career touches on many of the events and personalities who occupied the stage in this most important era of medical science. Abel was born on a farm near Cleveland, Ohio, on May 19, 1857. At the age of nineteen he entered the University of Michigan, where he took a course in physiological chemistry under Victor Vaughan and physiology under Dr. Henry Sewall. He received his Ph.D. degree from Michigan in 1883 and the following year worked in the Department of Biology of the Johns Hopkins University under Professor Newell Martin, the able pupil of Michael Foster. At the age of twenty-seven (1884), he decided to study medicine in Europe. During the next seven years he exhibited a remarkable ability to select as his teachers the most distinguished men of this period. From 1884 to 1886 he studied physiology in Leipzig under Ludwig and von Frey, histology under His, pharmacology under Bohn, pathology under Strumpell, and inorganic and organic chemistry under Wislicenus. The semester of 1886–1887 was spent in Strasbourg under Kussmaul in internal medicine and under von Recklinghausen in pathology and infectious diseases. The following semester he studied in Heidelberg with Erb in medicine and Czerny in surgery. The next year brought him back to Strasbourg, where he took courses under Naunyn, Hoppe-Seyler, and Schmiedeberg. It was from the latter that Abel's first interest in pharmacological research, particularly in its chemical aspects, was aroused. In 1888 he received his M.D. degree from Strasbourg, following which he worked in the laboratory of the outstanding Swiss biochemist, von Nencki, where he received his most important training in chemical research.

The time had come to return home, where he expected to carry on medical practice, since one had to have wide recognition to obtain a professorship and his funds were largely exhausted. Fortunately, in the late summer, while he was still in Berne, Vaughan, on Schmiedeberg's recommendation, offered him the chair of materia medica and therapeutics in the University of Michigan. The understanding was that he establish a modern department of pharmacology in the United States.

In January 1893 he received a letter from Osler inquiring whether he would be a candidate for the chair of pharmacology at Hopkins. When he learned that there would be adequate laboratory facilities, he accepted the offer and began work in the autumn of 1893 in Baltimore, assuming as well responsibility for the course in physiological chemistry.

It had been the custom to have pharmacology taught by practicing physicians who lectured and quizzed from textbooks. Abel used the original literature in the preparation of lectures. Some lecture-room demonstrations were given, but more emphasis was placed on the laboratory course, in which the students participated actively in the experiments. The laboratory course in physiological chemistry under Walter Jones was arranged in a similar way. From the time he arrived at Hopkins, Abel advocated an independent chair of biological chemistry. In 1908 he relinquished his responsibilities in this area to Walter Jones who had been made head of this new department.

Abel's attention was soon attracted to the problem of the isolation of hormones, an interest dating from 1895. He began to study the chemistry of the active principle of the adrenal medulla, a work to which he devoted himself with extraordinary vigor during the next ten years. The first paper published with Crawford in 1897 reported the isolation of a benzoyl derivative of the active principle. This was done as a means of separating the principal compound, on the assumption that the active substance contained phenolic groups. In a number of other experiments, the elementary composition of the base was established by the analysis of several derivatives including the sulphate, and was stated to be represented by the formula $C_{17}H_{15}NO_4$.

At this stage he was visited one day by the Japanese chemist Takamine, who after their discussions postulated that the process of Dr. Abel could no doubt be improved and simplified, with which Abel agreed. Takamine proceeded successfully to employ ammonia on very highly concentrated, though impure, extracts and immediately obtained the native base in the form of burr-like clusters of minute prisms in place of Abel's amorphous base. It became clear that Abel's epinephrine had contained a single hidden benzoyl radical. As Abel stated, taking this whole event stoically: "The efforts of years on my part in this once mysterious field of suprarenal medullary biochemistry, marred by blunders as they were, eventuated, then, in the isolation of the hormone, not in the form of the free base but in that of its monobenzoyl derivative." However, it was Abel's work which laid the foundation for the final triumph, and he will be remembered as the pioneer who clearly recognized the importance of the chemical isolation of hormones as the first step leading to their synthesis, rational pharmacological study, and therapeutic administration.

Abel's stoical personality was evidenced in an incident that occurred during the period in which he was working on epinephrine. On the evening of December 11, 1900, Dr. Auer relates that he heard an explosion in Dr. Abel's laboratory. Rushing there with Dr. Abel's helper, he found the professor at the sink, sluicing water over his face. Dr. Abel turned toward Auer and stated quite calmly, "My eye is gone, boys, I know it's gone." In spite of the loss of his eye, which represented a great handicap for him in his ensuing career, Abel diligently pursued his work and from then on never referred to this accident.

During the decade from 1895 to 1905, Abel, while deeply engrossed in his researches and in his teaching, still found time to participate in the founding of the first scientific journals and societies relating to research in the fields of his interest. In the fall of 1895 he indicated to President Gilman the need for an American journal covering the field of experimental medicine. After further consultation the *Journal of Experimental Medicine* was born, with William H. Welch as the editor-in-chief. The first issue appeared in January 1896. It has continued since that time to play an important role in the promotion of medical research. Abel was a founder of the *Journal of Biological Chemistry*, which first appeared in 1905 with Abel and C. A. Herter as its editors. At about this time Abel also assumed the leadership in the founding of the *Journal of Pharmacology and Experimental Therapeutics* and in the organization of the American Society for Pharmacology and Experimental Therapeutics, accomplished in 1908 with Abel as its first president.

It is not possible to relate all of the important research contributions of Dr. Abel. The story of his work on the pituitary and on the crystallization of insulin are well known. However, it is of interest to present in more detail three other areas in which his work and that of his colleagues ultimately had important clinical applications: the introduction of phenolsulphonephthalein as a test of renal function, the description of a method of renal dialysis, and the work which followed on plasmapheresis.

In 1909 Abel and Leonard G. Rowntree published their paper on the pharmacological action of phthalein derivatives. In 1884 Dr. Ira Remsen, professor of chemistry at the Johns Hopkins University, had described a new chemical compound, a purple dye, which he called by the formidable name phenolsulphonephthalein. He published an account in the *American Chemical Journal*, describing it as an interesting chemical for which there was no particular use, and then put it away on the shelf of his laboratory. Some years later a pupil of Remsen's, Sohon, described this substance as a bright red crystalline powder somewhat soluble in water, more so in alcohol, but insoluble in ether; its dilute alkaline solution he said is of a purer red than that of phenolphthalein, while a more strongly alkaline solution is purple. It is readily soluble in solution of sodium carbonate and has a stronger avidity as an acid than phenolphthalein. The object of the work of Abel and Rowntree was, firstly, to study the influence of substitution in various parts of the molecule upon pharmacological action, and secondly, to look for a purgative suitable for subcutaneous injection. A thorough study was made of the absorption and elimination of a series of phthalein compounds. No practical purgative resulted from the work, but Abel and Rowntree discovered that phenolsulphonephthalein was rapidly and completely excreted by the normal kidney without causing any evident renal damage. Rowntree recognized the importance of this observation, and with Dr. Abel's encouragement he further pursued the study of this compound. An interesting aspect of the story from this point on is told by Dr. Hugh Young in his autobiography. Rowntree, he states, presented his work on this drug at a meeting of the Interurban Surgical Society and indicated that it was eliminated more rapidly by a diseased than by a healthy kidney. Rowntree demonstrated this on a dog in which, under anesthesia, he had exposed the kidney and injected the renal artery with uranium nitrate, in order to produce a chemical nephritis. Then he divided the ureter and brought it out upon the skin, where he could collect the urine from it. The phenolsulphonephthalein (PSP) was injected intravenously, and urine from the right kidney collected through the ureter, which had been brought out upon the skin, while that from the left kidney was collected through a catheter in the bladder. It seemed evident that a larger amount of the purple dye was excreted through the kidney in which the artery had been injected with uranium nitrate than through the other presumably normal kidney. After the demonstration was over Young told Rowntree that he had a patient, with the same conditions presented by the dog, upon whom he had operated—the right ureter was blocked by a stone and all the urine was escaping through a sinus in the side. He suggested that it would be a good case in which to repeat upon a human being the experiment just carried out upon the dog.

The following day the dye was injected intravenously into Dr. Young's patient. Most of the drug was eliminated through the fistula leading from the right kidney. The correctness of Dr. Rowntree's test on the dogs seemed to be confirmed. However, a few days later the patient developed a fever, and a mass appeared on the left side. It was evident that there was a large pyonephrosis, which observation was confirmed at operation. Thus, Dr. Rowntree's interpretation was erroneous. Diseased kidneys eliminated the drug in less quantity than did healthy kidneys. Dr. Rowntree was joined by Dr. J. T. Geraghty in his studies, and a method was devised by which the exact percentage of the drug excreted could be read from a simple color scale. Then the degree of impairment of kidney function from prostatic obstruction could be determined. Rowntree and Geraghty's studies in the experimental animal as well as in man demonstrated the value of the phthalein test in clinical medicine. Among its advantages over other tests in use at that time were: firstly, its early appearance in the urine and the rapidity and completeness of its elimination by the kidney; secondly, quantitative estimation of the amount of drug excreted was simple and accurate; thirdly, elimination of the drug was decreased in both chronic parenchymatous and chronic interstitial nephritis. The test proved of practical value in prostatic obstruction, enabling the surgeon to select the optimal time for operation.

The use of the PSP test proved beneficial in the case of the great chemist who had originally discovered the compound but put it aside as valueless. Dr. Remsen, then president of the Johns Hopkins University, had been in poor health for a year. His mind became clouded, he resigned, and a successor was selected. Soon after this, Remsen came to Dr. Young, complaining of frequency of urination. He had only slight difficulty in voiding, but when a catheter was passed almost a quart of residual urine was obtained. The PSP test showed marked impairment of kidney function. With carefully controlled drainage his kidney function steadily improved until the PSP test was almost normal. Dr. Remsen became mentally alert and a prostatectomy was carried out successfully. He left the hospital entirely restored to health. He laconically remarked that had he known the cause of his infirmity, he would not have resigned the presidency.

In 1913 Dr. Abel visualized a method for the removal of diffusible substances from the circulating blood of living animals by dialysis (Fig. 1). Voegtlin in his excellent biography of Abel recounts how, before starting the work, Abel discussed his ideas and plans with his staff at the luncheon table. These informal daily meetings, which lasted throughout Abel's long career at Hopkins, were remembered by his associates as stimulating experiences. The basic idea of this proposal, which was to become known as "vividiffusion," was to provide means for the removal of substances detrimental to the animal body and to relieve the kidneys of this function in a variety of toxic conditions. The method, furthermore, was to serve the investigative purpose of isolating and identifying the multiplicity of diffusible substances in the blood. Marshall recalls that early in the fall of 1912 he was present at Dr. Abel's famous lunch table, when the professor proposed this "artificial kidney":

The blood from an animal was to pass from an artery through a series of collodion tubes surrounded by saline solution back into a vein. Small cylinders rolled from the

luncheon bread were used to illustrate the apparatus. The first experiment was performed on the afternoon of November 10, 1912, using a two-tube apparatus on a
rabbit. Abel talked of the clinical application of this machine for the treatment of
intoxications or to tide over when kidneys were not functioning. I admit, I considered
such talk visionary. However, in 1926, Haas of Giessen used an "artificial kidney" on
three patients, and twenty years later the "artificial kidney" was put on a workable
basis.

Associated with Dr. Abel in this work were Rowntree and B. B. Turner, who
later became professor of pharmacology at Indiana. That renal dialysis, which
has subsequently become of such widespread importance in the renal transplantation program, was in Abel's mind becomes clear from reading the first paragraph of the paper published in the *Transactions of the Association of
American Physicians* entitled "On the Removal of Diffusible Substances from the
Circulating Blood by Means of Dialysis":

There are numerous toxic states in which the eliminating organs of the body, more
especially the kidneys, are incapable of removing from the body, at an adequate rate,
the natural and unnatural substances whose accumulation is detrimental to life. In the
hope of providing a substitute in such emergencies, which might tide over a dangerous crisis, as well as for the important information which it might be expected to
provide, concerning the substances normally present in the blood, and also for the
light that might thus be thrown on intermediary stages of metabolism, a method has
been devised by which the blood of a living animal may be submitted to dialysis
outside the body, and again returned to the natural circulation without exposure to
air, infection by microorganisms, or any alteration which would necessarily be prej-
udical to life.

Abel and his associates were able to show that the elimination of salicylic acid
by this "artificial kidney" compared favorably with the elimination of this drug
by the natural kidney. Unfortunately Abel was ahead of his time, and the
effective application of this method to clinical medicine had to await over two
decades. However, they succeeded in isolating a number of blood constituents
from the dialysate. Of greatest interest was the identification of the amino
acids, alanine and valine, and indication of the presence of histidine and cre-
atinine. This isolation of amino acids was the first incontestable evidence of
their occurrence in normal blood, a fact of fundamental importance in the
study of protein metabolism. Shortly thereafter Abderhalden published his
work on the isolation of amino acids from deproteinized normal blood.

The first apparatus for vividiffusion was constructed with the help of
Abel's fabulous diener, Charlie Kamphaus, was found to function well, and was
demonstrated in 1913 at the International Physiological Congress in Groningen. Rowntree carried the apparatus to Europe, and as he was getting off the
streetcar in Groningen, a bicyclist knocked him to the ground. Fortunately, he
held the "artificial kidney" aloft and it escaped unharmed.

While they were engaged in the work of vividiffusion, these investigators
also carried out some experiments in plasmapheresis. The underlying idea was
to devise a more scientific method for venesection. Experiments on dogs
showed that large quantities of blood could be withdrawn repeatedly without

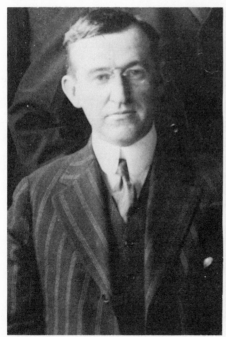

John Timothy Geraghty

From the Archives Office, The Johns Hopkins
Medical Institutions

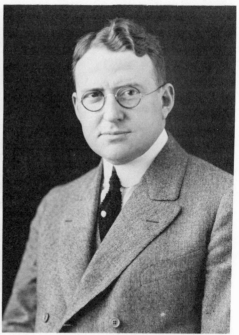

Leonard George Rowntree

From the Archives Office, The Johns Hopkins
Medical Institutions

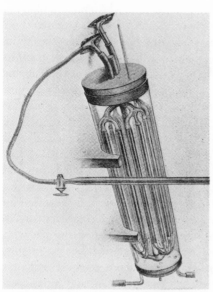

Fig. 1 Apparatus of "vividiffusion"

From *J. Pharmacol. Exp. Ther.* 5 (1913): 285

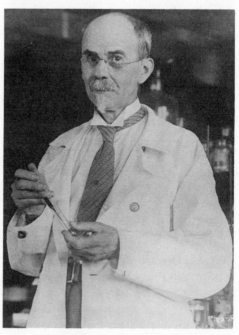

John Jacob Abel

From the Archives Office, The Johns Hopkins
Medical Institutions

apparent injury if the corpuscles, separated by centrifugation from the plasma, were suspended in Locke solution and reinjected. The paper dealing with this work, published in 1914, contains the following prophetic sentence: "In view of the fact that mammalian corpuscles retain their stability for three or four days when kept on ice, a supply of human corpuscles might possibly be kept in this manner in operating rooms for rapid injection in emergencies that would otherwise prove fatal." This is another striking example that Abel clearly perceived the practical applications of his work, although he was above all interested in the establishment of new fundamental principles.

One of the unforgettable stories relates to Dr. Abel's decision to carry out one of his plasmapheresis experiments on a patient in the hospital who had nephritis. The idea was to remove a pint of blood at a time, add an anticoagulant, bring it back to the laboratory, centrifuge it, replace the plasma with salt solution, return the blood to the patient and repeat the process as often as necessary. It was, of course, important to sterilize everything used for this work. However, a physical chemist's idea of sterility was a curious one. Everything was passed through a flame, some slowly, others fast, depending on their nature, until they were "about sterile." Having collected a supply of this "about sterile" apparatus, everyone repaired to the hospital. The patient was lying on an operating table with a donor next to him in case of accident. The surgical benches were filled with interested spectators. A surgeon asked Dr. Abel if he would not care to put on a cap and gown and take part in the experiment. Dr. Abel stepped up to the nurse and proceeded to get into his gown backwards, much to the consternation of the nurse. He finally got it on right side round, then his rubber gloves and, on top of all, one of his much-beloved operating caps, which he always wore. The professor went about on tiptoe, talking in a hushed voice and watching the drawing of the blood with the greatest interest. At first he walked about with both hands high in the air, his mind centered on asepsis. Then seeing someone in the stands to whom he wished to speak, he would go over, take hold of the iron railing with both hands and come back to the operating table again with his hands held high in the air. It was difficult for those watching the experiment to restrain themselves under these circumstances, but they did so extremely well. After the blood was drawn, Professor Abel rushed about in a very excited manner and in low, excited whispers gave directions to his assistants for carrying it back to the laboratory. When all was ready, he disappeared from the operating room, with both hands still high in the air. The moment the door was closed there was a sigh of relief, but not more than thirty seconds later the Professor came rushing back, still wearing his rubber gloves, his operating gown and cap, but with his derby hat stuffed on over it. He came up to the operating table, and stood there talking excitedly in whispers to the surgeon, while every few minutes he adjusted his derby hat with his rubber-gloved hands. Finally, he rushed out of the room. The spectators, peering out of the windows, could see him tearing up Monument Street with his gown flapping in the wind, his derby hat on the back of his head, and his rubber-gloved hands held high in the air.

During his earlier years, Abel was looked upon by many as somewhat of a visionary, but as the years passed his invaluable qualities were generally recognized. His colleague, Osler, in a letter written in connection with the reorganization of the Oxford medical school, paid Abel the following tribute:

The four lines of progress for our school are pharmacology, hygiene, the history of medicine and a clinicopathological laboratory in connection with the infirmary. Of these the first is a pressing need. Everywhere, I am sorry to say except in this country [England], the science of pharmacology is making rapid strides and the subject is universally recognized as one of the most important in university work. Moreover, it is one of the hopeful, progressive departments of medicine with great possibilities for public service. I can testify in the strongest possible way to the work of Professor Abel and his department of The Johns Hopkins Medical School. There are no classes more popular and the researches that have been carried on have been very valuable.

Abel was given many, many honors.

The tales about Abel and his eccentricities in the laboratory are numerous. One morning a young man came to Abel's laboratory from the Baltimore *Sun*, saying that he wanted a story on his work on sleeping sickness. Abel explained to the reporter that the work was in its infancy and had not gone far enough to justify publicity. He stated that when completed it would be presented to a scientific society and published in their journal. He then asked the young man for his card and promised to send him a reprint. After the reporter's departure, Dr. Abel explained to Rowntree that it was the young man's "job" to get a story if he could, but, he said: "I got rid of him without telling him a thing about our work and without hurting his feelings." Rowntree was quite impressed. However, that evening, in passing the Baltimore *Sun* building, he saw a great crowd around the bulletin board. It carried a story entitled "Hee-Haw Maude and Professor Abel." In reading the paper he found a badly distorted story of their researches. Naturally, the Professor investigated, and he found that a young lad who helped take care of the animals (including Maude the donkey) had graciously granted the reporter an interview and inadvertently filled him with misinformation. This laboratory assistant was really quite a lad and, as can be seen, "devoted beyond the call of duty." Needless to say, neither Abel nor Rowntree were accustomed to handling donkeys. Maude had been infected experimentally with a trypanosome that affects horses and cattle, and Abel and Rowntree were attempting to cure its disease with some new chemicals prepared by Dr. Abel. This necessitated intrajugular injections. The donkey was very fractious, so the Professor asked Rowntree to come down and help "steady the donkey" while he made the injections. This necessitated Rowntree's getting under the donkey's neck, putting his arm around the animal's shoulders, and holding it steady. But the donkey was incorrigible. Every time Abel started his injection, the donkey started to buck. After about a half-hour struggle Dr. Abel said "Now," but the donkey bucked again. But Rowntree that time saw something. The youthful helper, the lad who had given the interview to the press, was waiting for the crucial moment to jab a spike into the donkey's belly. Rowntree grabbed his hand, the professor saw the spike and arrived at the right conclusion. Though devoted far beyond the call of duty, the lad received no reward. He was dismissed then and there.

Another of the stories told about Abel and his curiosity related to the reception given for "Diamond Jim" Brady after he had left the money to found the Brady Institute. Brady lived up to his name and was ablaze with diamonds. Dr. Abel was introduced, and was captivated with his diamond stickpin. On leaving the line someone asked Abel about Mr. Brady's diamond ring. The Professor confessed that he had missed it, so he got in line, was introduced again and centered his attention on the huge sparkler. Then he was asked if he had noticed the diamond buttons on his coat. These he had also missed, so he was introduced again and took in the diamond buttons. Then some wag asked, "But did you see the diamond shoe buttons?" The Professor got in line, was reintroduced, centered his attention on Mr. Brady's shoes, and found to his chagrin that they were laced shoes with no diamonds to be seen.

Abel was first and foremost an investigator. His great enthusiasm and passionate devotion to research dominated his whole life. In one of his addresses, after discussing the training necessary for the medical investigator, wherein an extended chemical training is emphasized, he wrote:

But to what end is all this preparation for our young man? Is it solely that he may solve problems whose solution is of practical value to mankind? Is his mind to shape itself only to the insistent demands of utility? Even then our method of training will yield the largest profit.

But it does vastly more than that. Thus trained, our young scholar will be able to see beyond the immediately practical problem, even though it be as great a thing as the discovery of the cause and cure of the plague that decimates a people. *Greater even than the greatest discovery is to keep open the way to future discoveries.* This can only be done when the investigator freely dares, moved as by an inner propulsion, to attack problems not because they give promise of immediate value to the human race, but because they make an irresistible appeal by reason of an inner beauty.

Some of the greatest investigators indeed have been fascinated by problems of immediate utility as well as by those that deal with abstract conceptions only. Helmholtz invented the ophthalmoscope and thus made modern ophthalmology possible, and at the same time did work of the highest order in theoretical physics and wrote on the nature of mathematical axioms and the principles of psychology. Lord Kelvin took out patents on great improvements in the compass and on overseas telegraphy and also made contributions to our knowledge of the ultimate constitution of the atom and the properties of the ether.

From this point of view the investigator is a man whose inner life is free in the best sense of the word. In short, there should be in research work a cultural character, an artistic quality, elements that give to painting, music, and poetry their high place in the life of man.

Leonard George Rowntree

Leonard George Rowntree was an important collaborator of Dr. Abel in relating to the clinical application of his ideas. A Canadian born in 1883,

Rowntree, after finishing his internship in 1906, sought his medical future in the United States, first going into practice in Camden, New Jersey. This clinical experience ingrained in him a lifelong interest in patients and in their diseases. However, it soon became apparent to him that he needed more training. In the autumn of 1907 he enrolled as a voluntary student in the Department of Pharmacology at Johns Hopkins, and in the succeeding six years rose to be an associate professor under Dr. Abel. Rowntree's major contributions have already been related, but it is important that in his clinical exploration of his laboratory results, he always revealed his good judgment by inviting experienced physicians in the fields concerned to share in the human testing. When the first full-time department of medicine was organized at Johns Hopkins in 1914 under Dr. Theodore Janeway, Rowntree was invited to join the staff as an associate professor. In 1916 he accepted the professorship of medicine in the University of Minnesota, and spent the next sixteen years in the institution, the early years being devoted to work on the campus in Minneapolis and from 1920 to 1932 in Rochester at the Mayo Foundation and Clinic. His ability to stimulate clinical investigation found ample scope among the postgraduate faculty and the fellows of the clinic. In 1923 he first observed that a large intake of water caused serious intoxication which was an early stimulus to investigations of importance at the Mayo Clinic in regard to water and electrolyte problems. Rowntree was president of the American Society of Clinical Investigation in 1921, and he had a material part in establishing at Rochester, in April 1928, the Central Society for Clinical Research. During World War I he held a responsible executive position in the medical branch of the United States Air Service, and in 1940, when the National Selective Service was organized, Rowntree was appointed chief of the medical division, a post he held throughout World War II. He died in 1959.

John Timothy Geraghty

Dr. John Timothy Geraghty was for the last ten years of his life professor of clinical urology and assistant director of the James Buchanan Brady Urological Institute. Dr. Geraghty was born in St. Paul, Minnesota, on July 24, 1876, and spent his boyhood in that city. He was graduated from St. Thomas College in 1905 and two years later received his Ph.D. degree from the St. Paul Seminary in St. Paul. The next year he devoted to graduate work in chemistry and biology at the Johns Hopkins University, entering medical school in 1899. After graduation, he spent a year of study in Paris and Vienna. From 1907 to 1915 he was assistant, instructor and associate professor of genito-urinary disease at the Johns Hopkins Hospital. In addition he was a consultant urologist at Bayview Hospital and also engaged in private practice. He was a prolific contributor to various urological journals and an author of several books. His death on August 17, 1924, at an early age represented a real loss to the Division of Urology.

7 ❦ Neurosurgical Genius: Walter Edward Dandy

DISCOVERIES that are made by chance or by accident originate from an unintentional but hitherto unknown observation. The observation in itself does not constitute a discovery unless the observer recognizes its significance. It was in this connection that Louis Pasteur made the oft-quoted statement: "In the field of observation chance favors the prepared mind." An example is the discovery of ventriculography by the late Dr. Walter Edward Dandy, in which accident played a considerable part.

On January 3, 1917, a patient whose abdomen was about to be explored for intestinal perforation was sent for a chest x-ray on the way to the operating room. Dr. Frederick Henry Baetjer, the hospital radiologist who made the x-ray, included in it the upper abdomen, in which free air was seen under the diaphragm. Walter Edward Dandy, the surgical resident, operated on the patient and confirmed the presence of intraperitoneal air as well as the perforated typhoid ulcer through which it had escaped. This case probably crystallized for him what had been turning over in his mind as a result of the frequent comments by Dr. Halsted on the remarkable power of intestinal gases "to perforate bone," and his attention was finally drawn to its practical possibilities in the brain.

Striking gas shadows are present in all abdominal and thoracic radiograms. The stomach and intestines are often outlined by the contained air even more sharply than when filled with fluid and food. A perforation of the intestines may be diagnosed by the shadow of air that has accumulated under the diaphragm, as Dandy had already demonstrated. From these and other clinical and pathological demonstrations of the radiographic properties of air, as well as his earlier laboratory studies on hydrocephalus, it was but a step for this genius to conceive of injecting a gas into the cerebral ventricles, thus revolutionizing neurosurgery. In Dandy's studies air was used, and he found it necessary to remove at least more cerebrospinal fluid than the contents of one ventricle and to replace this fluid with an equal quantity of air. Before closure of the fontanelles he could readily make a ventricular puncture through the interosseous defect. After union of the sutures it was necessary to make a small opening in the bone. At the time of the first report he had put air into the cerebral ventricles at least twenty times and in some instances the process had been repeated. The amount of air injected varied from 40 to 300 milliliters, the larger quantities being in cases of internal hydrocephalus. Only once had there been any reaction, and in this instance the injection was made forty-eight hours after the first stage of an operation for cerebellar tumor. The report of Dandy's technique was published in a now famous paper entitled "Ventriculography Following the Injection of Air into the Cerebral Ventricles," which appeared in the *Annals of Surgery* in July 1918.

This discovery could also be considered the logical result of his experimental and clinical studies of the ventricles, the cerebrospinal fluid circulation, and hydrocephalus. It was not altogether a spontaneous and sudden inspiration. Dr. Samuel J. Crowe recalls that

in 1917 when Doctor Dandy was a house officer, he was very outspoken to his friends and associates about palliative brain surgery. A decompression, he said, relieves symptoms for a time, but when the cause is a growing tumor, the relief is not permanent. Early diagnosis, accurate localization and surgical removal are just as essential for the cure of a brain tumor as they are for a new growth in other parts of the body.

The first step in his search for an objective and accurate method to localize brain tumors at an early stage of their development, was to study with Heuer the x-rays of the skull of 100 patients with intracranial symptoms suggestive of new growth. In most of these patients the x-ray findings had been checked at operation or necropsy. It was found that brain tumors: (1) cast a shadow in only six percent of the cases, and in these the calcified areas alone were differentiated; (2) that local areas of thickening or atrophy of the skull may be due to an underlying cerebral tumor; (3) that destruction of the sella turcica may be a general pressure phenomenon, and finally that the skull changes shown by the x-ray always represent a late stage of the disease.

Dandy's next step was to test in the animal laboratory the possibility of filling the cerebral ventricles with a radio-opaque substance. He removed by ventricular puncture a part of the cerebrospinal fluid and replaced it with an equal amount of radio-opaque solution. The ventricles were then clearly outlined on x-ray. This procedure was repeated on animals with a simulated space-filling tumor, and as Dandy had predicted, the radiographs showed displacement of the ventricles. The drugs he used, however, were far too irritating to inject into the central nervous system of patients. Ventriculography was possible only by the substitution of a gas for the cerebrospinal fluid withdrawn.

As already related, the idea of using air was finally crystallized.

At the age of twenty-seven, Dandy, in association with Kenneth Blackfan, had published the first of a series of ten now-classic papers on hydrocephalus and the circulation of the cerebrospinal fluid. Prior to that time no satisfactory explanation of either existed. Dandy and Blackfan were able, in the dog, to produce dilatation of the lateral and third ventricles by obstructing the aqueduct of Sylvius and to produce distention of one lateral ventricle by obstructing its foramen of Monro. The latter could be prevented by previous removal of its choroid plexus. By separating the Pacchionian granulations from the great veins both over the vertex and at the base of the dog's brain, he demonstrated that hydrocephalus did not result and, therefore, that cerebrospinal fluid absorption did not occur in that manner, as had been widely believed, but, rather, directly into the blood vessels in the subarachnoid spaces. In the autopsy room an obstruction either at the aqueduct of Sylvius or at the foramina of Luschka and Magendie or along the basilar cisterns was demonstrated in every case of "idiopathic" hydrocephalus. This disorder was thus reclassified by these workers upon a solid basis of anatomical and physiological study and of clinical observation into communicating and noncommunicating types. The operations of choroidplexectomy and ventriculostomy were logical sequences of these discoveries.

Not long after Dandy's first publication in 1913, Professor Halsted, who was exceedingly proud of his very dynamic pupil, remarked: "Dandy will never do anything equal to this again [referring to his work on hydrocephalus]. Few men make more than one great contribution to medicine." In this instance it was repeatedly proven afterwards that the Professor's estimate was quite faulty. Among Dandy's many other contributions were his work on tumors of the nervus acusticus published in 1917, his extensive work on hypophysis, his work on Ménière's syndrome, on tic douloureux, on intracranial aneurysms, on head injuries, and on ruptured intervertebral discs.

In 1929 Dandy described two cases of "Loose Cartilage from the Intervertebral Disc Simulating Tumor of the Spinal Cord." The clinical picture was that of a cauda equina tumor, the preoperative diagnosis in each case having been metastatic malignancy. At operation it was found that a completely detached fragment of cartilage arising from an intervertebral disc was responsible, and histological study confirmed the operative impression that the fragments removed were not neoplastic. Dandy believed that the detachment was attributable to repeated minor trauma. Both patients had muscle spasm and tenderness over the vertebral spines. Dandy clearly pointed out that the early symptoms were those of localized vertebral pain plus bilateral sciatica—one side being affected more than the other. The later manifestations were those of rapidly increasing paralysis, sensory and motor, as well as loss of urinary and vesical control and of reflexes—all due to compression of the cauda equina. He stated clearly: "This lesion offers a pathological basis for cases of so-called sciatica, especially bilateral sciatica. The lesion is cured by operative removal of the cartilage." Here the question of intervertebral disc disease and the production of spinal cord pressure remained until 1934, when the classical article of Mixter and Barr appeared, which so clearly depicted the common form of small, laterally placed disc herniations with cervical and lumbar root compression symptoms.

Dandy was apparently unaware of the previous reports of herniation of an intervertebral disc, as he stated that search of the literature had revealed no cases similar to those which he reported. The first published report of a patient operated on for protrusion of an intervertebral disc into the spinal canal was that of Oppenheim and Krause in 1909. Their patient had a compression of the cauda equina by the third lumbar disc, similar to the two cases later reported by Dandy. The lesion was removed and the patient recovered. Middleton and Teacher in Scotland and Goldthwait in America reported cases in 1911. To Goldthwait belongs the credit for first suggesting that injuries to intervertebral discs might be a frequent cause of "lumbago" and "sciatica." He reported in 1911 the case of a patient suffering from a "right sacroiliac strain," who

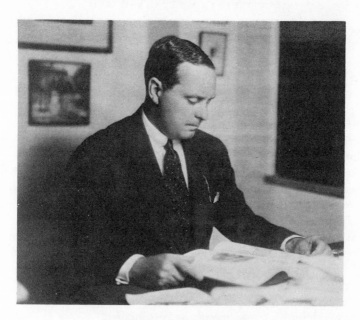

Walter Edward Dandy
Courtesy of Mrs. Walter E. Dandy

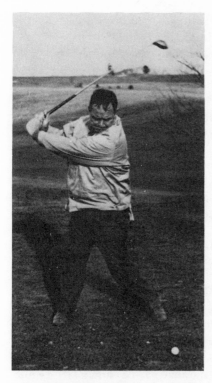

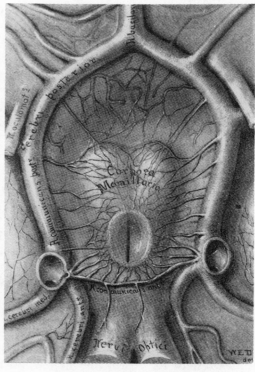

Walter Edward Dandy at play
Courtesy of Mrs. Walter E. Dandy

Fig. 1. Blood supply of the pituitary body
Fig. 2 from *Am. J. Anat.* 11 (1910): 142

CHRONOLOGICAL LIST OF THE CONTRIBUTIONS OF WALTER E. DANDY

1910   Described the blood supply of the pituitary gland.

1913   Experimental and clinical study of internal hydrocephalus with Blackfan.

1915   Studies on extirpation of the pineal body.

1916   Report of 70 cases of brain tumor with Heuer.

1918   Ventriculography following the injection of air into the cerebral ventricles. Refined technique for removal of choroid plexus.

1919   Air injection to visualize tumors of spinal cord.

1921   Devised an approach to the pineal region patterned after that used in his experimental removal of canine pineal glands. Treatment of hydrocephalus from occlusion of foramina of Magendie and Luschka.

1922   Third ventriculostomy for relief of internal hydrocephalus. Operation for the removal of cerebello-pontine angle tumors and removal of the choroid plexus. Operation for prechiasmal intracranial tumors of the optic nerves.

1923   First post-operative recovery room organized with Dr. W. M. Firor. Dye test for studying flow of cerebrospinal fluid on the operating table.

1924   Suboccipital drainage for suppurative meningitis.

1925   Operation for section of the sensory root of the trigeminal nerve at the pons. Description of intradural exposure of large basal tumors. Experimental studies of epilepsy.

1926   Advocated tapping cerebral abscess and letting the pus drip out.

1927   Operation for glossopharyngeal neuralgia.

1928   Surgical approach to the treatment of Ménière's disease. Introduced avertin anesthesia into neurosurgery.

1929   Description of protrusion of intervertebral disc. Operation for the cure of tic douloureux.

1930   Operation for the treatment of spasmodic torticollis.

1932   Paper on advantages of subcerebellar route for section of trigeminal nerve based on 250 cases.

1933   Monograph on benign encapsulated tumors in the lateral ventricle.

1935   Devised method of trapping a carotid arteriovenous aneurysm.

1938   Aneurysm of the internal carotid artery cured by operation.

1941   Monograph on orbital tumors; results following the transcranial operative attack.

1943   New method for handling cases of scaphocephaly.

1944   Monograph on the surgical treatment of intracranial aneurysms. Work on treatment of rhinorrhea and otorrhea.

1945   Summary of experience in treatment of strictures of aqueduct of Sylvius (causing hydrocephalus).

developed paralysis of the legs with bladder and rectal incontinence. A laminectomy was performed by Harvey Cushing, who found no lesion of the cauda equina except for "narrowing of the osseous canal at the lumbosacral junction." The patient made a slow, partial recovery following the operation. In the discussion of the case, Goldthwait reviewed the possible causes of the paraplegia. He dismissed tumor, hemorrhage and spondylolisthesis as possible factors and concluded that posterior displacement of the lumbosacral intervertebral disc with pressure on the cauda equina was the logical explanation. He suggested that other cases of paraplegia, lumbago, and "sciatica" might be the result of pressure on nerve roots from a displaced intervertebral disc.

In their article published in 1934, Mixter and Barr stated that Dandy in 1929 reported two cases from which he had removed loose cartilaginous fragments protruding extradurally into the spinal canal. They did not give Dandy as much credit as he deserved for recognizing the potential relationship between minor trauma, the production of herniation of disc material, and the appearance of sciatica. Dandy did not pursue the subject vigorously, although he noted in his article that since his two patients had appeared within a relatively short time, it was likely that such lesions were fairly common. It was only years later that he returned with his usual aggressiveness to this subject.

A comment by Professor E. A. Park on Dr. Dandy's personality seems particularly appropriate in relation to his work in a number of areas: "He seemed to the writer suddenly to be seized with intuitions; then almost as if possessed he would plunge forward with impetuous energy and boldness toward his goal. Another characteristic was his complete skepticism in regard to all accepted ideas." At first he appeared doubtful that the syndrome of the small lateral disc could be as common as it was soon being reported. Twelve years elapsed between the 1929 paper and his next publication on this subject. By that time he had as a result of his own experience become an enthusiastic convert. He was greatly impressed by the high degree of accuracy of preoperative diagnoses, particularly as recorded by Mixter and Barr, among others. He urged that myelography be abandoned in this connection as unnecessary and probably harmful.

Dandy might also have a claim as the originator of the intensive care unit. In the present setting of highly technical intensive care centers and elaborate recovery rooms for patients in the immediate postoperative period, it is noteworthy that perhaps the first organized unit was the postoperative recovery room adjacent to the old operating room in the Johns Hopkins Hospital, where neurosurgical patients were cared for around the clock by a special nursing group prior to returning to their rooms. It was located on the fourth floor of the old Surgical Building and consisted of three beds. This was in 1923 during the period (July 5, 1923–January 29, 1925) when Dr. Warfield M. Firor was Dandy's resident surgeon. When the Halsted and Carnegie buildings were built, the neurosurgical recovery room was moved to Halsted 7. It was the nearest room to the operating room and was adjacent to the doctors' quarters. It was staffed twenty-four hours a day with special recovery room nurses. This was the beginning of careful attention to airway care, temperature control, circulatory monitoring, fluid and electrolyte balance and observation of the state of consciousness of the patient. Interestingly, the new surgical intensive care unit is at present on the site of the old neurosurgical intensive care unit.

The life of a neurosurgeon is a difficult one, and his day is not always crowned with successes. One of Dandy's prominent patients was Thomas Clayton Wolfe, the novelist. Wolfe was born in Asheville, North Carolina, in 1900 and died in Baltimore, Maryland, in 1938 following an intracranial exploration by Dr. Dandy. Wolfe was, of course, a well-known writer to whom critics at one stage in his career compared to Whitman and Melville. Toward the latter part of his life, after publication of a collection of short stories, *From Death to Mourning*, Wolfe decided to set aside temporarily what he was doing while he wrote a different type of book—"a story about an innocent, gullible man discovering the harsh truths of life through disillusionment and trial. As he worked out the narrative, the original grandiose plan was scrapped in favor of a long chronicle about a new hero, George Webber." As the following three letters indicate, Wolfe did not live to see his new work completed. However, out of the vast manuscript which he left behind after his death, three books were eventually published: *The Web and the Rock* (1939), *You Can't Go Home Again* (1940), and *The Hills Beyond* (1941). Thomas Wolfe's books have maintained favor because of the richness of his work. As his biographer described, he evoked a poetic response with his rhythmical and lyrical passages; as a writer of narrative, at his best he achieved the brooding depths of Dostoevsky and the vivid portraiture of Dickens. His work was tempered with broad humor, which became predominantly satirical in his later work. Although his minor figures tended to caricature, his great characterizations displayed a full range of the strengths and weaknesses of human kind. If he had lived in a succeeding generation, this great novelist might not have met death at the age of thirty-eight.

The following three letters were made available by Dr. Walter E. Dandy, Jr.:

Neuro Surgical Clinic
902 Boren Avenue
Seattle

September 7, 1938

Dear Walter:

A patient, Tom Wolfe, is on his way to Baltimore and will consult with you and Bill Rienhoff. He has not been under my care. I saw him only in consultation just before he left. His sister will give you full details of the history of the case.

Briefly, he developed pneumonia about six weeks ago and when I saw him he appeared to have a frontal lobe abscess. His home is in South Carolina and his sister wanted to take him East. I advised him to stop off in Rochester in case his condition became alarming en route. Otherwise he should arrive in Baltimore about Saturday night. I will appreciate hearing what you find in this case. He is an author who writes for Harper's Magazine. Mr. Edward C. Aswell, 49 East 33rd Street, N.Y.C. is particularly interested in his case, so you might notify him as to your findings.

I was very much pleased to hear from Dean Lewis that you are going to Honolulu with us. I hope you can take the chairmanship of the Section on Neurosurgery. Frederick Reichert is anxious to have you do so and I also think it would be very fine. Did Dean Lewis, by any chance, give you a pipe that I sent by him. If he hasn't way-lay him and ask him about it. It is a pipe designed by the Professor of

Aeronautics, guaranteed to be the latest thing in proper drafts and disinfectant. Pipe smokers who have them are keen about them.

With kind personal regards, I am,

Sincerely yours,

George W. Swift

September 13, 1938

Dear George:

Mr. Wolfe arrived here in good condition but he was so ill that I immediately got busy. I must confess that my diagnosis was an intracranial metastatic tumor secondary to the lesion in the lung. I had Louis Hamman see him and he could not be sure whether it was a tumor or an abscess in the lung and consequently a secondary one in the brain. I must confess too that I expected the lesion was in the right frontal lobe because he had a left Babinski and because the eye ground on the right side was much more choked and contained many more hemorrhages than the left. I put air in and found that he had a tremendous hydrocephalus involving the entire ventricular system, the anterior half of the 4th ventricle showing in the dilatation. The ventricular fluid showed 230 cells, 75% of which were mononuclear. This, of course, practically made the diagnosis of an intracranial tubercle. I explored the cerebellum hoping to find the solitary tubercle and instead found myriads of them throughout the meninges. He must have a very extensive basilar meningitis because none of the air reached the subarachnoid spaces.

It was good of you to send me the pipe though I have not seen it—Dean is still away.

With all good wishes, I am,

Most sincerely,

Walter E. Dandy

September 20, 1938

Dear Doctor Dandy:

Thanks a lot for your letter of the thirteenth regarding Mr. Thomas Wolfe. As I told you in my letter I only saw him the night before he left for the East, at which time he was desperately ill. He had two men who are supposed to be the best tubercular specialists in Seattle treat him, but they did not think he had a tubercular meningitis. I advised his sister that the stiff neck, positive Kernig and left Babinski suggested the possibility of a brain abscess or a tubercular meningitis. I am sorry to have to send you such a hopeless case, but such is life ...

With kind personal regards, I am,

Sincerely yours,

George

Who was this extraordinary genius who for many years guided the destinies of neurosurgery at the Johns Hopkins Medical Institutions? Dandy was born in Sedalia, Missouri, on April 6, 1886, the only child of John and Rachel Dandy, who had emigrated from Barrow-in-Furness, Lancashire, England, only two years previously. John, a locomotive engineer, was a socialist and a member of the religious sect known as the Plymouth Brethren. Dandy attended the University of Missouri, where he came in contact with W. C. Curtis, the professor of zoology, who interested him in science. On graduation, because of his outstanding character, scholarship, and athletic ability, he was offered a

Rhodes Scholarship; at that time he was most eager to begin the study of medicine, and since in that era it was not possible to do so at Oxford, he declined the scholarship. In 1910 Dandy graduated from the Johns Hopkins Medical School, standing seventeenth in a class of eighty-five. He had attracted the attention of Halsted and was asked to spend his first year in the Surgical Hunterian Laboratory. Starting in 1911, he served as intern and later assistant resident, until 1916, when he was appointed chief resident, a post he held for two years.

In the Surgical Hunterian he came into contact with Dr. Harvey Cushing and the brilliant young group of surgeons including Heuer, Crowe, Goetsch, and Homans, who were investigating pituitary function. Dandy did his first scientific work on a study of the blood and nerve supplies of the canine and feline pituitary bodies, publishing two papers, one in 1911 and one in 1913. The beautiful drawings in these papers were made by Dandy himself, under the coaching of Max Broedel (Fig 1).

Dandy was Cushing's clinical assistant in the hospital during 1911–1912, the year preceding Cushing's departure to take up his duties as professor of surgery at Harvard. Doctor Cushing had invited Dandy to go to Boston with him. Both Cushing and Dandy were high-strung, temperamental individuals, and their personalities clashed on many occasions during the year in the Hunterian Laboratory. The following year in the hospital was not a happy one for Dandy. Incidents that aroused the ire of both men were frequent, and just before Cushing left for Boston he told Dandy that he had changed his mind and would not take him to Boston. Doctor Halsted had been told that Dandy was to go with Cushing, and he had filled all positions on his hospital staff.

Dandy was a very disappointed and despondent young man, not because Doctor Cushing had changed his mind, but because this change of mind had deprived him of his position on Halsted's staff. Doctor Halsted was away for the summer, but the director of the hospital, Doctor Winford Smith, was well aware of the potentials of this young man. He called Dandy to his office and said: "Dandy, I don't know whether you are on Doctor Halsted's staff or not. I am going to give you a room in the hospital, however, and sometime during the next year you will probably find out from Doctor Halsted what your status really is." At once Dandy and Kenneth D. Blackfan, resident in pediatrics, began to work in the Hunterian Laboratory on the origin, the circulation, the absorption of cerebrospinal fluid, and the causes of hydrocephalus. Dr. Halsted was much impressed by the originality of these experiments and promptly found a place for Dandy on his surgical staff. While a busy house officer, Dandy found time to extend and elaborate his studies of hydrocephalus.

Dr. Dandy possessed a marvelous combination of qualities: a clear-thinking brain, drive, a lively imagination, independence of thought and action, manual dexterity and a colorful personality. His was the genius to conceive of new and startling operative techniques with the courage to try them as well as the skill to make them successful. He is certainly one of the most outstanding men produced by Johns Hopkins.

8 ❦ Early Contributions to the Surgery of Cancer: William S. Halsted, Hugh H. Young, and John G. Clark

GALEN, BORN AT Pergamos in the year 131 A.D., eventually appeared in Rome as the private surgeon and medical advisor of the young Commodus. The malignant character of cancer was well known to him, and he contributed to the views of his day concerning its internal manifestations: "In the breast we often find a tumor in size and shape closely resembling the animal known as the crab, for as in the latter the limbs protrude from either side, so in the tumor the swollen veins radiate from its edges and give a perfect picture of the crab." Here stated for the first time was the reason for giving to neoplastic disease its peculiar name of "cancer." Galen was concerned also with its treatment, and while he considered cancer to be the product of black bile, was not opposed to operation. However, he gave this advice: "First get rid of the black bile by appropriate remedies and then attempt a cure by milder applications, since the more severe remedies merely increase the evil." Galen thus recognized that cancer possessed a malignancy peculiarly its own, for which reason he advocated the combination of medicine and surgery.

After Galen, medicine entered a period of quiescence, and in the subsequent centuries the operative treatment of cancer had its ups and downs. Even in the time of the Munros of Edinburgh, whose writings threw the operative treatment of cancer into grave repute, the failure of other remedies to fill the gap resulted in a revival of operations particularly for cancer of the breast, lip, and scrotum.

Two Germans, the surgeon Thiersch and the anatomist Waldeyer, showed by their careful microscopic studies that the concept of cancer as multicentric in origin was erroneous. Their results showed that cancer had its origin in a single primary focus, which if removed completely led to permanent cure. They demonstrated that tumor appearing in areas distant from the primary focus is the result of metastasis of small groups of cells which have dislodged from the primary focus and spread through the lymphatics and blood vessels.

Following their studies, surgeons attempted a more radical approach to the treatment of cancer, spurred on by the methods of Lister, which reduced the dangers of post-operative sepsis. As the significance of these studies and the enthusiasm engendered by the famous German surgeon, von Volkmann, took root, some order emerged from the previous chaos in the surgical management of patients with cancer. During this early period, members of the faculty at Johns Hopkins made important advances in the use of radical surgery for the attempted cure of cancer.

William S. Halsted and the Radical Operation
for Carcinoma of the Breast

The story of the evolution of the operative treatment of cancer of the breast is a fascinating chapter in the development of modern surgery. Although recognized throughout recorded history, no important advances were made in the treatment of breast cancer until Jean Louis Petit, a French surgeon of the eighteenth century, inaugurated a new era. Petit believed that the enlarged lymphatic glands in the axilla represented the roots of cancer of the breast, and that they, together with the breast tumor, and when necessary the pectoral fascia and muscle, should be removed. His work initiated an uninterrupted trend toward the development of the radical operation for cancer of the breast. Joseph Lister, the father of antiseptic surgery, was probably the first to expose the axilla by division of the pectoral muscle in cancer of the breast and must, therefore, have been the first to perform an adequate axillary dissection. Events thereafter moved rapidly, partly as a result of currently available studies in microscopic pathology. Von Volkmann in 1873 contributed the next progressive step when he advocated the routine complete removal of the breast, axillary dissection, and excision of pectoral fascia. Heidenhain extended Volkmann's operation and recommended removal of the superficial layer of the pectoral muscle.

However, these attempts among others were still short of the limits to which the surgical management of the disease could be carried out. The final step in the development of radical surgery of breast cancer was implemented in 1889 by William S. Halsted, who was particularly well equipped for this task. Halsted had already mastered the techniques of asepsis and the control of hemorrhage, and his skill in the gentle and meticulous handling of the tissues allowed him to carry out resections of a more extensive nature than others before him had attempted. His chief contribution can best be described by quoting from a letter he wrote to Dr. Welch, dated August 26, 1922, which read as follows:

You ask me to say something of my share in the development of the operation for cancer of the breast. This is pretty clearly stated in my first paper [*Johns Hopkins Hospital Reports*, 1895]. Volkmann had recommended stripping the fascia from the pectoralis major, "As for a classroom dissection," and Heidenhain [Kuster's assistant at Marburg] proposed cutting away the superficial fibers of this muscle. I advised and practiced the removal of the entire muscle, leaving in most instances the upper or subclavicular bundles [those above the cephalic vein]. I divided the pectoralis minor to further facilitate the cleaning of the axilla. A year or two later Willy Meyer advised removing the minor muscle as well as the major, and I, too, came independently to the conclusion that this might better be done. I insisted that all the tissues should be removed in one piece and upon the meticulous cleaning of the axilla and its estuaries [subclavicular and supraclavicular fossae]. I warned of the danger of excising pieces of malignant tumors for microscopic examination unless the operation followed immediately, and was, I think, one of the first surgeons in this country able macroscopically to make the diagnosis of the common tumors.

Halsted apparently began to work out his operation in 1882, published a brief note in 1890 and a fuller description of his work in 1894 and 1895.

Halsted's five-year cure rate rose from 20 percent to 45 percent and later to 72 percent when the disease had been treated before the axillary glands had become involved. At first he left a large wound which was allowed to heal under a moist blood scab, but later covered the wound with large skin grafts. He modified the primary incision so as to avoid a scar on the arm and across the axilla. Later he paid more attention to the reconstruction of the axilla in order to prevent the swelling of the arm after operation.

Baumgartner in 1913 made an evaluation of Dr. Halsted's work on cancer of the breast:

By combining and selecting the best suggestions offered by the most advanced operators (and adding many new and important details of his own) the American surgeon, Halsted, elaborated a surgical technique which gave a powerful impulse to a more radical and extensive extirpation of cancer of the breast. The operation he devised was quickly adopted, wholly or with variations, by the majority of surgeons the world over.... Halsted's operation or any other that approaches it, which is based upon the principles that govern it is amply justified by its (superior) results, as shown by all published statistics.

Dr. Joseph C. Bloodgood, to whom Halsted often expressed his obligation for efficiency and inexhaustible zeal in collecting the statistics of his operation year after year, further elaborated in 1908 the results of his chief as follows:

The statistics in Halsted's clinic at the present time show among 210 cases, in which three years and more have passed since the operation, that 42 percent are apparently well. If we consider the cases in which the axillary glands, studied microscopically, showed no evidence of metastasis, 61, or 85 percent are well. In cases in which the axillary glands showed metastasis (110) 30 percent recovered, being free from recurrence for 3 years. When the glands in the neck showed metastasis (40 cases), only 10 percent remained well for three years.

In all of these groups, metastasis has been observed after an interval of three years of apparent cure. Such late metastasis may take place up to eight years after operation. Excluding these cases of late recurrence, the number definitely cured in these three groups is reduced to 75, 25, and 7 percent respectively, or for all cases together, 35 percent.

A considerable body of surgical opinion holds today that removal of the entire breast with the axillary contents can be accomplished satisfactorily without resection of the pectoralis muscles. The radical mastectomy as described by Halsted was and continues to be an effective means of removing large tumors confined to the chest wall and axilla. One should remember, however, that Halsted's knowledge of breast cancer and its modes of spread was different from what is now known about the disease. The patient who came to his attention usually had large indolent tumors which remained confined to the chest wall and axilla for prolonged periods of time. All of his first fifty cases had axillary lymph node metastases. He was not aware that blood-borne metastases occurred, and based his operation conceptually on the idea that breast cancer only metastasized via the lymphatics. There is no evidence at the present time to support the concept that immediate mastectomy following a positive biopsy of breast cancer is necessary.

It is beyond the scope of this essay to discuss all of the other original contributions made by Dr. Halsted. These may be found in the two volumes of his *Surgical Papers*, published by the Johns Hopkins University Press.

The Halsted family lived in New York, was prominent financially and active in various philanthropic projects. Dr. Halsted entered Yale at the age of eighteen. His scholastic record was poor. He never borrowed any books from the Yale Library, as he elected to spend most of his time at various types of athletics. In his senior year he was captain of the Yale football team. While studying at the College of Physicians and Surgeons in New York, he became intensely interested in anatomy. After graduating with honors in 1877, he spent the next two years in Europe attending courses in anatomy as well as the clinics of Billroth, Mikulicz, von Bergmann, Thiersch, von Volkmann, and others. Here in Germany he observed the implementation of Lister's antiseptic surgery.

On his return to New York in 1880 he worked with Dr. Welch in pathology at Bellevue, and inaugurated at Roosevelt Hospital the first surgical outpatient department in New York. It was at this time that he became interested in Koller's discovery that the cornea could be anesthetized with cocaine. He experimented on himself and found that by injecting this drug into a sensory nerve he could render the whole area supplied by its branches insensitive to pain. Thus, he observed for the first time that the principle of nerve block could be utilized to obtain anesthesia for surgical purposes, a discovery promptly utilized in dental practice. He also demonstrated the blocking of the spinal cord with anesthetic drugs. It was not until April 1, 1922, only six months before Dr. Halsted's death, that his discoveries in local and regional analgesia were duly recognized by the American National Dental Association. It is interesting to note that fifteen years after Halsted's work, Cushing rediscovered the principle of nerve block and applied it successfully in operations on hernias. He was unaware that his chief had ever made studies on cocaine of any sort—so reticent was Dr. Halsted about this matter and so little did questions of priority interest him.

When Dr. Halsted was making these experiments on himself in 1885, it was not known that cocaine was a habit-forming drug. Through the aid and encouragement of Dr. Welch, he apparently overcame his addiction, but this episode radically changed his whole life. He returned to New York after his cure to a more thoughtful and leisurely existence, with time for reflection and study of the surgical problems that interested him most, a life far more fruitful than it could ever have been if he had continued the strenuous pace he had set for himself in the beginning. However, the problem with cocaine continued for the rest of his life.

In 1886 Dr. Welch invited Halsted to come to Baltimore. Halsted lived with Dr. Welch at 506 Cathedral Street and began his experimental studies in the pathological laboratory. Here he and Mall did their fundamental work on intestinal suture, and in the following year Halsted began his experimental work on basic questions of operative technique. He made histological studies of healing wounds and of the tissue reaction to various types of suture material. These meticulous studies led him to realize the importance of careful handling of tissues, the necessity of controlling bleeding with a minimum of crushing of tissues with forceps, and the value of transfixing vessels and ligating them with the finest silk. Three years of laboratory work were largely responsible for Dr. Halsted's appointment in October 1889 as associate professor of surgery and acting surgeon to the hospital. He was not made professor of surgery until April 1892, when he was forty years of age.

In 1919 Dr. Halsted began to have gallstone colic, for which a few weeks later he was operated on by Dr. Richard Follis. For several days he had complained to Dr. Welch of pain, but did not localize it or suggest a cause. Then one evening, when he and Dr. Welch were walking up the steps of the Maryland Club, Dr. Halsted stopped, and looking very serious and distressed, said: "Welch, I have found the cause for my pain. It's an aneurysm. Put your hand under my vest and see if you don't think I'm right." Dr. Welch was amazed to feel the violent, rhythmical pulsations and became very excited. Dr. Halsted had had a thin, rubber bag made, which he had fastened to his chest wall with adhesive. From the bag a small rubber tube ran to his pants pocket, where it ended in a bulb. While Dr. Welch was still palpating the "aneurysm," Dr. Halsted gave a great squeeze to the bulb and the bag exploded.

Insight can be gained into Halsted's qualities as a surgical technician by reading his paper, illustrated by Max Broedel, in the *Journal of the American Medical Association* in 1913. Here Dr. Halsted gives the most interesting account of the many methods which were peculiar to his clinic and which he had originated. He provides convincing reasons for his preference for fine silk over cat gut, for his use of gutta percha for the protection of granulating wounds, and for the prevention of adhesion of dressings and drains to the tissues (the present cigarette and cigar drains, so generally used, were of his making). The use of silver foil and a number of ingenious and original modes of suture are all described.

Most interesting is his summary of the development of the use of rubber gloves in surgery:

In the winter of 1889 and 1890—I cannot recall the month—the nurse in charge of the operating room complained that the solutions of mercuric chloride produced a dermatitis on her arm and hands. As she was an unusually efficient woman, I gave the matter my consideration and one day while in New York requested the Goodyear Rubber Company to make, as an experiment, two pair of thin rubber gloves with gauntlets. On trial these proved to be so satisfactory that additional gloves were ordered. In the autumn, on my return to town, the assistant who passed the instruments and threaded the needles was also provided with rubber gloves at the operations. At first the operator wore them only when exploratory incisions into joints were made. After a time the assistants became so accustomed to working in gloves that they also wore them as operators and would remark that they seemed to be less expert with the bare hand than with the gloved hands.

I think it was Dr. Bloodgood, my house surgeon, who first made this comment and that he was the first to wear them invariably, when operating. In the report which I made of the first year's work at the hospital, written in November and

December, 1890, and published in March 1891, I stated that the assistant who passed the instruments wore rubber gloves [*Johns Hopkins Hospital Reports*, vol. 6, pl. 12]. This assistant was given the gloves to protect his hands from the solution of phenol [carbolic acid] in which the instruments were submerged rather than to eliminate him as a source of infection. I do not recall having referred again, in my publications to the employment of rubber gloves. Dr. Hunter Robb in 1894, in his book on Aseptic Surgical Technique recommended that the operator wear rubber gloves. Dr. Robb was, at that time, resident gynecologist of The Johns Hopkins Hospital and had frequent opportunities to observe the technique of the surgical clinic.

This incidental reference by Robb in 1894 to the wearing of rubber gloves, and the fact that a photograph of an operation for breast cancer taken late in the year, 1893, shows that gloves were not regularly worn by us at that time, served to establish approximately the date of their definite introduction.

Dr. Joseph C. Bloodgood in his elaborate report on hernia makes the following statement with reference to the wearing of gloves: "The writer was the first as operator to wear gloves as routine practice in practically all clean operations. He began to wear gloves invariably in December, 1896. Before this date he had operated on 20 cases of hernia with four suppurations, all late infections. The wounds were closed with silver wire. Since wearing gloves he had operated on 100 cases of inguinal hernia. In one case (recent) the wound suppurated."

Thus, the technique of operating in gloves was an evolution rather than an inspiration or momentary thought. It is remarkable that during the four or five years when, as an operator, Halsted wore them only occasionally, he could have been so blind to the necessity for wearing them invariably at the operating table. This was something that he constantly asked himself: "We did not realize how slightly the sense of touch is obtunded by the rubber covering or how unessential it is in most operations that the greatest delicacy of finger perception be preserved." For example, he notes that in the early days of rubber gloves, he removed the glove from one hand, not infrequently, to palpate the common bile duct in search for stone. He ends by saying: "Furthermore, we are delighted with the results of healing already obtainable, so vivid were the memories of infections in the recent past."

Hugh H. Young and the Prostate Gland

Enlargement of the prostate has been since the beginning of time a burden to elderly men. Through the centuries the medical literature has been filled with expedients to combat this malady. It had been known for a long time that eunuchs do not develop prostatic enlargement, and in 1893 Dr. J. William White tried to capitalize upon this fact by removing the testes of men with enlargement of the prostate in an attempt to restore normal urine flow. However, the benefits of castration were only temporary and in a short time the operation fell into disuse, but not before thousands of testes had been sacrificed. Dr. Hugh Hampton Young, who is universally considered as the father of modern urology, knew well that the operations in vogue were too unscientific to be effective. While Dr. Young was a member of the surgical house staff, an elderly Negro was brought to the hospital in uremia, secondary to severe prostatic hypertrophy. It was impossible to pass a catheter, so an opening was made into the bladder by incision in the lower abdomen—a suprapubic cystotomy. The results were remarkable, for in a few days the uremia disappeared, the patient became conscious, and Dr. Young saw the dramatic improvement that could come from free drainage of the bladder (allowing free urine flow from kidneys that had become impaired by long-standing back pressure resulting from the prostatic obstruction). When the resident, Dr. Bloodgood, left for his vacation, Dr. Young stuck in his finger, felt the enormous mass and enucleated it, thus becoming one of the pioneers in suprapubic prostatectomy. His success in this case stimulated him to use the same technique in other patients. His results were much better than those previously obtained by others, whose operations were often incomplete merely because they had not thought, as did Dr. Young, to provide counter pressure against the prostate from below by a gloved finger in the rectum, thus pushing the prostate up so that it could be shelled out with the other index finger inserted into the bladder above.

As Dr. Young relates in his autobiography, he was stimulated to improve on the method of prostatectomy because in a number of cases the bleeding was profuse, and in some the post-operative infection so severe that death of the patient resulted. He discussed his problem with Franklin P. Mall, professor of anatomy, and prepared himself for a trial in patients by dissecting the perineums of scores of cadavers in order to improve an operation that had been initially tried in crude form by Proust.

At about this time a Mr. Samuel Alexander came from Hawaii with his doctor, daughter, and nurse, saying to Dr. Young: "Doctor, I've read everything I could get hold of on the prostate. I like what you have written and have come to you for relief, but I honestly think you have not yet got the perfect method. Could you give me something better?" Dr. Young had been working on a new method of attack, and told Mr. Alexander that if he were willing to wait, he would make the instruments with which the operation could be done more effectively and safely than ever before. This was accomplished, and Mr. Alexander, on October 2, 1902, had the first perineal prostatectomy done by Dr. Young's newly designed method. The enlarged lobes were easily shelled out from within the capsule of normal prostatic tissue that surrounded them. Then, with the finger working beneath the middle lobe that projected into the bladder, this was finally shelled out from the mucous membrane of the bladder that covered it and the whole hypertrophied mass consisting of three lobes was drawn out and removed. He had not removed the prostate, simply these enlargements which had grown within it, the extraction of which left a cavity within the prostate which soon contracted, and new mucous membrane eventually covered the defect. Dr. Young states that it was Mr. Alexander's insistence that brought action and started him on his remarkable career in prostatic surgery.

During the next fourteen months, he had fifty cases without a death at a time when the mortality from suprapubic prostatectomy was 20 percent. In

1908 he presented a paper entitled "Remarks on a Fatal Case after 128 Consecutive Cases of Prostatectomy Without a Death." This paper was on the program of a select society consisting of about fifty of Dr. Young's friends. He demonstrated the autopsy specimen and discussed at length the death that was due to an unrecognized disease of the kidney. When he sat down, Dr. E. L. Keys of New York said: "I, too, have had a death from prostatectomy," and sat down. Dr. J. Bentley Squire of New York rose and said: "I, too, have had a death from prostatectomy," and took his seat. Dr. Francis R. Hagner of Washington did the same, and so did six or seven others. White with rage, Dr. Young was getting up to vent his anger when Frank Watson, a dear friend, pulled him down and said, "Hugh, don't be foolish enough to reply to those rascals. They got together and concocted that scheme last night on the train just to torment you." In subsequent years, the operation was further improved from the technical point of view.

In 1903 after having developed the operation of perineal prostatectomy, Dr. Young encountered in the tissues of two prostates a small area of cancer, and he was struck by the fact that if the entire prostate gland had been removed with its capsule, it would have been possible to cure both these patients. He relates how on April 1, 1904, an elderly preacher arrived complaining of pain in the prostate which had not been relieved by a long course of osteopathic treatment. Four months previously an electrocautery operation had been performed to remove the obstruction to urination that had developed. On Dr. Young's examination, with his gloved finger in the rectum, he found the prostate to be enlarged, irregular, nodular, and hard, indicating that cancer was present. But as the disease had not progressed beyond the capsule, he was convinced that if an operation were done in which a wide berth was given to the cancer, the patient might be cured. In studying the literature, he could find that no such radical operation had ever been attempted. After making careful sketches of what he thought would be necessary and showing them to Dr. William S. Halsted, whose reputation was worldwide at that time because of his radical operation for cancer of the breast, it was decided to carry out the operation at which Dr. Halsted was to be his first assistant.

This operation was done on April 7, 1904, with success. In a paper published in October 1905 in the *Johns Hopkins Hospital Bulletin* entitled "The Early Diagnosis and Radical Cure for Carcinoma of the Prostate," being a study of forty cases and presentation of a radical operation which was carried out in four cases, he first reported the results of this new procedure. The conclusions which he drew from this study of forty cases were as follows:

Carcinoma of the prostate is more frequent than is usually supposed, occurring in about 10 percent of the cases of prostatic enlargement. An intralobular nodule in one or both lobes of the prostate in men past fifty years of age should be viewed with suspicion especially if the cystoscope shows little intravesicular prostatic outgrowth, and pain and tenderness are present.

The posterior surface of the prostate should be exposed as for an ordinary prostatectomy and if the operator is unable to make a positive diagnosis of malignancy, longitudinal incisions should be made on each side of the urethra (as in

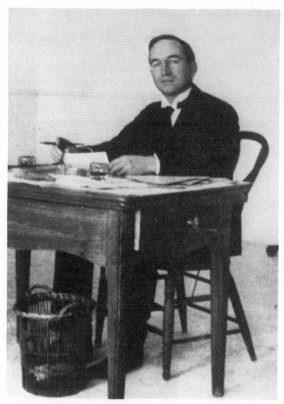

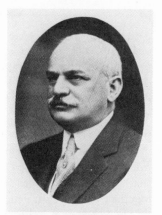

John Goodrich Clark
Courtesy of Dr. Francis C. Wood

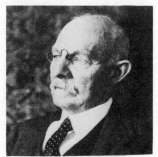

Hugh Hampton Young

From A. M. Chesney, *The Johns Hopkins Hospital and the Johns Hopkins University School of Medicine: A Chronicle*, vol. 2, *1893–1905* (Baltimore: The Johns Hopkins University Press, 1958)

William Stewart Halsted in 1922

From W. G. MacCallum, *William Stewart Halsted, Surgeon* (Baltimore: The Johns Hopkins University Press, 1930)

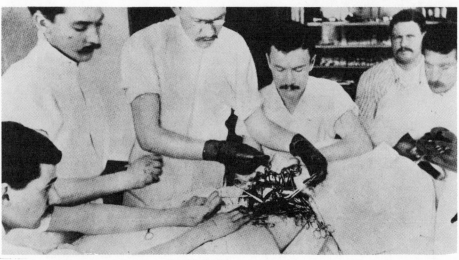

First surgical operation for which the operator wore gloves, 1893

The operator is William S. Halsted.
Photograph by James F. Mitchell. From *Ann. Surg.* 122 (1945): 902. Reproduced with permission.

prostatectomy) and a piece of excised tissue sent for frozen sections. If the disease is malignant, the incisions may be cauterized and closed and the radical operation performed. Cure can be expected only by radical measures and the routine removal of the seminal vesicles, vasa deferentia and most of the vesicle trigone with the entire prostate as carried out in these four cases.

These four cases in which the radical operation was done demonstrated its simplicity, effectiveness, and the remarkably satisfactory functional results.

In the following year Young published a monograph of 143 pages in the *Johns Hopkins Hospital Reports* (vol. 14), in which he assembled everything that had been written on cancer of the prostate in this county and abroad, together with a complete transcript of sixty-two cases of cancer of the prostate that had been seen in his clinic.

In December 1939 he stated that a careful analysis of the results obtained by his radical operation for cancer of the prostate was made. Over 50 percent of the patients followed for five years or more after leaving the hospital were apparently cured of cancer. These results compare favorably with those of any operation for cancer of deep-seated organs.

The prostate is only one area in which Dr. Young made highly significant contributions. The others are interestingly related in his autobiography.

Born in 1870 in Texas, the son of General William Hugh Young and Frances Kemper Young, he attended the University of Virginia, from which he also received his medical degree. At that time the university had no hospital, only a small dispensary for outpatients, and the only surgery Dr. Young saw was performed by Dr. William C. Dabney, who operated in the homes of his patients. Thus, when Dr. Young received his degree, although crammed full of "book learning," he knew nothing about the practice of surgery. He recognized his lack of sufficient training and he decided to go to the Johns Hopkins Hospital, which, although only five years old at the time, had already risen to the front rank.

When Dr. Young started his internship in surgery at the Johns Hopkins Hospital, there were fewer than three hundred beds. The operating room was small, with a wooden floor and inadequate ceiling lights. The operating table, which was of wood, had been brought from Germany by Dr. Halsted. It was a relic of the army hospitals of the Franco-Prussian War. It could not be tilted or turned. If one wanted the foot elevated, an orderly raised the board and put a saw horse under it, and a block of wood acted as a shoulder rest. To get the patient into a position with the thighs flexed and the legs in the air, two posts were stuck into holes on the side of the board and around these the legs were wrapped. Crude as it was, the finest surgery in America at that time was done on this table. This was before the days of sterile operating gowns and rubber gloves. Most surgeons put on short rubber boots without removing their shoes or trousers. Their sleeves were rolled up, a rubber apron tied on, and a small sterile towel fastened in front. Dr. Halsted made a great innovation at Johns Hopkins by insisting that his staff take off all their clothes, put on white tennis shoes, a duck suit with short sleeves and a little round skull cap. Although the instruments had been boiled for ten minutes, Lister's idea of infection from the air was still prevalent, and the instruments were kept immersed in 1:30 carbolic acid solution.

Dr. Young's autobiography makes exciting reading when he tells how he was given an opportunity by Dr. Finney to work in the surgical dispensary upon his first arrival in Baltimore and to take postgraduate courses being offered in the hospital at that time; how the occurrence of a vacancy in the resident staff gave him an opportunity to substitute for the man who was away; what mental anguish he went through because of Dr. Halsted's apparent indifference to his fate.

The story of how he was placed in charge of the genitourinary work of the Outpatient Department, however, can best be told by quoting his own recollection of the event.

In the Fall of 1896 I was transferred to the ward devoted to urological cases [those of the genital and urinary organs]. A patient had complained of frequency of urination for years. His bladder held only a tablespoon [15 cubic centimeters] and he had to void every fifteen minutes. It occurred to me that it might be possible by hydraulic pressure to increase gradually the size of the bladder. I rigged up a fifteen foot pole on which a source of fluid was suspended. By holding the nozzle tightly into the end of the urinary tract [penile urethra], by hydraulic pressure I was able to force the fluid through the urethra [the canal carrying urine from the bladder] and into the bladder. At first it was possible to introduce only 15 cc but by repeated dilatations several times a day the bladder became more tolerant and it slowly commenced to get larger. In a week the bladder held two ounces of fluid; in two weeks, three ounces. Simultaneously, the intervals between voidings increased to 40 minutes. At the end of a month, the patient was voiding about every three hours. In six weeks his bladder was half the normal size and he was voiding at intervals of four hours and eventually he was quite normal. This discovery was applied to other cases that appeared about this time and with equally good results . . .

The question arose whether hydraulic pressure might not cause fluid to pass up the ureters [ducts through which urine passes from kidney to bladder] into the kidneys and carry infection with it. To determine this it was necessary to conduct a series of experiments on animals and on cadavers and to search the world's literature on the subject. One day Dr. Welch was doing an autopsy. He had removed all of the abdominal organs except the urinary tract and I begged him to allow me to introduce a deep blue solution by hydraulic pressure through the urethra, as I had done in patients, to see whether any of the dye would pass up to the kidneys. The bladder became larger and larger, and the deep blue liquid could be distinctly seen within. A pint was introduced and then a quart and still the bladder continued to expand. It looked as if it might burst any minute. Dr. Welch and his staff beat a hasty retreat. When we opened the bladder we found that none of the fluid had gone beyond it. Hydraulic pressure could be employed without danger of fluids reaching the kidneys and setting up inflammation. These studies furnished material for a paper which I presented to the Johns Hopkins Medical Society with many charts and anatomical and pathological illustrations. . . .

While attending the genitourinary cases in Ward E, I became greatly interested in their bacteriology. One of these patients was a milkman who for eight years had carried the typhoid bacillus in the urinary tract, and probably had transmitted the infection to many of the homes where he carried milk. This case furnished the material for my first foreign publication which I presented to the Tenth International Congress in Paris on August 9, 1900. This case and additional ones afforded material for an extensive paper in Volume 8 of the Johns Hopkins Hospital Reports which under the editorship of Dr. Osler was devoted entirely to typhoid fever and its complications. I subsequently found the typhoid bacillus in the center of a stone taken from a kidney in a patient who had had typhoid fever many years before.

In my bacteriological studies I ran across some remarkable gonococcal infections and published several papers on them. I had the good fortune to be the first to demonstrate that chronic inflammation of the bladder and also of the kidney could be due solely to the gonococcus, and that the same organism could be responsible for a general peritonitis. These cases were published in extenso in an article contributed to a Memorial Volume to Dr. Welch by his students in 1900.

But all this time my interest was in general surgery. I almost never visited the genitourinary clinic conducted by Dr. James Brown and what urological work I had done was while I was an intern on Ward E. I had looked forward to being transferred to wards devoted to other forms of surgery. One day in October 1897 I was walking rapidly down the long corridor of the hospital. As I turned a corner, I ran into Dr. Halsted with force and almost knocked him down. I caught him just before he hit the floor and began to apologize profusely. Dr. Halsted, still out of breath, said: "Don't apologize, Young. I was just looking for you to tell you we want you to take charge of the Department of Genitourinary Surgery." I thanked him and said: "This is a great surprise. I know nothing about genitourinary surgery." Whereupon Dr. Halsted replied: "Welch and I said you didn't know anything about it but we believe you could learn."

How sound their estimate turned out to be. Dr. Young was one of the surgical titans of his time as well as a famous personality.

He became ill with coronary artery disease in 1945, but refused to limit his activities. On August 23, 1945, he had a fatal coronary occlusion. As stated by Miley B. Wesson in his obituary of Dr. Young: "He was a true son of the Lone Star State where men want to die with their boots on."

John Goodrich Clark and the Radical Operation for Carcinoma of the Cervix

Among the earliest attempts to cure cervical cancer was by simple amputation of the cervix. This became a common procedure in France in the early part of the nineteenth century, but in England there was considerable lag in its use, possibly because of Victorian modesty, which prevented vaginal examinations except in critical situations. Clearly it was not a satisfactory procedure and was soon displaced by simple hysterectomy. This, too, failed, and it became obvious that a more radical surgical approach would be necessary if the outlook was to be improved. In 1895 Emil Reis of Chicago developed a radical abdominal operation with pelvic lymph node dissection, which he performed on dogs and cadavers. However, it remained for Dr. John G. Clark to employ this radical technique in the operating room in 1895 while he was the resident gynecologist at Johns Hopkins. He gave this account of the undertaking: "After laying a plan before Dr. Kelly for the more complete extirpation of the uterus, the broad ligaments and a portion of the vagina and receiving his cordial endorsement and encouragement, I was granted the opportunity to put into effect the principles embodied in the proposed operation." Clark catheterized the ureters with bougies in order to obtain a better dissection of the broad ligament at the lateral pelvic wall, to facilitate ligation of the uterine vessels at their origin, and to enable removal of a large portion of the vagina without injuring the ureters.

Clark reported the first two patients on whom he used this procedure in an article entitled "A More Radical Method of Performing Hysterectomy for Cancer of the Uterus," which was published in the *Johns Hopkins Hospital Bulletin*. Three years later Wertheim of Vienna began to do the same radical abdominal type of hysterectomy, and popularized it in Europe and to a less extent in the United States. Wertheim's name has always been associated with this operation, although Clark was the first to perform it.

Some success was attained with this radical procedure when the disease was limited to the cervix; but when the process had spread beyond this stage, the outcome was usually unsatisfactory. The operation carried with it approximately a 10 percent mortality, and ureteral, vesical, and rectal fistulas to the vagina were common. Sampson, another gynecologist who was later to become famous for his work on endometriosis, did special work on the blood supply of the ureter with the intention of attempting to preserve it and thus avoid fistulas from the extensive lymph node dissection.

Realizing the shortcomings of operative cure of this disease, Kelly experimented with radium therapy. He and many gynecologists who followed his attempts attained greater success in the overall salvage of cervical cancer than had been attained by surgery.

John Goodrich Clark was born in 1867 and had his collegiate education at Earlham College and Ohio Wesleyan University. He received his M.D. degree from the University of Pennsylvania in 1891. From April 1892 until January 1895 he was an assistant resident gynecologist at the Johns Hopkins Hospital, and from January 1895 until February 1897 he was resident gynecologist. In 1898 he was made an associate in gynecology at the Johns Hopkins School of Medicine. In 1899 he became professor of gynecology at the University of Pennsylvania and gynecologist-in-chief to the University Hospital. As professor of gynecology he devoted his principal time and thought to the organization of his department, the securing and training of able personnel, and the equipment and conduct of his wards. He was noted for his wise and helpful guidance of students. One innovation of Clark's was widely imitated: "In the clinic the operating table was completely separated from the seats for students and visiting surgeons by a partition which can be raised or lowered. Behind this lowered screen preparations for operations were completed while to the audience in front of it was read an abstract of the case history followed by lantern slides demonstrating the steps of the proposed operation and the anatomy involved. The operation began at once when the partition was raised."

In his teaching, Clark largely discarded formal lectures, replacing them by conferences and clinical studies, which he enriched by a wealth of always apt and often amusing anecdotes and reminiscences; by lantern slides; by skillful, swiftly executed drawings; and by deft modeling with plastic material. Deeply interested in research, he founded the Undergraduate Medical Association at Pennsylvania, holding annually a one-day meeting at which all regular classes were suspended and papers were read and discussed, all based on the clinical studies and investigations of the students. He formulated definitely and authoritatively the indications and the limitations of radium in gynecology, and with Dr. Charles C. Norris published a monograph on the subject.

Dr. Clark was a member of the General Medical Committee of the Council of National Defense in 1917. He was president of the American Gynecological Society, in addition to many other honors which came to him.

Other important work in relation to carcinoma of the cervix has also come from the Department of Gynecology at Johns Hopkins. One of the notable contributions is that by Gerald A. Galvin, Howard W. Jones, Jr., and Richard W. TeLinde. Their classic paper, entitled "Clinical Relationship of Carcinoma In-situ and Invasive Carcinoma of the Cervix," appeared in the *Journal of the American Medical Association* in 1952. Several reports had helped establish the relation of carcinoma in-situ to the subsequent development of invasive carcinoma of the cervix. The first recorded histological picture of carcinoma in-situ appeared in T. S. Cullen's book on diseases of the uterus in 1900. However, it was this retrospective study of Galvin, Jones, and TeLinde, showing that in thirteen cases of carcinoma in-situ not treated, ten progressed to invasive carcinoma, one to seventeen years later, that firmly demonstrated that invasive cervical carcinoma is frequently preceded by carcinoma in-situ. TeLinde and Galvin had already established the histological criteria for the diagnosis of carcinoma in-situ and advocated total hysterectomy to prevent the development of invasive carcinoma.

Although Cullen had published an excellent picture of carcinoma in-situ, he had no conception of its significance. Others subsequently recognized similar lesions, but it remained for Schiller to light the first spark which generated the curiosity of TeLinde and his associates to investigate the condition further. They reasoned that in order to determine what microscopic picture actually represented early cervical cancer, it was first necessary to know what was not cancer. TeLinde selected eleven cases of questionable microscopic lesions and followed the patients for several years. None of these patients developed cervical cancer. They had lesions which have since been named "epidermidalization or squamous cell metaplasia," and are now universally recognized as benign lesions.

The practical aspect of the matter then lay in establishing whether there was a relationship between carcinoma in-situ and invasive carcinoma or whether carcinoma in-situ was simply a laboratory curiosity. Galvin and TeLinde undertook a study to try to establish this relationship. They had 11 biopsies in the laboratory about which there was considerable controversy. These biopsies had been taken because of a slight suspicion on inspection of the cervix, because of a history of intramenstrual bleeding with or without a suspicious-looking cervix, and in a few instances as a matter of routine at the time of curettage. On thorough studies of these sections they found absolute histological evidence of invasive cancer. From this microscopic study they strongly suspected that there was a relationship between this surface lesion and invasive cancer. However, efforts to convince their associates at that time failed. TeLinde was roundly criticized for making this suggestion, since in the words of one pathologist he had no right to an opinion because he was a clinician and not a pathologist.

TeLinde, Galvin, and Jones then decided to attack the problem from another angle. Among 723 patients with invasive cervical cancer treated in the Johns Hopkins clinic, there were 13 that had previous cervical biopsies from one to seventeen years before. This material from the previous biopsies was still available in the laboratory. On re-study of this material they found 11 with typical carcinoma in-situ. This study showed that invasive cervical cancer is frequently preceded by carcinoma in-situ and indicated that the lesion may be present several years before invasive carcinoma makes its clinical appearance, thus allowing ample time to effect a cure by hysterectomy. A later follow-up study by Galvin, Jones and TeLinde showed that the likelihood of subsequent development of carcinoma in-situ in patients whose biopsies showed cellular atypia was directly proportional to the degree of basal cell atypia. The practical importance of this finding was that when this atypia is found in a biopsy, the patient should be carefully followed with repeated cytologic smears and biopsies.

Shortly after TeLinde and associates had completed these investigations, cytology by smear became available. At first there was controversy concerning the relative merits of cytology and biopsy, but it soon became apparent that the two were complementary. It was obvious that one could not expect a practitioner to biopsy every cervix, and, indeed, he should not. But every practitioner could and should take smears. A positive or suspicious smear calls for biopsy and sometimes conization to determine the location and extent of the carcinoma. Thus, without cytology the work of TeLinde and his colleagues would have had limited value. But with cytology the importance of proper interpretation of the biopsy specimen becomes a very important link in the chain of evidence.

It is of interest that about 1905 Dr. Thomas S. Cullen wrote an article for lay consumption on the signs and symptoms of carcinoma of the cervix with the idea of educating women. It is difficult to believe, in the present-day framework in which education about the early signs of cancer is such a tremendous effort of the American Cancer Society and other organizations, that Dr. Cullen was almost thrown out of the Baltimore City Medical Society on the charge that this article represented undue publicity for the sake of enhancing his practice. Most people who knew Dr. Cullen recognized that he was not adverse to a little publicity, but it seems unbelievable that he could have been so severely criticized for a pioneering approach to preventive medicine—the education of the public about disease with the hope of early diagnosis and cure—an effort which subsequently has accomplished a great deal.

9 ❧ Fountainhead of American Physiology:
H. Newell Martin and His Pupil
William Henry Howell

H. Newell Martin
The First Professor of Biology

THE HEART is a remarkable organ that pumps five quarts of blood in a minute, seventy-five gallons in an hour, seventy barrels in a day, and 18 million barrels in seventy years. It does this by means of the most intricately woven muscle in the body, the anatomy of which was worked out in ingenious fashion by John Bruce MacCallum, the younger brother of William G. MacCallum, while a student at Johns Hopkins.

One of the most important problems in physiology was the mechanism by which the heart maintains its rhythmic beat. The ancients, during sacrificial rites, observed that the heart of an animal continued to beat for some time after it had been removed from the body. That the beat must originate in the heart itself was apparently clear to the Alexandrian anatomist Erasistratus, who lived in the third century B.C. However, anatomists ignored this evidence for the next twenty centuries because they were convinced that the nerves to the heart must generate the heartbeat. In 1881 Henry Newell Martin, a member of the original faculty of the Johns Hopkins University, first demonstrated that the heart of a mammal could be kept beating, although it was completely separated from the nerves, provided it was supplied with blood. We shall return to the laboratory and learn more of the ingenious experiments of this English-trained physiologist, but who was H. Newell Martin and how did he get to Baltimore?

When the Johns Hopkins University was organized, the most important problem was the choice of a faculty, and to this matter the trustees had given a great deal of thought. They wanted, in choosing a faculty member, to consider especially "the devotion of the candidate to some particular line of study and the certainty of his eminence in that specialty; the power to pursue independent and original investigation and to inspire the young with enthusiasm for study and research; a willingness to cooperate in building up a new institution, and the freedom from tendencies toward ecclesiastical or sectional controversies."

As related by John C. French, the first recruitment came about somewhat by chance. President Gilman was a member of the Board of Visitors of the U.S. Military Academy at West Point, and was invited to give the commencement address in 1875. While there he asked General Michie, the professor of physics at the academy, for advice as to the chair of physics at Johns Hopkins. The name of Henry A. Rowland, then an assistant instructor at the Rensselaer Polytechnic Institute, was mentioned. Gilman immediately interviewed him and was greatly impressed by the young man. On the advice of the trustees, Gilman took Rowland with him to Europe, where he was going in his search for additional faculty members. Gilman was thoroughly aware of the importance of providing for the sciences that were most closely related to medicine. In England he heard a lecture and was introduced to a young Irishman named Henry Newell Martin, who had served as assistant to both Michael Foster and Thomas Huxley. Martin was only twenty-eight at the time, and seemed, like Rowland and Remsen, to fit into Gilman's category of young men certain to be heard from.

Henry Newell Martin was born on July 1, 1848, at Newry, County Down, Ireland. He received his early education chiefly at home. Having matriculated at the University of London before he was sixteen, he became an apprentice to Dr. McDonogh in the Hampstead Road, London, on the understanding that the performance of his services as an apprentice should not prevent his attending the teaching at the medical school of the college and the practice at the hospital. In 1870 he obtained a scholarship at Trinity College, Cambridge. There he acted as the demonstrator of the newly appointed Trinity praelector, Michael Foster, whose right hand he continued to be during his whole stay in Cambridge. His energy and talents, and especially his personal qualities, did much to advance and render popular the growing school of natural science in the University.

In Cambridge, as in London, his career was distinguished. He gained the first place in the Natural Science Tripos in 1873. He proceeded to the degree of Doctor of Science, being the first to take that degree in physiology. His first publication on the structure of the olfactory membrane appeared in the *Journal of Anatomy and Physiology* for 1873.

In the summer of 1874 he assisted Foster in introducing into Cambridge the course of elementary biology, which Huxley had initiated at the Royal College of Science during the preceding year. He subsequently acted as assistant in the same course to Huxley himself, and in addition prepared, under Huxley's supervision, a textbook of the course. In 1874 he was made a fellow of his college, and was looking forward to a scientific career at Cambridge when he was invited to come to Baltimore.

Let us turn to one of his pupils, William Henry Howell, for insight into Martin's stature as a teacher and scientist from whose evaluation the following comments are drawn:

As a tribute to his work in Baltimore he was able to establish a broad-minded conception of the unity of the biological sciences which he derived from one of his own masters [Huxley] and the methods of scientific investigation in physiology which had been inaugurated in England by the other [Foster]. On the physiological side, these interests had been widened and vitalized into productive activity by the introduction of the experimental method as developed in the German-speaking countries. The new points of view were known to the leaders of botany, zoology and physiology in this country but their environment was not favorable to a change from the older to the newer methods of working and thinking. The timely establishment of the Johns Hopkins as an institution devoted chiefly to advanced instruction and research gave Martin an opportunity which he utilized fully to introduce the newer conceptions and methods into biological instruction. Most of the men who in the next two decades attained to prominence as teachers and investigators in the subject were his students and they helped to spread his influence in an everwidening circle.

As a teacher Martin thoroughly enjoyed introducing young students to the beauties and marvels of living structures and their adaptations. The story as he would unfold it came like a revelation, which startled his students into a new intellectual life. However, as a teacher of advanced students his method was entirely different. He seemed to utilize the sink or swim theory, and would show an extraordinary amount of indifference toward struggling research fellows floundering in the difficulties of their experimental work.

In his personal contact with his pupils, however, Martin exhibited a sincerity and a modesty which aroused a love for the subject and an affection for the teacher. His reticence in regard to his own work was remarkable. While keen to appreciate and publicly to praise the good work of others, he rarely, if ever, made reference before his students to his own investigations.

Martin's research was mainly in the field of animal physiology, and as an investigator he possessed unusual originality and insight. His best work was undoubtedly his brilliant series of experiments upon the physiology of the heart, already briefly mentioned, experiments that were made possible by his discovery of an entirely new method of studying the isolated heart. He published most of his research in the "Studies from the Biological Laboratory," which had a limited circulation. Years afterwards a distinguished German professor of physiology was disturbed to find that a long series of experiments published by him had previously been described by Martin both as regards results and methods. The principle of Martin's method for studying the mammalian heart in isolation was widely used for many years in experimental medicine in relation to studies in cardiac physiology, pharmacology, and pathology. Martin himself saw clearly the value of his discovery and hoped that it would be designated in the physiological literature as the "Baltimore method." However, the originator of the idea is not remembered in connection with it.

The genesis of this new method for studying the heart can best be related in Martin's own words:

In the course of experiments made in conjunction with Dr. W. T. Sedgwick on blood pressure in the coronary arteries of the heart I was impressed that the mammalian heart is no such fragile organ as one is inclined to assume but possesses considerable power of bearing manipulation. But I knew of various unsuccessful attempts to isolate the mammalian heart and study its physiology apart from the influence of extrinsic nerve centers such as used for physiological investigation on the heart of a cold-blooded animal. The mammalian heart, however, always died before any observation could be made. It occurred to me that the essential difference lay in the coronary circulation. In the frog there are no coronary arteries or veins, the thin auricle and spongy ventricle being nourished by the blood flowing through the cardiac chambers. But in the mammal the thick-walled heart has a special circulatory system of its own and needs a steady flow through its vessels and cannot be nourished by merely keeping up a stream through the auricles and ventricles. The greater respiratory needs of the heart of the warm-blooded animal also need consideration. The lungs ought either to be left connected with it or replaced by some other efficient aerating apparatus.

Martin's work at first was confined to the study of heart and lungs living together when the rest of the body of the animal was dead. His first experiments were made with cats. The animal was narcotized, tracheostomised, and a cannula put in the left carotid artery. The thorax was opened and artificial respiration was started. The innominate artery was tied beyond the origin of the left carotid but proximal to the point where the right subclavian and right carotid separate. The left subclavian was ligatured near its origin and the aortic arch tied immediately beyond the origin of the left subclavian. Finally, the superior and inferior cavae and the root of one lung were tied. The cannula in the left carotid artery was connected with the manometer of the Kymographion and tracings taken in the usual manner. Under these circumstances the course of the blood was left auricle, left ventricle, aortic arch, and the ligatured arterial stumps connected with it, the coronary vessels, the right auricle, the right ventricle, the pulmonary circulation through one lung and back to the left auricle. All circulation was cut off from every organ in the body except the heart and lungs. Yet the heart went on beating with considerable force and regularity for more than an hour.

Martin's original method still left much to be desired. He wanted to keep the heart alive much longer. After several attempts an apparatus was devised and found to answer admirably. With it he kept a heart, isolated physiologically from everything except the lungs, beating with beautiful regularity for more than five hours, and he had no doubt he could keep it considerably longer should that be necessary. He states:

It is, I think, clear that by this plan of work the study of the physiology of the mammalian heart is made possible to an extent never before attainable; I have now made a considerable number of observations which show that for at least four hours and often for considerably longer, great regularity and power in the heart's beat can be maintained. To investigate the direct action of any drug on the heart one would have only to inject it by hypodermic syringe into the cardiac end of the tube as in the usual manner of injecting curare into a vein. By altering the temperature of the chamber one can readily study the effect of various temperatures on the pulse rate, arterial pressure being kept at a given level while the tracings are being taken by altering the outflow through the stopcock if necessary; between the readings a uniform flow is kept up irrespective of arterial pressure. By keeping the temperature constant and altering the stopcock the direct influence of various arterial pressures on the pulse rate can be readily observed [Fig. 1].

Since his work involved experiments on animals, he was attacked by the antivivisectionists. A particularly outspoken critic was J. Rendel Harris, former fellow and lecturer of Clare College, a specialist in New Testament manu-

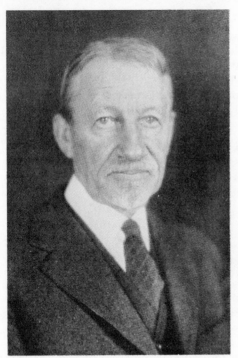

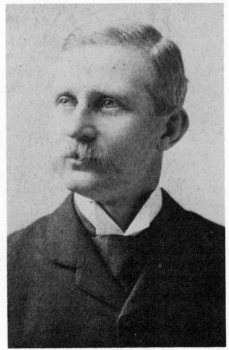

William Henry Howell
From *Bull. Johns Hopkins Hosp.* 68
(1941): 291

H. Newell Martin
This photograph was taken in 1876, Martin's first
year in Baltimore.
From the Archives Office, The Johns Hopkins
University

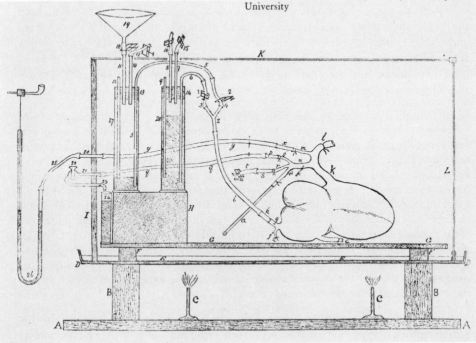

Fig. 1. New method of studying the mammalian heart

Plate 1 from *The Physiological Papers of H. Newell Martin* (Baltimore: The Johns Hopkins University Press, 1895)

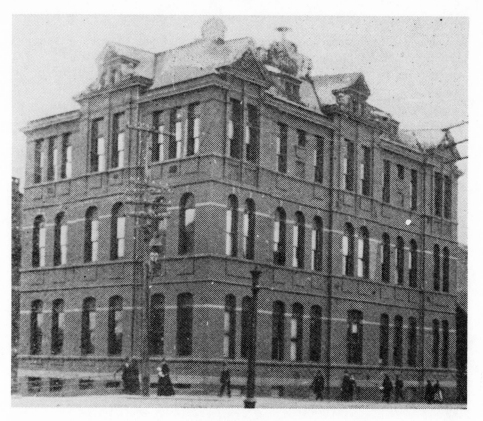

Biological Laboratory.

Occupied in 1883, it is said to be the first building in the United States devoted to research and instruction in biology.

From J. C. French, *A History of the University Founded by Johns Hopkins* (Baltimore: The Johns Hopkins University Press, 1946)

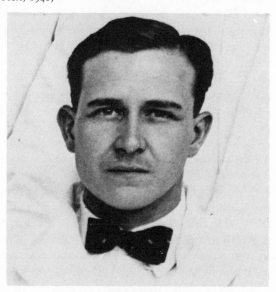

Jay McLean

From the Archives Office, The Johns Hopkins Medical Institutions

scripts, and then associate professor on the Johns Hopkins faculty. His objections led to his resignation in 1885, explained by President Gilman with this statement in his report: "In matters which pertain to another department he was not in accord with the policies here pursued."

A university planning to open a medical school in the near future could not have been more perceptive than to appoint as its first professor of biology a man who defined the mission of his department as follows: "To advance our knowledge of the laws of life and death; to inquire into the phenomena and causes of disease; to train investigators in pathology, therapeutics and sanitary science; to fit men to undertake the study of the art of medicine—these are the main objects of our laboratory. I do not know that they can be better summed up than in the words of Descartes, which I would like to see engraved over its portal: 'If there is any means of getting a medical theory based on infallible demonstrations, that is what I am now inquiring'."

Martin was appointed as the first professor of physiology, but unfortunately he was never to teach in the School of Medicine. Failing health forced his resignation in 1893, just before the medical school opened its doors. He returned to England after his resignation and died shortly thereafter at the age of forty-five.

William Henry Howell, one of his pupils, was appointed to succeed him, and because of this relationship Martin deserves a place on the honor roll of those who successfully launched this milestone in the development of medical education and research in this country.

William Henry Howell
The First Professor of Physiology

William H. Howell, who died in Baltimore on February 6, 1945, was the last of that "galaxy of clinical and scientific talent" entrusted with the organization of the departments of the medical school of the Johns Hopkins University prior to the opening of its doors to students of medicine in 1893.

Howell was born in Baltimore, February 20, 1860, the son of George Henry and Virginia Magruder Howell. Both parents were natives of Maryland, coming from families that had lived since 1751 in the southern counties of the state. The whole of Howell's formal education was acquired in Baltimore in the public grade and high schools and in the Johns Hopkins University. Howell's interest in science was aroused at age sixteen, at which time he became a student assistant to the professor of physics and chemistry in the City College. The professor encouraged him to carry on his own experiments, and Howell remembered with pride how he repeated Wohler's classic experiment of converting ammonium cyanate to urea—the first conversion of an inorganic to an organic compound. It was this among other things that led Howell to study medicine. He was greatly interested in the newly founded Johns Hopkins University and decided to take its chemical-biological course as a preparation for a career in medicine. When he applied at the office of the university, the registrar, Thomas Ball, an old friend and schoolmate, suggested that he see President

Gilman. Howell demurred as it did not seem to him that the president of a great university would care to waste his time upon an inconspicuous, totally unknown candidate for entrance. Ball insisted, however, and Howell was escorted into the president's office. Mr. Gilman received him in the kindest possible way, and they talked for half an hour or more. Howell explained his previous preparation, and Gilman extracted from him all his hopes and ambitions for the future and gave him helpful advice in regard to his courses in the University. This was the beginning of a friendship which lasted until Gilman's death.

Howell embarked on the chemical-biological course in the autumn of 1879. Since the course in general biology was given by the head of the department, Henry Newell Martin, Howell came in contact at once with that brilliant individual who undoubtedly exerted a great influence on his subsequent career. Howell obtained his A.B. degree after two years of study during which he completed major courses in biology and chemistry and minors in physics, German, and philosophy. The commencement exercise was held on June 6, 1881, and sixty years later Howell said of that occasion:

Never have I experienced such an all-pervading, quiet, but deep sensation of satisfaction as on that day when I received my bachelor's degree in arts. It seemed to me that I was being admitted into that goodly company of scholars I so much admired—and in fact that proved to be the case, for since that time my associations have been mainly with scholars, meaning by that term men and women who have a love of learning and the desire and ability to promote it.

Upon graduation as a bachelor of arts, Howell was awarded a graduate scholarship for one year. He was short of money and was thus enabled to continue his education. Years later Howell remarked: "In this way my original intention to become a practitioner of medicine was diverted and I entered upon the career of a teacher and investigator." Surely no scholarship bestowed by the Johns Hopkins University has ever returned more to the institution itself than the one awarded to William Henry Howell.

The Johns Hopkins Department of Biology, when Howell was a graduate student, consisted of William K. Brooks, associate; William T. Sedgwick, associate; Henry Sewall, associate; and Edmund B. Wilson, assistant. All four of these men achieved eminence in their chosen fields as time went on, and together with Martin constituted an inspiring group. It was during Howell's last year as a graduate student that the new biological laboratory of the Hopkins was opened. This was a three-story building situated at the southeast corner of Eutaw and Little Ross streets. Howell moved into this new building when he accepted the post of assistant in biology offered him upon his receiving the degree of Doctor of Philosophy in 1884. His thesis was on the subject of "The Origin of Fibrin Formed in the Coagulation of the Blood."

The study and teaching of physiology was the keystone of the Department of Biology, and it was in that environment that Howell, now twenty-four years of age, began his career as a teacher. In spite of his heavy teaching duties, Howell found time to conduct his own investigations, and three papers were published by him during the five years in which he was in the Department of Biology. In 1887 Howell married Miss Ann Janet Tucker of Baltimore, and in the following year he was appointed associate professor of biology. In 1889 he was called to the University of Michigan to take the chair of physiology, which his friend and former associate at Hopkins, Henry Sewall, was leaving because of failing health. In 1891 the laboratory course in physiology became a requirement for all medical students at Ann Arbor, the first laboratory course in physiology to be required in any medical school of the country. Howell's stay at Ann Arbor was brief, for in 1892 he accepted an appointment as associate professor of physiology under H. P. Bowditch at the Harvard Medical School. Before the termination of that year, Mr. Gilman made the trip to Boston to tell Howell of the plans for the new medical school in Baltimore and to offer him the chair of physiology. Howell accepted at once without discussion, for, as he put it, "I had a deep affection for the University that had done so much for me, everything, in fact, so far as my career was concerned."

Howell, among those who first headed the four preclinical departments at Johns Hopkins, was the only one without extensive experience as a worker in foreign laboratories. When Mall and Abel came to the school, they were given laboratories in two extra stories hastily added to the old Pathological Building, while Howell carried on the teaching of physiology in the biological laboratory some two miles across town. It was not until the old Physiology Building was occupied toward the end of the century that the medical group became unified and all the teaching was carried on in East Baltimore.

The thirty-eight active years Howell spent at Johns Hopkins were divided between the medical school proper, which had the lion's share of twenty-five years, and the School of Hygiene and Public Health, which had the rest. During this period he was dean of the medical school for twelve years, and first assistant director and then director of the School of Hygiene and Public Health, from 1918 until his retirement in 1931. His address on "The Medical School as Part of the University," given at the Harvard Medical School in 1909, illustrates his thinking on the broad subject of medical education. He arrived at the conviction that the heads of the major clinics should be made, as the preclinical chairmen already were, fulltime university professors. It is historically significant that in Dr. Howell's last year as dean of medicine, in 1911, the discussions began in the medical faculty which two years later were to usher in the second great reformation in medical education in America first put into effect at the Johns Hopkins—namely, fulltime clinical chairs.

Dr. Howell's strong influence as a teacher and investigator extended far beyond the boundaries of Johns Hopkins. When the American Physiological Society was founded in 1887, he was an original member, and at the initial meeting of the society in Washington in 1888 he read one of the scientific papers. His activities in that society remain unequaled. He was a member of the council for almost a quarter of a century, and he was its president for six successive terms. Also, he was the society's choice as president of the International Physiological Congress when it met for the first time in America in Boston in 1929.

Howell's research accomplishments were many. He published five papers during his Ann Arbor–Harvard period. Three deserve special mention. In one, there was a description of particles in red corpuscles that take nuclear stains, today known as Howell-Jolly bodies. The other two papers, which were awarded the Weir Mitchell prize, dealt with nerve degeneration. During Howell's period at Johns Hopkins, he published some fifty-five papers, only a few of which can be mentioned here. He was the first investigator to suggest that the two lobes of the pituitary gland are functionally different, and he presented this concept in a paper read by invitation before the first Congress of American Physicians and Surgeons. He described experiments showing that the circulatory effects of extracts of the pituitary gland were the result of substances derived entirely from the posterior lobes. Since that time a clear distinction has been made between the functions of the two lobes.

Howell's interest in salt action suggested to him the possibility that cardiac slowing resulting from vagus stimulation might occur because of the liberation of diffusible potassium. Guided by this hypothesis, he demonstrated that potassium is liberated during vagus stimulation and in amounts sufficient to stop the heart. Otto Loewi found that acetylcholine is liberated during vagus stimulation, that atropine stops the action of acetylcholine but not that of potassium, and consequently concluded that acetycholine is the inhibitor. Later it was shown by Lenhartz that acetylcholine liberates potassium but not in the presence of atropine. Therefore, Howell was the first investigator to suggest the chemical nature of the nervous influences which control the heart rate. How many cardiac surgeons of today who employ potassium to induce cardiac arrest realize that they owe to Howell the fundamental knowledge of the effect of inorganic ions upon the heart?

After 1909 Howell's interest was devoted almost exclusively to the study of blood coagulation. At that time another worker in this field had said of the subject of blood coagulation that "it is now in a state of anarchy." Howell was fully aware of the difficulties. He realized that the process of clotting involved chemical and physical-chemical reactions among substances whose nature and properties were known only imperfectly and that a complete explanation of the details of the reactions must await a better comprehension of the chemistry and physical chemistry of the blood. Yet he devoted an immense amount of time and effort to the isolation and purification of the components involved in the coagulation process. If he had had available the present techniques of approach to this problem, his progress undoubtedly would have been much faster. Even so, his contributions won for him the designation as the greatest American pioneer of blood coagulation.

At the time Howell began working on this subject there were at least five factors known to be concerned with the clotting process, most of which had been described by Alexander Schmidt of Dorpat. In his papers published between 1861 and 1895, Schmidt showed that a soluble blood protein, fibrinogen, is converted into the insoluble fibrin of the clot through the action of thrombin, which he regarded as an enzyme, and that the thrombin is not present as such in normal blood but is formed in shed blood from a precursor, prothrombin, through the action of a "zymo-plastic substance" secreted by the white cells of the blood. In 1890 Hammarsten and Arthus and Pages showed independently that calcium plays a role in the conversion of prothrombin into thrombin.

To these established findings, Howell's work resulted in the addition of a sixth factor. His earlier experiments (1884) in this field had led him to the correct conclusion that the normal plasma of the terrapin does not contain thromboplastin—the plasma of carefully drawn blood does not clot unless that factor is added. However, as a result of his studies in 1912 he found that the mammalian plasma differs from that of other vertebrates in that it contains within itself an available source of thromboplastin, derived, most likely, from constantly disintegrating blood platelets. Further work led Howell to conclude that intravascular mammalian blood does not clot, though it contains all the necessary factors, because of the presence of an "antithrombin."

Some three or four years after he had expressed these ideas, he assigned a second-year medical student, Jay McLean, the problem of isolating from heart and liver certain "phosphatides" which were believed to induce clotting. In the process a product was obtained, presumed to be a phosphatide, which instead of inducing clotting actually retarded it. From this point on Howell continued the investigation of his "anticoagulant," which he named "heparin" because it was derived from the liver. Howell and his co-workers succeeded in purifying heparin to the point where 1 milligram prevented the coagulation of 100 milliliters of blood for 24 hours at 0° centigrade. Having demonstrated its presence in normal blood, he early designated it as a "physiological" anticoagulant. Justification for thus regarding it had been supplied by the finding by others that heparin is normally present in certain cells in the walls of blood capillaries, whence it can readily gain access to the blood.

Jay McLean, the second-year medical student who first isolated heparin, was born in San Francisco in 1890. He had his first year of medical education in California, came to Baltimore in 1914, and was admitted to the medical school in 1915. He received his M.D. degree in 1919. After his graduation from Hopkins he was a member of the surgical house staff from 1919 to 1921 and an instructor in surgery from 1921 to 1924. After that he became an instructor in surgery at the University of California. Later he was appointed associate professor of experimental surgery at Ohio State University, remaining there for four years, from 1943 to 1947. In 1947 he became director of the Bureau of Cancer Control of the District of Columbia. Later he was director of radiation therapy and consultant in malignant disease at the Savannah Cancer Center. He died on November 14, 1957. Concerning the discovery of heparin, he stated: "The discovery of heparin came as a result of my determination to accomplish something by my own ability. It was this determination to become a physiologically based surgeon, rather than an anatomy-based surgeon that led to the discovery of heparin." In 1963 a symposium, Symposium on Bleeding in the Surgical Patient, was held in New York City at the New York Academy of Sciences in honor of Jay McLean. At that time a plaque was presented to the Johns Hopkins University which read as follows: "Jay McLean, 1890–1957, in recognition of his great contribution to the discovery of heparin in collaboration with Professor William H. Howell, this plaque is presented to The Johns Hopkins Medical School by the Conference on Bleeding in the Surgical Patient —New York Academy of Science—May 3, 1963." McLean published his paper on the thromboplastic action of cephalin in the *American Journal of Physiology.* In this paper the following paragraph appeared:

The heparphosphatid on the other hand when purified by many precipitations in alcohol at 60 degrees has no thromboplastic action and in fact shows a marked power to inhibit the coagulation. The anti-coagulating action of this phosphatid is being studied and will be reported upon later. Cuorin and heparphosphatid when dry have no odor, but when moist with warm alcohol have a characteristic odor common to both. It is possible that on further purification, the heparphosphatid may be shown to be identical with cuorin.

As Emmett Holt described it when he came to Baltimore in the fall of 1916, the physiological course was glamorous above all others. It was the best-taught course in the medical school, and also the most important. One very bright student whom Holt knew had actually penetrated the department and was working on a mysterious substance known as metathrombin. This student was Arnold R. Rich. Holt went to see Dr. Howell and asked to participate in the activities of the laboratory. Howell told him that the interest was principally in blood clotting, and if he would like to work on that he could. Jay McLean had left the laboratory and Holt was assigned the task of purifying the anti-coagulant liver fraction. He spent hours reading German monographs on phosphatides, extracting dog livers, precipitating and re-extracting and purifying heparin. In subsequent years Dr. Howell obtained purer, phosphorus-free preparations of heparin and identified carbohydrate groups in it. Its final constitution was established by Jorpes in Sweden. Holt notes that in preparation for a talk about Howell in 1961 he looked up the article on blood coagulation in what had once been *Howell's Physiology* and was still listed as the eighteenth edition of *Howell's Physiology* in the subtitle. It was a good article, but Holt was somewhat shocked to find no mention of Howell in it and no reference to any of his painstaking work, which extended over a period of thirty-five years. Certainly Howell's work was not in vain. Many of his concepts remain and much of his work provided solid building stones for those who came later. He made real progress in purifying and identifying a number of clotting factors, developed the first practical method of measuring prothrombin and antithrombin, and identified cephalin as the important thromboplastic constituent of brain tissue. He developed the concept that circulating anticoagulants were responsible for keeping the blood fluid in the blood vessels and demonstrated the presence of two of them, antithrombin and heparin, in normal blood. Thus, with the newer tools of today, Howell's scientific contributions are gradually being buried by new knowledge, a fate that is reserved for all but a few epoch-making discoveries.

After Howell became assistant director of the Hopkins School of Hygiene and Public Health, most of his research was devoted to the problem of hemophilia. His observations on this disease were made possible mainly through the rare opportunity which presented itself when three hemophilic brothers served both as dieners in his laboratory and as his principal subjects. These studies began in 1914, and although he was not able, because of the state of the art at that time, to unravel the true nature of hemophilia, it rekindled his interest in the nature of thromboplastin. While Howell was engaged in these investigations, he began having minor attacks of chest pain. On Thursday, February 1, 1945, he had one more severe than usual and was ordered by his physician to remain at home for a week. Disregarding these instructions, he went to his laboratory on Monday, the fifth. Early Tuesday morning he had a very severe attack and died within half an hour, fourteen days before his eighty-fifth birthday.

Howell had a deep interest in the spirit of investigation and the deportment of investigators. He stated, for example, that in Martin's laboratory: "The spirit of research was in the atmosphere. There was no pressure of any kind to produce results and there was no expectation that anyone was going to make a great discovery or even an important discovery. The sole animating motive was that he had the privilege of adding something new to the state of physiological knowledge." At a later time he remarked, "In medical research at present [about 1927] there is a keen, almost cruel competition to secure results that will attract attention. It has its good side, no doubt, in stimulating productivity but it does tend to distort values and set up standards that give to scientific research something of the low motives of commercial warfare." In 1915 Howell wrote, "Investigators by nature are men who cannot refrain from following out their ideas. They are driven constantly to such work by interest or by irritation. Either stimulus is sufficient. I fancy that among our greatest investigators it is the irritative impulse that predominates."

At no time did Howell display more than a quiet enthusiasm in discussing his researches, although he was always ready to defend his findings. Yet one wonders whether this outward calm did not conceal this same drive. Howell was not a trained chemist, but toward the end of his career he is said to have remarked, "I'd get along faster if I got an expert organic chemist to work with me, but it is more fun to do it myself." Howell was chemist enough to determine almost completely the composition of heparin, to recognize cephalin as a thromboplastic agent, and to devise a quantitative test for prothrombin which with slight modifications was used for many years. He could easily have secured the collaboration of a trained chemist and so speeded his work, but the drive was there to do it himself.

The Story of Franklin P. Mall, Florence R. Sabin, and John B. MacCallum

Franklin Paine Mall

FRANKLIN P. MALL was probably the least known to the public of the original department heads of the Johns Hopkins Medical School. He was never acclaimed as a brilliant discoverer, but his colleagues almost without exception believed that he was the leader of them all. Florence Sabin described Mall as a man of power, yet modest, unassuming, even shy. Always youthful in appearance, he was often mistaken for a student; nevertheless, he was one of the outstanding educators of his time. In an era when scientific research in medicine was taking root in this country, he contributed greatly to its development. When he came on the scene, the ancient science of anatomy had no real status and was no more than a handmaiden to surgery. He left anatomy on a sound foundation with a school of outstanding disciples. He was a leader who foresaw the opportunities for the development of a sound educational and scientific base and helped set the stage for it. His vision was the creation in this country of a university of scholars in the European sense.

Mall was born in Belle Plaine, Iowa, September 28, 1862, and died in Baltimore, November 17, 1917, at the age of 55, following an operation for gallstones. At the age of eighteen he entered the medical department of the University of Michigan. In that year, 1880, the standards of admission at the medical school were raised. No student was admitted under the age of 16, and every candidate who could not show a certificate of graduation from a respectable high school, academy, or college had to pass an examination. This seems meager enough now, but at the time it was a real advance in medical education in this country, since in the 1860s and 1870s there were essentially no requirements for admission to our medical schools. To secure admission, a young man had only to register his name and pay a fee.

Also in 1880 the medical course at Ann Arbor was upgraded, and for the first time in any institution it was extended to three years. Mall's comments on the medical school at that time are quite revealing:

During this transformation it was necessary to introduce much new work both in the laboratory and in the lecture hall to occupy the students during the increased time they now had to study medicine. Old instructors filled their share of the additional time by requiring the students to attend their lectures a second time in order that they might remember better the many facts presented to them. Yet there was considerable vacant time to be filled, which thus gave opportunity to new instructors to come to the front with new ideals and methods to enrich the medical course.

It was this second group of instructors that made the greatest impression on Mall. Foremost among them were Professors Victor C. Vaughan and Henry Sewall. They gave pertinent information at first hand, and from the beginning made it clear that they had mastered their respective subjects.

They dealt little with the opinion of others, but instead produced trustworthy facts and demonstrations, as well as laboratory experiments for the students, upon which to build. The principle involved appeared to be the development of the student while presenting the subject matter, and now it is plain to me that no one but an investigator in his subject can do this. These high ideals were shared to a greater or less extent by other instructors, and were acceptable ... to only a minority of students. The majority of students were seeking a certain quantity of knowledge, and preferred to have it drilled into them. Little did the solving of problems and the development of reason appeal to them, and it naturally followed that they mistook versatility for power. An educational institution of highest order must carry on perpetual warfare against drilling trades into inferior students, in order to retain its high position.

It appeared to Mall that the change beginning to take place in the medical department at Michigan in 1880 was toward training thinking physicians with an underlying foundation composed of recent medical research as well as accepted facts; in other words, its goal was toward the university stature.

Mall went to Germany for clinical work, as so many young doctors were accustomed to doing, without any particular interest in research. It was his contact with His and later with Ludwig which opened his eyes to the sciences of anatomy and physiology. This was the golden age of the German university, and here Mall passed directly from what he had termed "the medical high school" into the freedom of university life. Here he found mature students, better trained than he in planning their own education. This he was keen to do, and his notebooks show that he planned his own course and worked with tremendous energy. A great dissatisfaction with medicine as it was currently practiced besieged him, and compelled him to find out what the nature of research was like.

The first problem His assigned to him was in embryology. Mall made pertinent observations, which clarified an obscure field, and came to conclusions directly opposed to those of his mentor. There thus arose between the two men, one a respected professor of years and the other a young student with his first problem, a scientific controversy rarely surpassed in its high plane of intellectual fairness. Mall found evidence that the thymus came from the endoderm of the pharynx rather than from the ectoderm of the third gill cleft, as expounded by His. Subsequently, His found that Mall was right, and made the correction of this matter in the form of an open letter to Mall published in the same journal in which their articles had appeared. The history of Mall's approach to this first problem reveals his ability. It is clear that he went to Leipzig without preliminary training in embryology, that in a brief year he acquired the technique of serial sections, and then by the new methods of reconstruction he mastered the complex forms of the gill arch region in the embryo chick, putting his finger on the crux of the differences of opinion regarding the origin of the thymus. As Sabin points out, his series of articles might serve as a model to the medical historian for a study of the growth of medical thought, for they show how problems arise, how they depend on the development of methods, and how they are based on previous work.

In October 1885 Mall entered the laboratory of Professor Carl Ludwig, whose influence was the most dominant in Mall's life. Under Ludwig's tutelage, Mall studied the blood vessels of the intestine. He showed that the vasculature developed in such a way that every segment of the organ had an equal supply of blood and that the pattern of these vessels could really be expressed as a simple branching of one artery into five different orders. Subsequently Mall showed that this simple concept of five different orders of arteries for an organ had a general application to the vascular supply of all organs. Between Mall and Ludwig there developed a rare friendship, and in the companionship of these two men, both in the laboratory and in Ludwig's home library, there was revealed to the younger man a strong sense of idealism and a devotion to scientific research. When Mall said good-bye to Ludwig and tried to thank him for all he had done for him, Ludwig said: "If you feel this way about it, pass it on." This is the key to Mall's devotion to the cause of medical education and research, which was to mean so much to the development of American medicine.

From 1886 to 1889 Mall was first a fellow and then an assistant in pathology under William H. Welch. Mall's excellent study of the stomach was done during this time, with the same thoroughness displayed in his study of the blood and lymphatic supply of the intestine in Ludwig's laboratory. Mall also continued his physiological studies of the intestine, being interested in the types of contractions and their influence on its circulation. Further, he studied the distensability of the intestine on the basis of its connective tissue coats and the nature of its contractions on the basis of its muscular coats, working out the arrangement of the various components as they were adapted to aid the muscles in changing the lumen of the intestine. During these studies, Mall realized that surgery of the intestine depended upon the properties of the submucosa. Halsted stated in later years that it was Mall who made this suggestion. Thus, in Welch's Department of Pathology in those early years there were examples of joint research at its best, for Halsted worked out his methods of intestinal anastomosis, while Mall both assisted with the operations and studied the results from the structural standpoint. The histological work published later by Mall showed that the best results were obtained when the sutures entered but did not penetrate the submucosa. The submucosa with its predominance of white fibrous tissue was the only layer strong enough to hold the sutures; the muscle coat, of course, not only allowed the sutures to pull out, but additionally, when the needle penetrated the muscularis mucosa, posed two dangers: one of infection along the sutures and, failing that, when the muscularis mucosa was torn, the second danger of a marked new growth of the glands into the zone of the submucosa.

In his study on intestinal contraction, Mall made wide use of the work of previous observers. He saw that intestinal contraction had to be studied in connection with the blood supply, for on contraction the intestine invariably became paler, harder, and shorter. From his own studies he found that there are three types of contractions to be considered. The first is the rapid peristaltic waves so frequently seen after the death of an animal, which contractions pass quickly over the intestine and may go in either direction. The second form is the normal peristalsis of digestion. This wave is always in one direction, which Mall proved by getting Halsted to create surgically a reversal of an intestinal loop. After recovery from the operation, these animals were well for a short time but then became ill. At post-mortem it was found that the reversed loop was dilated most markedly at the proximal end, where there was a piling up of intestinal contents and an ulceration of the mucosa. This demonstrated that the mechanism of normal peristalsis lies within the wall of the intestine itself and that this wave is irreversible. The third type is local rhythmic contractions, later shown by the work of Cannon with x-rays and the fluoroscope to be significant in the breaking up of food and the mixing of it with digestive fluids. In his final summary Mall said, "To conclude, we may state that with this arrangement each contraction of the muscular wall of the intestine not only propels the contents of the intestine downward, not only aids in mixing the chyle, but also expels blood from the intestine into the portal vein, makes room for new blood, and thus acts indirectly upon the liver."

Mall studied the various materials making up the intestinal coats, including the white fibrous coat (submucosa) and the elastic membranes. He realized that reticulum was important and discovered that the reticular network not only constitutes the framework of the lymphoid tissues but also forms the supporting tissues of all the organs. This work is considered to have established the fact that the reticular framework of organs is independent of cells. Mall showed that reticulum is so labile a framework that it adapts itself to and supports all of the functioning cells of each organ. Thus, Mall was interested not only in morphology but in function.

In the spring of 1889, Mall accepted the position of adjunct professor of anatomy at Clark University in Worcester, Massachusetts. Thus after years of training in embryology, physiology, bacteriology, and pathology, he finally chose anatomy, basing his decision on his interest in structure and on his talents as Ludwig had seen them. It was during this period that Mall's attention focused on embryology, and he began to write short articles to be distributed to doctors about the preservation of the valuable human material that came into their possession. Mall's own studies on the nervous system with specific reference to the development of the eye began during this period.

Mall soon developed remarkable insight into the problems of the histogenesis of the central nervous system, a subject then in its infancy. Schleiden and Schwann had postulated that the nerve fiber is an outgrowth of a nerve cell. This concept was made more likely through the discrimination of axone and dendrite by Deiters, as well as by the then well-known methods for specific staining of neurons devised by Golgi and Ramon y Cajal. Many years later, in 1907, this concept was conclusively established in Mall's department, by Ross G. Harrison, by watching the outgrowth of the fiber in tissue culture, a method Harrison devised for the specific study of this problem. In 1893 Mall, judging that the balance of evidence at that time was in favor of the neuron doctrine, developed the concept that there was a specific polarity of the developing neuron in that the receiving pole of the cell always pointed to the surface of the ectoderm or toward the central canal of the central nervous system. Mall described the pattern of each of the sense organs, from the simplest one in the olfactory nerves to the most complex one in the retina, on the basis of this polarity. Mall clearly foreshadowed Kappers' theory that throughout the central nervous system each group of developing neurons is oriented in the lines of the incoming sensory impulses. Thus again one sees the originality of Mall's mind, for in taking up a new field, neurology, he made observations which have stood the test of time. Mall sensed their meaning and judged the force which directs the path of the growth of neurons.

In 1892 Mall left Clark University for the University of Chicago, but in the spring of 1893 he was offered the professorship of anatomy at the Johns Hopkins University, which he accepted. He was then thirty-one years old.

Mall's mature years were spent in Baltimore. He had a profound influence on medical education and a share in the founding of several anatomical journals. He exerted leadership in scientific societies and finally established a research institute for embryology. His effect on medical teaching in this country was the result not only of the originality of his ideas on education but also of the power of his example. However, he continued to exert his major efforts in research. His research work in Baltimore can be classified under three headings: embryology, the structure of organs in the adult as adapted to their functions, and a beginning in anthropology. His embryological studies included the development of the diaphragm, the ventral abdominal walls, the body cavities, and the loops of the intestines in human embryos. From the study of the early stages of the development of the liver, Mall was led to a consideration of the whole development of the body cavities and the loops of the intestines. Both of these projects he followed by means of three-dimensional wax models. Of this work, His wrote that it was the first time that the development of any organ had been carried from its early stages through the transition forms to its condition in the adult which he regarded as a great advance.

There was a slaughterhouse near the laboratory in Baltimore from which an abundant supply of embryo pigs in every stage could be obtained in fresh state with the hearts still beating. Using this material, Mall became interested in the development of the blood vessels, a problem he assigned to a number of his research fellows, including J. B. MacCallum, H. M. Evans, G. L. Streeter, and Florence Sabin. To the latter group he suggested the problem of the origin of the lymphatic system, while the growth of the lymphatics in amphibian forms was to be followed by E. R. and E. L. Clark. Their studies led to the fundamental concept that blood vessels come from cells, that is, angioblasts, and that endothelium is the primary tissue of the vascular system. The work on the lymphatic system likewise led to a concept of the fundamental nature of the endothelial cell.

Mall's best known work of his mature years was that on the spleen, the liver, and the heart. He discovered that the veins of the splenic pulp have an incomplete endothelial lining, a discovery often credited to Mollier. This established the fact of an open circulation in the spleen. By means of injections with asphalt, Mall showed that the route from artery to vein was through the pulp spaces. Mall made what he regarded as the crucial experiment for demonstrating the circulation through the spleen. He tied the splenic veins at the hilus in two dogs and then returned the spleen to the body cavity for half an hour. At the end of this time, when the spleen showed maximum distention, he tied the arteries in one animal, removed the spleen and fixed the organ in formalin for twenty-four hours with the capsule intact. In frozen sections, he found the pulp spaces engorged with blood. In the other animal he cut the veins, watched the contractions of the organ, which took a few seconds, and produced a spleen entirely free of corpuscles. His work on the framework showed how the spleen was constructed in order to bring about the emptying of the pulp spaces into the veins of the pulp. Thus, the spleen is an organ in which blood readily flows into the tissue spaces, the so-called pulp; but unlike other organs, it has an efficient mechanism, the smooth muscle of the trabeculae, for speedily bringing the blood back into the circulation. These concepts of the open circulation were subsequently confirmed by physiological work, especially that of Bancroft.

Mall's paper on the structure of the liver is another good example of his superb work. In this paper Mall stated one of the fundamental generalizations to come out of his laboratory: "The anlage, then, of the vascular system is the capillary; artery and vein are secondary and are differentiated out of them by the flow of blood set in motion by the heart." Mall thought that throughout the vascular system, including the lymphatics, endothelium is the essential tissue. Muscle coats and connective tissue coats are accessories, or as their names suggest, adventitial. He, attempted to determine the nature of the structural unit in the liver. By means of corrosion of the hepatic and portal veins, he reconstructed the pattern of this organ and determined that the so-called lobule with its center at the hepatic vein cannot be considered as a structural unit, since the lobules vary so greatly in size. On the other hand, the portal units meet all the conditions of a structural unit, since all of them are of the same size. Portal units also have the artery and bile ducts as well as the portal vein in the center, and their size is determined by the length of the capillary bed of the organ. To obtain a three-dimensional picture of the portal units of the liver is so difficult that it probably cannot be gained from pictures alone; but the study of the corrosions of the vessels which Mall left in his laboratory makes this possible. Mall showed that this concept was essential in following the development of the liver. In this study of the liver, Mall brought to its fullest fruition the concept of structural units, which he had first formulated in the study of the intestinal villus in Ludwig's laboratory, that is, there is a structural unit for each organ which is a unit of function.

Florence Rena Sabin

On April 25, 1925, the National Academy of Sciences elected a woman to its membership for the first time in the sixty-eight years of its existence. She was Dr. Florence Rena Sabin, professor of histology in the Johns Hopkins Medical School, the first woman to be a full professor in that institution and also the first woman to be president of the American Association of Anatomists. By her extraordinary scientific talents and personality, Florence Sabin demonstrated to university administrators of this country that a woman can be the equal of a man in academic pursuits. More than anyone before her, she opened the doors of our medical schools and hospitals to women seeking to devote themselves to a career of scientific investigation.

Florence Sabin was born on November 9, 1871, in Central City, Colorado. Her grandfather had practiced medicine, but her father gave up his leanings in this direction in 1860 to become a mining engineer. In January 1885 Florence began studies at Vermont Academy and four years later entered Smith College. A course in zoology aroused her interest in biological sciences. While she was still in college, the plans for a Johns Hopkins University School of Medicine were being discussed, but its opening was delayed for lack of sufficient funds. In 1890 a group of women headed by M. Carey Thomas and Mary E. Garrett, both daughters of trustees of the university, founded the Women's Fund Committee to obtain money for the endowment of Johns Hopkins, provided women should be admitted to the school on the same terms as men. By 1893, the year of Florence's graduation from Smith College, half a million dollars had been raised; most of this was furnished by Miss Garrett, and the Johns Hopkins Medical School was opened to both women and men. In all likelihood the possibility of entering this medical school of high standards on an equal footing with men influenced Miss Sabin to decide upon medicine as a career. She did not have the necessary funds at that time, but finally entered Johns Hopkins in 1896. At Hopkins she came under the influence of Dr. Franklin P. Mall, whose attitude toward the teaching of anatomy imbued the best type of student with the excitement of original discovery. In her biography of Mall she stated, "The writer worked for twenty years under Mall, four years as a student, one as a fellow and fifteen years on his staff. Her start in research as a medical student and her opportunity for a career in scientific medicine she owes wholly to him." While a student under Mall, she began her first investigation into the structure and function of the medulla and the midbrain. In this work models were constructed from serial microscopic sections of these regions of the central nervous system of a newborn infant. Reproductions of these models were used for years in several medical schools, and shortly after her graduation she published her first work, "A Model of the Medulla Oblongata, Pores and Midbrain of a Newborn Babe." This excellent work is thought to be one of her best contributions.

After graduation she received one of the greatest opportunities for a woman physician at that time, an appointment as an intern at the Johns Hopkins Hospital. During her internship she realized that research and teaching held a greater appeal for her than the practice of medicine, but there were no medical school positions at that time for women. However, the same group of women in Baltimore who had raised the money which permitted the medical school to open its doors provided funds for a fellowship in the Department of Anatomy for Dr. Sabin. Soon her work led to the prize of the Naples Table Association, which maintained in the zoological station at Naples a position or table for the promotion of scientific research by women. Within four years Dr. Sabin was promoted successively to the rank of assistant, associate, and associate professor of anatomy. During this period a series of published papers established her reputation as an investigator of the first rank. In 1917 she was appointed professor of histology.

The road to success in her research career was not easy. Her work began at a time when the anatomy of the smallest lymphatic channels and their relationship to the tissue spaces was poorly understood. In her own words,

When I began my work it was the accepted theory that lymphatics arose from the tissue spaces and then grew toward the veins, although both Langer and Ranvier had expressed the view many years before that the lymphatic plexus grows outward from the veins by means of extensions of endothelium. However, their work had been done with relatively large pig embryos, and their views were not generally accepted, since the lymphatic system in pigs of that size is so well developed that it might almost be considered as adult in form.

Therefore she studied the development of the lymphatic channels in small pig embryos. She succeeded in injecting these vessels with colored or black materials in embryos as small as 23 millimeters in length. These preparations showed that lymphatics arise as buds from the veins and grow outward as continuous channels by a process of further budding. To clear up the opposing views, Dr. Sabin combined the injection method with the technique of reconstruction from serial sections. For example, after the right jugular lymph sac and the lymphatics leading to it were filled with colored materials, the lymphatics in an embryo pig 27 millimeters in length looked like continuous channels extending outward from the jugular sac. Next, reconstructions were made from serial sections of this injected plexus and also from similar sections of the same area of the other side of the embryo, a region which had not been injected previously. The plexus that had been filled with colored material could be almost completely reconstructed and showed lymph channels connecting with each other. The reconstruction of the uninjected side showed what appeared to be unconnected lymphatic spaces. The tiny connections between the uninjected and consequently empty lymphatics of the second reconstruction had failed to show in the serial sections, whereas when these channels were previously filled with colored material, the connections were rendered visible. By this and other studies, Florence Sabin demonstrated that the lymphatics arise from veins by sprouts of endothelium, so that the entire system is derived from already existing vessels. Further, she showed that the peripheral ends of the lymphatics are closed and that they neither open into the tissue spaces nor are they derived from them. Her views met with much opposition, and although the controversy

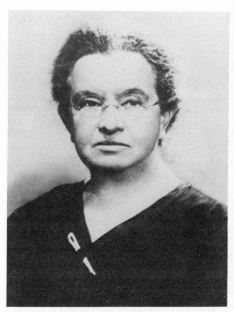

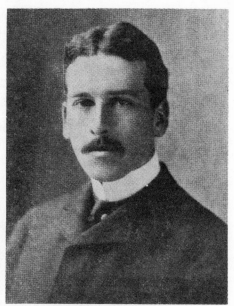

Florence Rena Sabin

From the Archives Office, The Johns Hopkins
Medical Institutions

John Bruce MacCallum

From A. Malloch, *Short Years: The Life and
Letters of John Bruce MacCallum, 1876–1906*
(Chicago: Normandie House, 1938)

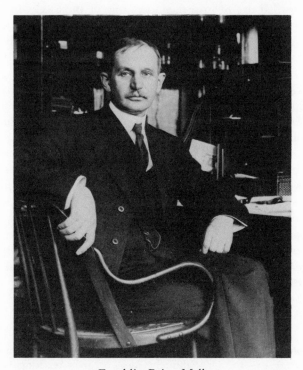

Franklin Paine Mall

From the Archives Office, The Johns Hopkins Medical
Institutions

became sharp, her views prevailed because of the accuracy of her observations. Through it all she showed herself as willing and able as any man to fight for her cause.

Dr. Sabin next embarked on a study of the origin of endothelium. For this she used living tissue and the method of tissue culture devised by Ross Harrison. She was able to watch cellular growth in the hanging drop preparations and to see under the microscope the development of the earliest blood cells in explanted bits of blastoderm of the chick embryo. She reported that on the second day of incubation of such cultures only red cells could be seen coming from the endothelial walls of the blood vessels. By the third day white cells appeared, arising partly from new cells that differentiated from mesenchyme without becoming part of the vessel's lining.

She later developed various techniques for the study of preparations of living cells by staining them with certain innocuous dyes. These methods of supravital staining became useful research tools, employed by laboratory workers throughout the world. The characteristic difference in the intracellular distribution of the dyes enabled workers to identify many of the cell types and to study some of their functions under normal and diseased conditions. Among these cells appeared certain mononuclear units termed "monocytes." Her experiments indicated that these cells were involved in tissue reactions against infectious agents, particularly the tubercle bacillus. Accordingly, she turned her attention to the cellular defenses of the body against disease. Her work with living monocytes led her to investigate the role of these cells in the defense of the body against infections, a subject which carried her to a second career in pure research, unburdened by teaching, and forty years later to her third career as a reformer of the public health laws and a fighter against tuberculosis in Colorado.

By 1925 Dr. Sabin had reached a position of great distinction. However, when Dr. Mall died, the position of professor of anatomy and head of the department was not offered to her but to one of her former students. By this time her cellular studies had led to an increased understanding of the bodily defenses against infectious diseases, notably the monocytic cells in the defense against the tubercle bacillus. Dr. Simon Flexner, the director of the Rockefeller Institute for Medical Research, who had long been interested in the humoral rather than the cellular mechanism of defense against infections, concluded that investigation of both mechanisms was desirable. Accordingly he urged Dr. Sabin to accept a position as a full-time member of the Rockefeller Institute. She was the first woman to become a full member of that institution.

Her career as a teacher was well summarized in 1951 at the dedication of the Florence R. Sabin Building for research in cellular biology at the University of Colorado School of Medicine. In his address Dr. Grover F. Powers, then professor of pediatrics at Yale University, said in part:

Dr. Sabin is a great teacher. The impact of her teaching upon pupils is to inculcate a love of scholarship, a high regard for learning, a fostering of the spirit of inquiry and of intellectual curiosity—for Dr. Sabin the ideal of great teaching is stimulation of the student to the love and pursuit of knowledge—kindling of the mind—upsurging of the spirit! It occurred to few students entering medical school shortly after the turn of the century that a great teacher was other than one who presented information and facts in an interesting and entertaining manner. The first vigorous and disquieting impact of Dr. Sabin upon pupils was to dispel that concept. Soon, however, as a result of her teaching and example, it was found by many that minds kindled and intellects awakened were more to be desired than minds well-stocked with information, interesting and useful though it might be. In her own teaching career Dr. Sabin perfectly exemplified the characterization she herself gave of one of her own teachers and colleagues. Using her own tribute to Franklin P. Mall we say of Dr. Sabin: "Her contempt of slovenly or dishonest work, her admiration of rigidly perfected technique, her encouragement of objectivity in study, her insistence upon familiarity with the bibliographic sources, her emphasis upon the duty and pleasure of extending rather than merely acquiring knowledge, her impatience with inaccuracy and with stupidity, her unanswering loyalty to the highest ideals of natural science—all these were qualities that made her a working companion of inestimable value to the young men and women who entered the Johns Hopkins Medical School." And thus in very truth is characterized the great teacher we salute today.

Florence Sabin received many honors, including the honorary degree of Doctor of Science from Smith College. Four years before leaving Baltimore, she was asked to speak as a representative of American Women of Science at a reception for Madame Curie held at Carnegie Hall in New York. In 1945 she received the Trudeau Medal of the National Tuberculosis Association.

Each state in the Union may be represented in the National Statuary Hall in the Capitol in Washington by two statues. The first from the state of Colorado is a bronze statue of Dr. Florence Sabin by Mrs. Joy Buba of New York City. It was formally presented by the state of Colorado to the United States of America on February 26, 1959.

Johns Hopkins Had Its Keats: John Bruce MacCallum

"And folly does it seem to blindly live
The few short years that light us to the grave"—J.B.M.

John Keats, in 1810, was apprenticed to a surgeon and later served as a dresser at Guy's Hospital under Mr. Lucas. Sir Astley Cooper took an interest in this young man, who was a diligent medical student. Poetry, however, was his real vocation, as during this period he wrote his famous sonnet "On Reading Chapman's Homer." His career in medicine was short, as was his life.

Johns Hopkins also had its medical student poet—John Bruce Mac-Callum. His story is a poignant one, as he, too, was seized with tuberculosis in the prime of his life. This younger brother of Dr. William G. MacCallum was one of the most creative and talented people ever to enter the Johns Hopkins School of Medicine. After John's death, William G. MacCallum turned over to Archibald Malloch hundreds of letters written by John to his family and to others, including some to "Miriam" and the "Poetess," and a collection of his poetry. It is unusual for a scientific investigator to leave behind such a wealth of material. These letters and poems reveal in heartrending detail the story of this sensitive young man whose career in many respects paralleled that of John

Keats. But while Keats's few years were best spent as a creative poet, Mac-Callum's were best spent as a creative scientist. Malloch wrote an excellent biography, which in large part allows John Bruce MacCallum to tell his own story. This essay, which presents in abbreviated fashion the man and his contributions, is based entirely on the book written by Malloch entitled *Short Years: The Life and Letters of John Bruce MacCallum, 1876–1906.*

John was born in Dunnville, Ontario, on June 8, 1876, two years after his brother, William G. MacCallum. Thus, the two men had a similar childhood environment in which their practitioner father, Dr. George A. MacCallum, played a formative role. In addition to being a physician, their father was an authority on birds and other areas of natural history in that part of Ontario. It was evident from his early years that John was an extremely intelligent young man, but one who had frequent periods of severe depression. While attending the University of Toronto he began to write short, and more often than not, melancholy poems. During the summer of 1894 he first exhibited his scientific ability by collecting material from an unused limestone quarry near Dunnville, which he studied in a small laboratory at home. These efforts resulted in a paper entitled "The Fresh-Water Cladocera," which was read before the National Science Association of the University and was published in the *University of Toronto Quarterly* in 1895. In the autumn of 1895 he began his last year at Toronto, and among his fellow students was Jack McCrae (John McCrae, the author of "In Flanders Fields"). It was during this autumn that John MacCallum decided to enter the Johns Hopkins University School of Medicine. His severe depressive moods can be appreciated from the words he wrote just before leaving for Baltimore: "When I open my eyes and look into the long mirror at the end of the hall, I see only a grey, long face, with dim sad eyes, with nothing of beauty or grace, inspiring no love except that which is born of pity. My heart sinks to that sickening ache which fills up so many of my moments now." But later one finds him writing the following sentences which indicate that his hope lay in the prospect that scientific work would be his salvation: "If one can work with a great zeal and a true enthusiasm half of the secret of happiness is won. . . . No law is a simple one, but the keeping of it makes up the great force that has ruled the world for centuries. It is not a law to most men, it is a religion—a science of being happy—whose great master word is contentment and whose master is work."

Thus, in the fall of 1896 John MacCallum came to Baltimore to study medicine. During the first year he lived with his elder brother and his two friends, J. L. Nichols and C. R. Bardeen, at 1200 Guilford Avenue. One of the highlights in his life was his introduction to Dr. Franklin P. Mall, one of the first teachers with whom he came in contact and who more than any other influenced his subsequent career. In Mall's system of teaching, a student could choose to a large extent what aspect of anatomy he wished to study. How such good results could be obtained by such a method of teaching at that time would cause one to wonder, but the students were handpicked. Each student had a college degree and had to possess a reading knowledge of French and German as well as a background in physics, chemistry, and biology.

Even with this stimulating atmosphere that MacCallum found in Baltimore, his severe melancholic tendencies did not entirely leave him. However, he was able at times to find outlets that gave him moments of pleasure. The first Christmas Eve in Baltimore he found himself alone, as his brother was working in the hospital and his other two roommates had gone home. Desiring some excitement, he went down to Lexington Street and joined in the Battle of Tin Horns that took place in those days on Christmas Eve. In his own words he describes this:

It was the craziest thing I was ever in and I felt somewhat like an idiot when I got home. The Baltimore people go a little mad on occasions like this and hardly know what they are doing, so the only thing for a foreigner to do is to go mad too. Everyone goes downtown and this one street is simply packed with people all with tin horns. All the girls in the place were there, I guess, and the object of the thing seemed to be for the girls to blow their horns in the men's ears and for the men to get the horns away from the girls and vice versa. As you may imagine, no introductions are needed and men and girls talk and scrap in the most unconventional way possible. It is the queerest sight I ever saw. Men with silk hats on and dressed in their best and girls decked out in all their finery, pulling at different ends of a tin horn and talking and scrapping as hard as they could although they had never seen one another before. I quite enjoyed it after I had gotten a little practice. There wasn't a soul there I knew but before I left I became tolerably familiar with a great many of the prettiest ones. I don't expect the acquaintance to last very long though. It was exactly like the description of the carnival in that book of Hans Christian Andersen called *Improvisatore*.

Nowhere else in America could MacCallum have done the work that he completed during his first year in medical school. Obviously he was a creative genius born to make discoveries, and undoubtedly this would have been expressed anywhere in the course of time. However, with his excellent training in biology and the stimulation of Dr. Mall, he promptly became proficient in methods of cutting and staining microscopic sections, so that in a very short time he made impressive observations on the histology and histogenesis of the heart muscle cell. These contributions promptly marked him as an accomplished anatomist and embryologist at twenty-one years of age, when his medical student friends were struggling to remember anatomical names and the origins and insertions of muscles. It is not possible to summarize thoroughly the nature of this work, but he concluded his paper as follows: "It is to be emphasized, then, that in the protoplasm of the adult heart muscle cell, there are columns of fibrils which run longitudinally surrounded by sarcoplasm, in a way that each bundle is surrounded by a varying number of small sarcoplasmic discs, the horizontal, separating partitions of which are continuous with Krause's line [the narrow striation across the fibrils] on the fibril bundles." His schematic drawings, beautifully executed in pen and ink, showed sarcoplasmic discs piled in columns like counters used in games, one on top of the other with the sides of the columns touching one another. Malloch points out that this paper illustrates MacCallum's great ability to think in three dimensions.

In his second year MacCallum entered the study of pathology, and in

November 1897 he wrote as follows: "I should like very much to give the lecture (in anatomy) on heart muscle but I guess Dr. Barker will do it. They have two days' work on 'my discoveries' which is pretty good, I think, considering that I was in their place last year." It was characteristic of MacCallum that he began his work in pathological anatomy also with an original investigation —a study of the nature of the changes which occur in fragmentation, segmentation, and fibrosis of the heart muscle. His earlier work on the development of the heart muscle cell led naturally to this investigation. In speaking of it, he said: "Dr. Simon Flexner has been most obliging about the work I am doing under him. He does all the staining and hardening of my preparations and I simply cut them and study them. I think it will be a very important piece of work if it comes out right. It will be a basis for all the pathology of heart muscle for there is little known about it at present.

How well known MacCallum had become as a result of his creative accomplishments is reflected in the following statement from his notebook:

I had been working in the pathological laboratory and Dr. Cohn was demonstrating to me. We had heart muscle fatty degeneration that day and Dr. Cohn hadn't quite reached that when Dr. Flexner came over and asked me if I had looked at the section yet. I told him no and he said, "You look at it. Tell me where you think those fat particles are." And then as Dr. Cohn turned around, Dr. Flexner said, "You know MacCallum knows so much more about heart muscle than anyone else who has written on it." Cohn looked surprised. Flint said afterwards that Flexner just did that to keep Cohn from making an idiot of himself by demonstrating heart muscle to me. This, however, is vanity, the kind that tastes sweet without being sickening—for after the long lean years it is good to have the fat ones.

During the winter of 1898 MacCallum continued his work under Flexner. He presented a paper before the Johns Hopkins Hospital Medical Society on June 6, 1898, and a synopsis of it, entitled "On the Pathology of Fragmentatio Myocardii and Myocarditis Fibrosa," appeared in the *Johns Hopkins Hospital Bulletin*. The full paper, also illustrated by his own excellent pen and ink drawings, was published in the *Journal of Experimental Medicine*. This was the work that Dr. A. E. Malloch, an old friend of MacCallum's father, referred to when he said in introducing John to some young girls one summer day in Ontario: "This is the man who has proved that you can really have a broken heart."

MacCallum's next paper was also an anatomical one, and a natural sequence to his work on the development of the heart—an investigation of the nature of voluntary muscle. This paper, "On the Histogenesis of the Striated Muscle Fiber and the Growth of the Human Sartorius Muscle," was published in the *Johns Hopkins Hospital Bulletin*. He did most of this work during the winter of 1898, using human embryos ranging in size from 10 to 200 mm. He found that the changes during the course of development of striated muscle are similar to those in the various stages of development of the human heart muscle cell. As a result of this work, he made the suggestion that: "Hypertrophy of the heart is due to growth in the size of the fibers rather than to any increase in their numbers."

MacCallum's classmates found him a delightful companion, but nevertheless were unable to establish a real understanding or relationship with him. He had frequent periods of great detachment, and at these times was definitely inaccessible. Osler affectionately called MacCallum "Saint John," which seems to have been immensely perspicacious. The following verses in MacCallum's notebook were probably written sometime in the year 1898.

DEATH

Strong men have trembled at thy name, O Death,
And Nations lifted up their hands in prayer
To crave the senseless boon that Thou wilt spare
Their little lives, their wasted suppliant breath.

But I here on the borders of thy land
With cold damp winds against my aching brow
Am not afraid of thee, for in thy hand
I see no gift but rest, and only thou
Canst comfort me, for thou dost understand
O Death, and I await thee even now.

The third year of the medical course brought him in close contact with William Osler, although not for the first time, since he had already been invited to Osler's house. His description of the work in medicine is of interest: "It is all dispensary work and clinics which I suppose are the best things for us. Dr. Osler's clinics are splendid though. It is nice to hear him talk to patients. He has a joke for everyone and some good advice for everyone else. He sits on the table and swings his legs and talks. The patients don't know exactly what to make of it, but for us it is the nicest part of the course."

In his final year of the medical course his desire to carry on his scientific work burned as strongly in him as ever. The "Pithotomy" of which he was now a member had taken a house on Jefferson Street near the Johns Hopkins Hospital, and there he lived very happily with a number of others. Here is how he described his medical clerkship: "As I think I told you before, I am on the medical side and am clinical clerk in Ward E. My duties there are not very arduous although I have to get up early in the morning. Rounds are made at 9:00 by Osler and I have to have the blood examinations made and all the others and the charts ready each morning before Dr. Osler comes. I have six cases now so I am kept pretty busy." It was during this year that he first consulted Dr. Osler because he was not feeling well. In November 1899 Dr. Osler examined him and found nothing abnormal. However, later in the year he developed a pleurisy with effusion.

Another of MacCallum's outstanding contributions appeared in the volume *Contributions to the Science of Medicine Dedicated by His Pupils to William Henry Welch on the 25th Anniversary of His Doctorate*. This was published in May 1900 by the Johns Hopkins University Press in Baltimore. This article, describing the discoveries he made in 1899 on the heart, is perhaps MacCallum's most important anatomical work. The arrangement and course of the muscle fibers of the heart are very difficult for the student to understand.

The heart is a muscular pump, and when the heart muscle (or myocardium) contracts, blood is squeezed out of its chambers. That much the student knows, and he can see that the heart muscle has several layers and that in each layer the fibers run in the same direction. However, he can see little order as he attempts to trace their course, for they seem to run in almost every direction. Every muscle has an origin (one place of attachment) and at the other end an insertion (the site of attachment), but the student has difficulty in making them out in the case of the heart muscle. It is representative of his genius that young MacCallum unraveled these complex arrangements. The full paper appeared in the American Journal of Anatomy and was entitled "On the Muscular Architecture of the Ventricles of the Human Heart." Some ten years later his teacher, Franklin P. Mall, wrote of this work as follows:

He did succeed in unrolling the wall of the left ventricle into a single sheet or scroll of muscle fibers. His presentation of the architecture and growth of the ventricles of the heart marks a milestone in this study, the like of which is found only in Gerdy's some 75 years before. Both Gerdy and MacCallum studied the heart muscle as a whole and did not deal with it in fragments. MacCallum, as Gerdy, did his work while still a medical student but unlike him presented his work in a masterly way. His paper is comprehensive. If we recall that MacCallum unravelled the heart musculature of the fetal pig in the brief period of a week, conceived his illustrations in a second week, and wrote his beautiful paper in a third week, we realize that he was possessed with genius of a very high order.

The chief points of his discoveries can be paraphrased from his own recapitulation of his paper.

Nearly all of the several layers of muscle begin in the auriculoventricular ring surrounding the valve on either side of the heart, and end in the papillary muscles [which act through the chordae tendinae on the free edges of the segments of the valves] of the other ventricle. Those fibers which begin near the outside of one ventricle end near the inside of the other ventricle. After the thin superficial muscles are removed, the left ventricle can be unrolled so that its cavity and papillary muscles are exposed. This shows it to be a flat band of muscle continuous with the muscle fibers which cross over in the septum (the wall between the two ventricles) from the right ventricle. Grouping these layers together, it is plain that the heart in the embryo is a scroll-shaped band of muscle with tendons at each end. As it grows older the layer of muscle passing over in the septum from the right to the left ventricle remains comparatively thin, while the ventricular walls increase greatly in thickness. The places of most active cell growth are near the inside of the ventricular walls, and they are, therefore, at the two ends of the band of muscle making up the heart.

MacCallum was able to show this latter point by knowledge gained through his discoveries on the histology and histogenesis of the heart muscle. It was clear to MacCallum that his work was merely the first of a series of studies to be made before a full knowledge of the heart's growth could be gained. Mall, in his introduction to the paper noted above, refers to this and says: "Ill health checked MacCallum's studies in this direction and his untimely death brought them to an end. However, the problem and his spirit of work have lingered with us and it was Knower who showed that what MacCallum had found in the fetal pig's heart could be confirmed in the human adult."

From Baltimore, MacCallum went for a period to Germany but was harassed during his stay by recurring difficulties with his illness. On Dr. Osler's advice, he went back to Canada, and there his health rapidly improved again. It was obvious to MacCallum and his family that it would be impossible for him to return to Baltimore to work again under his great friend Mall. After considering a variety of possibilities, he packed his trunk and set off to practice medicine in Denver. His description of the process of obtaining a license to practice is amusing: "I got my license to practice without any trouble and they all seemed very curious about the Johns Hopkins diploma—nobody had seen one before. I had to swear that it was mine before a notary public and it turned out to be a most attractive young party—for girls can do everything here, vote, and be lawyers and everything. I made some jocose, irrelevant remark in the middle of my swearing and she made me swear all over again and then said she didn't believe it was my diploma at all." He took an office and read Osler's *Textbook* in the event patients should come. A little notebook remains in which he wrote out doses of drugs and prescriptions for all sorts of ailments. He did earn enough to pay his expenses. He tried his best to become a "practical" man, for he wrote that at Johns Hopkins he had "systematically avoided all practical things." But soon the chance came to go to California in the Department of Physiology under Loeb. His time, however, was short.

MacCallum's philosophy is revealed in the many letters that he wrote. One is particularly of interest.

Flint is a very fortunate man as usual [Flint was a fellow student of his at Hopkins]. He gets the best of things more than anyone I ever saw. Someone said that he is the kind who buys standing room in a theater and before the play is over is sitting in the boxes. Still, I can't complain about anything. I've had a good mixture of the good and bad things of the world and if I had the chance, I would gladly live over the last few years I have lived. The evil of them was more apparent to outsiders than the good. After all, a person's happiness depends much more on himself than on what happens to him. The great secret of it all is to develop resources within yourself that will make you independent of other people and other things that may happen and those months I had of simply sitting and looking at the sunshine made me much better able to go cheerfully through the rest of my days.

His final illness was in 1905, and on April 6, his life of less than thirty years ended. Professor Loeb summed it up well in the brief sketch which was printed at the beginning of MacCallum's monograph, "On the Mechanism of the Physiological Action of the Cathartics":

MacCallum belonged to that type of scientists whom we may designate as discoverers. His results were obtained quickly, were made secure beyond doubt, and were put into such shape that they could easily be demonstrated by him. . . .

In his work as well as in his life he was a calm thinker, the reverse of a hustler. He conceived his experiments in the spirit of an artist and the realization of his ideas was the poetry his work put into his life. He did not work for outside success, nor did he pose as a benefactor of mankind. . . .

11 ✤ Johns Hopkins—The Birthplace of Tissue Culture: The Story of Ross G. Harrison, Warren H. Lewis, and George O. Gey

Ross Granville Harrison

THE TECHNIQUE of successfully growing tissue *in vitro*, which had its beginnings in the latter part of the nineteenth century, has been highly perfected during recent years. This phenomenal research tool is of major importance in many fields of scientific investigation, including cytology, histology, embryology, virology, cancer research, radiobiology, molecular biology, and biochemical genetics. The development of important new knowledge through the use of tissue culture techniques has become so extensive that it has been designated by many as the greatest technical advance in medical science since the invention of the compound microscope.

Attempts to culture tissues *in vitro* were made by Roux as early as 1885, but Ross Granville Harrison was the first to devise successfully a simple technique by which explanted tissue fragments could be grown outside the body. It was in 1907 that Harrison, working in the Department of Anatomy at Johns Hopkins, first published the results of his experiments on the cultivation of animal tissues outside the body. His classic paper did not appear in toto until 1910.

While studying the embryonic development of the nervous system, Harrison came to grips with a basic question in the field at that time: By what means does the embryonic animal body construct the individual fibers of the nerves that connect its various parts? Some embryologists supported the view that each fiber grows out from its cell, even to great lengths; others were equally certain that the fibers are formed from short lengths built by local cells which somehow join end to end. But there was no critical experimental proof of either of the two suggested answers, both of which seemed highly improbable to many investigators.

Ross Harrison solved the problem by actually watching nerve fibers as they grew, unobscured by other tissue elements. This he did by cutting out a bit of spinal cord from a frog embryo and placing it in a clear drop of coagulated lymph on a hollowed-out microscope slide. In these preparations, the first successful cultures of animal tissue, Harrison watched the living fibers sprout from nerve cells at the edge of the explant and grow out day by day as far as the clot allowed them to spread. Thus, he showed that these fibers, whether long or short, develop from one particular nerve cell in the brain, spinal cord, or outlying ganglion. The following passages regarding this discovery are taken from Harrison's paper, published in the *Anatomical Record*, entitled "Embryonic Transplantation and Development of the Nervous System."

According to Held the peripheral nerve fiber does not grow out free into spaces between the cells, but it can grow only into the protoplasmic bridges or plasmodesmata which have already been formed by other cells. To translate his own words: "The nerve paths arise through the transformation of plasmodesmata into neurodesmata." Striking as Held's preparations are, it does not seem to me that they prove the essential nature of the protoplasmic bridges. In fact, it is not even proved that these so-called plasmodesmata are not to a considerable extent coagulation products, and even if they are actually present in the living embryo just as seen in preserved specimens, their extremely fine structure would seem almost to preclude the possibility of distinguishing whether the nerve fibers actually grow within them, or whether they entwine themselves amongst them as a vine growing upon a lattice.

That the material upon which Held bases his views is quite capable of another interpretation is evidenced by the fact that Ramon y Cajal, who has studied the same question, upon similar material, making use of the same methods as Held, emphatically supports the outgrowth theory in its original form. The conclusions drawn from such preparations, however, definite as they may seem, appear, therefore, to be nothing more than a matter of interpretation.

In order to reach a final settlement of this question it thus became necessary to devise a method by which to test the ability of a nerve fiber to grow outside the body of the embryo, where it would be independent of protoplasmic bridges. At first a number of futile attempts were made to cultivate pieces of embryonic nerve tissue in various physiological salt solutions and within the cavities of the normal embryonic body. It then seemed that the outgrowing nerve might be stereotropic, and hence unable to leave a solid mass of cells to grow into a perfectly fluid medium. As the most suitable solid medium in which it would be possible to envelop embryonic tissue and observe its subsequent development, fresh lymph was chosen, first, because the fibrin threads which are formed on clotting might simulate mechanically Held's "plasmodesmata," though they could not be supposed to actually transform themselves into the nerve fiber; and, secondly, because the serum of the lymph would presumably afford a natural culture medium for the embryonic cells. Small portions of various tissues of the embryo were dissected out and removed by a fine pipette to a cover slip upon which was placed a drop of lymph freshly drawn from one of the lymph sacs of an adult frog. The cover slip was then inverted over a hollow slide and sealed on with paraffin. These manipulations were carried out as far as possible under aseptic precautions. The lymph clots almost immediately and holds the transplanted tissue in place. The specimen can then be readily observed under high powers of the microscope from day to day.

It has been found possible to keep such preparations alive for more than five weeks, and during the first week at least, differentiation takes place in a manner characteristic of each tissue. Cells taken from the muscle plates differentiate into muscle fibers with striated fibrillae, and when small pieces of spinal cord with portions of the muscle plates attached are taken, twitching movements of the muscle fibers may often be observed on the following days.

Let us now observe how the nerve tissue under cultivation in the lymph behaves. It must be borne in mind that when this is taken from the embryo it consists entirely of rounded cells without any signs of differentiation into fibers. Examined after a day or two of cultivation, fibers are found in a considerable number of cases extending out from the mass of tissue into the lymph clot. An early stage of this development is shown in Figure 22, which represents a cell that has become detached from the main mass of tissue. This cell is still gorged with food yolk, but at one pole it has sent out a hyaline protoplasmic process, which was observed to undergo distinct changes in form. . . . [Fig. 1.]

The foregoing observations show beyond question that the nerve fiber begins as an outflow of hyaline protoplasm from cells situated within the central nervous system. This protoplasm is very actively amoeboid, and as a result of this activity it extends farther and farther from its cell of origin. Retaining its pseudopodia at its distal end, the protoplasm is drawn out into a thread, which becomes the axis-cylinder of a nerve fiber. The early development of this structure is thus but a manifestation in a marked degree of one of the primitive properties of protoplasm, amoeboid activity. We have in the foregoing a positive proof of the hypothesis first put forward by Ramon y Cajal and von Lenhossék, who based it upon the consideration of the cones of growth found by the Golgi method at the end of the growing fiber.

Thus, by this simple but elegant experiment, Harrison not only invented a magnificent research tool but also solved one of the fundamental problems concerning the neurone theory. The demonstration of the nerve origin of the axone changed the whole line of thought in neurology.

Over the years the question has been raised as to why Harrison did not receive the Nobel Prize for such an outstanding discovery. The following account appears to resolve the issue:

For the study of growth during embryonic development, the method of cultivating animal tissues outside of the body that was introduced in 1907 by R. G. Harrison has been of great value. From frog embryos Harrison took fragments of the tissue of different parts of the body and placed them in a drop of clotted frog lymph. The tissue remained alive and even continued to grow. Harrison found that shoots grew from the edge of pieces from the medullary tube and that, in certain cases, they were outgrowths of nerve cells. They grew rapidly, branched out and ended up with the typical growth cones. His method has since been improved and has been widely used by experimental biologists. In 1917 a majority of the Nobel Committee recommended that the Prize should be given to him "for his discovery of the development of the nerve fibers by independent growth from cells outside the organism." The Institute, however, decided not to award the Prize for that year. When Harrison's work was again submitted to a special investigation in 1933, opinions diverged and, "in view of the rather limited value of the method and the age of the discovery," an award could not be recommended.

This clearly demonstrates the difficulty of forecasting the progress of science, since in 1956 a Nobel Prize was awarded for the growth of poliomyelitis virus in cultures of kidney cells (the Harrison method), which made possible the large-scale production of poliomyelitis vaccine. At present, Harrison's method is more universally used in experimental biology and medicine than almost any other approach to a variety of basic problems. Its application in the field of medicine has been unbelievably successful.

It is further of interest that in 1933 the Nobel Committee had the difficult

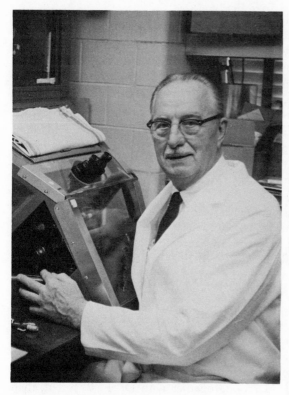

George Otto Gey
From the Archives Office, The Johns Hopkins Medical Institutions

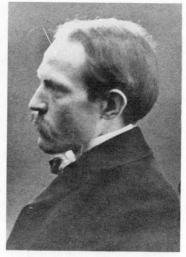

Ross Granville Harrison
From the Archives Office, The Johns Hopkins Medical Institutions

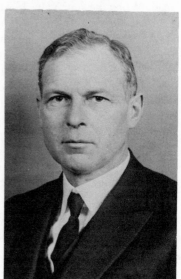

Warren Harmon Lewis
From the Archives Office, The Johns Hopkins Medical Institutions

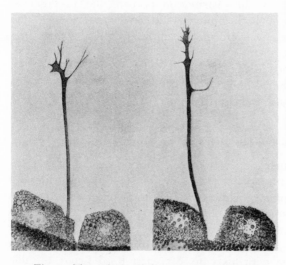

Fig. 1. Two views of the same nerve fiber, taken 50 minutes apart

From R. G. Harrison, "Embryonic Transplantation and Development of the Nervous System," *Anat. Rec.* 2 (1908): 385

choice between Harrison's work on asymmetry, which was being pursued vigorously at that time, and the outstanding studies of Thomas Hunt Morgan. Both of these men had been students in the Department of Biology at Johns Hopkins under H. Newell Martin. In 1933, however, the rebirth of Mendel's observations was in progress and genetics was on the ascendancy. The award for 1933 was given to Morgan, the first native-born American to receive the Nobel Prize. However, Harrison received many other honors. In 1913 he was elected to both the National Academy of Sciences and the American Philosophical Society. In 1925 he received the John Scott Medal and Premium of the City of Philadelphia "for the invention of devices for tissue grafting and tissue culture," and in 1947 the John J. Carty Medal of the National Academy of Sciences.

Harrison was born in Germantown, Pennsylvania, in 1870, studied biology at Johns Hopkins and medicine at Bonn, where he received his M.D. degree in 1899. After a succession of research and teaching appointments at Johns Hopkins under Franklin P. Mall, he moved to Yale in 1907 to become Bronson Professor of Comparative Anatomy and head of the Department of Zoology. He was the first editor of the *Journal of Experimental Zoology*, producing no fewer than 104 issues of this important periodical before his retirement in 1946. When he left Yale, Harrison became chairman of the National Research Council, serving from 1938 to 1946. Under his leadership, the National Research Council, formerly a simple adviser on request to government agencies, became an operating agency which coordinated scientific research during the critical period of World War II. Harrison, together with Dr. F. B. Jewett, then president of the National Academy of Sciences, played a major role in developing national research policy during this important period. His administrative capabilities are seen in his appointment of Dr. Chester Keefer, a Hopkins graduate who successfully oversaw the distribution of penicillin in order to provide for the critical needs of both military and civilian personnel, and Robert D. Coghill, who successfully overcame the difficulties of the mass production of penicillin.

"Wherever Harrison touched medicine, whether by advice, teaching, research, training anatomists or the administration of problems directly related to medicine, his input was always wise and fruitful."

Warren Harmon Lewis

Warren H. Lewis was an extraordinary man, continuously active at his research bench for more than fifty years. His many outstanding contributions include basic work in two separate fields: investigations concerning the embryology of the eye, which provided important facts related to the modern theory of embryonic induction; and observations on the structure and behavior of living cells in tissue cultures, which he began and continued for more than forty years in close collaboration with his wife, Margaret Reed Lewis, an able scientist in her own right.

In the fall of 1896, Warren H. Lewis became a member of the fourth class to enter the Johns Hopkins Medical School. He developed a strong attachment to Dr. Mall's Department of Anatomy, of which at that time Charles R. Bardeen and Ross G. Harrison were senior members. Immediately after graduation in 1900, Lewis and his equally famous classmates, Florence R. Sabin and John B. MacCallum, became assistants in that department.

In 1901 Lewis published his first paper—a description of the pectoralis major muscle and some of its variations—in the *Johns Hopkins Hospital Bulletin*. In the same year, the *American Journal of Anatomy* was established from Mall's department, and the first article in the first issue was a joint paper by Bardeen and Lewis. This paper, on the development of the muscles of the limbs and trunks, handsomely illustrated and based on skillful dissections and reconstructions, remains the classical monograph on the subject.

The following summer Lewis had the privilege of working in the laboratory with the great physiologist Jacques Loeb. This experience opened his eyes to the exciting possibilities of experimental cytology, and in the ensuing years he did his important work on the embryology of the eye. During these years Lewis was a valuable member of Mall's department, and when Harrison left for Yale in 1907, Lewis became Mall's senior colleague. In 1914 the university took the then unusual step of creating for him a second chair in the Department of Anatomy, with the title of Professor of Physiological Anatomy.

In 1910 there was an important change in the direction of Lewis' experimental work and also in his personal life. In that year he married Margaret Reed, a graduate of Goucher College and an accomplished experimental biologist who had received her research training under Thomas Hunt Morgan.

As related earlier, Ross G. Harrison devised his method of tissue culture in 1907. In the following year Margaret Reed, while working in Berlin, observed the experiments of Dr. Rhoda Erdmann, who was cultivating amoebae on nutrient agar, made with physiological salt solution. Margaret Reed explanted a small piece of bone marrow from a guinea pig into a tube of this medium. She observed that after a few days in the incubator the bone marrow cells formed a membrane-like growth on the surface of the agar and that some of the nuclei exhibited mitotic figures. In other words, the cells were living and multiplying. This was probably the first *in vitro* culture of mammalian cells.

Harrison's experiments with explanted nerve tissue immediately attracted the attention of Alexis Carrel, of the Rockefeller Institute, who had been successful in transplanting whole organs of laboratory animals. Carrel's objective, of course, was maintaining human organs and tissues which might be used to replace similar structures destroyed by disease or removed by surgery. In 1909 Carrel sent his assistant, Montrose T. Burrows, to Harrison's laboratory to learn the new methods and to adapt them to the tissues of warm-blooded animals. Carrel and Burrows almost immediately succeeded in cultivating cells from chick embryos in sterile chicken blood plasma.

The Lewises had begun independently in the fall of 1910 to cultivate bone marrow cells from guinea pig embryos in the blood plasma of older embryos. This was clearly a follow-up of Margaret Lewis's 1908 observation. They utilized Harrison's new method, except that the culture medium they used was mammalian blood plasma instead of frog lymph. In spite of early failures, the report of Carrel and Burrows encouraged them to renew their efforts. Their second attempt involved material from embryonic chicks with explantation of discrete bits of tissue instead of a few cells as before. They obtained growth and multiplication of the cells of many organs. However, they recognized, which Carrel apparently had not, that most if not all of the proliferating cells were types common to all tissues, namely, connective tissue cells and the endothelial cells of blood vessels.

For the next decade and a half, all tissue culture workers concentrated their efforts on discovering what kinds of cells could be grown and what were the best culture media. Carrel's long-range hope was to maintain organs while the Lewises wanted mainly to study the microscopic structure of individual cells, for which they needed very clear media. Having been successful with a simple mixture of Locke's solution, agar and bouillon, they then tried clear salt solution alone and found that connective tissue cells, endothelium, and nerve fibers would spread out into the fluid from the explanted bits. This was the first attempt to grow cells in a solution containing only chemically definable constituents. It was premature, however, as little was known at that time about factors important in the regulation of growth such as vitamins, trace elements, and so forth. Since then, of course, great strides have been made in the use of defined media. The Lewises were some fifty years ahead of their time. In the Locke-Lewis solution, with or without the supplement of bouillon or plasma, cells of a basic type such as fibroblasts and macrophages migrated out from the explant and flattened themselves on the undersurface of the cover slips. They could then be observed under high magnification, an arrangement ideal for the study of cytological details.

Thus, by 1915 the Lewises were in a position to present a comprehensive description of the living cell, including its nucleus, cytoplasm, and mitochrondria, and of the segregation vacuoles which the cell formed around phagocytized particles. Later (1917) they observed various physiological activities of the cell, including the locomotion of leukocytes, the contraction of smooth muscle cells, and the budding of striated muscle fibers.

After the death of Franklin P. Mall in 1917, the Lewises joined the Carnegie Institute under the direction of Dr. George Streeter. By courtesy of the university, Warren Lewis retained his professorial rank and title. At this time they had difficulty in terms of wide variation in survival time and rate of growth of their cultures, but they were beginning to appreciate, as many biologists were at the time, the physiological importance of hydrogen ion concentration. Using W. Mansfield Clark's newly available indicators, Margaret Lewis and a young colleague, Lloyd D. Felton, studied the effect of pH in the growing tissue culture and found the proper value for optimal results. The Lewises were then in a better position to study the functional behavior of living cells. They observed the transformation of fibroblasts into flattened mesothelial layers similar to those lining the peritoneal cavity, and the development of macrophages, epithelioid cells, and giant cells from mononuclear cells. Warren Lewis noted the similarity of the cells thus formed to those observed in the lesions of tuberculosis. These and other studies served to clear up the hazy phylogeny of the monocyte-macrophage-epithelioid cell-giant cell series. In contrast to the thoughts of their colleague, Florence R. Sabin, the Lewises showed that the monocytes and the macrophages are not two distinctive cell types but are different physiological stages of the same cell.

In 1923 Warren Lewis became interested in the changes in the cells of malignant tumors, and his first venture into this field of cancer research was made with a young colleague, George O. Gey. They studied certain cells which are found among the spindle cells of a mouse carcinoma, and which Carrel had assumed to be the malignant elements. Lewis and Gey soon demonstrated that these cells were macrophages and that the spindle cells themselves were the malignant elements. They showed that tumor cells are permanently altered from the normal state, retaining a malignant pattern of growth through many successive cultures. In his observations from 1933 to 1948, Lewis described in detail the cytological features by which the living malignant cell of connective tissue origin differs from its normal counterpart, the fibroblast.

In 1929 Lewis began the use of motion pictures to record microscopic observations. He soon found that he could learn much more about cell mobility and other physiological changes by this technique than by direct observation. The use of time-lapse cinematography enabled him to speed up on the screen activities far too slow in their time course to be understood by direct observation. An immediate result was the discovery, in 1931, of a type of cell activity which Lewis labeled "pinocytosis" (drinking by cells). He observed cells to actively enfold and engulf drops of fluid from the surrounding medium. Lewis's moving pictures of living cells of higher animals in physiological activity, of mammalian ova in the process of division, of blastocyst formation, and of the development of the zebra-fish egg won widespread attention when they were exhibited at various meetings. These films were widely disseminated, and thousands of students all over the world thus had a vivid impression of the structure of the living normal and malignant cells of the blood and connective tissues, of cell division, phagocytosis, pinocytosis, and other cellular functions.

Warren Lewis was elected to membership in the National Academy of Sciences in 1936 and in the American Philosophical Society in 1943. Both he and Margaret Lewis were awarded the William Wood Gerhard Gold Medal of the Pathological Society of Philadelphia in 1958.

George Otto Gey

Last but not least in this long line of contributions to science by means of tissue culture is the work of George O. Gey. His fruitful association with Warren and Margaret Lewis began in 1922. After a period of six years as a cancer research fellow at the Columbia Hospital in Milwaukee, Wisconsin (1923–1929), he returned to Johns Hopkins as director of the tissue culture laboratory in the Department of Surgery. Born in Pittsburgh in 1899, he received his B.S. degree from the University of Pittsburgh and later served there as instructor of zoology. He received his M.D. degree from Hopkins in 1933.

George Gey worked with tissue culture techniques for a period of forty-seven years, during which time he was responsible for many new developments in relation to organoid and cell culture, intracellular and membrane cytology, and *in vitro* investigations related to endocrinology, cancer, and virology. The introduction to his Harvey Lecture of 1955 reveals in part the tremendous breadth of his interest:

For a number of years we have dedicated our efforts toward the isolation and maintenance of normal and malignant or otherwise diseased tissues as temporary or stable organoids or as derived cell strains. These have provided us with controllable living cell systems which may be used in various studies: one, of their nature and functional competence; two, of their stability and variability; three, of their metabolic behavior; four, of their comparative constitution; five, of their proliferative behavior; and six, of their responses to altered environments or to various agents.

There are so many innovations that came out of Gey's laboratory that one can only list them: (1) the maintenance *in vitro* of organoid and hormonal tissues (thyroid, parathyroid, placenta, chorio-carcinoma); (2) the "roller tube" technique (which was used by Enders and his group in their Nobel Prize–winning experiments on the cultivation of poliomyelitis virus in nonnervous system tissues); (3) the continuous maintenance of both normal and malignant human and rat cell lines; (4) flat-sided tubes and "flying cover slips" for cytological studies; (5) collagen as a natural, often crucially important, substrate for fastidious cells and organoids; (6) the growth of cells suspended in agitated fluid media; (7) the nutrition of cells in tissue extracts and body fluids and their specific requirements for trace metals, amino acids, proteins, lipids, and carbohydrates; and (8) the sterilization of biological media by fast electrons. There were also many discoveries in the field of virology, including the different susceptibilities of normal and malignant cells as hosts for eastern equine encephalomyelitis virus; the simultaneous propagation of cells and viruses over long periods of time (HeLa and the eastern equine virus for thirteen years); and viral particles in normal chick embryo cells. In the field of cancer research major accomplishments include the manifold differences between a great variety of malignant cells and their normal prototypes; the emergence and loss of malignancy in cell lines *in vitro*; and the derivation of cell lines that have served as international work horses in studies on cell nutrition, virology, and malignancy.

George Gey's best-known contribution, the HeLa cell culture, resulted from an interest of the Department of Gynecology in carcinoma-in-situ of the cervix. A number of studies, already referred to in an earlier chapter, had helped to resolve the problem, but in the early 1950s Richard TeLinde interested George Gey in trying to grow these cells with his roller-tube technique in order to study the growth characteristics of normal cervical epithelium, intra-epithelial carcinoma, and invasive cancer. Dr. Ward Coffman, an assistant resident gynecologist, began to collect specimens for Dr. Gey, but none of these specimens would grow in culture. However, on February 1, 1951, a thirty-one-year-old woman, complaining of intermenstrual spotting, was seen by Howard

Jones. Her cervical lesion was biopsied and revealed carcinoma. This patient, Henrietta Lacks, is permanently enshrined in medical literature, as the cells from her biopsy grew out in Gey's cultures and this cell line has since been known as the HeLa (abbreviation of patient's name) cell. This was the first established cell line, and it has contributed enormously to subsequent studies in the field of molecular and cell biology. Cultures of this cell line have been used for studies of the nutritional requirements of cells in culture, of viral growth, of protein synthesis, of drug effects and of somatic cell genetics, including genetic control mechanisms, mutations at the cellular level, and many others.

Gey's genius for synthesizing mechanical and optical means to investigate the living behavior of normal, malignant, and infected cells yielded untold benefits in terms of the usefulness of these techniques for many investigators as well as the basic information which he himself contributed. His time-lapse, phase-motion photographs, supplemented with interference and electronmicroscopy, revealed the almost unbelievable activity of the plasma-gel layer in producing membranous pseudopods, microfibrils, and spicules that contribute extracellular matrix; the continuous role of streaming hyaloplasm in intracellular nutrition and communication; the ways in which pinocytotic and inclusion droplets become associated with mitochondria and the cytocentrum; the bizarre mitoses and the increased pinocytosis, feeding habits and metastatic potential of malignant cells; and the degenerative damage caused by polio and eastern equine encephalomyelitis viruses. These magnificent photographic records alone would have been a monumental contribution for almost any investigator.

In 1947 Gey was appointed director of the Finney-Howell Cancer Research Laboratory and in 1958 was promoted to the rank of associate professor of surgery. He received many honors, including a Harvey Lectureship in 1955, the Catherine Berken Judd Award for Cancer Research in 1954, and the Wien Award for Cancer Cytology in 1956.

Margaret Koudelka Gey was his closest collaborator. Trained as a surgical nurse, she helped to create the high standards of excellence which were the hallmark of the laboratory. She worked with George Gey to bring about the establishment of the W. Alton Jones Center for Cell Science at Lake Placid, New York.

Thus, the story of these five pioneers in the use of the tissue culture technique is one of the most dramatic and important in the history of research at the Johns Hopkins Medical Institutions. The original observation of Ross Granville Harrison ranks among the outstanding scientific contributions of the twentieth century.

12 ⚛ Creators of Clinical Medicine's Scientific Base: Franklin Paine Mall, Lewellys Franklin Barker, and Rufus Cole

FROM THE TIME that the Johns Hopkins Hospital opened in May 1889, Dr. Osler enthusiastically emphasized the importance of the work of the clinical laboratories in the medical clinic as an indispensable adjunct of the work on the medical wards. Since the laboratories, which were situated under the medical wards, were quite small, this work at first consisted of routine examinations; the more difficult studies, thanks to the courtesy of Dr. Welch, were carried out in the pathological laboratory.

After the opening of the medical school, an urgent need became manifest for better physical facilities in which to instruct the medical students in laboratory methods, and additional rooms were built near the wards for this purpose; the idea was to give every third- and fourth-year student his own work space and to teach the essentials for microscopical, chemical, and physical work on materials derived from patients on the wards. In the third year each student was given a systematic training in the use of modern laboratory methods. In the fourth year, as a clinical clerk, the student practiced these techniques on the individual patients assigned to him. Such instruction was a major innovation in the education of medical students at that time.

As valuable as this early work was, opinion soon developed that it should be supplemented by experimental studies in order to evolve new methods and to allow investigation of the problems presented by the diseases observed in the clinic. Although this viewpoint had the sympathy of Dr. Osler, it appears that he thought such work should be conducted in the Departments of Anatomy, Physiology, Pharmacology or Pathology. Representing the best nineteenth-century British tradition of medical teaching, Osler was a master of observation and description of disease and a great diagnostician, but he did not undertake nor did he vigorously promote studies of the fundamental nature of disease. He was first and foremost an eminent physician, and this was reflected in his conception of the aims of medical education and the role of the professor of medicine. Major emphasis was placed on teaching students the techniques and skills necessary for observing and interpreting the manifestations of disease in patients, less on the investigation of underlying disease processes. As Dr. Arthur Bloomfield stated it: "Osler, I have been told, felt strongly that those things which are Caesar's should be rendered unto Caesar—in other words, laboratory research should be done in the pathological and physiological laboratories and not in the medical clinics by clinicians." In part Osler's attitude may be attributed to the lack of adequate facilities for such study, but he, together with most of his contemporaries in America, did not fully comprehend how rapidly physiology and chemistry were progressing or the potential they had to form the base for important advances in clinical medicine. On the other hand, at this stage in the development of American medicine, the investigators in the basic sciences such as physiology, biochemistry, pharmacology, anatomy, and pathology believed that medical research could be carried out only in their departments and that clinicians had neither the time nor the training for such activity.

A monumental step toward changing this situation was taken by Lewellys Franklin Barker who assumed the post of professor of medicine when Osler left Baltimore in 1905 to become the Regius Professor of Medicine at Oxford. Unlike Osler, Barker came to the professorship of medicine at Hopkins by the route of a professorship of anatomy and with considerable experience in laboratory research. A graduate of the University of Toronto, Barker interned for one year in Canada and came to Baltimore for the first time in 1891 to work in the newly opened Johns Hopkins Hospital. After spending a year in Osler's clinic, Barker was made a fellow in pathology under Welch. He then joined Mall in the anatomical laboratory, and for the first time felt the thrill of discovery by demonstrating the presence of iron in eosinophil cells. Barker advanced to the position of associate professor of anatomy and in 1899 was appointed associate professor of pathology. Thus, for a space of eight years, he worked in close association with Osler, Mall, and Welch. In 1895 he spent six months in Leipzig under von Frey. Here he carried out a detailed study of the localization of the sensory points in the skin of the arm, using for this purpose his own arm, in which sensation was disturbed owing to the presence of a cervical rib. When he returned from Germany, Barker wrote a large illustrated book, *The Nervous System and Its Constituent Neurons*. A pioneer in this field, he soon became an authority. In 1899 Barker and Simon Flexner led a commission to study the diseases of the Philippine Islands. Shortly after his return to the United States, Barker accepted the position of professor of anatomy at the University of Chicago, although he had "always hoped and expected to work in internal medicine." While in Chicago, he translated and edited Spalteholz's *Anatomy*.

In 1903 he was given a leave of absence to work in Munich with the famous German clinician Frederick Müller and in the equally famous chemical laboratory of Emil Fischer. During this period he witnessed the vigorous pursuit of research both in the laboratory and in the clinic, a joint endeavor characteristic of German medicine. The impact of this experience on Barker is evident in an address he delivered in 1903 entitled "Medicine and the Universities," in which he made a plea for the reorganization of the clinical departments in medical schools. He believed that they should rank with the other departments of the university and should emphasize research into the problems of human disease as well as teaching. To do this, he stressed, professors would have to be relieved of the necessity of carrying on private practice. Mall had already pointed out that such a change was necessary—an idea which he apparently got from his mentor, the great German physiologist, Ludwig. Such a step followed logically from the changes which had already been made in the preclinical departments with such brilliant results. Mall clearly understood that clinical medicine had to change, had to add to the art of healing all that science could contribute toward greater skill in diagnosis and treatment. Mall understood disease as the price of ignorance and worked continually behind the scenes to introduce the methods and the trained investigators who would make the clinics more scientific. During his early years in Baltimore, Mall discussed this goal with his staff and students. Among this group was Lewellys Barker, who was responsible for the course in neuroanatomy. The fact that the articulate Barker had to be his spokesman demonstrates one of Mall's characteristics. Few of the medical community know even yet how great a role he played, as his work was always done quietly. Whatever the origin of the idea, however, Barker was the first to outline such a plan in detail and to give it wide publicity.

When Barker assumed the post of professor of medicine, he wanted it to be on a full-time basis, but the university did not have sufficient endowment to put this plan into effect. Nevertheless, he took the important step of organizing research divisions within the department to provide opportunities for investigation into the nature of various disease processes. Of course, scientific investigations in departments of medicine did not begin with the opening of these laboratories, but the *institution of laboratories for this specific purpose* started a movement which has not only greatly influenced the character of university clinics but started a chain reaction in the evolution of clinical investigation that was to play a major role in creating the scientific base of modern medical practice.

Barker wrote of the need for these new research laboratories in the medical department as follows:

Technology has demonstrated how necessary it is for the promotion of the individual arts to secure investigators trained in the so-called sciences of physics, chemistry and biology who will devote themselves to the application of the methods and principles of these sciences to the solution of the special problems by which those who wish to advance the industrial arts are concerned. One has only to recall the tremendous advances in metallurgy, in brewing and in electrical engineering ... to realize how fundamentally significant the interest of men trained in pure science in the solution of so-called practical problems has been for the more strictly utilitarian domains.

Barker pointed out that von Ziemssen in Germany had recognized the need for similar applications of the fundamental sciences to the solution of the special problems of diagnosis and therapy and founded clinical research laboratories in Munich.

In the beginning, under Barker's chairmanship of the Department of Medicine, there were three research divisions: the Biological Division, under the direction of Dr. Rufus Cole; the Physiological Division, under Dr. Arthur D. Hirschfelder; and the Chemical Division, under Dr. Carl Voegtlin. There was also a general clinical laboratory for instruction and research, under Dr. Thomas

R. Boggs. A psychopathological laboratory for the investigation of the emotional aspects of the patients in the medical wards was projected, but no funds were available.

The Physiological Laboratory

The physiological laboratory was organized in October 1905 to study diseases from the standpoint of disturbance in function. There was one laboratory in the new surgical building of the hospital for the clinical study of patients by the special methods in use in physiological laboratories, particularly the graphic methods; a second laboratory was in the Hunterian Building of the medical school, which was well equipped for animal experimentation and where disease conditions seen in the medical wards could be reproduced in animals and studied by physiological methods. It was the aim in this laboratory "to bring the studies upon the patient as closely as possible into relation with the findings upon animals and mechanical models and to turn these results to practical use."

In 1907 the *Johns Hopkins Hospital Bulletin* published an issue containing an article by Barker describing the organization of these clinical research laboratories and also a series of papers describing original work carried out in them.

Three of these papers came from the Physiological Division of the Medical Laboratory and were presented by the director, Arthur D. Hirschfelder. In the first paper, entitled "Some Observations Upon Blood Pressure and Pulse Form," Hirschfelder discussed the Strasburger method for the determination of minimal blood pressure and pointed out its inaccuracies. In this method, the pressure in the cuff upon the upper arm was gradually increased while the observer palpated the pulse at the wrist and determined the point at which the volume of the pulse was maximal. On careful estimation, Hirschfelder found the error to be only 5 to 8 millimeters. The method had been put into use in the Johns Hopkins Hospital during the preceding year for routine blood pressures taken by medical students. For them it was found quite unsatisfactory, the discrepancy lying mainly in the lack of uniformity of pressure exerted by the palpating finger upon the radial artery. This could be eliminated by taking the precaution of simply laying the tips of the index and middle fingers upon the lower end of the radius, just lateral from the artery and palpating the pulse with the balls instead of with the tips of the fingers. Hirschfelder also made observations on the dicrotic pulse in typhoid fever, concluding that it was the result of the coincidence of very marked peripheral dilatation with somewhat increased heart action.

In the next paper, Hirschfelder discussed "Some Variations in the Form of the Venous Pulse." He encountered a slight variation of form occurring in the diastolic portion of the cardiac cycle, which might well be confounded with disturbances in conduction or with atrial extrasystoles. The wave referred to occurred after the collapse following the V wave, and at the end of the subsequent rapid filling of the vein, and gave rise to a small elevation closely resembling that produced by an atrial contraction. He presented evidence to justify the conclusion that this wave was to be regarded as an event in the normal diastole, more pronounced in some hearts than in others.

The third paper was entitled "The Rapid Formation of Endocarditic Vegetations." Hirschfelder, working with Dr. H. A. Stewart, showed that in some cases the cauliflower-like form of the vegetations of verrucose endocarditis may be determined by the thrombotic deposit which collects upon the valve immediately after the production of the lesion. They produced lesions in dogs by means of a blunt button-pointed probe introduced into the left carotid artery and thrust through the aortic valve. At autopsy in these cases, it was found that the puncture through the valve had become plugged with fresh yellow fibrin and blood platelets, which in one instance had assumed definite cauliflower-like outlines. This vegetation, really a thrombotic deposit, was absolutely fresh and non-adherent. Such a rapid temporary repair might play a large part in the recovery from spontaneous rupture of an aortic valve after overexertion and perhaps also in staying the course of the leak in acute endocarditis.

These papers document what primitive techniques were available for application to clinical problems at the turn of the century.

More exciting events, however, were on the horizon. Barker had an interest in the clinical methods of investigating cardiovascular conditions, and this was the subject of his Jerome Cochran Lecture before the Alabama State Medical Association in 1909. In this paper he discussed the development of electrocardiography, citing the original work of Waller in 1889, in which he demonstrated the possibility of galvanometric registration of the action current emanating from the human heart. As the currents generated are extremely small, their detection was so difficult that a clinical application seemed out of the question until the Dutch physiologist, Einthoven, first applied the capillary electrometer and later devised his thread-galvanometer for this purpose. Edelmann in Germany developed and manufactured a complete instrument for the recording of the electrocardiogram in man, and Barker announced in this lecture that one of Edelmann's instruments was being installed (1909) in the Johns Hopkins Hospital. Similar instruments were being set up simultaneously at Presbyterian and Mount Sinai hospitals in New York City. While spending the summer of 1909 in Europe, Barker had visited the laboratories in which the electrocardiograph was being used. Impressed by its value in the study of irregularities of rhythm of the heart, Barker ordered the small type of instrument from the Edelmann firm in Munich for the Johns Hopkins Hospital. When he returned to Baltimore, he asked Dr. George S. Bond to review the German literature and to make preparations for the arrival of the Edelmann machine. It arrived about the first of October 1909 and was possibly the first operating electrocardiograph machine in the United States. Drs. James and Williams at Presbyterian Hospital in New York had one for use in that clinic, but according to Bond's information, it did not become operative until several months after the one at Hopkins. Dr. George Bond, then, played an important role in the introduction of electrocardiography into the Johns Hopkins Hospital.

Bond was born in Richmond, Indiana, in 1884, the son of a prominent physician. He received his M.D. degree from the University of Michigan in 1908. After graduation, he applied to Dr. Barker for an opportunity to work in the medical clinic at Johns Hopkins. He was accepted as a volunteer worker and assigned to study under Dr. Hirschfelder in the Physiological Division. Bond's laboratory was in the basement of the clinical building, behind the elevator; this location was chosen because it was on the ground floor and as free from vibration and noise as possible. Bond and Hirschfelder worked with the small Edelmann machine for about six months and concluded that it was too small for satisfactory clinical work. They then ordered from Edelmann the large type, with electromagnetic galvanometer, which arrived in late October 1910. The two instruments were set up in the same laboratory, and Figure 1 shows the arrangement existing in 1911. On the near side is the original galvanometer, and on the far side, the large new galvanometer. These converged so as to throw both filament shadows on the camera in the rear. The large one was used for taking electrocardiograms (Fig. 2), and the small one for taking pictures of the heart sounds (Fig. 3). These could be taken simultaneously. The switchboards for handling both these circuits were on the table at the left. By this time, they had discarded the unsanitary tanks of salt solution in which the patient immersed his arms and legs and were simply fastening salt soaked pads to the extremities with metal electrodes, which could be changed with each patient. In the far rear of the picture are the cabinets and tables that had to do with the development of films. On the right hand wall is a telephone switchboard designed for remote control. Three leaden wires and a telephone were connected from the heart station to each of the medical wards. Thus it was possible to call and ask the nurse to connect the electrodes to the patient on that ward, and the tracing was recorded in the heart station. The telephone allowed conversation while this was being done. The plan was soon abandoned, however, because it was found that a patient could be sent to the heart station more quickly than a nurse could perform this activity on the ward.

Their method of taking heart sounds is also of interest. Since there were no microphones or amplifying circuits, the engineers of the Bell Telephone Company in Baltimore changed the spring tension in one of their telephone transmitters to make it quite sensitive. This was in turn mounted inside a heavy lead box and suspended by springs. It was connected to a stethoscope bell by soft rubber tubing, and then to a regular telephone circuit in which the galvanometer acted as the receiver. In this way the investigators were able to obtain good tracings of heart sounds.

After serving on the staff of the Johns Hopkins University for six years, Dr. Bond returned to Indiana in 1914 to become assistant professor of medicine in the Indiana School of Medicine. His first assignment there was to set up a heart station for Indiana University. In 1936 he was made professor of cardiology, a post he held until 1956. He was the second president of the Indiana Heart Association, and from 1957 to 1960 he was a member of the

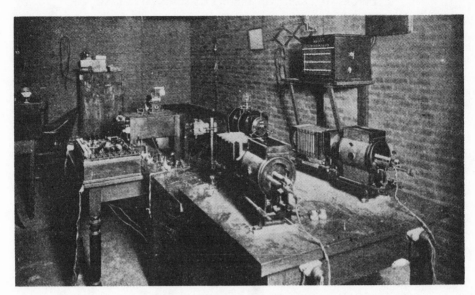

Fig. 1. The heart station, 1909
Courtesy of Dr. Kenneth Kohlstaedt

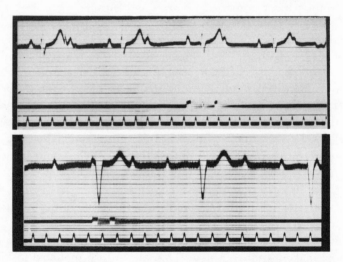

Fig. 2. Electrocardiogram, complete heart block

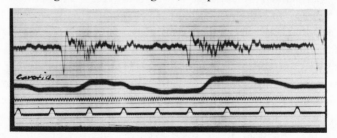

Fig. 3. Phonocardiogram, systolic murmur
Cardiograms courtesy of Dr. Kenneth Kohlstaedt

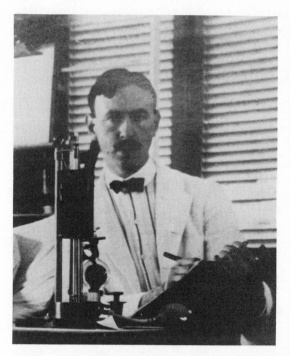

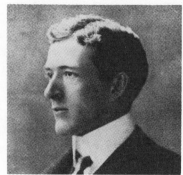

Lewellys F. Barker

From A. M. Chesney, *The Johns Hopkins Hospital and the Johns Hopkins University School of Medicine*, vol 2, *1893–1905* (Baltimore: The Johns Hopkins University Press, 1958)

Arthur D. Hirschfelder

From the Archives Office, The Johns Hopkins Medical Institutions

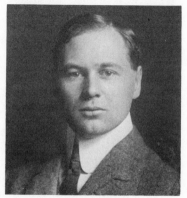

Carl Voegtlin

Courtesy of Dr. Paul Talalay

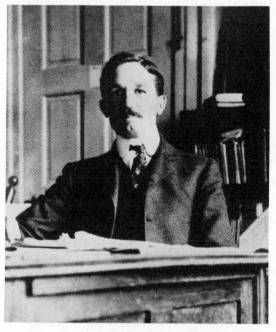

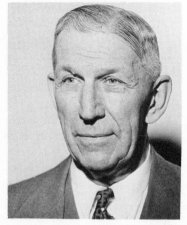

Rufus Cole

From Chesney's *Chronicle*, vol. 2

George S. Bond

Courtesy of Dr. Kenneth Kohlstaedt

board of directors of the American Heart Association. In 1967 he received the Distinguished Service Award from the Indiana Heart Association.

Arthur D. Hirschfelder, a graduate of the Hopkins school (1903), was born in San Francisco in 1879. After graduation, he studied abroad at the Pasteur Institute in Paris and at the University of Heidelberg. When he returned to the United States, he entered the Johns Hopkins School of Medicine. He served as resident house officer in Baltimore for a year and then went to San Francisco, having been appointed assistant in medicine in Cooper Medical College, where his father was a member of the faculty. He remained there for only one year, at which time he returned to Johns Hopkins as a voluntary assistant in medicine.

While Hirschfelder was in charge of the physiological laboratory, the principal problems under investigation dealt with disturbances of the heart and the circulation. During this time Hirschfelder published a book entitled *Diseases of the Heart and Aorta,* which went through two editions. In 1913 he resigned to become professor of pharmacology at the University of Minnesota, where he remained until his retirement. He died on October 11, 1942.

The Biological Laboratory

The biological laboratory was quite primitive in comparison with the facilities for research in infectious diseases available in clinical departments today. The division occupied three small rooms in the southeast corner of the second floor of the Surgical Building until the completion of the Carnegie Building in 1927, when the laboratory was transferred to the sixth floor of that building. The equipment included a small centrifuge and a larger one, which revolved 25 cubic-centimeter tubes at a speed of 3,000 revolutions per minute—necessary in precipitating bacteria from suspensions. Sterilizers and all the apparatus necessary for routine bacteriological and biological investigation were at hand, and there was an animal house for holding a limited number of small animals. The purpose of the laboratory was to investigate biological methods of diagnosis and treatment, and the facilities were available to members of the medical staff and to postgraduate students working in medicine.

Dr. Rufus Cole, the director, was the first to develop the technique of direct blood cultures, and he demonstrated the value of this procedure in a paper published in 1902. Cole's pioneer studies of typhoid bacilli in the bloodstream constituted the first systematic clinical laboratory research done at the Johns Hopkins Hospital.

Among the first problems studied in this laboratory was the mechanism of recovery from infection with bacteria. At that time there was considerable interest in the so-called "opsonic" theory as an explanation of the ability of the body to recover from the invasion of disease-producing microorganisms. Among other areas of interest was the treatment of infection by the use of specific vaccines.

It is of more than passing interest that Dr. Frederick F. Russell, who was then an officer in the Medical Corps of the United States Army and who was later to introduce with great success the practice of vaccination against typhoid fever in the army, began his work with typhoid vaccine while working in Cole's laboratory. Russell also studied opsonins and treated cases of osteomyelitis with autogenous vaccines, but without remarkable results. When he returned to the U.S. Army Medical School in Washington, he continued his work on typhoid vaccine. After the inoculation of one thousand soldiers, he informed the Surgeon General that he was ready to start his complete vaccination program. Antityphoid vaccination was made compulsory in the U.S. Army in 1911, thereby reducing the incidence of typhoid fever during both world wars to an exceptionally low figure when compared with the incidence among American troops during the Spanish-American War.

The Chemical Laboratory

The third new laboratory was the chemical laboratory, under the direction of Dr. Carl Voegtlin, a native of Switzerland. Voegtlin had obtained his Ph.D. degree in chemistry from the University of Freiburg in 1903 and had studied at the Victoria University in Manchester, England, before migrating to the United States to take a post at the University of Wisconsin. Barker learned about Voegtlin through a University of Wisconsin postgraduate chemist whom he met during a visit to the laboratory of the celebrated Emil Fischer in Berlin. Dr. Barker invited Voegtlin to take charge of the Chemical Laboratory; he accepted and was appointed assistant in medicine. This laboratory and its equipment were made possible through the generosity of Dr. Osler, who asked the trustees of the university to allocate for the purpose a gift of $1000 which he had made to the university during the course of a fund campaign. This the university trustees agreed to do, and the trustees of the hospital then added $1,100 for the same purpose. Dr. Barker also received a gift of $1,000 from his brother-in-law, R. T. H. Halsey of New York, and this amount was used to pay Voegtlin's salary during his first year as head of the laboratory. The division was located in a large room on the second floor of the Surgical Building, and was modeled after the arrangements in the first chemical institute in Berlin.

One of the first problems tackled in this laboratory was the value of a high caloric diet in the treatment of typhoid fever. This was an important subject at that time, since the disease was rampant in some cities along the Atlantic seaboard, including Baltimore, and there was as yet no specific remedy which would cut short the long duration of the disease and its very depleting effect. It was demonstrated that there was value in a high-caloric diet containing large amounts of carbohydrates, but the results were not published. Voegtlin also studied the role of inorganic ions in the metabolism in certain disease states; and it was while he was in charge of this laboratory that he and William G. MacCallum made the important discovery of the role which the parathyroid gland plays in the control of calcium in the animal body. Voegtlin did not remain long in charge of the chemical laboratory, and after two years he transferred to the Department of Pharmacology in order to fill the post vacated by Arthur Loevenhart. Upon Voegtlin's transfer, J. M. Johnson, who had just obtained his Ph.D. degree in chemistry from the Johns Hopkins University in June 1908, was appointed to take charge of the Chemical Division, with the title of Associate.

Thus, Barker's innovation—the creation of research divisions in the Department of Medicine—was successful and set the pattern which has been followed in essentially all American medical schools since that time.

All three of the original directors of these research divisions led a successful career, but one of them, inspired by his combined experience as chief resident physician for both Osler and Barker, was to carry the torch of clinical science as a basis for medical teaching and practice to even greater heights. Rufus Cole, in addition to his talents as a physician and an investigator, had the good fortune to be on the scene at a time when important events were in the making. After graduation from the Johns Hopkins Medical School in 1899, Cole became an intern on Dr. Osler's medical service. He saw at first hand the great skill of Osler as a clinical observer and diagnostician, as well as the importance of the graded system of residency training which Osler had established at Hopkins. He saw as well Barker's determination to follow the German example by making the investigation of disease a major obligation of the Department of Medicine.

The next important step in his career was taken after John D. Rockefeller authorized, in February 1907, the preparation of plans for a hospital for clinical investigation to be associated with the Rockefeller Institute for Medical Research. By June 1907 the outlines of a fifty-bed hospital equipped with laboratories independent of those already existing in the institute were presented. Although Cole had just been offered the professorship of medicine at the University of Michigan, when given the opportunity, he decided to stake his future career on this small clinical research hospital in New York, which at that time was unbuilt and unendowed. On October 10, 1908, he was elected a member of the Rockefeller Institute in charge of scientific and medical conduct of the hospital, and on November 28 was named director of the Rockefeller Hospital. This was a momentous occasion for the future of medical education and medical research.

Cole visualized in the activities of this hospital an opportunity to develop a program of intensive medical investigation in an environment pervaded by the research spirit, free from the ordinary routine of practice and of the teaching of medical students. Here he could train young men and women who would later carry the new methods and the new scientific approach to clinical medicine to other medical schools and teaching hospitals. This multiplier effect was most successful, and had a tremendous influence in providing the scientific base for medical practice as we know it today.

The plan which Cole presented to the Board of Directors concerning the organization of the hospital staff was a combination of what he had learned from Osler of the advantage of a fulltime graded residency training program and from his second chief, Barker, of the crying need for fulltime clinicians trained for and devoted to clinical investigation. His plan called for a resident staff of young physicians proven capable of doing independent research. Rather than being simply assistants to the physician-in-chief and his senior associates, each would have full control of a group of patients suffering with a disease in which he was particularly interested. Each resident would be provided with enough assistance to leave him time for research, and adequate facilities for laboratory tests and animal experimentation would be at his disposal. Thus, the new hospital would be an independent department in which Cole and his staff would be an organized group comparable to the existing departments of the institute.

The directors voted unanimously in January 1909 to approve Cole's plan, and one month later John D. Rockefeller, Jr., announced that his father would provide for the proposed salaried hospital staff in the general endowment of the new hospital. The Hospital of the Rockefeller Institute was officially inaugurated on October 17, 1910—a truly red-letter day in American medicine. Cole made a monumental step in advancing the concept that the diagnosis and treatment of disease should go hand in hand with their study in the laboratory —the ultimate basis for the principle of fulltime academic medicine, particularly in clinical departments. In Cole's own words:

As soon as the work was underway, I realized that owing to conditions then existing in medical teaching, the hospital should have at least one other function besides the investigation of disease. The idea of so-called university departments of medicine was in the air and it was evident that this idea would soon reach concrete expression in a number of places. The new hospital appeared to be the logical place in which leaders of this new movement could be trained, be given opportunities to work and be fired with the spirit of investigation which could thus be disseminated throughout the projected clinics. It seemed that the hospital should not adopt a policy of a splendid isolation but should play its part in the reorganization of medical teaching in this country.

That Cole succeeded admirably in this role is evidenced in part by the fact that by 1938, of the 179 people who had been on the hospital staff during its twenty-eight years of existence, 112 or 62.5 percent occupied fulltime academic positions, and many more had university affiliation of some type. Thus, in large measure due to the vision of Mall, Barker, and Cole, a new member of the medical family came into being—the clinical scientist—who serves as a vital link between the practicing physician and the basic scientist.

Cole's career teaches another very important lesson: to mold one's research interest in depth around one major field of interest rather than to make superficial attacks in many different areas. Cole is an outstanding example of persistence in the study of the mysteries of a single important problem in medicine. With dogged tenacity, he attacked the problems of pneumonia, and he and his colleagues solved one problem after another as it arose. The long series of contributions to our knowledge of pneumococcal pneumonia are important not only with reference to the disease itself but also to our knowledge of the fundamental concepts of immunochemistry and heredity.

Cole began work on pneumococcal pneumonia while in Baltimore. This disease was so common in the nineteenth century that Osler called it "the captain of the man of death," using the phrase John Bunyan had applied to tuberculosis. This type of pneumonia was due to the pneumococcus discovered by Louis Pasteur in 1880. Cole's objective was to produce an immune serum agaisnt the pneumococcus by inoculating horses with gradually increasing quantities of the germs, thus eliciting in the horses' blood antibodies capable of neutralizing the effects of the pneumococcus. Cole and his two co-workers, Dochez and Marks, ran into real difficulties, as pneumococci isolated from patients represent several strains differing in virulence. By the end of 1912, Cole and Dochez had developed a serum for use against type I and were working toward one for the other types.

One of their major contributions was to develop a method for the typing of pneumococci. Further efforts to control pneumonia depended on detailed knowledge of the slight chemical differences that gave each strain of pneumococci the ability to elicit its own particular antibody. To tackle this problem, an investigator was needed who had a thorough knowledge of bacteriology and a background in chemistry. Cole chose Oswald T. Avery, who joined the staff of the hospital in 1913 and spent the rest of his career investigating the chemistry of pneumococci.

Avery and his associates soon located the specific immunity-inducing substances in the capsule that surrounds the bacterium, which is composed of polysaccharides—that is, sugar linked into very complex compounds, differing slightly in the various strains of pneumococci.

As Corner has pointed out, the attack on lobar pneumonia begun by Cole and carried on by Avery and Dochez was one of the most elegant performances from the standpoint of theory and technique in the history of bacteriology. As far as the cure of the patient is concerned, much of the work was made obsolete by the discovery of the antibiotics; but the use of immune serum was the only specific treatment of lobar pneumonia for many years and is credited with saving thousands of lives the world over. However, as is so often the case in research, these studies of the pneumococcus opened up unpredicted areas of research in the chemistry of immunity and of heredity.

In 1923 Walther F. Goebel came to the Rockefeller Institute to join Avery and Heidelberger in their study of the specific antigens and the capsular polysaccharides of the pneumococcus. He participated in the discovery that these are complex sugarlike substances, which in their native state are probably combined with the proteins of the bacterial cell. His work led to the establishment of the important principle that the immunological specificity of a carbohydrate depends upon its precise molecular structure.

By 1929 Avery and Goebel were able to produce an artificial antigen that would elicit antibody formation not only against itself but also against virulent pneumococci. By 1935, using a synthetic sugar derivative, Goebel produced an artificial antigen so close to that formed by living pneumococci that when injected into rabbits, it protected them against infection with the highly virulent type III organisms. This triumph of immunochemical skill gave final proof of the concept that had been developed over the past twenty years: the antigenic specificity of the pneumococcus resides in the polysaccharides of the bacterial capsule. This is one of the foundation stones of immunochemistry.

When Rufus Cole retired as director of the Rockefeller Hospital in 1937, Oswald T. Avery was still deeply involved in the investigation of the chemistry of the pneumococcus which he had begun long ago at Cole's suggestion. This work had gone far beyond the practical aim of finding means to control this one organism and, as we have seen, resulted in the discovery of much of the basic knowledge of immunochemistry. Avery retired in 1943, but continued to work in the laboratory for several more years. His later years were marked by a great discovery that was to link together some of the basic phenomena of immunity and heredity.

The story of the transforming factor begins in 1928 with a report by a British pathologist, Fred Griffith. When Griffith inoculated mice with a mixture of a harmless strain of living pneumococci and the dead remains of a virulent strain, the mice, to his astonishment, died from infection with live organisms of the virulent type. Since he could not believe that the killed bacteria had come to life, he had to assume that something in their dead bodies had transformed the living harmless strain into the virulent one. This excited Avery's interest, and he asked Martin Dawson to study this phenomenon. Dawson was able to reproduce it *in vitro* rather than in a mouse. In 1932 J. L. Alloway of Avery's group took the matter a step further by using as transforming agents not whole dead cells, but a cell-free extract made from them. This indicated that the transforming agent was a chemical substance. Avery himself now entered the investigation, working with Colin MacLeod and later with Maclyn McCarty. These investigators extracted and systematically broke apart the chemical constituents of virulent type III pneumococci, testing the transforming power of each fraction. In 1944 they arrived at an essentially pure substance possessing the transforming power in very high concentration. This proved to be a nucleic acid of a type which Levene and Jacobs had first identified years before at the Rockefeller Institute, deoxyribonucleic acid (DNA). It was difficult to exclude the possibility that the transforming action of DNA might be due to a small amount of protein contaminant. McCarty was able to prepare the enzyme which destroys DNA, and he showed that when treated with this substance, the pneumococcal extract lost its transforming power. The demonstration that a nucleic acid was the effecting agent in inducing a heritable change in a living organism was unexpected, since nucleic acids had generally been thought to be chemically undifferentiated and rather inert biologically. Other investigators showed that DNA, which exists in chromosomes of higher animals, is a constant and characteristic ingredient of genes. The work of Avery's group on bacterial transformation pointed to a striking similarity of the chemical mechanism of heredity throughout the biological scale from bacteria to mammals.

Thus, not only did Cole create a clinical investigation unit which was to exert a major influence on the future of medical education, research, and practice in the United States, but the persistence of his group in the study of a single outstanding problem in medicine—the nature of pneumococcal pneumonia—led to one of the most fundamental discoveries in biology.

This story is replete with valuable lessons. It traces one of the most important facets in the evolution of clinical science and the birth of a new member of the scientific community—the clinical investigator. This new member of the scientific family circle serves as a vital link between the practicing physician and the basic scientist. He is unique in that he alone is trained in the methodology of science and works with human disease. The problems which interest him in the clinic and the conclusions he reaches are not only useful to the practicing physician but may result in discoveries basic to our understanding of biology.

13 ❦ Compleat Clinician and Renaissance Pathologist: Louis Hamman and Arnold R. Rich

Louis Hamman

LOUIS HAMMAN was a warm, intelligent, and able clinician whose wit and personality endeared him to patients and colleagues alike. His greatness lay in his uncanny ability to gather clinical facts, organize them effectively, arrive at the correct diagnosis, and thus have the best basis for the management of the patient's problem. During his life he published some seventy-five papers, all of which contributed important new knowledge for better medical practice and provide pleasant and delightful reading. The best of his work emphasized prognosis based on correct diagnosis, which he summed up in a 1938 paper in the *New England Journal of Medicine* on "The Diagnosis of the Causes of Heart Failure": "The aim of medical practice is the prevention and cure of disease. Its highest accomplishment is prognosis. Its foundation is diagnosis. The function of diagnosis is to direct and guide treatment." As pointed out by J. C. Harvey in his excellent survey, Dr. Hamman's writings illustrate "the points the patients make." All of his investigative work was done on normal volunteer subjects or on patients. He never worked with experimental animals, although he followed the work of others and used the information effectively in his practice.

Dr. Hamman was born in Baltimore in 1877, attended local schools, and ultimately entered Rock Hill College. He received his M.D. degree at the Johns Hopkins School of Medicine in 1901 and then joined the resident staff of New York Hospital. He returned to Baltimore in 1903, and his first assignment as head of the new Phipps Tuberculosis Clinic is referred to in a letter from Dr. Osler to Dr. Thayer: "Hamman seems an A-1 fellow. We can recommend him in September though probably all the new nominations should come before the Trustees in June." Later in the same letter he says: "Mr. Phipps has promised another $10,000 when needed. We must take this chance to get the Outpatient Department remodeled and a separate tuberculosis clinic established. I dare say Mr. Phipps will do anything we ask."

In February 1905 the Phipps Tuberculosis Clinic opened. With Dr. Samuel Wolman, Dr. Hamman undertook a series of investigations on the use of tuberculin in the diagnosis and treatment of tuberculosis. Their pioneer investigations in the clinical use of tuberculin were ultimately compiled in a book entitled *Tuberculin in Diagnosis and Treatment,* published by Appleton in 1912.

Another of Dr. Hamman's original contributions resulted from a study of blood glucose. A report by Jacobson in 1913 on the hyperglycemia followed a normal individual's ingestion of starchy foods suggested to Dr. Hamman that with "the use of a similar method to study carbohydrate tolerance, perhaps the character of the curve might be altered in different diseases, and the test therefore yield important data." Estimation of a patient's ability to dispose promptly of a certain amount of glucose taken at one time into the stomach, known as the "glucose tolerance test," has definite clinical value. His experiments with the administration of glucose were reported in May 1916 at the meeting of the Association of American Physicians. A full report of the work appeared in the *Archives of Internal Medicine* in November 1917. The principle of the glucose tolerance test was clearly delineated by Dr. Hamman, and he described the blood sugar response to a second dose of orally administered glucose several years before Staub and Traugott, who are generally credited with this observation. J. C. Harvey points out that the present-day concept of the glucose tolerance test is credited to work done by Janney and Issacson, reported by them first at a meeting of the Society of Experimental Biology and Medicine in February 1917 and published in April 1918—a year after Dr. Hamman's paper appeared. Thus, Hamman and his co-worker, Hirschman, should be given the credit for the concept of the glucose tolerance test and for the so-called Staub-Traugott Effect.

Dr. Hamman published a number of excellent papers on diseases of the heart, particularly on coronary artery disease. He brought order to the symptomatology of coronary occlusion, delineating the immediate reaction associated with the anginal seizure, including pain, shock, and suppression of urine; the appearance next of symptoms of myocardial dysfunction such as chronic passive congestion, gallop rhythm and rapid pulse; and finally symptoms of infarction (fever, leukocytosis, and pericarditis).

He and Dr. Arnold Rice Rich conducted clinical-pathological conferences which were eagerly attended by students and faculty alike. It was here that the students received much of their fundamental conception of the clinical skills necessary in the practice of medicine. Dr. Hamman developed an approach to differential diagnosis, which is still useful and forms the basis of a textbook on differential diagnosis written by Harvey and Bordley. His view of the clinical-pathological conference, which he conducted with such skill, was as follows:

As a method of instruction, it has great advantages over the bedside clinic, not it is true, to the physician discussing the problems but certainly to his hearers. At the bedside an able and experienced physician supported by the weight of reputation may make almost what he pleases of the clinical facts before him. None will be so rash as to openly dispute his conclusions and nearly all will go away convinced of his skill and erudition. But his position at a Clinical-Pathological Conference is quite different. Here all the advantage is on the side of the hearer for though physicians may be supported by reputations to equal Osler's and by the honors of all the Academies, there sits the smiling pathologist ready and sometimes even eager to administer the coup-de-grace to his reputation, erudition, and elegance. What he may say is to be judged immediately and irrevocably. He is no longer the glorious high priest of medical science introducing novices to her mysteries, but the very humblest suppliant prostrate at her feet.

One of the outstanding examples of his keen clinical perception and ability to reason logically about the clinical information available is exemplified in the story of the diagnosis and cure of a patient who had a streptococcus viridens bacteremia arising from infection on a traumatic arteriovenous aneurysm. This "clinical adventure" was published in the *Bulletin of the Johns Hopkins Hospital* in 1935, in collaboration with Dr. William F. Reinhoff, Jr., who operated on the patient. An interesting personal account of this event has been kindly provided by Dr. Benjamin Baker.

In 1934 while I was a patient in Marburg having had a radical sinus procedure, Dr. Hamman, who was my partner in practice, came into my room, sat down and lit a cigarette. I was still a little drowsy from the morning anesthesia and sedation. He told me that he had come over not only to see how I was but to see a new patient that had been admitted that afternoon. It was Dr. Hamman's custom to discuss his patients with his colleagues, giving them the benefit of following his successful clinical analysis. He told me about the patient that he had come to see. It was a man who had been shot in the leg, following which he developed an arteriovenous aneurysm in the popliteal space. Subsequently, he began to have chills, fever, and other evidences of infection. Dr. Hamman, in his delightful way, said to me: "Now, Ben, what in the world do you think this man could possibly have?" I remember replying, probably a little deliriously, "Oh, Dr. Hamman, that is a very simple situation. The man has an arteriovenous aneurysm with vegetations on it." Whereupon Dr. Hamman threw his head back, clapped his hands together in a fashion which no one else could imitate, and said: "Oh, you young whippersnappers in medicine, particularly when you're drugged up with anesthesia and sedatives, you do have the wildest ideas and it takes people of my age to keep you boys in line." Of course, this was exactly what I needed under the circumstances when I was a little down and out over my surgery. I am perfectly certain that Dr. Hamman had already made the diagnosis within a short period of hearing the patient's story, but he directed my thinking by leading questions to the answer. This was his way of cheering me up and giving me something to think about. The association between us, however, and our thoughts running in somewhat the same vein, mine deliriously or not, were stimulating to me.

The moment that the aneurysm was removed, the organisms disappeared from the bloodstream and the patient's temperature fell as quickly to normal as in a patient with pneumococcal pneumonia treated by penicillin. This was the first reported case of infection of an arteriovenous aneurysm, and certainly the first cured by an operative procedure. The basic clues to Dr. Hamman were the finding of the arteriovenous aneurysm, the positive blood culture, and the absence of any signs of heart disease. This was a clinical first, representing diagnostic skill at its best.

Another fine example of his ability to solve problems was the "clinical adventure" published in the *Bulletin of The Johns Hopkins Hospital* in 1939, describing the condition now known as "Hamman's disease"—spontaneous mediastinal emphysema. Dr. Benjamin Baker also relates this story:

As far as I know, I was probably the first case of spontaneous mediastinal emphysema with anything close to recognition of the underlying process. The event occurred when I was an assistant resident working in the heart station. While bending over the desk making routine electrocardiographic measurements, I suddenly noticed a vague discomfort in my chest which did not disturb me greatly. However, I was surprised and perplexed to hear a strange noise within my own thorax. I found that by leaning back in my chair the noise would disappear and on leaning forward it would return. This occurred over and over. I then called my colleague, Dr. Donald MacEachern, who leaned over the desk with me and agreed that he could also hear the noise in certain positions. We listened with a stethoscope and heard a strange crunching sound over the precordium which disappeared when I leaned back in my chair. I was in the midst of a minor respiratory infection with a little tracheitis and cough at the time this happened. Our explanation was that there was an emphysematous bleb against which the heart beat in certain positions and made the strange noise. Drs. Longcope, Thayer, and Carter took this strange situation under advisement for several days without arriving at any definitive diagnosis. Subsequently, when I went into practice with Dr. Hamman, we frequently discussed various clinical experiences, and I remember telling him about this. We speculated about its mechanism.

On February 12, 1933, Dr. Hamman was called to Washington to see a robust, vigorous, fifty-one-year-old physician who had suddenly developed an intense pain in the chest. The electrocardiogram was normal and the patient felt quite well. However, when a stethoscope was placed over the apex of the heart there could be heard with each contraction an extraordinary crunching, bubbling sound, the like of which Dr. Hamman had never heard before. The peculiar sound disappeared after a few days, and Hamman did not connect it with the episode that he had discussed years before with Dr. Baker. About four months later Dr. Hamman, having put the matter aside in his mind, saw a young boy in whom he heard the same sound under circumstances which left no doubt as to how it had been produced. There was also subcutaneous crepitation over the front of the neck, clearly indicating the presence of mediastinal emphysema, although there had been no trauma. Thus came the term "spontaneous mediastinal emphysema." Subsequently he saw additional cases and concluded:

From these observations it seems that not infrequently pulmonary alveoli must rupture, allowing air to escape into the interstitial tissues of the lung. If only a small amount of air escapes no symptoms may appear or perhaps only localized pain. This condition may account for some of the many transient pains in the chest of which patients complain and for which no cause can be discovered. If a larger amount of air escapes, it may travel along the interstitial bands to the pleura and there form a vesicle. The pleural membrane over the vesicle is stretched and often ruptures. This seems to me the most reasonable explanation for the recurrence of spontaneous mediastinal emphysema. The symptoms produced may be severe and may closely simulate those of coronary occlusion or pericarditis. Once familiar with the condition we may recognize it easily by the following peculiarities: one, the absence of the usual constitutional symptoms which accompany coronary occlusion and pericarditis and the absence of shock and myocardial weakness; two, the presence of the peculiar crunching, crackling, bubbling sound heard over the heart with each contraction. Often this sound is heard in certain positions, not in others; three, the area of cardiac dullness may be diminished in extent or replaced by a hyperresonant percussion note; four, roentgenograms will often demonstrate the presence of air in the mediastinum; five, the detection of crepitation in the subcutaneous tissues of the neck makes the diagnosis obvious.

Dr. Hamman was very gentle and kind in his relationships with patients. His patients in turn responded with kindness and generosity to him. The following account of a visit with Dr. Hamman was given by Dr. John Romano. At the time (1941) Dr. Hamman was on a visit to Peter Bent Brigham Hospital in Boston as physician-in-chief *pro tempore*:

While I had known of Hamman for years, I had never had the opportunity to know him well, and we talked together on many matters. He was of tremendous help to us at that difficult time [Dr. Soma Weiss, the professor and chairman of the Department of Medicine at Harvard and Peter Bent Brigham Hospital, had recently died suddenly of a subarachnoid hemorrhage] and did much to reduce the anxiety and the uncertainty of those of us left in the hospital. One day we were speaking about how much one did learn from patients. In that setting he told me this story:

"It happened to me many years ago. I had just finished the residency in medicine and Dr. Thayer, who was then professor of medicine at the Hopkins, called early one morning to ask if I would take his professorial rounds at the Hopkins that day. Thayer had been called on an emergency basis to see a VIP in Washington and he did not have time to make other arrangements. I was delighted and very honored and quite anxious but finally succeeded in shaving without cutting my throat and did appear at the proper time at the hospital floor, where news of my coming had been spread. There faced me a semicircle of faculty, students, nurses, and peers with that same leer on their faces that a substitute fifth-grade teacher finds as she enters the room. I can assure you those facial expressions did not help and, to make matters worse, as I walked toward the first patient on the left, the crowd surrounded me completely. I shall never forget, nor fail to be eternally grateful to that first patient. For when I leaned over to examine him, he whispered in my ear, 'Heart's on the left side.' "

Can you think of anyone's being kinder than that?

For many years, Dr. Hamman was an associate professor of medicine, and for a year during World War I he was acting head of the Department of Medicine. As he approached the statutory age for retirement from the active university staff, it troubled him. In the words of Dr. Charles Wainwright, another colleague of his in practice:

He did not resent his increasing years for he was active in body, his judgment and his mind agile and ever receptive to that which proved to be good. It marked the termination of his active participation in the training of youth. He loved youth—its enthusiasm, its eagerness, its boldness and he was never one to stifle these traits. However, he did feel called upon, in so far as his influence lay, to stress the fundamental truths, to clarify the thinking of youth, and to aid in sifting the wheat from the chaff. In this simple straightforward way he stood out as a teacher of medicine few could equal and none excel.

His clinical skills made his opinion sought after by his fellow physicians, and his advice and guidance were an inspiration to his patients. He was truly the . clinician's clinician. He died in 1946 of coronary thrombosis.

Renaissance Pathologist: Arnold Rice Rich

During his career, Arnold Rice Rich, Baxley Professor and director of the Department of Pathology, carried out many important investigations closely related to the problems of clinical medicine. The results of one of these investigations appeared in the *Bulletin of The Johns Hopkins Hospital* in 1942 in a now classic article entitled "The Role of Hypersensitivity in Periarteritis Nodosa as Indicated by Seven Cases Developing During Serum Sickness and Sulfonamide Therapy." In this report Rich noted that before the introduction of sulfonamide therapy, it was a rarity for a case of serum sickness to come to autopsy in the Johns Hopkins Hospital. However, once sulfonamide therapy came into use, autopsies on patients with serum sickness or on those who had had serum sickness shortly before death became more frequent. Even in ultimately fatal cases of infection, the sulfonamides, used in conjunction with antiserum, prolonged life sufficiently to permit serum sickness to occur before the patient died from his infection.

None of the patients reported had any symptoms suggesting periarteritis nodosa prior to their terminal acute illness for which the serum or sulfonamide was administered, and the vascular lesions were fresh. Rich concluded that these cases indicated that vascular lesions of this type could be a manifestation of the anaphylactic type of hypersensitivity, and suggested the importance of a search for the inciting antigen in cases of periarteritis nodosa that would come under clinical observation.

Because of the infrequency of autopsies on patients with serum sickness, the first of these cases was examined with particular interest. It was with surprise that fresh lesions of periarteritis nodosa were encountered. This was regarded as a coincidence until the second case that had had an urticarial serum reaction came to autopsy, and again marked lesions of periarteritis nodosa were present. These cases were first presented at a clinical-pathological conference in March 1941, with the suggestion that since periarteritis nodosa is an uncommon disease, the combination of serum sickness with the arterial lesions in patients who had been well before the fatal lobar pneumonia for which they were treated might be more than a coincidence. Clinical interest was aroused, and when a fifth patient who had received antiserum for pneumonia developed serum sickness followed by symptoms suggestive of periarteritis, a biopsy was performed. In the small piece of biceps muscle tissue obtained, a marked periarterial inflammatory infiltration of polymorphonuclear and mononuclear cells was found. Later in the same year, Rich described a case of a patient who received no serum, in which periarteritis nodosa developed as a result of an anaphylactic type of hypersensitivity reaction due to sulfathiazole. He then reported cases following reactions to iodide and to penicillin. Thus he

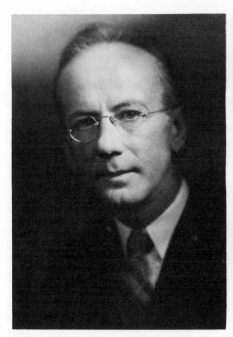

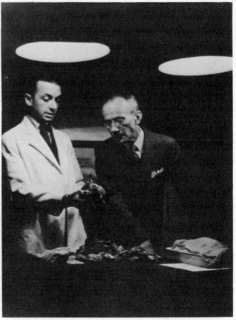

Louis Hamman

From the Archives Office, The Johns Hopkins
Medical Institutions

Arnold R. Rich and Louis Hamman
conducting a clinical-pathological conference

From T. B. Turner, *Heritage of Excellence: The
Johns Hopkins Medical Institutions, 1914–1947*
(Baltimore: The Johns Hopkins University Press,
1974)

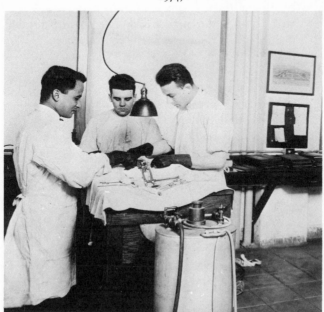

Arnold R. Rich at work in his laboratory

Courtesy of the Department of Pathology, The Johns Hopkins School
of Medicine

developed extensive clinical and pathological evidence that periarteritis nodosa is a manifestation of anaphylactic hypersensitivity.

Experiments were carried out in the laboratory in conjunction with Dr. John E. Gregory, in which typical visceral periarteritis nodosa was produced by the intravenous injection of a single large dose of foreign serum into the normal animal, thus providing the opportunity for a protracted circulation of antigen while hypersensitivity developed.

Over sixty years ago Clemens von Pirquet, the first fulltime professor of pediatrics at the Johns Hopkins School of Medicine, was first to suggest that the immune system might sometimes be responsible for injurious effects. Von Pirquet observed that in "serum sickness," a disease which may follow injection of foreign blood serum, the blood of the patient contained the foreign protein and the antibody against it. Von Pirquet concluded that the combination of antibody with the foreign protein (antigen) produced a "toxic" substance that gave rise to hives, rash, pain in the joints and, in severe cases, death due to serum sickness. He also suggested that an immune response to viruses might cause disease, and that an interaction of antibodies with the viruses of smallpox and measles might be the basis for the skin eruptions characteristic of these diseases. These suggestions lay fallow until the 1950s, when Wallace P. Rowe, a graduate of the Johns Hopkins Medical School, proved the validity of von Pirquet's hypothesis while studying the virus of lymphocytic choriomeningitis (LCM). At first his infected mice showed no sign of illness, although the virus multiplied rapidly in many organs. On the sixth day, however, the mice showed an immune response to the virus, developed meningitis, and died. Rowe crippled the immune response of the mice by exposing them to x-rays and then infected both the treated mice and untreated controls with the LCM virus. The irradiated animals did not develop meningitis, although the virus replicated in their tissues just as rapidly as in the control mice.

Later, Donald H. Gilden, Gerald A. Cole, Andrew A. Monjan, and Neal Nathanson, working in the Johns Hopkins School of Hygiene and Public Health, took Rowe's studies a step further. It was known that the immune system responds to foreign substances in two ways: (1) mediated by antibodies; and (2) mediated by lymphocytes. The immune lymphocytes recognize antigens on the surface of foreign cells and thereby destroy tissues such as tumors or skin grafts. Gilden and his co-workers used drugs to suppress the immunological response in mice. They infected them with LCM virus and then divided the animals into three groups. One group received injections of anti-LCM antibody, the second was given anti-LCM lymphocytes, and the third received normal lymphocytes. The animals receiving the antibody or normal lymphocytes remained well, but those given the immune lymphocytes developed the symptoms of LCM disease and died. In the case of LCM it was the combination of immune lymphocytes and the virus that produced the disease. Thus, the immune response to viral antigens on the surface of infected cells can cause tissue injury.

Von Pirquet's studies in the early 1900s on serum sickness suggested another mechanism: one involving the combination of antigen and antibody. In the 1950s Frederick G. Germuth, Jr. and his co-workers in the Department of Pathology at Johns Hopkins, as well as Frank J. Dixon and his colleagues at the University of Pittsburgh School of Medicine, found that they could produce serum sickness in rabbits by injecting combinations, prepared in the test tube, of foreign protein and antibody. Their studies showed that these injected complexes circulating in the rabbits' blood became trapped in the capillaries of the kidneys and led to changes resembling the human disease known as "glomerulonephritis." Thus, the disease which Arnold Rich had produced was shown to be caused by an antigen-antibody complex and was called "immune complex" disease. Although the immune complex syndrome could readily be produced in animals in the laboratory, the fact that it could also occur in response to viral infections in man had to await the development of new techniques for the recognition of virus-antibody complexes. A group at the National Institutes of Health working with the lactic dehydrogenase virus (LDV) devised a very sensitive technique for detecting virus-antibody combinations. Using this technique, they observed that the infected mice were making antibody to LDV. Other investigators demonstrated that infectious virus-antibody complexes were characteristic of several of the chronic infections and that some of these chronic infections ended in glomerulonephritis. In addition, the polyarteritis that occurs in mink infected with the Aleutian virus and in man infected with the hepatitis virus is associated with circulating immune complexes. The possibility that viruses and the immune response may also be involved in diseases such as rheumatoid arthritis and systemic lupus erythematosus is being investigated in many laboratories. It has already been demonstrated that an antigen-antibody complex of DNA and anti-DNA antibody is concerned in the pathogenesis of the glomerulonephritis seen in patients with systemic lupus erythematosus.

Arnold Rice Rich was born in Birmingham, Alabama, in 1893. He spent three adolescent years at the Bingham School in North Carolina, a military school with old traditions. He entered the University of Virginia, then a relatively small institution, and enjoyed the intellectual atmosphere there. When time came to choose a career, Arnold, having developed an interest in zoology, finally chose medicine. Much of his last year in Charlottesville was spent in the Department of Zoology working on his first research problem—the reactions of the proboscis of a flatworm, *Planaria albissima Vejdovsky*. The proboscis containing the mouth of the worm was apparently a very extraordinary structure. When detached from the body of the worm, it would swim around freely ingesting everything, regardless of its food value. Only when the worm's nervous connections were intact would it be selective in its choice.

During his years at the Johns Hopkins Medical School, Rich spent much of his time in the research laboratory. In his first year, he came under the spell of Dr. William H. Howell, and like all of Howell's pupils, became interested in blood clotting. Rich studied the nature and properties of metathrombin, a compound of thrombin and antithrombin that has been ignored by modern students of coagulation, and he described the process of clotting as observed under the dark field microscope.

When the United States entered World War I in the spring of 1917, Arnold Rich was finishing his third year in medical school. Rich's part in the war was described by Emmett Holt in his presentation remarks when the Kober Medal was awarded to Arnold Rich in 1958:

All of us students wanted to do our bit but we were told we could be much more useful if we finished up our course and served as doctors. The Army thought so too, but they felt that army training and medicine should go hand in hand. So, in the fall of 1918 the Students' Army Training Corps, Johns Hopkins Unit, was organized. The medical students were put into ill-fitting uniforms and housed in improvised barracks. We marched, we drilled, we scrubbed the floors, we did guard duty, and we were disciplined. Rich, because of his military school experience was sergeant. For a time patriotism sustained us but it was soon apparent that military duties were seriously interfering with our medical education. There was a remedy for this situation, however—sick leave, and better yet, transfusion leave. Anyone who sold blood could be relieved of military duty for days—even longer if one would be immunized with streptococcus viridans—it was in the days when immune transfusions for subacute bacterial endocarditis were in vogue. The happy blood donor slept late while his comrades in arms rose early and drilled. They could eat when and where they chose. They were privileged characters and they now had time to study. The armistice came, and in the weeks that followed the morale of the Johns Hopkins troops deteriorated sadly. The numbers of the sick and the blood donors increased. I do not recall that Sergeant Rich was among the latter, but I do seem to remember that his health suffered to some extent during this period.

It had been Arnold Rich's plan to go into experimental surgery, but on the advice of Dr. Halsted he had decided to take a preliminary year in pathology with Dr. MacCallum. During this year it became clear to him that pathology offered an extraordinary opportunity to study the problems of disease. Rich's request to be relieved of his commitment to surgery was granted, and he remained thereafter in the Department of Pathology at Johns Hopkins, ultimately succeeding Dr. MacCallum as director of the department.

Rich's experimental work for more than forty years in the Department of Pathology covered a wide range of subjects. For many years he worked on jaundice and bile pigment metabolism. Little was known at that time about the mechanism and sites of hemoglobin breakdown. Rich and his co-workers showed that the pigment formed from hemoglobin in hemorrhages, known as hematoidin, was in fact bilirubin, and that this was formed not by extracellular enzymes or bacteria, but within the cells of the reticuloendothelial system. The final demonstration of this was in tissue culture, where reticuloendothelial phagocytes were allowed to engulf red cells, bilirubin appearing intracellularly as the hemoglobin disappeared. In further studies he clarified the role of the liver in the different types of jaundice and worked out a classification of jaundice with two main types: retention and regurgitation jaundice.

In the late 1920s he became interested in bacterial allergy and immunity and the relationship between them. In those days the hypersensitivity response was thought of as a protective one, even though it might result in tissue necrosis. The exaggerated inflammation was thought necessary to wall off the noxious agent. In tuberculosis the dictum of the day was "the individual is as resistant as the shell of his tubercle." Rich and his collaborators showed, however, first in tuberculosis, then in syphilis and then in other infections, that although hypersensitivity and immunity might develop simultaneously, they were independent phenomena. They dissociated the two in a variety of ways. Hypersensitivity might decrease while resistance remained, and cellular barriers were easily penetrated when resistance was low. It was antibodies rather than cell walls that checked the spread of bacteria.

Rich's studies on tuberculosis led to other studies on the nature of resistance to tuberculosis in general. He later wrote a monograph and an epochmaking textbook on this subject. One of his most fundamental contributions was the observation that bacterial allergy was a cellular phenomenon. The cells themselves were sensitized and would retain this property when grown in tissue culture. This was in sharp contrast to anaphylactic hypersensitivity, in which the ability to respond, as is well known, can be transferred with the serum.

His later studies, already described, showed the role of anaphylactic hypersensitivity in disease and demonstrated that periarteritis nodosa could result from hypersensitivy to drugs. In all of these studies, including his experimental observations on polyarteritis and acute nephritis resulting from experimental hypersensitivity, Rich always stressed that the findings did not prove identity of etiology or pathogenesis.

Although the central theme of Arnold Rich's work followed a consistent pattern in the area of hypersensitivity and immunity, he was, simultaneously, contributing important work on a host of different problems. For example, there were papers demonstrating the role of trypsin in the pathogenesis of the vascular lesions in hemorrhagic pancreatitis; the first experimental production of nodular cirrhosis of the liver by dietary deficiency, and its prevention by a factor in the diet; and the production of whooping cough in chimpanzees. Rich identified the Gaucher cell as a mononuclear phagocyte by injecting colloidal iron *in vivo*. He found patterns of cell motility in tissue culture distinguished between the early myeloid and lymphoid cells. By this means it was shown that the cells of previously questionable origin that appear in the spleen in acute infections are lymphoid in type. These studies also showed that this type of alteration and proliferation of lymphoid cells was the first visible response to the presence of a soluble antigen, pointing to the possible participation of these cells in antibody formation.

Rich's many experimental contributions, however, were only part of what he contributed that had an important relationship to clinical medicine. At a time when most people assumed that observation of stained sections of autopsy material had contributed all that it was able to, Rich discovered something new in morphological pathology almost every year. For example, Rich described a peculiar renal lesion characteristic of syphilis, a fatal type of interstitial fibrosis of the lung (in collaboration with Hamman), a characteristic lesion of the spleen in sickle cell anemia, the tubular degenerative lesion of the adrenal cortex in infections associated with circulatory collapse, and the subpinal focus responsible for tuberculous meningitis.

As a teacher, Rich was unsurpassed. His staff clinical-pathological conferences and his teaching in the small student groups in pathology and for the resident staff were models for their clarity and incisiveness. Rich also was the prime mover of a small group of research scientists who formed the Johns Hopkins Research Club. They met periodically to discuss their own work and occasionally to hear an invited guest. On one occasion an outsider had been invited to demonstrate his professed ability to freeze fish without killing them by using a quick-freezing technique. After a great deal of practice with goldfish, the visitor informed Dr. Rich, who was to preside at the meeting, that the demonstration would not work and that he would not come. The audience was all anticipation and it seemed a pity to disappoint them, so Rich decided to fake it. Two frozen fish—and they were well frozen—were displayed to the expectant scientists, who all agreed that they were frozen. The fish were then ostensibly placed in a teapot full of water, though in fact they were slipped up Dr. Rich's sleeve. The teapot contained two live goldfish, but nobody had investigated its contents in advance. When it was later examined and found to contain two actively swimming fish, there was great excitement. The entire group of observant Johns Hopkins scientists had been completely taken in.

To Arnold Rich, academic life meant everything. He described it vividly in his Kober Medal acceptance speech:

The attraction of an academic life in medicine consists, of course, in the character of the opportunities that an academic environment provides, and in the leisure for the satisfying enjoyment of these opportunities—leisure for trying to know one's field well, and opportunities for using that knowledge helpfully; leisure for trying to decrease the vast area of the unknown in health and in disease; leisure for association with the fresh young minds of students; and leisure for the enjoyment of one of the great charms of academic life—communion with one's colleagues young and old, in all fields, who are animated by these same pleasures and are interested in each other's interests. For the enjoyment of these leisures the 1920s and 1930s, like the decades immediately preceding them, were halcyon days in academic medicine, days when in most university medical schools there were few of the encroachments upon scholarly leisure that one hears so much about today, and which tend to increase with an increase in institutional size and organization. It had not yet become necessary to think seriously about the farsighted concern of Daniel Gilman, the wise first president of Johns Hopkins, who, early in the present century, warned universities against the danger of losing the elements of repose, the quiet pursuit of knowledge, the friendship of books, the pleasures of conversations, and the advantages of solitude.

One of the happiest memories for all students of Johns Hopkins from the 1920s through the 1940s were the clinical-pathological conferences which Dr. Rich conducted first with Dr. William Sydney Thayer, then with Dr. Louis Hamman, and finally with Dr. A. McGehee Harvey. Thayer and Hamman had been Rich's teachers who later became colleagues, with whom he worked in close association. He stated that: "Apart from the particular facts and the skills of which each was a master, by their unpremediated example they taught an art of life, of which each was also a master in his own individual way."

Arnold Rich, during his long and distinguished career, received many honors at home and abroad. He remained a nonconformist all his life. He avoided exercise religiously. He had a lively distaste for everything routine and refused to adapt himself to the customary time schedules of his fellow men. He never arrived at his office much before noontime, but he always worked late and did most of his writing between 2:00 and 4:00 A.M., when the world was at its quietest. Perhaps that is one of the reasons, says Emmett Holt, why his medical writings were such classics. Rich had, however, many interests besides those in medicine. He was a composer, a poet, an engraver, and a fly fisherman. He was also the father of the well-known poet Adrienne Rich. In spite of his many activities and his intense devotion to his work, Rich was always able to find time for any of his colleagues, young or old, who wanted to discuss their problems with him. These sessions were always brisk, with ideas tossed about, dissected and resynthesized so that one always came out with a clearer understanding of the problems and with a firm knowledge of what needed to be done as the first step toward solving them. This is why Arnold Rich was such a stimulating force in the Johns Hopkins Medical Institutions during the entire period of his career there.

It was Thomas Sydenham (1624–1689) who first gave clinical observation its place of honor as a scientific method—one which for those who cultivate it is still a basic asset of the complete physician. Sydenham's great contribution was to direct attention from the general to the specific. Previously, physicians had been studying man, as well as illness, in the most general terms. With inadequate methods and techniques they could not solve the problems of general pathology. Sydenham emphasized the importance of special pathology. He concentrated on the study of specific diseases and tried to discern how they made themselves perceptible to the physician in the individual patient. "Where Hippocrates wrote the histories of sick people, Sydenham wrote the history of the individual."

Sydenham improved the existing nosology by reviving and developing two taxonomic concepts, which are referred to as "cluster" and "temporal correlation." In the concept of cluster, often used medically to designate a syndrome, several individual manifestations of illness are combined to form a single entity or disease. In the concept of temporal correlation, a "disease" is named not just according to its immediate manifestations, but according to the correlated pattern of its evolving clinical course. As examples, Sydenham descriptively separated the clustered temporal pattern of gout, with its self-limited episodes, from the individual entities that had been called "rheumatism," and the cluster of measles, with its nonrepetitious transiency, from what had been called "exanthemata." A disease had been recognized for the first time as an entity in which specific clinical manifestations caused by specific anatomical abnormalities could evolve in a specific course and might be cured by a specific therapeutic agent.

Much has been added since Sydenham's day, and there is still more to be revealed to the alert clinician in his daily practice. This chapter will tell the story of the classical observations of Sir William Osler, Warfield T. Longcope, Thomas P. Sprunt, Frank A. Evans, Chester S. Keefer, and Augustus Roi Felty, each of whom described new clinical entities which through the years have remained classical descriptions of disease.

William Osler

In 1874 Sir William Osler was a student in Vienna. Some thirty-four years later he revisited Vienna, at which time he sent home a letter, intended for the

American medical profession, describing the influence of the Vienna school on American medicine. In this letter he commented that while the Vienna school still maintained a great reputation, it could not be denied that the Aesculapian center had moved from the Danube to the Spree. He continued:

But this is what has happened in all ages. Minerva Medica has never had her chief temples in any one country for more than a generation or two.... Not until she saw in Johannes Müller and in Rudolph Virchow true and loyal disciples did she move to Germany, where she stays in spite of the tempting offers from France, from Italy, from England, and from Austria.

In an interview most graciously granted to me as a votary of long standing she expressed herself very well satisfied with her present home, where she has much honor and is much appreciated. I boldly suggested that it was perhaps time to think of crossing the Atlantic and setting up her temple in the New World for a generation or two. I spoke of the many advantages of the absence of tradition—here she visibly weakened as she has suffered so much from this poison—the greater freedom, the enthusiasm, and then I spoke of missionary work. At these words, she turned on me sharply and said, "That is not for me. We gods have but one motto—Those that honor us, we honor. Give me the temple, give me the priests, give me the true worship, the old Hippocratic service of the art and of the science of ministering to man, and I will come. By the eternal law under which we gods live, I would have to come...." Doubtless she will come, but not until the present crude organization of our medical clinics is changed, not until there is a fuller realization of internal medicine as a science as well as an art.

No one, perhaps, did more to lay the groundwork for Minerva Medica's move to the United States than Osler. How did his talents to bring this about develop? From what directions did his innovations in clinical teaching and organization come? One influence seems to have been the International Medical Congress of 1881, which Osler attended when he was just beginning his career as a physician and teacher of medicine. This congress was held in London under the presidency of Sir James Paget. Other illustrious men in attendance included Virchow, Pasteur, Donders, Charcot, and Lister. The importance of clinical demonstration of cases was never better illustrated than at this congress, when this technique was used more effectively than at any previous time. In his essay "On the Educational Value of the Medical Society," Osler emphasized that no meeting should be arranged without clinical demonstrations. Further, in a letter to the editor of the *Canadian Medical and Surgical Journal* describing the congress, Osler wrote:

Sir, the seventh session of this Congress concluded last evening by an informal soiree at the Crystal Palace.... The sight of above three thousand medical men from all parts of the world drawn together for one common purpose and animated by one spirit quickened the pulse and roused enthusiasm to a high pitch. The presence of the Prince of Wales and the Crown Prince of Prussia gave great satisfaction and added a flavor of royal patronage which even science—republican though it be—seemed thoroughly to enjoy....

One of the most instructive parts of the Congress was the museum held in the Geological Society's rooms. This consisted of illustrations of disease in the living subject as well as a large assortment of rare and interesting prepared specimens. Among the former, Dr. William Miller Ord exhibited a remarkable set of cases illustrative of the disease described by Sir William Gull and himself to which they gave the name myxedema from the mucoid degeneration of the connective tissues which produces the general swelling of the skin. The cases are usually in women and the affection is progressive. The patients exhibited by Dr. Ord showed the various stages of the disorder and his lucid description left no doubt in the minds of his peers that a definite pathological entity was before them.

Mr. Jonathan Hutchinson had a number of cases each morning and his demonstrations on leprosy, rheumatic arthritis, and inherited syphilis attracted large audiences.... The walls of the rooms in which the specimens were collected were covered with colored drawings. Among the most remarkable of these was a set of water colors by Sir Charles Bell illustrating gun shot and other wounds seen by him after Waterloo. Mr. Hutchinson's enormous collection attracted particular attention and illustrated most of the special departments in which he has become famous. What struck me as most remarkable among them was a set illustrating eruptions due to iodide and of bromide of potassium, particularly two portraits of a man the subject of an extensive eruption of tuberous masses on the skin, many of them ulcerated. The iodide had been given for ten weeks in increasing doses up to 20 grains for a swelling in one iliac fossa....

Osler's background was very broad, encompassing physiology, pathology, and all of the branches of clinical medicine. He developed keen powers of observation, and from his experiences gained a deep appreciation of the value of clinical demonstration of patients as a basic teaching method. He loved to teach the students on the wards and at the bedside. He abolished didactic lectures and made the student an integral part of the hospital organization. He said modestly, "I hope my gravestone will bear only the statement: 'He brought medical students into the wards for bedside teaching.'" In addition, he made the students responsible for the history of the patient's illness, for a complete physical examination, and for the simpler laboratory examinations. All of this seems commonplace now, but in the late nineteenth century it took vision, courage, and faith to assign such important tasks to students. Osler himself was beset by the haunting fear that these innovations would be fought by the public and spurned by the medical profession. To his genuine relief, their acceptance by both was immediate, and they survive today as important keystones in medical education.

When Osler arrived in Baltimore in 1889, his capacities as a clinical observer and his ability to ferret out and describe new clinical syndromes were at their peak. What were some of the new clinical syndromes he recognized during his Johns Hopkins period?

In spite of his many exacting duties, he found time to continue his work in infectious endocarditis, and in 1893, the year that the medical school opened, he published a paper in which he noted the protracted course of the disease in two patients. In this paper he drew attention to the main features of what is now known as subacute bacterial endocarditis. In 1908 Osler described the ten cases he had observed since delivering the Gulstonian Lectures, a contribution that attracted wide attention. He characterized these cases as "not marked especially by chills but by protracted fever, often not very high, but from four to twelve months' duration."

The best-known observation that he made in these patients concerns the cutaneous lesion which now carries his name. His attention was first called to this manifestation by Dr. Mullin of Hamilton, Ontario. Osler described these lesions as follows:

The spots came out at intervals as small swollen areas, some the size of a pea, others a centimeter and a half in diameter, raised, red, with a whitish point in the center. I have known them to pass away in a few hours, but more commonly they last for a day, or even longer. The commonest situation is near the tip of the finger, which may be slightly swollen. Spots of this character occurred in seven of the cases and in three at least they were of importance in determining diagnosis. Thus, in the case of Dr. Carroll, the well-known American Army surgeon, the collaborator with Dr. Reed in the brilliant work on yellow fever, the presence of these spots appeared to me to clinch the diagnosis. They are not beneath, but in the skin and they are not unlike an ordinary wheal of urticaria. I have never seen them hemorrhagic, but always erythematous, sometimes of a very vivid pink hue, with a slightly opaque center.

He stated that the symptom was known to the French, who termed it *Nodosités cutanées éphémère*. In a paper published in the *Interstate Journal of Medicine* in 1912, describing a case of "chronic infectious endocarditis" with an early history like that of splenic anemia, Osler again spoke of these lesions and stated that he believed them to be pathognomonic. It was F. Parkes Weber who in 1913 wisely suggested calling these lesions "Osler's spots" and "Osler's symptom" because it was Osler who had first called general medical attention to their full diagnostic importance and had distinguished them from the ordinary eruptions not rarely met with in cases of malignant endocarditis. They are most commonly referred to as Osler's nodes.

In commenting on Osler's recognition of polycythemia vera, Wintrobe says:

Although the concept that patients might be overburdened with blood was held by Galen and his predecessors, as well as by those who followed him, as late as 1889 the hematologist Hayem stated that he did not believe in the existence of a plethoric state which could be ascribed to an increase in red cells. In writing in 1892 "Sur une forme speciale de cyanose s'accompagnant d'hyperglobulie excessive et persistante," Vaquez attributed the condition to congenital heart disease even though there were no ausculatory signs. Failure to find evidence of congenital heart disease at autopsy made Vaquez's case more mysterious. Russell in 1902 recognized that these cases perhaps represented a new classical entity and by the time Osler's report was published, it was becoming clear that there were two classes of polyglobulism: relative, in which the condition was due to a diminution in the quantity of the plasma of the blood; and true, in which there is an actual increase in the number of blood corpuscles. Vaquez and his pupil, Quiserne, in 1902 had clearly defined true polycythemia and included the disease first described by Vaquez under this head together with conditions in which there is difficulty in proper aeration of the blood, as in high altitude or in heart disease, congenital and otherwise.

Osler first gave his report on polycythemia vera before the Association of American Physicians in May 1903. He accented the supposition of Saunby and Russell that the condition was a definite clinical entity and clearly described the syndrome. He presented four patients who typified completely the picture of polycythemia vera: the incidence in middle or late life; somewhat greater frequency in males; high incidence in Jews; presence of symptoms such as headache, vertigo, constipation, weakness, and vascular disturbances; the finding of splenomegaly in many cases; and the occurrence of leukocytosis in addition to polycythemia. Osler made it quite clear that priority of description rested with Vaquez. Osler's paper entitled "The Chronic Cyanotic Polycythemias with Enlarged Spleen," which appeared in the *British Medical Journal*, distinguished this syndrome from that caused by primary tuberculosis of the spleen. Little has been added since that time to Dr. Osler's clinical presentation.

In the *Johns Hopkins Hospital Bulletin* for November 1901, there appeared a paper by William Osler entitled "On a Family Form of Recurring Epistaxis, Associated with Multiple Telangiectasis of the Skin and Mucous Membranes." In this article he presented three cases of hereditary telangiectasia and stated that he had been able to find only a single report in the literature describing this condition (*Rendu-Gaz.* Des Hôpitaux, 1896, p. 1322): a man, aged fifty-two, whose father had had repeated attacks of melena and whose mother and brother had been subject to epistaxis, was admitted in a condition of profound anemia, having had for three weeks a daily recurrence of epistaxis. In the three patients that Osler described, two belonged to a family in which epistaxis had occurred in seven members. Both of these patients had had bleeding of the nose from childhood and both presented numerous punctiform angiomata on the skin of the face and the mucous membranes of the nose, lips, and tongue. The third patient had suffered from recurring epistaxis, and the telangiectases were most abundant over the body but numerous also on the mucous membranes. The condition, Osler pointed out, has nothing to do with hemophilia, with which the cases had been confounded. This, again, represented a classical description of a clinical syndrome which has scarcely been improved upon since Osler's time.

Osler was known as a therapeutic nihilist, but this designation does not tell the whole story. It is true that he had no sympathy for random polypharmacy and relied a great deal on "mother rest and father time." He was fond of quoting Oliver Wendell Holmes that if the entire pharmacopeia were dumped into the ocean, it would be good for the patients but very bad for the fishes. That he was interested in the development of new approaches to the effective management of diseases is illustrated by his report in 1896 of "Six Cases of Addison's Disease, with the Report of a Case Greatly Benefited by the Use of the Suprarenal Extract." Osler pointed out that recent studies had rendered it very probable that the original view of Addison was correct—namely, that the symptoms of the disease were caused by loss of function of the adrenals. Thus, the disease was analogous in all respects to myxedema and was caused directly by the loss of the internal secretion of the gland. He pointed out that the analogy would be complete if it were found that in suitable cases the use of suprarenal extract cured Addison's disease in the same remarkable way that thyroid extract relieved myxedema. Case 6, who had pulmonary tuberculosis and then gradually developed asthenia with deepening pigmentation, was treated for eight months with suprarenal extract, following which there was rapid disappearance of the serious symptoms, marked and persistent improvement in the general condition, but no change in the pigmentation. The patient was William H., age forty-six, a sailmaker admitted to the Johns Hopkins Hospital May 3, 1895. The patient had classical Addison's disease. On May 16 the treatment with suprarenal extract was started. Thirty-six pig's suprarenals were obtained at the time of slaughtering, cut up fine, thoroughly powdered with pestle and mortar, and to this mass about 6 ounces of pure glycerin added. (In commenting on this case years later, Dr. George Thorn pointed out that glycerin is the best solvent for preserving the active hormone in the suprarenal cortex.) The mixture was then filtered several times through a fine-meshed gauze. The filtrate consisted of a syrupy, reddish-brown fluid of a rather disagreeable odor. After it was filtered, there were 38 drachms of the extract so that 1 drachm corresponded to 1 adrenal capsule. The patient began with half a drachm of the extract three times a day. Dr. Thayer noted on May 24, eight days after use of the extract was begun: "The patient looks brighter and says he feels better. The pulse which had ranged from 120 to 140 is now 100. He has gained three pounds in weight."

On June 6, the amount of the extract was increased to the equivalent of three glands daily. During the week ending June 16, the patient gained 5½ pounds, a gain of 9½ pounds since the use of the extract was begun. The patient continued to take the equivalent of three glands daily. The treatment was continued throughout July and August, and in spite of the hot weather the patient improved progressively. He left the hospital on September 10. His weight on discharge was 118 pounds, a gain of 19 pounds. His condition on January 15, 1896, was recorded as follows: "The color was good. To me his face looks a little less pigmented but Dr. Thayer, who had the patient in charge during the summer while he was in the ward does not think that there is any material change in the face but thinks that discoloration is less intense on the trunk. The change in the patient's general vigor is remarkable. He walks briskly, is active, energetic, in very good spirits, and says that he is as well as he ever was in his life."

The story of Sir William Osler is too well known to consider in detail. He was born in 1849 at Bond Head, at the then edge of Ontario's wilderness, twenty-five miles from Toronto. He was the youngest boy of nine children of an Anglican missionary who served numerous parishes in twenty townships, traveling always on horseback. The mother who reared these nine children under the primitive conditions of the frontier lived not only to celebrate her one-hundredth birthday but also to see three of her sons achieve international fame, in law, banking, and medicine. Here one detects one of Osler's key possessions, superior genes. Young William came early under the salutary guidance of a Reverend Mr. Johnson, who introduced him to the wonderful world to be seen under a microscope, and before the age of twenty he had written three papers on the diatomaceae, the infusoria, and the polyzoa found in Canadian waters. Although originally directed toward the clergy, he graduated from McGill medical school in 1872 and spent the next two years in Europe studying under Virchow, Rokitansky, Jenner, and Burdon Sanderson. On his return to Montreal at the ripe age of twenty-five, he was made professor of medical institutes at McGill, which involved the teaching of physiology, pathology, and histology. The students dubbed him "the baby professor." A year later he was made pathologist to Montreal General Hospital, and in the next nine years he performed over nine hundred autopsies, the protocols of which filled five volumes written in his own hand, carefully correlating the clinical picture with his own observations at the autopsy table. On the title page of one of these volumes he wrote, "Pathology is the basis for all true instruction in clinical medicine." These exacting and instructive experiences in the postmortem room, many times repeated, undoubtedly provided the basis for the uncanny clinical sense which he displayed in later years.

In 1884, at the age of thirty-five, he was made professor of medicine at the University of Pennsylvania, then considered the highest post in medicine in this hemisphere. It is interesting that when Osler attended the International Medical Congress in London in 1881 he met there Samuel Gross, Jr., who was representing his father, the famous Philadelphia surgeon, who was too ill to attend the congress. At this time it so happened that there was a committee in Philadelphia searching for a new professor of medicine. Dr. Gross was so entranced with Osler that he immediately wrote a letter to the committee urging in the strongest terms that they consider this outstanding young man for the position. (This letter has recently come into the possession of the College of Physicians of Philadelphia.) Osler, of course, later married the widow of Samuel Gross, Jr., Grace Linzee Revere Gross. After a few years in Philadelphia, Osler came to Baltimore in 1889 and joined Dr. Welch and others in creating the new medical school, Johns Hopkins.

Warfield Theobald Longcope, Clinician and Investigator

In his remarks upon being awarded the George M. Kober Medal of the Association of American Physicians, Dr. Longcope said:

But all of us who have spent much time in the wards of a hospital are subject to the irresistible temptation of describing rare forms of disease, or of recounting the clinical features presented by a group of patients suffering from a malady that has not previously been clearly defined. Though information gained from this type of simple observation, in which I must confess to have indulged, still has some place in clinical medicine, we all know that the most fertile field of work lies in the investigation of the fundamental processes that form the basis of disease in man.

Dr. Longcope was one of the pioneers in applying the methods of laboratory research to the problems of clinical medicine. At the same time, however, he was still the "dean" of American clinicians, who by his keen observation at the bedside and his broad knowledge of medicine made several important new descriptions of disease.

Warfield Theobald Longcope was born in Baltimore, Maryland, on March 29, 1877, the son of George von S. and Ruth Theobald Longcope. He came from a distinguished line of physicians. His great-great-grandfather was Nathan Smith of Dartmouth and Yale, who treated typhoid fever in the latter part of the eighteenth century by hydrotherapy. His mother's brother was Dr. Samuel Theobald, the first professor of ophthalmology at the Johns Hopkins Medical School. In Baltimore he attended a private school under the direction of Dr. Deichman and received his undergraduate education at the Johns Hopkins University, graduating with an A.B. degree in the class of 1897. He received his M.D. degree from Johns Hopkins in 1901. In 1915 he married Janet Dana. They had four children; one of them, Christopher, has followed his father into medicine and is now doing excellent research in endocrinology.

Although he had no way of anticipating such an appointment, Dr. Longcope's training prepared him admirably for the fulltime chair of medicine that was soon to be his at the Johns Hopkins University. As Dr. Tillet pointed out in his biography of Dr. Longcope: "It is very informative to follow Dr. Longcope's career after graduation since his growth reflects what was taking place in relation to medical education and the preparation for academic medicine during that period."

During his four years in medical school he had close contacts with Welch, Halsted, Osler, Mall, Howell, and Kelly. Dr. Mall, in particular, opened a door that let him see both the rewards and difficulties of medical research. How he reacted is indicated by the fact that in 1901, the year he graduated, he published three papers. When Longcope left Baltimore at the age of twenty-four, "he took with him not only the best that this country had to offer in medical education, but also a warm and friendly graciousness in the technique of living which Baltimore can teach a receptive student." From Johns Hopkins he went to Pennsylvania Hospital in Philadelphia as resident pathologist. It seems paradoxical that this great American clinician took no internship. After ten years in Philadelphia, working first in the laboratory and later in both the laboratory and the wards, he went to New York as an associate professor at the College of Physicians and Surgeons. At that time there was a great deal of verbal conflict between clinicians and laboratory men. Dr. Longcope solved this problem by being both.

At the time Dr. Longcope went to Philadelphia, experimentation in clinical medicine was almost unheard of. Observations made at the bedside with very simple forms of apparatus, inquiries into the etiology of disease carried out by rather crude bacteriological techniques, and pathological examinations of material obtained at autopsy formed the bases for clinical studies. Venapuncture for bacteriological culture was such an innovation that he recorded, "as a daring novice trembling with apprehension I made the first blood cultures ever performed at the Pennsylvania Hospital."

While working under the direction of Simon Flexner in the Ayer Laboratory at Pennsylvania Hospital, Dr. Longcope began his studies in immunology and in the etiology of disease. Later, with David Edsall, he learned the necessity of employing chemical methods in clinical research. The story of his experience in the Ayer Laboratory is a particularly important one because here Dr. Longcope developed the combination of clinical activity and laboratory study that serves as a model of the full-time academic medical scientists who populate university departments of medicine at the present time.

The previously existing clinical laboratory of Pennsylvania Hospital was described as "a dark and evil-smelling corner in the basement, mostly reserved for urine examination." It was understandable that no clinicians had any prime interest in the activities of the laboratory. However, in 1898 the new Ayer Building was completed, equipped with new apparatus, and with it the harbinger of a new place for the laboratory in clinical medicine had arrived. Dr. Longcope at that time was looked upon by his colleagues as somewhat "wacky" for spending so much time in the laboratory when he might have been practicing clinical medicine. Furthermore, the bacteria with which he was working in the laboratory were still somewhat "theoretical" in practical medicine. As a result, he was known by the students and others in medical circles in Philadelphia as "Bugs" Longcope. However, his activities in the Ayer Laboratory included work in pathology, biochemistry, bacteriology, and serology. He also visited the wards frequently and gave valuable advice about diagnosis and treatment of patients. In 1909 he received an additional appointment as assistant professor of applied clinical medicine at the University of Pennsylvania.

In these efforts Dr. Longcope became one of the first Johns Hopkins graduates to extend to another medical school the teachings and point of view in internal medicine that Osler had initiated at the founding of the Johns Hopkins School of Medicine. When he finished his term of service at Pennsylvania, he emerged as a uniquely trained academician who set a new standard of learning in several different scientific disciplines, all merging in a broader approach to the problems of disease and an understanding of the nature of disease both etiologically and pathologically.

Longcope's reputation soon spread, and in 1911 he was appointed associate professor of medicine. At the age of thirty-seven he became Bard Professor of Medicine and director of the medical service of Presbyterian Hospital in New York City. His career was interrupted by duty in Washington during World War I, and he also later served overseas. After the war he returned to Columbia, but in 1922 he made his final change of position when he became professor of medicine at the Johns Hopkins School of Medicine.

Longcope's investigative work over the years in relation to glomerulonephritis and its pathogenesis represents classical studies, which he outlined well in his remarks at the award of the Kober Medal. He made contributions in many other fields in terms of his laboratory background and interest. A notable one was the excellent study with BAL (British Anti-Lewisite) during World War II for use in the treatment of metallic poisoning by such substances as arsenic and mercury. These reports were models of clinical investigation. His first important article on the kidney, entitled "The Production of Experimental Nephritis by Repeated Protein Injections," was published in 1913. His interest then shifted to the problem of acute hemorrhagic nephritis and its relationship to hemolytic streptococci.

To his many students, his outstanding characteristics were his powers of observation and the clinical discipline which he exhibited at all times in his visits on the wards and in his handling of patients. This led him to contribute in many areas to the better understanding of disease and its variety of clinical manifestations. Three of these major clinical contributions will be briefly presented here.

His now classic paper written in collaboration with Dr. Walter A. Winkenwerder, and entitled "Clinical Features of the Contracted Kidney Due to Pyelonephritis," was published in the *Bulletin of the Johns Hopkins Hospital* in 1933. Here for the first time the fully developed clinical picture of chronic nephritis due to bilateral pyelonephritis with shrunken kidneys was clearly described and its importance emphasized. At that time there was essentially nothing in the textbooks, or indeed in English medical literature, about this not uncommon clinical entity. It had been recognized by Lohlein in 1913, for in his article on "Schrumpfnieren" he clearly separated the pyelonephritic type as a special form of secondarily contracted kidney. Longcope and Winkenwerder described nine patients, five of whom had died in uremia and had been examined at autopsy. They described the disease as occurring most frequently in women. Its course was often characterized by attacks of pyuria accompanied by lumbar pain and sometimes by fever. In some patients the course was virtually symptomless until uremia suddenly appeared. Pyelograms showed irregularities of various types in the size and shape of the kidney, pelvis, and calyces. Evidences of impairment of renal function appeared sometimes years before death and occasionally progressed to a remarkable degree without serious symptoms.

Another disease, generally designated as "sarcoid of Boeck," was first described and pictured as an affection of the skin by Jonathan Hutchinson some ninety years ago. Hutchinson termed the condition "Mortimer's malady," thus perpetuating the name of his female patient. In 1899 Boeck published an account of cases in which histological examination of the lesions in the skin had been made, and he later added much information concerning the character of the disease and its tendency to involve not only the skin but the lymph nodes and the internal organs. After Boeck's paper, the literature on the subject grew, but it appeared principally in dermatological journals, and internists paid no attention to the condition.

This situation changed dramatically in 1936, when Longcope read a paper at the meeting of the Association of American Physicians entitled "The Generalized Form of Boeck's Sarcoid." Dr. Longcope had been collecting observations on patients affected with Boeck's sarcoid for many years. He became interested at first because of the peculiar form of lymph node involvement, but later he noted eight examples of the generalized form, making a total of seventeen cases. He described patients who revealed all of the classical manifestations of this disease. He also noted that the miliary collections of epithelioid cells in the lymph nodes were arranged in much the same form as tubercles, and he pointed out that necroses were rarely seen and no large areas of caseation were ever observed. This paper was followed by a fuller description of

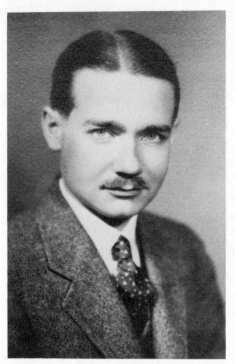

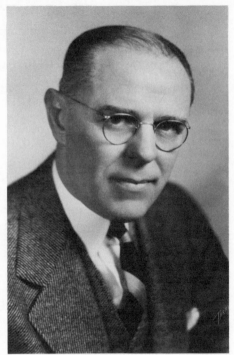

Augustus Roi Felty
Courtesy of Dr. Jean Felty Kenny

Frank Alexander Evans
Courtesy of Dr. Frederick R. Franke

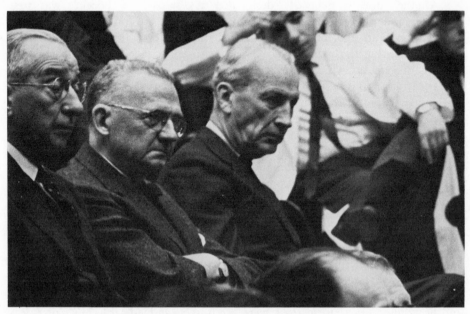

Chester Scott Keefer (*center*)
To Keefer's right is Dr. Lewis Flinn; to his left, Dr. Brownley Hodges.

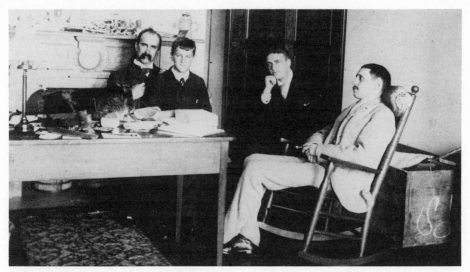

Left to right: William Osler, W. W. Francis, William S. Thayer, and H. A. LaFleur
(Osler's first resident)

This is an interesting and amusing photograph, which was sent to Dr. Ester Rosencrantz by W. W. Francis. It had been sent to Francis by Dr. John Fulton. Francis sent the following note of thanks to Fulton on January 17, 1936: "I was delighted to have the photograph. Some years ago Thayer sent me the one on William Osler's knee. It was published as a frontispiece to the February issue of the Bulletin of the Institute last year, but without warning me. They say it was William Osler's office in the year 1890. It was taken in LaFleur's living room, and I think the year was 1891. At any rate LaFleur was just packing up to return to Montreal. Notice the cat on the table and also what remains of the top hat. If I remember rightly, William Osler decided that the latter was not fit to be taken back to Montreal and started a football game with it."
From the Archives Office, The Johns Hopkins Medical Institutions. I am indebted to Dr. Earl Nation for the legend to this picture.

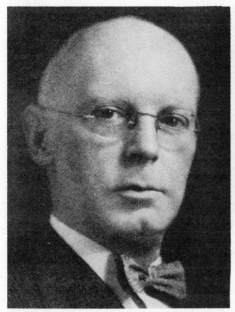

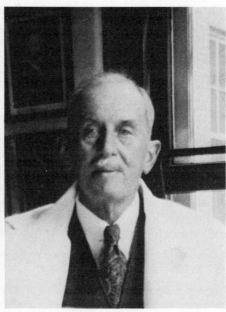

Thomas Peck Sprunt
Courtesy of Dr. Katherine Sprunt

Warfield Theobald Longcope

these cases by Warfield T. Longcope and J. William Pierson entitled "Boeck's Sarcoid [Sarcoidosis]," which appeared in the *Bulletin of the Johns Hopkins Hospital* in 1937. This paper contains the fully documented, classical description of the manifestations of sarcoidosis. One of Dr. Longcope's last papers on sarcoidosis was published in collaboration with David G. Freiman, of the Massachusetts General Hospital. This monograph was entitled "A Study of Sarcoidosis Based on a Combined Investigation of 160 Cases, Including 30 Autopsies from The Johns Hopkins Hospital and the Massachusetts General Hospital." Since the publication of these classic studies by Dr. Longcope, sarcoidosis has become a disease familiar to all practicing internists.

The third example of Longcope's brilliance at clinical observation is evident in his article, published in 1940, entitled "Bronchopneumonia of Unknown Etiology (Variety X): A Report of 32 Cases with Two Deaths," which appeared in the *Bulletin of The Johns Hopkins Hospital*. Although others had noted that there was apparently a new type of bronchopneumonia appearing sporadically in various cities of the United States, Longcope's findings provided the most thorough report of the disease. It commonly appeared in mild form, but at times it produced a serious illness or caused death. In many individuals the acute phase of the disease was preceded by a day or two of malaise with a cough which was usually unproductive but which increased in intensity. The patient's temperature was usually high; however, pulse rate and respiration were not proportionately elevated. Examination of the lungs during the first few days of illness did not disclose any conspicuous abnormality. One feature of the disease in its early stages was a moderate leukopenia. The clinical characteristics were sufficiently well defined to allow one to recognize it as a clinical entity. Longcope thought that the disease was communicable and that it had occurred in localized epidemics. For want of a better name, he called the syndrome "variety X." This keen description undoubtedly applies to what is now known as mycoplasma pneumonia, which has been shown to be associated with agglutinins to streptococcus m.g. Probably of greater diagnostic value than the streptococcus m.g. agglutination is the appearance, late in the illness, of cold agglutinins for human type O red cells, a phenomenon first described in 1918 by two members of the medical house staff—Ina Richter and Mildred Clough (*Johns Hopkins Hosp. Bull.* 29 (1918):86).

Dr. Longcope knew full well, since he had been one of the pioneers in clinical research, that the study of the mechanisms and causes of disease were to be given a higher priority than classical descriptions of new clinical syndromes. However, he was one of that generation of renaissance physicians who had the ability to perform skillfully both in the clinic and in the laboratory, an ability which is still important if one is to maintain leadership in the training of young physicians who may ultimately find their career pattern in clinical medicine as well as in research medicine.

The Classical Description of Infectious Mononucleosis

An illness characterized by enlargement of the cervical lymph nodes, failure of the glands to suppurate, and hepatosplenomegaly, which appeared in children in epidemic form and ran a favorable course, was described by Emil Pfeiffer in 1889 in a paper entitled "Glandular Fever." Following Pfeiffer's publication, similar cases were described in various parts of the world, including the United States. Attention was called to an increase in the small mononuclear elements of the blood by Burns, who reported an epidemic in the children's ward of the old Union Protestant Infirmary in Baltimore in 1909.

Articles began to appear describing a sporadically occurring infection which was thought to be related to the "glandular fever" of Pfeiffer. In 1907 Turk recorded his surprise at the recovery of a young man in whom he had made the diagnosis of acute leukemia and whose family had been told that death would soon follow. Other cases were being reported as examples of acute leukemia with spontaneous cure.

The first complete description of infectious mononucleosis and recognition that it occurred in adults as well as children came with the classic paper of Dr. Thomas P. Sprunt and Dr. Frank A. Evans, from the Division of Clinical Pathology of the Medical Clinic of the Johns Hopkins University and Hospital, published in November 1920 in the *Johns Hopkins Hospital Bulletin*. Four of the six patients whom they described were students in the medical school, three female and one male. They pointed out that the close similarity in symptomatology, in physical findings, and especially in the hematological findings made these cases a clear-cut entity. The blood picture, described accurately for the first time, was essentially the same in all of the cases, with only minor variations. The small lymphocytes, and to a lesser extent the cells of the large mononuclear-transitional group (the granular mononuclears of normal blood), were increased, but the chief change was the presence of those cells designated "large lymphocytes." Under this heading, Sprunt and Evans included all of the mononuclear-transitional group. They noted all types of pathological lymphocytes in the blood smear. They were not able to determine the significance of these cells, but concluded that they were lymphoid in origin.

Sprunt and Evans stressed that a better appreciation of the syndrome was desirable not only for the sake of accuracy in diagnosis, but also because in this relatively benign affection, with the early disappearance of fever and the more gradual return of the blood picture to normal, a favorable prognosis may be given. They also emphasized that because of the resemblance in many instances of this disease to acute lymphatic leukemia, caution should be exercised in making the latter diagnosis prematurely.

It is of interest that Dr. Walter Baetjer first used the term "infectious (or infective) mononucleosis" in 1915, when he and his colleagues, R. A. Ireland and John Rührah, described a case of lymphatic leukemia with apparent cure.

Warfield T. Longcope, with slight reservations, accepted the identity of the two diseases (in children and in adults) in his report presenting ten case histories of sporadic infectious mononucleosis with particular emphasis on the hematological abnormalities and microscopical appearance of excised lymph nodes.

The serological era in the historical development of infectious mononucleosis was ushered in by the fortuitous observation, published in 1932 by Paul and Bunnell, that the blood serum of patients with the sporadic form of this disease may contain antibodies against sheep erythrocytes in concentrations far above a normal titer, an observation made accidentally in the course of a study of nonspecific serological reactions in a variety of clinical conditions. This test soon became firmly entrenched, and was a major advance in the clinical confirmation of the diagnosis.

John R. Paul was born in Philadelphia in April 1893. After graduating from Princeton in 1915, he enrolled in the Johns Hopkins University School of Medicine. His summer vacation between his freshman and sophomore years was spent working in Dr. Grenfeld's mission in Labrador. The following year he went overseas as an enlisted man in the first American base hospital, where he worked with Walter Cannon in his investigation of shock and with Hans Zinsser on wound infections. In 1919 he received his M.D. degree from Johns Hopkins, and he stayed an additional year as assistant pathologist under Dr. W. G. MacCallum, whom he accompanied to Peru to study Oroya fever.

The late Dr. Alan Bernstein, a Johns Hopkins doctor of medicine, while an assistant resident on the Osler service, was one of the first to extensively employ the Paul-Bunnell test in the clinic. His studies were reported in the *Journal of Clinical Investigation* in 1934. Dr. Bernstein published his classic monograph on the subject of infectious mononucleosis in 1940; in it he made a plea for wider routine performance of the Paul-Bunnell test. He pointed out its usefulness as a confirmatory procedure in infectious mononucleosis as well as its value as one of the diagnostic agglutination tests performed in patients with fever of unknown origin.

One of the important conclusions of Drs. Sprunt and Evans concerned the specificity of the mononuclear cell reaction. The suggestion had frequently been made that "glandular fever" was not a clinical entity at all but, rather, a peculiar individual reaction to a number of different infectious agents. One of Sprunt and Evans's patients developed tonsillitis three months after the attack of infectious mononucleosis, but this time, instead of a mononuclear reaction, he developed the usual polymorphonuclear response. Dr. Bernstein observed a similar case in a twenty-four-year-old medical student.

Dr. Thomas Peck Sprunt was born in South Carolina in 1884. Following his graduation from Davidson College, he entered the Johns Hopkins School of Medicine, receiving his degree in 1909. He remained in Baltimore and on the staff of the Johns Hopkins Hospital thereafter, his residency in medicine being taken at the Baltimore City Hospitals under Thomas R. Boggs. In 1917 he became associated in practice with Lewellys F. Barker. Dr. Sprunt was an assistant professor of medicine at the Johns Hopkins University, and after 1922 he also taught at the University of Maryland School of Medicine. During World War II he was made acting head of the Department of Medicine in that school during Dr. Maurice C. Pincoff's period of active duty in the armed services. Sprunt was a scholarly clinician who not only gave to his patients the benefit of his years of study, investigation, and clinical experience, but also took a gentle, kindly, and sincere interest in their welfare. He died in 1955.

Frank Alexander Evans was born in Pittsburgh in 1889. He graduated from Washington and Jefferson College in 1910 and received his M.D. degree from Johns Hopkins in 1914. He interned at Hopkins and had his residency training in pathology at Presbyterian Hospital in New York. He then returned to Hopkins as an instructor in medicine associated with Dr. C. G. Guthrie in the clinical laboratory. During World War I he served in the U.S. Army Medical Corps and was attached to the first Gordon-Highlanders, British Expeditionary Forces. He was awarded the military cross. Later he returned to the Johns Hopkins Hospital Unit in France and subsequently to Baltimore, where he again took up his duties in the medical department and in the clinical laboratory. In 1922 he returned to Pittsburgh for the remainder of his distinguished career as an internist, becoming in 1924 an attending physician on the staff of Western Pennsylvania Hospital in Pittsburgh and in 1931 its physician-in-chief. In 1926 Dr. Evans published a monograph on pernicious anemia. In later years he jokingly referred to the fact that Minot's epoch-making study of liver therapy in pernicious anemia was reported at the meeting of the Association of American Physicians in the same year (May 1926). Thus, Evans' book, appearing at the same time, made no mention of this vital discovery. Nevertheless, it was a worthwhile contribution to the clinical features of the disease. Dr. Evans died in 1956.

A Case of Malta Fever Originating in Baltimore

On the eighteenth of October 1922 a nineteen-year-old white male technician who worked for Dr. Florence Sabin in the laboratory of histology was admitted to the Johns Hopkins Hospital complaining of fever and chills for three weeks. The onset of his illness was gradual, with evening fever, chills, headache, and arthralgias. Physical examination revealed only slight evidence of loss of weight, pallor, and a low-grade fever. The cause of his illness was an enigma until the answer was arrived at by an intern, Dr. Chester Scott Keefer.

In those days the medical interns rotated through the biological laboratory and did all the bacteriological work for the inpatient service, including blood cultures. Dr. Keefer kept the blood cultures on this patient in the incubator for more than the minimum length of time and noted that they became positive. On smearing out the organisms he found that they were Gram-negative, so small, in fact, that he thought they were cocci. He leafed through the bacteriology texts of the day to find out what the organism might be and finally decided that it fit the description of the bacillus melitensis. The organism was sent to the Hygienic Laboratory in Washington, where Dr. Alice Evans, who had been working with the bacillus melitensis, identified it as belonging to the abortus group.

By this time there was great excitement on the service. Dr. Charles Wainwright, who was on the house staff at the time, recalls that on a Saturday afternoon the tubes to look for agglutinins in the blood were set up, and on Sunday morning all of the interns gathered as a group to examine the results. There was clearly a positive agglutination, so that confirmation was complete— this was the first case of bacillus abortus infection in Baltimore.

The next question was: Where did the patient acquire the infection? At this stage Dr. Keefer could find no definite explanation, but since the man ate a great deal of cheese, he postulated that the patient had acquired the infection by eating cheese made from goat's milk. After Dr. Evans made the final identification of abortus strain, the matter was left to rest. However, Dr. Keefer, in his report of the case in the *The Johns Hopkins Hospital Bulletin*, identified the infecting organism as a porcine strain, since it grew readily in air, a characteristic of infections acquired from pigs.

A further review of the history disclosed that the technician made frequent trips to the abattoir to secure animal material for teaching and for research. The specimens he obtained frequently came from swine, and it became clear that this was the source of infection. Subsequently, a number of other porcine brucella infections were traced to this same abattoir. In Keefer's original case report, he had concluded that the origin of the infection was probably bovine and not caprine because it belonged to the abortus group. He stated that this was the first recorded case of a disease in man corresponding to Malta fever due to an organism belonging to the abortus group. As related, it turned out that it was the first reported case in this country of a human infection with the porcine organism.

Keefer published several other worthwhile papers while he was a member of the resident staff. A number of them were prepared in collaboration with Dr. William Resnick, a fellow resident. The most important was their classical analysis of the pathogenesis of angina pectoris. Although this paper was presented at the New York Academy of Medicine on April 17, 1928, after Keefer had joined the faculty of the University of Chicago, the ideas expressed were generated while these two friends were both members of the Johns Hopkins house staff. Their conclusions, which represented a basic advance in the understanding of coronary artery disease, were as follows:

A critical analysis of the theories that attribute angina pectoris to coronary spasm, to disease of the aorta, or to myocardial exhaustion demonstrates that these views are open to such serious criticism that they become unacceptable; on the other hand, it can be shown that anoxemia of the heart ... explains every characteristic of angina, including the likelihood of sudden death, which must be considered an integral feature of the condition.... The angina pectoris of Heberden has but one cause, anoxemia of the myocardium.

Dr. Chester Scott Keefer was born in Altoona, Pennsylvania, on May 3, 1897. After graduating from Bucknell University in 1918, he entered the Johns Hopkins School of Medicine and received his M.D. degree in 1922. During the next four years his medical training as intern and assistant resident at the Johns Hopkins Hospital launched his academic career, a most distinguished one both as teacher and as investigator, with an extraordinary production of excellent papers for one so young. From Baltimore he went to Chicago as resident physician at Billings Hospital, University of Chicago Clinics, from 1926 to 1928. In that year he married Jean Balfour, a Hopkins nurse. Together they embarked for China and Peiping Union Medical College, where he was associate professor of medicine until 1930. He was then recruited by Francis Weld Peabody to join the Thorndike Memorial Laboratories at Boston City Hospital as associate physician and assistant professor of medicine at the Harvard Medical School. Here, in the company of George R. Minot, Soma Weiss, William B. Castle, Henry Jackson, and their associates, he became one of an extraordinary group of "medical greats" who carried on Peabody's ideals of excellence in patient care, research, and training.

It was during this period that the author first met Keefer, while making rounds on his service in 1932 as a third-year medical student. These rounds were the most popular medical event in the Boston area. During his ten years at the "Thorndike," Keefer taught many fellows who later became distinguished contributors in the field of infectious diseases, including Wesley Spink, Lowell Rantz, and Charles Rammelcamp. In 1940 he left Harvard to accept a position at Boston University as professor and chairman of the Department of Medicine and as physician-in-chief and director of the Evans Department of Clinical Research and Preventive Medicine at University Hospital. For over twenty years he maintained an active role in these positions, and in 1955 he was made dean of the medical school and in 1959 director of the Boston University Medical Center. At this time he resigned his other titles to assume the position of university professor and Wade Professor of Medicine Emeritus, remaining very active in medical education and administration until his death in 1972.

During World War II, Keefer was assigned the role of monitoring the distribution of the extremely short supplies of penicillin for both military and civilian needs. He was very rigid but fair in his execution of these responsibilities, and was known as the "penicillin czar" by the press. For his outstanding services he was decorated with both the U.S. Medal of Merit and His British Majesty's Medal for Freedom. In 1953 he became Special Assistant for Medical Affairs to the first Secretary of Health, Education, and Welfare.

Keefer viewed the modern medical center as the institution best suited for total education in the medical profession. As stated by Dr. Robert Wilkins, his successor as professor of medicine: "Both by his acceptance of the position of director of the Boston University Medical Center and his refusal over the years to accept numerous offers from elsewhere to be a department head, a dean, a college president, and the like, he showed his devotion to the medical center concept and to the Boston University Medical Center in particular which he himself established."

Dr. Keefer was primarily a teacher, and as I can testify from personal experience, one of the best that this country has ever produced. He enjoyed personal bedside clinical teaching and warmly supported others in their efforts to learn medicine. Dr. Keefer lived not only to see the impressive Chester Scott Keefer Auditorium erected in his honor at the new Evans Building, but also to participate in the dedication ceremonies, at which time he said: "The discoveries made here—and no one can doubt that they will be made in abundance—will promote the gift of life: a longer, better, happier life, free of pain and misery for people everywhere." Throughout his career Dr. Keefer maintained a very active interest in and loyalty to the Johns Hopkins Medical Institutions, and he is certainly one of its most illustrious alumni.

There is an interesting sequel to Keefer's study of the technician who contracted Malta fever. In 1923 the method of staining blood cells with supravital dyes was applied by Florence Sabin to the study of developing blood cells in the embryo chick. Two years later she pointed out that this technique was so simple that it was readily applicable to the study of clinical cases. In an article published in the *Johns Hopkins Hospital Bulletin* entitled "Studies of Living Human Blood Cells," she described her observations on normal human blood cells when utilizing this method. It was evident that there were in the blood two strikingly different types of cells belonging to the monocytic strain. Indeed, she pointed out that they were so different in appearance as to require some proof that there are only two phases of life in a single cell. The first form corresponds to the large mononuclear form of Ehrlich, a cell entirely different from the large lymphocyte; the second is the transitional cell of the Ehrlich classification.

Sabin had the opportunity in her clinical studies to study Keefer's case of Malta fever, in which the findings made it clear that these were merely two phases in the life cycle of the same cell. Her observations were made before and at intervals after the administration of an autovaccine given at intervals of four to five days. In the pretreatment differential count 27 percent were large mononuclear cells and 18.5 percent transitional cells. After the second dose of the vaccine, all of the monocytes were of the transitional form. After the third dose, there was a very marked increase in the stainable substance of the transitional cells, the cytoplasm being completely filled with large stained vacuoles. That they were actively phagocytic was evident from the red blood cells that were found engulfed in them. After the fourth dose, there was a brilliant demonstration of the fact that the transitionals were merely older, more active, large mononuclear forms. The entire life cycle of the monocytic strain, from the youngest to the dying cells, could be seen in one preparation. The patient being studied was discharged from the hospital on December 10, 1922, but it was not until April of the following year that the staining reaction of the monocytes became normal.

Sabin concluded her paper as follows:

In these studies of white blood cells it has been shown that there is much evidence to favor the view that the large mononuclear cell is the young form of the monocytic strain and that the large lymphocyte is the young stage of the lymphocytes. The method offers a chance to distinguish cells that have been stimulated from those which are degenerating. I am convinced that this method opens a new phase in the study of the physiology of the white blood cells.

This is an example of how the careful study of disease in man can provide fundamental information not obtainable in the examination of the normal preparation.

Felty's Syndrome

When Dr. Augustus Roi Felty, on the Medical Service at Johns Hopkins, observed a patient with chronic arthritis associated with splenomegaly and leukopenia, he knew that he was dealing with an unusual clinical syndrome. He was familiar with the fact that slight splenic enlargement in association with arthritis had been noted by various observers. Leukopenia, he also knew, was occasionally present in arthritis, but the association of all three conditions was distinctly a new observation. He searched the hospital records for similar cases and unearthed four. This led to a study, which he reported in the *Bulletin of The Johns Hopkins Hospital* (1924) in an article entitled "Chronic Arthritis in the Adult, Associated with Splenomegaly and Leukopenia: A Report of Five Cases of an Unusual Clinical Syndrome." Little did he realize that as a result his name would be perpetuated forever in medical literature, for this syndrome has since been known as "Felty's syndrome."

Little has been added to the description given by the young assistant resident physician some fifty years ago. Felty pointed out that the syndrome occurred in individuals of middle age, the average age being fifty years. He noted that the arthritic process was distinctly chronic, the average duration of the joint involvement being four and one-half years. He observed that, in striking contrast to the prolonged course of the disease and the ubiquitous distribution of the pain which was the presenting symptom in all of the patients, the objective findings both by physical examination and roentgenographic studies were neither widespread nor indicative of a very damaging or destructive process. Rather, he was impressed by the relatively benign nature of the involvement when compared with the typical case of chronic deforming arthritis of equal duration and extent. In every one of his cases the spleen was palpably enlarged, firm but not tender. In all of the cases except one there was a slight anemia, but most striking was the leukopenia, with counts ranging from 1,000 to 4,200.

It is now recognized that this syndrome is a variant of rheumatoid arthritis, appearing in less than 5 percent of the cases coming to medical attention. The basic disease is usually deforming in nature, accompanied by subcutaneous nodules and characterized by the presence of rheumatoid factor in the serum of higher titer than is seen in patients without splenomegaly. Other manifestations of systemic rheumatoid disease such as pericarditis, episcleritis and peripheral neuropathy are often present.

Dr. Augustus Felty was born in Abilene, Kansas, on August 27, 1895. His father, John W. Felty, together with his uncle, had a general medical practice in that town. For reasons that are somewhat obscure, John W. Felty chose to relocate his practice in Hartford, Connecticut when Augustus was still quite young. Augustus attended the elementary and high schools in Hartford, where he was recognized for scholarship in Latin and Greek. He entered Yale College in 1912, intending to become a professor of Latin and Greek. However, while he was in college he had the opportunity to hear a lecture by Sir William Osler, an experience which, among other things, influenced him to enter the study of medicine. He majored in chemistry at Yale, graduating seventh in his class in 1916. He was elected to both Phi Beta Kappa and Sigma Chi. He entered the Johns Hopkins Medical School that same year and graduated in 1920, second in his class and having been elected to Alpha Omega Alpha. He interned on the Osler service in 1920–1921, and the following year he spent at Columbia Presbyterian Hospital in New York as a research fellow, during which period he studied the electrolyte and acid-base derangements in dogs during experimental pyloric obstruction. He then returned to Johns Hopkins, where he served as an assistant resident in medicine from 1922 to 1924, during which time he described Felty's syndrome.

Although he was interested in a career in academic medicine, his father urged him to return to Hartford to join him in practice. He did this somewhat reluctantly, "out of filial obligation." He practiced internal medicine with success in Hartford until 1958, when he retired to Old Saybrook, Connecticut. Felty was on the consulting staff of a number of Connecticut hospitals and was very active in the American College of Physicians. In November 1963 he had a stroke, and he died suddenly on February 4, 1964. He was married in 1926 to Alice Bryce, a Johns Hopkins nurse. They had three daughters, one of whom, Jean, is a graduate of the Johns Hopkins Medical School and an assistant professor of pediatrics in the School of Medicine at the University of Pittsburgh.

Dr. Felty's first scientific paper was published in the *American Journal of Medical Science*. It was concerned with the preparation and ionization of dialkyl-phosphoric and benzene disulphonic acid, and was written while he was majoring in chemistry at Yale. His second paper, written while he was a medical student, described an unusual double kidney he had found in a cadaver while studying anatomy. His most prolific period was 1923–1924, when he published a number of papers in association with Dr. Arthur Bloomfield and Dr. Chester Keefer, who was his lifelong friend. These papers were concerned with various subjects in the field of infectious disease and epidemiology.

15 ❦ The Second Professor of Gynecology and the Department of Art as Applied to Medicine

The Blue Umbilicus—Cullen's Sign

On March 21, 1918, a thin, wiry woman was admitted to the Church Home and Hospital. Although only thirty-eight, she had the appearance of a woman of sixty. She was the mother of seven children. For three weeks she had had pain in the right lower abdomen with intermittent attacks of abdominal distention. One week after the onset of her symptoms the umbilical region suddenly became bluish-black, although no injury had been incurred.

Thomas S. Cullen described what happened next:

With the patient asleep the uterus was found to be slightly enlarged. To the right of the uterus was a freely movable mass about 8 cm long and 5 cm broad. I was instantly reminded of a case reported by Dr. Joseph Ransohoff of Cincinnati and referred to at length on page 307 of my book on "Diseases of the Umbilicus." Dr. Ransohoff was called to see a man of 53 who presented an obscure abdominal condition. This was associated with jaundice of the umbilicus and of the umbilical region. At operation rupture of the common duct was found and the abdomen contained a large quantity of free bile. Bearing this case in mind, I dictated the following note prior to opening the abdomen: "The bluish-black appearance of the navel unassociated with any history of injury together with the mass to the right of the uterus makes the diagnosis of extrauterine pregnancy relatively certain, although the patient has not missed any period and although there has been no uterine bleeding." On opening the abdomen, I found it filled with dark blood, and attached to the fimbriated end of the right tube was an extrauterine pregnancy.

It so happened that in 1918, the year in which this operation took place, Dr. Osler's pupils and colleagues were preparing a volume of their original contributions to medicine, which was to be presented to Osler as a seventieth birthday gift. As his contribution to the volume entitled *Contributions to Medical and Biological Research, Dedicated to Sir William Osler, in Honor of His Seventieth Birthday, July 12, 1919, by His Pupils and Co-workers,* Tom Cullen prepared a paper on his case of the "blue navel," which was illustrated in color by Max Broedel (Fig. 1). From that time on, Cullen's sign had a secure place in gynecological teaching. Moreover, its use was not limited to the diagnosis of ruptured ectopic pregnancy, as illustrated by a letter to Cullen from Captain J. Mason Knox in November 1944 from the 60th Field Hospital of the U.S. Army in Europe: "One of the boys was shot in the abdomen and there was considerable discussion as to whether there was internal bleeding. I insisted he was bleeding because he had a positive 'Cullen sign' and, sure enough, when I explored I found he was hemorrhaging from the liver and stomach."

In 1893, while waiting for his promised residency in gynecology, Cullen was assigned to pathology. Little work had been done in this area in relation to gynecology. As Cullen stated, "The field was unworked, and we were among the first in it. There is nothing better than that. I know how a lumber man feels when he comes on a stand of first-growth timber or a prospector when he hits the gold-bearing rock. But this was more like placer mining. We panned everything, picked out the nuggets and added the general run to the records." Tom Cullen found life very exciting in the backwater of the pathological laboratory, where he worked in a small room on the first floor. This was the first laboratory of gynecological pathology, and its accomplishments have been both numerous and excellent. Many men who trained there later established similar laboratories elsewhere, and the field of gynecology has been greatly enriched by the new knowledge gained.

Early volumes of the *Johns Hopkins Hospital Reports* and *Bulletins* are a vivid record of the achievements of those years and from 1894 on, Cullen's share in these achievements grew steadily. In the *Johns Hopkins Hospital Bulletin* for April 1895, he published a paper on the possibility of developing a rapid method of making permanent specimens from frozen sections by using formalin. If this could be accomplished, a more accurate pathological diagnosis could be made promptly in patients undergoing operation than could be made by frozen section alone. If tissue could only be hardened more quickly for immediate examination in cases of suspected cancer, for example, surgical treatment of the majority of cases could be completed in one operation, thus relieving the suspense and fear of the necessity of a second operation in many instances. The need being recognized, a hunt for a quick and practical method of hardening tissue began in nearly every pathological laboratory. It was Cullen's good fortune to find such a method in his second year in the laboratory, recording this as a first in print. Describing the event, he stated:

I tested the formalin method I had worked out on every sort of tissue and in every way I could think of. Then I went upstairs showing one of my sections to Dr. Welch and told him how I had hardened it and how long it had taken me. He looked at it and listened. Then he handed me a piece of tissue that Schutz [Dr. Welch's diener] was about to prepare for him. "Take this and prepare it your way," he said. "If you make me a satisfactory specimen, I will be convinced." I took the tissue and made a specimen and brought it back. Popsy looked at it, looked at his watch and said, "Publish it." So I did. I wrote up the method and took my paper to Dr. Hurd, who was then editor of the *Johns Hopkins Hospital Bulletin*, the same night, but it was nearly too late. Dr. Hurd said he was sorry, but the last copy for the next issue of the *Bulletin* had gone to the printer and mine would have to wait a month. I was going away on that comment, but he called me back and asked me how much space I would need to describe my hardening method. I said half a page, and he said "go ahead and write it then." "It's written," I said, and gave it to him, and it was in print in the *Bulletin* two days later.

Thomas Cullen was born in Bridgewater, Ontario, Canada, on November 20, 1868. He received his medical education at the University of Toronto, graduating in 1890. While an intern at Toronto General Hospital, he assisted at an operation performed by Dr. Howard A. Kelly, and was so impressed with Kelly's surgical skill that he decided at once to go to Baltimore and work under him. This opportunity was made available, and he began his duties as a member of the hospital staff in January 1892. Although he was promised a residency position to replace William Wood Russell, who had planned to leave the hospital in the summer of 1893, when Cullen returned from pathological work in Europe in October 1893, he found that the position was no longer open. This was a fortuitous quirk of fate, as he then took up an assignment in gynecological pathology, with the excellent results already described. In 1896 he became resident gynecologist, serving in that capacity for a year, and then resigned from the resident staff to enter private practice in Baltimore. He retained his connection with the hospital as a member of the visiting staff and as an active teacher in the school. When Kelly retired in 1919, gynecology was made a subdepartment of the Department of Surgery, and Cullen was placed in charge as professor of clinical gynecology, a post he held until his retirement in 1939.

Among Dr. Cullen's many important contributions to Johns Hopkins— including his work on endometriosis, which will be discussed later—was his role in raising money for the endowment of a new department, the Department of Art as Applied to Medicine. This provided a secure place for Hopkins's first medical illustrator, Max Broedel, and led to the training of many talented medical artists whose accomplishments over the years have been a credit to the Hopkins Medical Institutions.

Art as Applied to Medicine—The Fabulous Max Broedel

There appeared in the September 1911 issue of the *Johns Hopkins Hospital Bulletin* a one-page article entitled "The New Department in The Johns Hopkins University: Art as Applied to Medicine." The article was by Max Broedel, associate professor of art as applied to medicine, and in it, Broedel pointed out that the illustrations of medical publications were as a rule far below the standard set by other publications, both in regard to the correctness of the pictures and their artistic merits. The reason for this, he believed, was that there were no schools of instruction in this important branch of art, and all medical illustrators were self-taught. The illustration of medical books is a highly specialized form of art, requiring on the part of the artist not only reliable draftsmanship and adequate technique, but also a thorough understanding of medicine in most of its branches. To bridge the gap between art and medicine, the Johns Hopkins University had created a department under the general title "Art as Applied to Medicine." Here a new generation of medical illustrators could be trained, sparing them the years of trial and disappointment that their self-taught predecessors had endured. Instruction was designed to

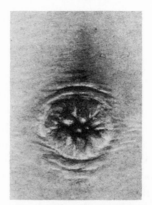

Fig. 1. The "blue navel"

Drawing by Max Broedel for Cullen's article in *Contributions to Medical and Biological Research* (New York: Paul B. Hoeber, 1919), p. 420. (Broedel Collection, Department of Art as Applied to Medicine, The Johns Hopkins School of Medicine)

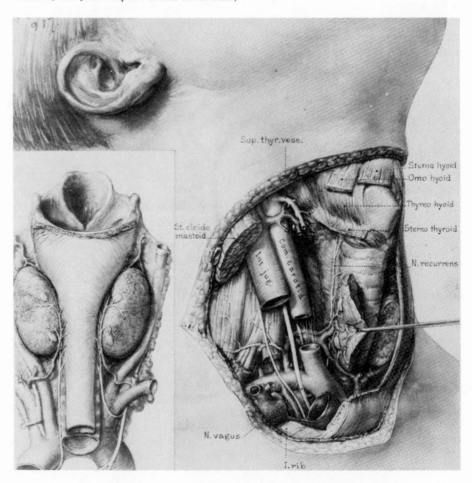

Fig. 2. The operation for exophthalmic or hyperplastic goiter

Drawings by Max Broedel, 1917. Plate 84 from W. S. Halsted: *The Surgical Papers*, vol. 2 (Baltimore: Johns Hopkins University Press, 1952)

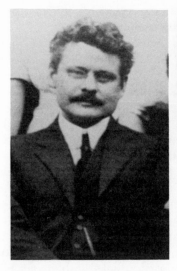

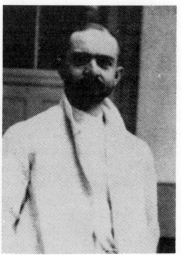

Max Broedel

From the Archives Office, The Johns
Hopkins Medical Institutions

Thomas S. Cullen

From A. M. Chesney, *The Johns
Hopkins Hospital and The Johns
Hopkins University School of Medicine: A Chronicle*, vol. 2, *1893–
1905* (Baltimore: The Johns Hopkins University Press, 1958)

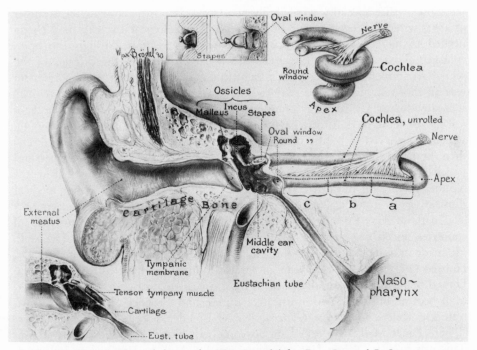

Fig. 3. Drawing of the ear by Max Broedel for Drs. Samuel J. Crowe
and Stacey Guild

From the Broedel Collection, Department of Art as Applied to Medicine, The Johns Hopkins School
of Medicine

meet the needs of two groups, medical students and art students, and course work for the two groups was outlined in the announcement.

Max Broedel, a kindly, curly-haired man who was one of the greatest medical illustrators up to that time, was himself self-taught. He considered his early attempts in the medical field to be unsuccessful, recognizing that his early training had not fully qualified him as a medical artist. From 1885 to 1890 he attended the Gewerbe Schule and Kunstakademie at Leipzig, where he first studied the basic principles of all artistry, copying originals, then drawing from the cast and finally from life. He also studied lithography, and he later attributed to this early training in the graphic arts his uncanny ability to draw medical illustrations with such technical accuracy. He remembered vividly the many weary months spent in the lithographic department; the hand stippling required in chromolithography was particularly trying. It seemed useless to him to spend many days placing on stone millions of little dots, the aggregate of which represented the yellow plate of a landscape, a color so faint that it hardly showed in the print. Then came a gray, a blue, and so on through twelve to twenty colors, each on a separate stone and each stippled in by hand. His friend Horn, who sat at the adjoining desk, also found the work very trying, but both artists later realized that the exercise taught them the patience necessary for a prolonged task such as that involved in reproducing a microscopic picture. They also acquired a steadiness of hand and a control of line that were useful assets in medical drawing.

Until 1893, Broedel had no ambition to become a medical illustrator; his selection of that specialty was wholly accidental. It came about in the summer of 1888, when Professor Carl Ludwig of the Physiological Institute in Leipzig needed to have a color microscopic picture of a section through the brain enlarged about 150 times. His artist was not available, and the director of the school recommended Broedel as a substitute. To make such an enlargement was an enormous task, for it required the portrayal of all the cells in a strip six inches wide and a yard long. There was no camera lucida or any other mechanical aid in those days. Broedel worked many years to make that first drawing, which he believed to be the most difficult he ever attempted. He did not know then, he later stated, that the only way to plan a picture is to leave paper and pencil alone until the mind has grasped the meaning of the object. It was a blunder to rely on faithful copying alone. "Copying," he said, "is not medical illustrating; in a medical drawing full comprehension must precede execution."

In those days Ludwig's laboratory was the mecca for medical men of all countries, and it was there that Broedel first met Dr. Welch and later Dr. Mall. He made drawings of the reticulum for Dr. Mall and drawings of goiter for Dr. Halsted (Fig. 2). After two years of careful thought, he decided to come to the United States for a few months, or at most a year, to work for Mall. However, Mall became busy with administrative duties, and Broedel undertook to illustrate Dr. Kelly's *Operative Gynecology*. As Broedel described this event later: "There I met Mall, who asked me to come to Chicago and illustrate for him. This was in 1891. When I accepted in 1893, Dr. Mall had moved to Baltimore to organize the new anatomical department at the Hopkins. He was too busy to utilize the services of an illustrator and glad when Dr. Kelly offered to take one off his hands."

When he arrived in Baltimore on January 18, 1894, he was greeted at dockside by Cullen. He was a bit dismayed by the city, which he found unattractive, but was soon enamored with its kind inhabitants and challenged by his work, which he found totally different from anything he had ever done. He began his work by using a series of photographs, taken by Anthony Murray, illustrating the various steps of operations, but he soon realized that emancipation from the camera was an absolute necessity for the medical illustrator. After a few months, he completely rejected photographic aid, realizing that independence of judgment and originality of conception were only to be gained by original study. So, with Dr. Kelly's permission, he systematically dissected and studied the anatomical regions with which their work was concerned. Broedel found that in making dissections or by watching operations, he automatically obtained a series of vivid mental pictures that served admirably as guiding images during the subsequent task of drawing. Broedel's approach to medical illustration is best described in his words:

In order to function effectively, the artist must originate a different type of picture; one that shows far more than any photograph could ever do. He must first fully comprehend the subject matter from every standpoint: anatomical, topographical, histological, pathological, medical and surgical. From this accumulated knowledge grows a mental picture from which he crystallizes the plan of the future drawing. Therefore, the planning of the picture is the all important thing, not the execution. There is where we learn from Dr. Kelly. He had a way of making little modest outline sketches when he explained his operative procedure to his illustrators. He invented diagrams to show variations of form and relationship, motion, pressure, tension, rupture, the sequence of operative steps, the placing of sutures, etc. In short, every clinical phenomenon, every operative procedure flowed in simple eloquent lines from the end of his pencil. Few medical men can do that. We understood his diagrams; they were eloquent. In this way Dr. Kelly taught his artists the secret of the correct conception of an illustration, which is the very basis of all creative drawing. This is one great debt we owe to Dr. Kelly.

While making a drawing, the conscientious artist has a way of discovering gaps in contemporary knowledge; so when knowledge was lacking and the literature silent on the subject, Dr. Kelly always permitted the artist to make original investigation to clear up the obscure point. That meant temporary cessation of illustrative output until the question could be answered. Few authors of medical books will do that. Without his sympathetic attitude, we could not have learned our trade as we did.

When Broedel first arrived in Baltimore, there were no other artists at Hopkins. As one might well imagine, Dr. Kelly was asked from time to time by members of the hospital staff to lend them his artist. Thus, Broedel also did illustrations for Barker, Cullen, Clark, Crowe, Cushing, Dandy, Halsted, Heuer, Mall, Russell, and others (Fig. 3). He was obviously very busy, but about a year after his arrival, Hermann Becker, an old friend of his from Leipzig, came to assist him at Hopkins. The only difference in their training was that Becker had studied wood engraving. Becker became a master in his specialty, which was particularly fitted for microscopic drawings, and he contributed illustrations to Cullen's work on cancer and Kelly's and Hurdon's work on the appendix. In 1898 another old colleague, August Horn, arrived, having had the advantage of several additional years of study in Munich and in Italy. He soon proved his worth by his watercolor drawings of breast tumors for Drs. Halsted and Bloodgood. For the next several years these three men, Becker, Horn, and Broedel, worked together closely, each interested in his own field and method, but benefiting from criticisms of each other's drawings. They all worked on Kelly's publications, and the success of one proved an inspiration to the others. Each made many important technical contributions to medical illustration in the thousands of drawings they prepared for the various books and articles written by the faculty and staff of the Johns Hopkins University School of Medicine and Hospital. The fantastic results of their work are known throughout the world.

But Broedel was not only a marvelous artist, he was also a true investigator. For example, Cullen related that on one occasion Dr. Kelly wanted some anatomical data about the blood supply of the kidney. Broedel went to the autopsy room, obtained a normal-looking kidney, and attaching it by a tube to the tap, washed the blood out of it. He then filled the arteries of the kidney with red dye, the veins with blue dye, and the ureter with yellow dye. Next, he dissected the kidney, using the method he had seen Mall employ in Ludwig's laboratory in Leipzig. The vascular portions of the kidney reminded him of the branches of an apple tree, and all over these branches were minute apples—the glomeruli, or filters, of the kidney. Broedel pointed out the avascular area in the kidney and suggested opening the kidney along this line when exploring it for stones. Before finishing this kidney investigation, he developed a suture which could be used to "stitch up the kidney that had fallen down." This suture is still referred to as "Broedel's suture." It is triangular, and so placed that a piece of kidney will tear out before the suture will give way.

Cullen also related an interesting story of how vivid Broedel's illustrations really were. In February 1923 Cullen underwent a gall bladder operation, with the removal of many stones. Max Broedel was present at the operation and took the gallstones to his studio, where he made a facsimile in color of Cullen's name with the date and also a frame for the picture patterned after the large and irregular stones. So graphic was the picture that when one of Cullen's special nurses saw it, she immediately put out her hand to pick off one of the gallstones from the frame; she really thought that the large stones had been glued to the picture.

Max Broedel believed that the training of other artists was just as important as his own artwork. Therefore, he always gave much time and thought to the instruction of anyone, artist or amateur, who was interested in medical illustrating. He found talented pupils not only among artists but also among the medical faculty and students (Fig. 4). Beginning in 1905, while he was still in the employ of Dr. Kelly, he conducted a class in general technical sketching for histology, gross anatomy, and pathology, and he devoted several hours each week to teaching research workers in various departments. He also gave special

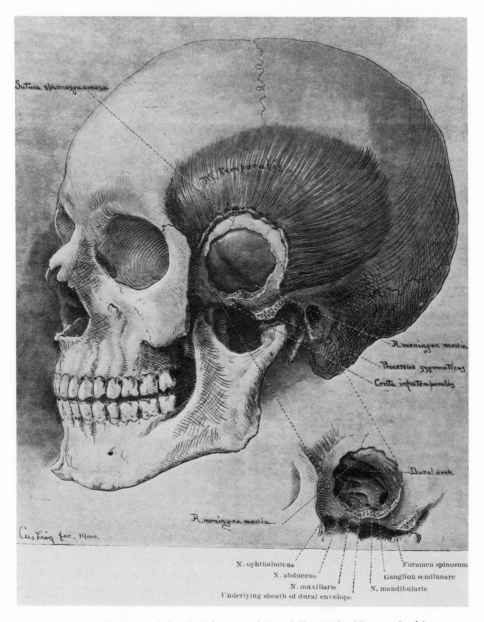

Fig. 4. A drawing of the skull by one of Broedel's pupils, Harvey Cushing

From the Broedel Collection, Department of Art as Applied to Medicine, The Johns Hopkins School of Medicine

instruction to a few exceptionally talented medical students. Horn and Becker, on the other hand, continued to produce excellent illustrations, but neither became involved in teaching activities.

In 1909 Horn became ill, and after a lingering illness he returned to Germany, where he died in 1910. Becker's health unfortunately also became impaired, and he was obliged to abandon his work temporarily. In December 1910 Broedel's work for Dr. Kelly was completed, and he was faced with the possibility of severing his connections with Johns Hopkins. This he was loath to do, knowing that if he left, much of what he had started would probably be abandoned. He did, however, receive an urgent invitation to join the staff of one of the big private clinics in America.

Cullen was worried sick about the possibility of Broedel's departure. In thinking over what he could do to prevent this, Cullen "dreamed of a Department of Art as Applied to Medicine at The Johns Hopkins Medical School." Here artists who wanted to make medical art their lifework could get specialized training for two or three years. Medical students could be taught how to make charts and blackboard illustrations, and the head of the department could use his spare time to illustrate articles published by members of the faculty.

Just four days before Broedel had to give his answer, Cullen successfully enlisted the aid of a hardheaded businessman who had a deep interest in art, Mr. Henry Walters, in establishing such a department. To that end, Walters promised the school $5,000 a year for three years. On receipt of Walters' letter, Cullen invited President Remsen and the trustees of the university to luncheon at the Maryland Club on forty minutes' notice, since prompt action was necessary. The letter was read, and the trustees at once accepted the generous offer; thus, the Department of Art as Applied to Medicine came into being. (The correspondence between Walters and Cullen is deposited in the Incunabula Room at the Walters Art Gallery.)

In the spring of 1937, R. W. Green, of the W. B. Saunders Company of Philadelphia, told Cullen that his company wanted to honor Max Broedel. Cullen suggested that they do this by having Broedel's portrait painted and presented to the Johns Hopkins University. It was painted by Thomas Corner, and in the late afternoon of March 4, 1938, a host of Broedel's friends met at the Barkley Hotel in Philadelphia, where they were joined by leaders in medicine and surgery from all over the country. Howard Kelly and Maurice Fishbein, the distinguished editor of the *Journal of the American Medical Association*, told of Broedel's profound influence on medical illustration. Henry Mencken described the celebrated Saturday Night Club, which he and Max Broedel had started in 1910. Lawrence Saunders then presented the Corner portrait of Max Broedel to the university.

Max Broedel, in revolutionizing medical illustrating, placed it on a very high plane, and his pioneer work in the field was of inestimable value to medicine and surgery. His own description of his work and of his department is given in a paper entitled "Medical Illustration," which appeared in the *Journal of the American Medical Association* on August 30, 1941. Broedel was made an honorary member of the Medical and Chirurgical Faculty of Maryland in 1909; he was the first layman to be given this honor.

The Department of Art as Applied to Medicine has trained students uninterruptedly since 1911, and now offers the degree of Master of Arts in medical and biological illustration, as well as producing excellent illustrations and offering exhibit services. What a fitting memorial to the outstanding medical illustrator of all time, Max Broedel!

Endometriosis

Members of the Department of Gynecology of Johns Hopkins, beginning with Thomas S. Cullen, have played an important role in the development of our knowledge of endometriosis. Endometriosis is divided into separate clinical and pathological types, which appear to be essentially different diseases. One is internal endometriosis, more often called "adenomyosis," which is the involvement of the myometrium by endometrium from within the uterine cavity. The other is external endometriosis, which is the involvement of tissues outside the uterus or the uterine serosa.

Adenomyosis was first described by Rokitansky in 1860. Sporadic reports appeared until 1896, when von Recklinghausen established it as a definite pathological entity. In 1897 Thomas S. Cullen reported his first case of "adenomyoma" of the uterus, and in 1908 he published his classic monograph on this disease, reporting ninety-two cases. He also recognized "diffuse adenomyoma of the uterus," now more properly designated as adenomyosis. It was von Recklinghausen's contention that the intramural endometrium was derived from Wolffian tubular rests. Cullen, however, offered the most generally accepted theory that the tissue is of Müllerian origin and is a direct downgrowth from the uterine cavity. He was able to show by serial sections in cases of diffuse adenomyosis a direct continuity between the basalis of the endometrium and the endometrial islands within the areas of adenomyosis.

External endometriosis, or ectopic endometrium growing elsewhere than in the uterine musculature from within, is of clinical importance more frequently than is adenomyosis. Endometriosis of the ovary was first described by William Wood Russell, associate in gynecology at Johns Hopkins, in a paper read before the Johns Hopkins Medical Society on April 4, 1898. His paper, entitled "Aberrant Portions of the Müllerian Duct Found in an Ovary," was published the following year in the *Johns Hopkins Hospital Bulletin*. In the specimen he described, there was a collection of glands in a groove on the surface of the ovary. The epithelium covering them was continuous with a single layer of columnar cells at the margin and extended a short distance over the surrounding surface. Russell stated: "Thus we have direct proof that the germinal epithelium is capable of producing glands analogous to those of the uterine mucosa." Russell's findings were beautifully illustrated in the accompanying drawings by Max Broedel (Fig. 5).

William Wood Russell was born in Minneapolis on July 29, 1866. His

PLATE I

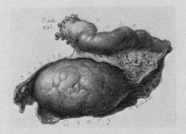

Fig. 1.—Natural size, showing normal tube with patent fimbriated extremity. Ovary posterior view with portion of adventitious capsule.

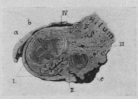

Fig. 2.—Longitudinal section through centre of ovary.

I. Space partially surrounding corpus luteum (b) lined with epithelium, in which on lower side glands were present.

II. Groove, at bottom of which is a wedge of tissue made up of glands and interglandular tissue covered with a single layer of epithelium continuous with that on the surface.

III. Space lined with columnar epithelium and surrounded by mucous membrane of the uterine type and non-striped muscle.

IV. Point beneath adhesions, (a) where germinal epithelium was preserved. (c) Cystic follicle.

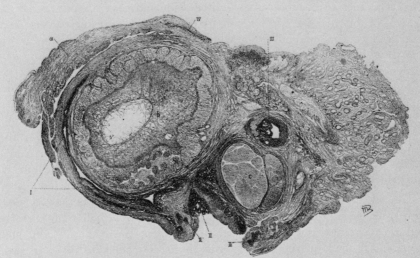

Fig. 3.—Longitudinal section through ovary and hilum posterior face. (Magnified four times.)

I. Corresponds to I, Fig. 2. In the lining of the space toward the centre of the ovary is seen distinct gland formation.

II. Corresponds to II, Fig. 2, in which the glands can be plainly seen, some of which are cystic.

II'-II''. Groups of glands near surface of ovary surrounded by distinct stroma of uterine type.

III. Space surrounded by mucous membrane and muscle, an exact prototype of the uterine mucosa and muscle, some of the glands cystic, corresponds to III, Fig. 2.

IV. Germinal epithelium in adhesions. (a) Adhesions forming capsule. (b) Corpus luteum. (c) Cystic Graafian follicle. Right corner of section represents vascular zone of hilum, entirely free from glands.

Fig. 5. Aberrant portions of the Müllerian duct found in an ovary

Drawings by Max Broedel for W. W. Russell

From *Johns Hopkins Hosp. Bull.* 10 (1899): 8

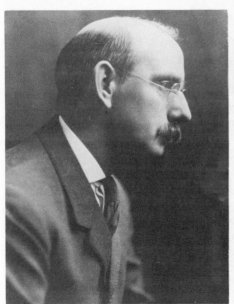

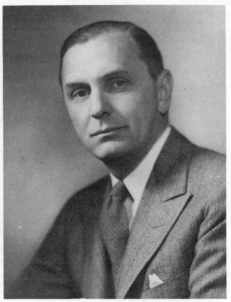

William Wood Russell
Courtesy of Mrs. Stewart Lindsay

Richard W. TeLinde
Courtesy of Dr. Richard W. TeLinde

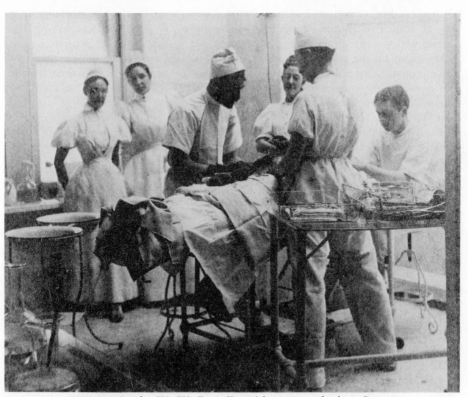

An operation by W. W. Russell, resident gynecologist, 1894–95

Left to right, facing camera: Miss Gross, sister of Mrs. J. M. T. Finney; Miss Carr (Mrs. Iglehart);
Dr. Russell; Miss Cooke, later head nurse at Dr. Kelly's clinic
Courtesy of Mrs. Stewart Lindsay

family was among the first settlers of St. Anthony's Falls, later Minneapolis. Russell received his degree in civil engineering at the Pennsylvania Military Academy in 1887. He then entered the University of Pennsylvania Medical School, receiving his M.D. degree in 1890. He served as an assistant resident gynecologist at the Johns Hopkins Hospital from April 1891 through January 1894 and as resident gynecologist from February 1894 to February 1895. The next year he studied at Göttingen and Berlin, and visited other leading European universities. In April 1899 he became an associate in gynecology at Johns Hopkins and gynecologist at the Union Protestant Infirmary, the Church Home, and the Woman's Hospital. He was a founder of the American College of Surgeons and a member of the Southern Surgical Association and of numerous other societies. He developed a large private practice in Baltimore, but was forced to retire in 1921 because of failing health. He moved to California and died on July 11, 1923, in Colorado Springs.

Russell's observations lay fallow for a number of years, until in 1921 Albertson Sampson published the first of a series of twenty-one papers on a condition for whose recognition and study he became internationally famous, namely, endometriosis and "chocolate" cysts of the ovary. His most important contribution was his theory of implantation, which he described as follows:

Ovarian and other forms of peritoneal endometriosis arise from the implantation of bits of Müllerian mucosa, of either uterine or tubal origin, which, having been carried with menstrual blood escaping through patent tubes into the peritoneal cavity, have lodged on the surfaces of the various pelvic structures. The ectopic mucosa in these implants, regardless of their size or situation, may become additional foci for the spread of the endometriosis by direct extension and also by the implantation of bits of Müllerian tissue which escape from them during their reaction of menstruation. This latter phenomenon is most spectacular in the ovary where ectopic endometrial cavities may attain a much larger size than elsewhere, forming the well-known endometrial cyst of that organ.

Sampson operated on many patients at the time of menstruation and frequently observed blood coming from the ends of the tubes. He fixed and sectioned this blood and demonstrated the presence of uterine mucosa, which he believed to be viable.

Cullen stated that "those who were associated with Sampson during his years as intern, assistant resident and resident gynecologist at The Johns Hopkins Hospital will never forget that quiet, earnest, and reliable man who by his intimates was known as 'Sammy.'" Born in Troy, New York, on August 17, 1873, he received his A.B. degree from Williams College in 1895 and in the same year entered the Johns Hopkins Medical School. Whereas his first medical paper, published in January 1902, was on flat feet, in the four years from 1902 through 1905, while he served as an assistant resident and resident in gynecology, he published seventeen papers on gynecological subjects. In 1905 he opened an office in Albany, New York, and soon became associated with the Albany Medical College, on whose faculty he served until 1945, when he retired from the professorship of gynecology and as gynecologist-in-chief of the Albany Hospital.

Interesting as Sampson's observations were, it was not until recently that clear experiments were done to show whether or not the cast-off particles of menstrual endometrium are capable of implantation and growth. In 1950 Roger Scott and Richard TeLinde reported some experimental work which seemed to demonstrate the capability of growth of desquamated menstrual endothelium. The uteri of ten rhesus monkeys were divided from their vaginal attachments and rotated on their ovarian axes to allow intraperitoneal menstruation to occur, spilling the menstrual flow in the cul-de-sac or upward toward the diaphragm. Six of the ten animals developed typical areas of endometriosis within the peritoneal cavity. Growing evidence also came from the Department of Gynecology at Johns Hopkins in 1959, when Ridley and Edwards collected the menstrual flow of ten women through a cervical cannula for twelve hours. This material was centrifuged and the sediment injected into the rectus muscle of the same patient, who was to have a laparotomy 90 to 100 days after the single injection. One of these patients had a definite area of endometriosis 175 days after injection, and another had an area suggestive of endometriosis at 110 days. Three of the women had a noncommunicating horn of a double uterus; the only exit of the menstrual flow from the noncommunicating horn was through the fallopian tube, and each woman developed endometriosis in the ovary on the side of the rudimentary horn.

TeLinde's contributions to our knowledge about carcinoma-in-situ of the cervix have already been noted in an earlier chapter, but he also made a notable observation relating to the pathogenesis of endometriosis. Richard TeLinde was born in Waupum, Wisconsin, on September 2, 1894. He graduated from the University of Wisconsin in 1917 and from the Johns Hopkins Medical School in 1920. From 1920 to 1925 he remained in residency training in gynecology at Johns Hopkins. He entered practice in Baltimore, and in 1939 he was appointed professor of gynecology and gynecologist-in-chief of the Johns Hopkins Hospital. He served in these positions until his retirement in 1960. Dr. TeLinde is still active in the practice of gynecology some fifteen years after his retirement from the chairmanship of the Department of Gynecology.

TeLinde has made many important contributions to gynecology in addition to his work on carcinoma-in-situ and endometriosis. He is also the author of a text on operative gynecology which has become a classic in that field. In 1953 he was elected president of the American Gynecological Society.

16 ❧ John Whitridge Williams—
His Contributions to Obstetrics

J. WHITRIDGE WILLIAMS, affectionately known as "the Bull," was chief of the Department of Obstetrics of the Johns Hopkins Hospital and professor of obstetrics in the Johns Hopkins University for thirty-two years. Born in Baltimore on January 26, 1866, he was the son of Dr. Philip C. and Mary Cushing Whitridge Williams. His father, who came from Winchester, Virginia, had graduated in medicine from the University of Pennsylvania in 1850, studied in Paris, and finally settled in Baltimore to practice. He was a man of high reputation with a keen and logical mind, and in 1867 he was president of the Medical Faculty of the District of Baltimore. A medical career seemed natural to J. Whitridge Williams, for in addition to his father's career, members of his mother's family had practiced medicine in America for more than 160 years and in Baltimore for over 110 years.

After three preparatory years at Baltimore City College, Williams entered the Johns Hopkins University, where he became interested in chemistry under the stimulating influence of Ira Remsen. He graduated in 1886, the first and only student to take the A.B. degree in two years. Two years later, at age twenty-two, he received his medical degree from the University of Maryland and went at once to Vienna and Berlin for general courses in bacteriology and pathology.

The following year he joined the gynecological-obstetrical staff of the newly opened Johns Hopkins Hospital as a voluntary outside assistant, helping with the operations in the morning and working up the operative material in the pathological laboratory in the afternoon. He was the youngest member ever admitted to the American Gynecological Society (1892), with a thesis on tuberculosis of the female generative organs.

Although Williams had planned to establish his career in gynecology, he switched to obstetrics because of the unusual opportunity for developing this field at Hopkins. In 1894 he went abroad for another year, first to Leipzig to study obstetrics. Then, while working in Chiari's laboratory in Prague, he produced a fine monograph on sarcoma of the uterus. After a visit to Paris, he returned to become associate professor of obstetrics at Johns Hopkins until 1899. In that year Howard A. Kelly was made head of gynecology, and Dr. Williams became professor of obstetrics in the university and obstetrician-in-chief to the hospital. However, throughout his life, Williams had a strong conviction that gynecology and obstetrics should constitute a single department. He voiced this opinion firmly in May 1914 in an address as president of the American Gynecological Society: "I hope I may live to see the day when the term obstetrician will have disappeared and when all teachers, at least, will unite in fostering a broader gynecology, instead of being divided as at present into knife-loving gynecologists and equally narrow-minded obstetricians who are frequently little more than trained man-midwives." Williams was well ahead of his time in this belief, and also in recognizing that the methods of science must be applied to the study of the day-to-day problems seen in the clinic by the gynecologist and the obstetrician.

The year 1911 found Williams dean of the medical school, a position he held with distinction until 1923. In 1919 he became chairman of the first full-time department of obstetrics in the country. He had been among those who strongly supported the creation of fulltime clinical posts, and after his appointment he was able to give himself more fully to research and to the service of his new clinic. With J. Hall Pleasants, he was also responsible for a major reorganization of Bay View (Baltimore City Hospitals). Full-time staffs in pathology, medicine, and surgery, with representatives from Welch's laboratory as visiting and resident pathologists, were established, and free access to the clinics there was accorded to students from all Baltimore medical schools.

During the height of his career, Williams was a prolific contributor to obstetrical and gynecological pathology, although he advocated the use of other approaches and laboratory methods, especially physiology and chemistry. The early creation of a chemical laboratory promoted the study of the metabolism of pregnant women as a basis for creating a better understanding of the abnormalities which might appear during pregnancy. Howard Kelly, in a review of Williams's scientific contributions, was astounded at the amount and regularity of his output and above all at the fairness with which he consistently handled his material. After a preliminary surgical paper in 1890 reporting attempts to fasten the retroflexed uterus to the abdominal wall without opening the abdomen, he published in 1891 four communications of significance: "two on obstetrics and two on pathology." His early studies dealing with bacteriology and pathology were carried out in the pathological laboratory of Dr. Welch. Later on, after accumulating a great deal of material, Williams began statistical studies which continued without intermission during his entire period as head of obstetrics. Between 1891 and 1926 he produced seven careful analyses of contracted pelves and their effect upon labor. His notable early publications concerned with pelvic pathology include "Papillary Cystoma of the Ovary" (1891) and "The Deciduoma Malignum" (1895). Studying particularly the pelvic outlet, Williams demonstrated the importance of the funnel-shaped pelvis due to a narrowing of the diameter between the tubera as a common cause of dystocia. He also collected a great deal of material leading to the publication of a monograph on spondylolisthesis (1899). The investigation of the toxemias of pregnancy (begun in 1905, continued with Slemons in 1907) was a major interest for him and for his staff, and these studies added a great deal to the knowledge of the clinical course and treatment of toxemia. Among his monographs on pathology were elaborate investigations of chorio-epithelioma, hydatidiform mole, placental infarcts, syphilis, tuberculosis, and many other subjects. The work on premature separation of the placenta demonstrated the effectiveness of careful correlation between the pathological and clinical material. He found that the lesions, frequently not limited to the placental site, included hemorrhages of variable size into the uterine musculature. The resultant impairment, modifying the contractions in labor and subsequently, was responsible for hemorrhage requiring hysterectomy. In all, Dr. Williams's contributions to the literature comprised some 120 papers and his famous textbook.

One unusual but very searching paper was his presidential address in 1914 before the American Gynecological Society, in which he asked the question: "Has the American Gynecological Society done its part in the advancement of obstetrical knowledge?" To find the answer, he carefully tabulated an analysis of 1,010 papers that had been read before the society during the previous thirty-eight years. Of these, 664 were on gynecological subjects and 346 on obstetrical topics. He classified the 346 obstetrical papers according to his estimates of their merit. In his words:

With as little bias as possible, I have attempted to form a judgment as to the value of the papers, and I have designated as good or creditable those in which the subject under consideration was presented in a useful and attractive manner, but without adding anything new, and as excellent such papers as had contributed, even to a slight extent, to the sum total of obstetrical knowledge. Judged by these criteria, I have placed 42 papers in the former and 27 in the latter category, 12 and 8% respectively. Consequently it would appear that on the average less than two creditable papers have been contributed each year and that only two [truly original] contributions could be expected in three years. Surely this is not a showing of which our society can be proud.

He was greatly surprised to find a complete dearth of papers on certain important subjects, such as the biological and biochemical aspects of pregnancy. It was his opinion that the main reason for the failure of the society to advance obstetrical knowledge was the complete absence in this country of true university departments of obstetrics and/or gynecology in the sense that chemistry, physics, and biology were true university departments. In those sciences full-time faculty members devoted all their time to teaching and research; and so, relieved of the burden of earning a living by any kind of extra-departmental activity, were in a position to advance knowledge. To quote Williams again:

There is no doubt in my mind that the professorial chairs in the university medical schools need to be filled by broadly trained scientific men who are prepared to give their time to their duties. Such a development, however, is scarcely to be expected until the universities are prepared to equip and maintain women's clinics somewhat similar to the "Frauenkliniks" of Germany, but more liberally provided with laboratories for the anatomical, chemical, pathological, and physiological investigation of gynecological and obstetrical problems. In this event the director must be an accomplished scientific man in addition to being a competent clinician, who will devote the major portion of his time to the conduct of his department. Institutions of this character will also require the services of a large staff of well-trained and enthusiastic

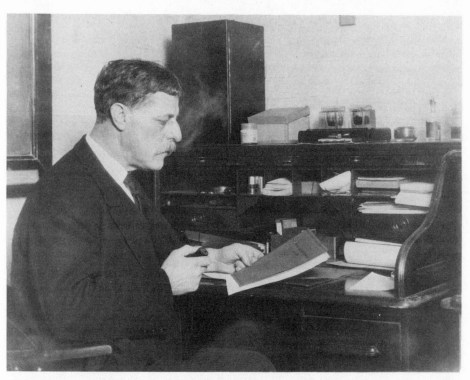

J. Whitridge Williams
From the Archives Office, The Johns Hopkins Medical Institutions

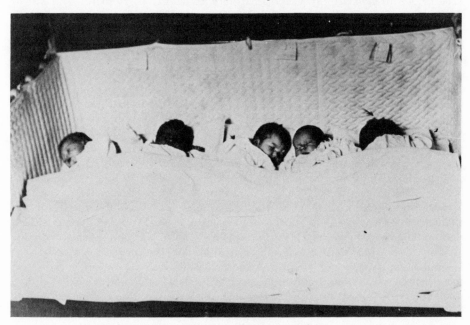

The nursery in the Department of Obstetrics, 1903
From the Archives Office, The Johns Hopkins Medical Institutions

assistants.... Large endowments or state aid will be necessary for the support of such institutions, but I can conceive of no better expenditure of funds if it leads to fuller knowledge of the many unsolved problems connected with women and to the development of a body of men competent to undertake their investigation.

Fortunately, the late Alan Frank Guttmacher recorded his reminiscences of John Whitridge Williams. He pointed out that while much had been written about his scientific contributions, it was equally important to describe the man himself. Williams made basic contributions to the study of the abnormal pelvis and also to the physiology and pathology of the placenta. He was also in large part responsible for the establishment of adequate prenatal care in this country. In addition his book on obstetrics went to six editions in twenty-seven years and sold well over 100,000 copies. In Guttmacher's opinion, however, these measures of distinction are negligible when compared to the power, the force, and the intelligence of the man:

He was a large, dignified and handsome man well over six feet in height. His huge head with its big, virile features was made even more manly by a heavy, nicotine-bleached, drooping mustache. As he sat before his class he would look over the top of his eyeglasses bending his large head on a thick powerful neck. This gave him a very formidable appearance leading the students to aptly nickname him "the Bull." This comparison was further enhanced by his deep rumbling voice. He was so strong and vigorous that the force of his sneeze fairly rocked the building. Dr. Williams was a man who deified punctuality, system and routine. His days were all the same, six days a week. At 9:04 he greeted his resident with the usual morning salutation— "Well, whom did you kill last night?" He then drank a full glass of ice water, and stood before his class at 9:05. Class lasted until 10, and from 10 to 10:30 he visited the interesting patients on the ward and then his private patients. From 10:30 until 1:30 he worked in the laboratory, studying the material from the operating room and from the autopsy table and teaching those of his staff who chanced to come in. He ate lunch in the staff dining room from 1:30 until 2:00 and at 2:00 answered his mail, saw visitors and private patients. If time sufficed, he returned to the laboratory until about 5:30. He then bade everyone a hearty good-bye, "See you tomorrow, God willing." He took the streetcar home and dined at 7 o'clock. After dinner he went to his library where he read and studied medicine. His publishers bound him a special copy of his textbook, each page being interleaved with a blank page. On these blank pages he jotted down a resume of each important obstetrical article that he read. He made the notation on the blank leaf opposite the page of the textbook to which it applied. He occupied himself with this type of work while reading in the general fields of medicine and science each evening from 8 until 10. Because of this method of summarizing the current obstetrical literature it was relatively simple for Dr. Williams to get out a new edition of his obstetrics every five years. He also had a rigid routine about his pipes. He always smoked a dollar pipe and spurned the more expensive ones which were so frequently given him. He would soak a new dollar pipe in alcohol for twenty-four hours to remove all the varnish. When it had dried completely he would put a tight fitting cork in the bowl and another in the opening where the stem articulates. Then he would immerse the whole thing in molten paraffin. He took it out of the paraffin and after removing the excess, rubbed the bowl on his hand until it attained a wonderful lustre. He then took the jackknife which he always carried and carved a roman numeral in the wood. He would discard his old pipe which was similarly numbered and substitute the new one. He kept seven pipes in constant circulation using the pipe numbered for the particular day of the week.

Williams was the most popular teacher in the medical school at that time. His celebrated course in anecdotal midwifery was elaborated by his inexhaustible supply of stories, which he told in a rare Rabelaisian vein, completely disdainful of the fact that half a dozen women medical students were present. A good example of his milder stories was one about the dignified parson who brought his new and elderly wife to consult Dr. Williams. The parson knew that first labors were usually protracted and difficult in women approaching forty, and the old fellow was sincerely concerned. After examining the patient, Dr. Williams assured them that pregnancy and labor would be quite normal. They left, but a few moments later the parson's wife returned alone. She firmly shut the door to Williams's consulting room and sat down beside him. She said, "Dr. Williams, I have something to tell you." The professor replied, "There is something I can tell you. Some years ago you were indiscreet and had a child." "Yes, that's it," she said, "but what shall I tell the reverend?" Dr. Williams thought for a moment and then replied: "Parsons are hard people. I wouldn't say a word about it or he'll kick you out." The reverend's lady left, grateful for the practical advice. After the usual number of months the parson's wife went into labor, and the poor parson had an exaggerated case of nervousness. He was fearful that his wife would have to go through a terrible and prolonged ordeal. Just the reverse occurred. After a very short labor—only two hours— she was delivered of a large boy. Dr. Williams came down to the sitting room where the anxious fathers await their progeny and broke the good news to the divine. The parson was jubilant. "Wasn't that marvelous, Dr. Williams, and the whole thing only took two hours—two hours, mind you, in a woman of forty with her first baby. Dr. Williams, that is another incontestable proof of the efficacy of prayer, for I have been praying for nine months that my wife should be delivered speedily."

Another of his favorite stories was about a young, wellborn couple who came to him with a three-month pregnancy a few weeks after their marriage. They were terrified at the disgrace which was in store for them, and asked Dr. Williams's help and advice. He told them not to worry, that he would take care of the situation. When the woman was seven months married and nine months pregnant, she fell into labor. Dr. Williams notified the delivery floor that he expected a premature baby and requested that they get the crib warmed up and that they prepare a layette for a premature infant. The woman delivered a nine-pound girl. Dr. Williams winked—he had a very informative wink—and the nurses cut and tore the premature jacket so that they could squeeze the baby into it. Then he went out and told the assembled grandparents that their granddaughter was a delicate seven months' baby and that her chances for survival were very poor. He asked their cooperation and requested them not even to look at the baby, for such puny premature infants are especially susceptible to respiratory infections, and he feared that the grandmothers might breathe some germs on it. The family willingly acquiesced, and the baby was whisked into the nursery in a covered blanket. After two weeks Dr. Williams informed the family that the child had established a world's record, it had grown from four pounds to ten—truly a marvelous thing—and he asked their permission to report the case at a medical meeting. It is evident that many of his stories did not teach much in the way of obstetrics—his textbook did that. However, Dr. Williams was a humanist in the broadest sense.

Williams made it clear to the students that obstetrics was an old art but a new science. Perhaps his greatest contribution was the men that he trained, many of whom later became professors of obstetrics. The long list includes such names as Francis C. Goldsborough, J. Morris Slemons, Frank W. Lynch, Clarence D. Ingraham, Arthur H. Morse, Herbert Thoms, Karl M. Wilson, Everett D. Plass, Thomas O. Gamble, John W. Harris, Tiffany J. Williams, Henricus J. Stander, Robert Gordon Douglas, Daniel G. Morton, John L. McKelvey, Andrew A. Marchetti, and Herbert F. Traut.

Dr. Williams had great confidence in his ability to judge men—and lineage was not the least of the points by which he judged them. (Williams had a distinguished lineage on both sides of his family, and family data and associated records were of such interest to him that he preserved them with extreme care in a well-known tin box.) If a man was wellborn and/or the son of a distinguished parent, Dr. Williams would accept him in the medical school even though his entrance grades were quite low. First, however, he would send for the man and tell him that he was being accepted because of his "blood" or because of a distinguished relative. Dr. Williams then told the student that he would have to justify the confidence placed in him by doing better than average work. If his work was only average he would be asked to leave the school. Many of these men proved to be excellent students, and only occasionally was Williams disappointed.

Williams's devotion to science never lessened his sympathy for the patient. Indeed, every aspect of the organization in the clinic was directed toward the understanding of the processes of childbirth and the relief of the attendant pains and perils, and every effort was made to lower the mortality of both the mother and the infant. It was well known that no assistant could remain on the staff who was harsh or discourteous to any of the patients. Williams made the fees moderate, so that the service might be available to the largest number, recognizing also a limit to the value of professional services, irrespective of the individual. Dr. Williams was literally loved by his patients—especially the ward patients, to whom he was always thoughtful and gallant. One evidence of this was the several score of Whitridge Williams Smiths and Joneses who grew up in East Baltimore.

Although his contributions to medicine may not achieve immortality for him, nevertheless Williams gave to all who were associated with him incomparable training in the art and science of obstetrics, as well as a "way of life" which served them well throughout their careers. For over three decades he exerted a dominating influence on the development of academic obstetrics in the United States.

17 ❧ The First Full-time Academic Department of Pediatrics: The Story of the Harriet Lane Home

Pediatrics in the Early Period
(1889–1910)

IN 1889 THE STAFF of the Outpatient Department or Dispensary of the Johns Hopkins Hospital was organized as follows: chief of the dispensary, William S. Halsted, M.D.; Department of General Medicine, William Osler, M.D.; Department of Diseases of Children, William Osler, M.D., and William D. Booker, M.D.

William David Booker was born in Prince Edward County, Virginia, on November 11, 1844. After graduating from Hampton-Sydney College in 1862, he enlisted as a private in the Third Virginia Cavalry, C.S.A., and served until the end of the Civil War. In 1867 he took his M.D. degree at the University of Virginia. He married Julia T. Manning of Baltimore and became a practitioner in that city. When the Johns Hopkins University opened in 1876, he enrolled as a graduate student in the Department of Biology, which was under the direction of Henry Newell Martin. Martin's laboratory soon became a center of physiological research, attracting a number of young men interested in investigation who were destined to play an important role in American medicine. Along with other young Baltimore physicians, Booker also attended classes in physiology and enrolled in Welch's first course at Hopkins, a series of nine lectures on "Micro-organisms and Disease," given during the winter of 1886.

Booker's major field of interest was the summer diarrheas in children. His work, carried out in the pathological laboratory, concerned the colon bacillus. In 1888 he wrote a paper on "The Bacteria in the Dejecta of Infants Afflicted with Summer Diarrhea" and subsequently one entitled "Bacteriological and Anatomical Study of the Summer Diarrheas of Infants," which appeared in 1896.

Dr. Booker became professor of physiology and dean of the Woman's Medical College of Baltimore, also serving as professor of diseases in children in that institution from 1886 to 1893. In March 1896 he was nominated by the medical faculty as Clinical Professor of Diseases of Children in the Johns Hopkins University. This title, however, did not mean that the hospital authorities regarded "diseases of children" as an independent specialty. The field was considered a part of medicine, and was organized, therefore, as a subdepartment under the guidance of Dr. Osler. It remained in that status for a number of years partly because, as outlined by Chesney, the hospital had insufficient facilities for the care of children. Thus, pediatrics was largely an outpatient activity until the Harriet Lane Home for Invalid Children was opened in 1912. Booker remained in charge of the Division of Diseases of Children until 1909, when he was succeeded by Clemens von Pirquet of Vienna.

The Role of Booker and Osler in the American Pediatric Society

One of Booker's most notable contributions was his role in the organization of the American Pediatric Society. The only documentation of this event is a statement by Booker, who was made temporary secretary at the organizing meeting of September 18, 1888: "After the adjournment of the Pediatric Section of the Ninth International Congress, September 9, 1887, a meeting was held by a few members of the section, and on motion of Dr. W. D. Booker of Baltimore, seconded by Dr. I. N. Love of St. Louis, it was decided to organize the American Pediatric Society. Dr. J. Lewis Smith of New York was elected temporary chairman, and Dr. W. D. Booker of Baltimore, temporary secretary."

In the late 1880s American pediatrics in any organized sense was in the doldrums. It was represented only by the Section on Diseases of Children of the American Medical Association (AMA), which was in a deteriorated state. The need to separate pediatrics from obstetrics and gynecology had not been recognized by the general membership of the AMA, and was actually opposed by those two sections. The excellence of the program at the Pediatric Section of the International Congress brought home the necessity for separating pediatrics as an organized branch of medicine. Dr. Booker's statement continued as follows:

The chairman was authorized to take such measures as he saw fit to secure the cooperation of some of those physicians who had taken a special interest in the advancement of the study of diseases of children and when advisable to appoint five of those to act with the chairman and secretary as a council to arrange for the permanent organization of the Society. Notices were sent to a limited number of physicians who had become known through their interest and work in promoting a more scientific study of diseases in children asking for their views in regard to the propriety of establishing the Society and inviting cooperation.

Among the physicians to whom notices were sent were several members of the Association of American Physicians. Of the original members of this association at the time of its organization in 1885, six became founding members of the American Pediatric Society, including William Osler. Thus, the Association of American Physicians gave impetus to the formation of the American Pediatric Society and served as its model. The relations between the two societies were remarkably close, and of the forty-three founders of the American Pediatric Society, fourteen were then, or later became, members of the Association of American Physicians. Six became presidents of the Association of American

Physicians (Busey, Pepper, Osler, Jacobi, Vaughan, and Forchheimer), and three became presidents of both societies (Osler, Jacobi, and Forchheimer).

The first scientific meeting of the American Pediatric Society was held in Washington, D.C., on September 20, 1889, and on the following day in the newly opened (May 8, 1889) Johns Hopkins Hospital. Presented at the scientific session were two elaborate bacteriological studies of the stools in the diarrhea of infants; one of these was given by William Booker. Booker isolated some nineteen varieties of bacteria, designated A to S, including proteus, which was the most frequent organism. Feeding experiments on rabbits and other young animals were inconclusive, and Booker stated that, on the whole, "this work is too incomplete to admit of positive conclusions."

At the third meeting of the society held in Washington, D.C., on September 22–25, 1891, there was a symposium on the diagnosis of pneumonia. The presentations at this meeting illustrate the almost complete dependence on signs and symptoms that characterized so much of clinical medicine in those days. One of the papers was given by Osler on "The Diagnosis of Pulmonary Tuberculosis in Children." Osler divided pulmonary tuberculosis in children into three categories: acute, subacute and chronic ("protracted") forms, of which the first two could only be distinguished from nontuberculous pneumonia with difficulty and uncertainty. Of the last, ulcerative phthisis, he stated: "The diagnosis is rarely doubtful—here, too, we have an opportunity such as rarely happens in other cases of examining in the vomit portions of the expectoration and discovering the tubercle bacilli. On several occasions I have been able to do this, and it certainly should be practiced whenever possible." This is perhaps the earliest description of the value of examination of the gastric contents in the diagnosis of tuberculosis.

The fourth meeting was held May 2–4, 1892, in Boston, Massachusetts, under the presidency of William Osler. In his presidential address Osler offered his famous "Remarks on Specialism," describing himself as "one whose work has lain in the wide field of general medicine"; he admitted the necessity of "limitation of work" resulting from "the extraordinary development of modern medicine." However, he went on to emphasize the equal necessity of preliminary training for the specialist in other and broader fields such as physiology, anatomy, and pathology and cited the Socratic dictum that the physician should apply his methods "to the whole body, and try to treat and heal the whole and the part together." This sentence, Osler said, "embodies the law and the gospel for specialists." Here was perhaps, as noted by Faber and McIntosh, the earliest known formulation of what today we call our concern for appraisal of "the whole child." Osler noted that pediatrics was the last specialty to separate from general medicine, "not because of any extreme of differentiation, but rather because the pediatrician is the vestigial remnant of what was formerly in cities the general practitioner.

"That which has been is that which shall be." Thus Osler reminded his audience that medicine seemingly began with specialization and that "the tail of our emblematic snake has returned into its mouth, for at no age has specialism been so rife as at present." It was regarded as a very timely address on an important topic, and Osler had the courage to say that "no more dangerous members of our profession exist than those born into it so to speak as specialists." However, he went on to acknowledge the unquestioned advantage of division of labor in the profession and made the following remarks: "Specialism is not, however, without many advantages. A radical error at the onset is the failure to recognize that the results of specialized observation are at best only partial truths, which require to be correlated with facts obtained by wider study. The various organs, the diseases of which are subdivided for treatment, are not isolated, but complex parts of a complex whole and everyday's experience of the truth of the saying, 'When one member suffers, all the members suffer with it.'"

At the seventh meeting at the Virginia Hot Springs on May 27–29, 1895, Osler presented an excellent paper on a case of what was later called "Pick's syndrome," including a detailed autopsy report by Simon Flexner entitled "On the Association of Enormous Heart Hypertrophy, Chronic Proliferative Peritonitis and Recurrent Ascites with Adherent Pericardium." Pick's paper appeared more than a year after Osler's, and of the two Osler had the better claim to eponymic credit.

The thirteenth meeting was held at Niagara Falls, New York, on May 27–29, 1901, under the presidency of William D. Booker. His address, "The Early History of the Summer Diarrheas of Infants," dealt with a subject that was not only of importance to pediatricians in general but also to bacteriologists. The scholarly address included information about the disease to about 1833. Faber and McIntosh quote one passage as follows:

About the middle of the 18th Century there occurred in the towns and cities along the Atlantic Coast of the United States of America, a serious disease among infants which had not been observed before. Its incidence was limited to the summer months, and it appeared each year in an epidemic form with such regularity that it was looked for as an annual visitor—"the dread of parents and the opprobrium of physicians." It was thought to be peculiar to America. It was unknown to the aborigines of our continent; and the first settlers of the colonies have left us no record of its existence. It was not until the people began to collect in towns and villages that the disease was engendered, and it had no local habitation or name until it was described by Benjamin Rush in 1777, in a paper entitled "An inquiry into the cause and cure of the cholera infantum."

This was a fitting contribution by the first clinical professor of the diseases of children at Johns Hopkins in view of the fact that later investigations conducted in the Harriet Lane Home contributed so much to the understanding and treatment of the summer diarrhea of children. Booker, who died from pneumonia on March 15, 1921, at the age of seventy-six, thus helped Baltimore play an impressive role in the early history of pediatrics in this country.

The Flowering of Biochemical Research in Pediatrics

During the first decade of the twentieth century the foundation of biochemical investigation in pediatrics was laid by L. Emmett Holt, who established well-equipped laboratories at the Babies' Hospital in New York in 1910 and 1911. Holt accomplished this under the aegis of the Rockefeller Institute for Medical Research, which he had been instrumental in founding.

In 1912 one of Holt's associates, John Howland, came to Baltimore as full-time head of the pediatric department at Johns Hopkins, the first such appointment in America. It was during the fifteen years following Howland's arrival in Baltimore that pediatric biochemistry flowered. Much of the basic work in pediatrics during this period was done by Howland and the remarkable group of young men associated with him in the Harriet Lane Home.

John F. Howland was born in New York City on February 3, 1873, the son of Judge Henry E. Howland, a Yale graduate. He was the direct descendant of another John Howland, who on December 21, 1620, disembarked from the *Mayflower* at Plymouth. Judge Howland, a well-known figure in the social life of New York City, moved in fashionable circles but retained a freshness and simplicity which also characterized his son John. Howland's mother, Sarah Louise Miller, was an accomplished pianist. Howland was an example of the best in New England inheritance, possessing a strong sense of duty, a desire for constant improvement, and complete intellectual and moral integrity. He entered Yale in 1894 at the age of seventeen. He became an editor of the *Yale News*, was elected to Skull and Bones, the famous senior society of which Dr. William H. Welch was also a member, and was an intercollegiate tennis champion. On graduation at the age of twenty-one he ranked in the upper fourth of his class scholastically and was the sixth-ranking tennis player in the country and a member of the United States doubles team.

Howland decided to study medicine while a sophomore at Yale. He attended the New York University School of Medicine, which was apparently a rugged institution at the time. For example, at a surgical clinic given there by Dr. Percy Bolton, an ex-Harvard crew man, the students behaved so offensively that Bolton stopped the clinic, took off his coat, rolled up his sleeves, and defied the ringleader to come down into the pit and have it out. Bolton thereafter had no trouble. Undoubtedly, New York University had the lowest scholastic standard of the three New York medical schools. Howland chose it because it gave the degree in one less year, and he thought that all any of the three schools really accomplished was to hand out the degree of Doctor of Medicine. When he graduated, he obtained the coveted internship at Presbyterian Hospital, winning over students of four years' training. After two years at Presbyterian, he interned for a year at the New York Foundling Hospital. Howland's contact there with the dynamic personality of Dr. L. Emmett Holt probably was responsible for his choice of pediatrics. After Howland had become firmly established at Hopkins, the chair of medicine there became vacant upon the death of Theodore Janeway. Howland would have been given this post had he been willing to change to medicine. When Edwards Park once asked Howland why he didn't change, Howland replied that he was too old, but added that if he were just beginning, he would enter internal medicine.

After his internship at the Foundling Hospital, Howland studied in Europe, first at the University of Berlin and then in Vienna. It was this trip to

Europe that gave him the inspiration to become an investigator of disease rather than a practitioner. When he returned to America in 1902, Howland was made assistant to Dr. Holt, attending physician at the Willard Parker Hospital, and instructor and associate in pediatrics at the College of Physicians and Surgeons. In 1903 he married Susan Morris Sanford, daughter of the leading general practitioner of New Haven.

As a result of his investigative work and his remarkable promise, Howland was elected professor of pediatrics in the reorganized fulltime medical school at Washington University in St. Louis in 1910. In preparation for this appointment he went to study under the most distinguished pediatrician of the time, Czerny of Strasbourg. Here he developed his interest in the nutritional disorders of children and learned of the possibilities of chemistry as a research tool. Most important, he saw a great German clinic in which the advancement of knowledge was the prevailing motif. He returned in 1911 but he was in St. Louis only six months when he was invited to succeed von Pirquet as head of pediatrics at Johns Hopkins. Howland assumed his duties at Hopkins in 1912 and remained there until his death in 1926. His final illness developed when he was traveling in Greece, where his brother was charged with the repatriation of the Greeks from Turkish territory. After this tour, the Howlands went to Paris. While there, he had a profuse gastric hemorrhage and was operated on with the expectation that an ulcer would be found. However, the condition proved to be hopelessly advanced cirrhosis of the liver. He died shortly after the operation. In 1921 Howland had had an attack of jaundice, after which Dr. Thomas Brown found that his liver and spleen were enlarged. He had no history of alcoholism or "catarrhal jaundice," but as a young man had used chloroform in the laboratory to produce experimental liver disease.

When Howland came to Baltimore, there was no pediatric department at Hopkins. Although von Pirquet had been professor since 1910, there was no hospital building designated for pediatrics. Von Pirquet worked in two small rooms in the medical dispensary, and it was he who designed the Harriet Lane Home on the basis of some pre-existing plans. In 1911 he returned to Germany on leave of absence and while there accepted the chair of pediatrics in Breslau.

Howland also found no pre-existing pediatric staff. He selected his own group, and as stated in Genesis, "There were giants on the earth in those days and they became mighty men—men of renown." Practically every one of Dr. Howland's original staff later became the head of a pediatric department in a medical school. Dr. Edwards A. Park joined him as chief of the Outpatient Department Service. Park had become interested in rickets while at the New York Foundling Hospital and had gone to Germany in the summer of 1912 to study the pathology of that disease under Professor M. B. Schmidt in Marburg. While there, he received a cablegram from Howland offering him the post of assistant in pediatrics at Hopkins. Park, who had already committed himself to work as the office assistant to Dr. Theodore Janeway in New York, declined. However, Janeway heard about the offer and released Park so that he could go to Baltimore. Kenneth Blackfan (who had been Howland's chief resident in St. Louis) was appointed chief resident on the inpatient service. Grover Powers

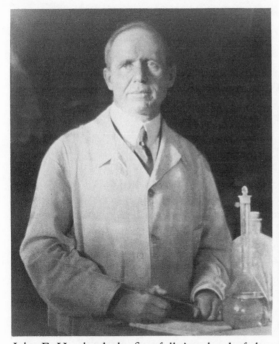

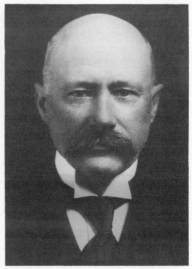

John F. Howland, the first full-time head of the Department of Pediatrics

From the Archives Office, The Johns Hopkins Medical Institutions

William David Booker, the first clinical professor of the diseases of children at Johns Hopkins

From the Archives Office, The Johns Hopkins Medical Institutions

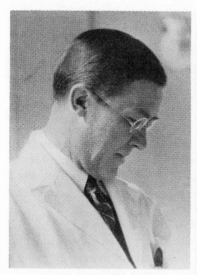

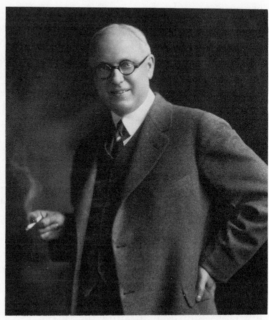

Kenneth D. Blackfan

From D. Riesman, ed., *History of the Interurban Clinical Club*, *1905–1937* (Philadelphia: John C. Winston Co., 1937)

William McKim Marriott

Courtesy of Dr. David Kipnis

then joined the group in 1913, McKim Marriott in 1914, and James L. Gamble in 1915. In 1916 Marriott left to become professor of pediatrics at Washington University, and the following year Benjamin Kramer took his place. Frederick Tisdall arrived in 1918, sent from Toronto by Dr. Allen Brown to get a foundation in pediatrics.

Howland, along with the resident staff, took sole care of the children on the wards, and he personally had charge of all private patients. He did not want his resident staff to have any duties except the care of children, and demanded that they be at his beck and call at all times. The members of the research staff were allowed to work in the dispensary but were not given ward privileges. Marriott was so essential to Howland in the laboratory that he had the greatest difficulty in obtaining consent even to work in the dispensary. The same situation developed later in Kramer's case. Park thought that Howland's method of organization of the department was not the best for its fullest fruition. "We underlings," he said, "were never allowed experiences essential for the development of ideas and we had no opportunity to carry out the ideas which we did have. With the exception of the clinic for the treatment of congenital syphilis, Howland would not allow any special clinics or the formation of any subdepartments. However, his policy kept the department completely under his immediate control; and his system was conducive to successful research."

As an investigator, Howland was an opportunist. In general he chose subjects for his studies in which from the beginning he could see the end. The projects chosen for his earlier studies appear to have been as chance offered, but later, when he became interested in rickets, they had a continuity. He was extraordinarily keen in perceiving possible openings and a superb judge of their value. In his studies with the calorimeter he worked alone, but in almost all other cases he worked in collaboration with someone else. The collaborator might be chosen because his problem appealed particularly to Howland, but more often because of some special knowledge or ability which Howland lacked. In general the collaborators whom he chose were most unusual men. A. N. Richards was an early collaborator, and later work was done chiefly with Marriott and Kramer. Park believed that Howland did not have what might be called an imaginative or creative mind—that he was unusually dependent on others for ideas. The great asset which he did possess, and its importance cannot be overemphasized in a department head, was his almost unerring judgment. He was, for example, among the first to perceive the importance of chemistry for the investigation of disease in children.

Dr. Howland did not provide technicians in the chemical laboratory. He insisted that investigators must gain, through experience, resourcefulness in the use of the required methodology in order to have full faith in their results. Marriott, however, did manage to provide himself with a technical assistant by an illicit arrangement. In the course of working out a method for measuring beta-hydroxybutyric acid, he became very bored setting up a battery of distilling flasks and then titrating the distillates. There was a bright fifteen-year-old girl in the laboratory whose assignment was to wash the glassware. Marriott taught Topsy to perform the distillation procedure, and he boasted gleefully that none of "you chemists" could measure so near the mark as Topsy. Although Howland had little knowledge of theoretical chemistry, he was remarkably skillful in technical procedures. Shohl observed that Howland was the best "spinal cord" chemist he had ever seen.

Howland had also become an ardent golfer, having given up tennis when he entered medical school. He played not by the round but by the day. If after eighteen holes in the morning and again in the afternoon there was daylight left, he would play some more. Because of John Howland's interest, many trips were taken to Pine Valley, New Jersey, for interludes of golf between the preparation of papers and their presentation before the "Young Turks" in Atlantic City each spring. These trips were made in Dr. Gamble's 1915 Cadillac touring car which "was loaded on the return trip through Philadelphia with laboratory equipment purchased with the yearly unexpended balance that otherwise would be returned on June 30 to the University."

Edwards A. Park described vividly the man and the stimulating environment created by him in the Harriet Lane:

What a joyous place the Harriet Lane was in those early days under this virile man. We were all young, our chief not much older than we, certainly not older in spirit, a happy family in which each had his duty. There was not a discordant soul amongst us—all was fresh, hard work was a delight and each day brought the new experiences and excitement of creative work. It must be remembered that this pediatric oasis was set in the larger oasis of Johns Hopkins, then still in its early glory, filled with interesting and distinguished men, engaged in important work and having wide outlooks. At the time of his death Howland was the most distinguished figure in American pediatrics and had he lived he would have received every honor which could have been bestowed. He was twice lecturer before the Harvey Society. He was a member of the Board of Scientific Directors of the Rockefeller Foundation for Medical Research, and of the Council of Pharmacy and Chemistry of the American Medical Association; a Director of the Russell-Sage Institute and a member of numerous societies and organizations. In pediatrics he had become a world figure as the result of his investigative work and also his editorship with Dr. Holt of the famous textbook of Pediatrics. Abraham Jacobi was the pioneer in pediatrics. Dr. Holt established pediatrics in this country as a special branch of medicine, defining it, putting it in order and assigning it the welfare of the child in health as well as in disease. John Howland, on the other hand, modernized pediatrics. He changed the course of pediatrics by substituting for bedside observation and conjecture, the study of disease through laboratory methods and experiments. He caused pediatrics to become a rapidly expanding subject. He did this by example—by the development of a model clinic; model from the point of view of administration, medical care, teaching, research and spirit. The Harriet Lane Home became known all over the world. He created and sent out missionaries, his pupils, filled with his ideas and his spirit. A new era in medicine founded on the application of scientific methods to the study of clinical problems was coming anyway. The Rockefeller Institute, for example, was founded in 1901 but Howland started the movement in Pediatrics and the Harriet Lane Home under his guidance was the first fulltime university clinic to win complete success.

The Acidosis of Infantile Diarrhea

Howland's first great accomplishment in the Harriet Lane Home was proving that an acidosis existed in children with diarrhea. The selection of the problem was Howland's. The development of a better method for the recognition of the acidosis was Marriott's contribution. Presented at the twenty-seventh meeting of the American Pediatric Society in May 1915, this paper by Howland and Marriott on severe diarrhea in infancy was a landmark in the history of pediatrics. It offered an explanation different from the existing one for the symptoms of what was called "alimentary intoxication"—marked dyspnea without signs of respiratory obstruction, plus restlessness, stupor, and coma. Finkelstein had ascribed these manifestations to the toxic effects of intermediary products of metabolism; Howland and Marriott showed that they were the result of loss of base, producing acidosis. The evidence was clear and convincing: they demonstrated a marked increase of urinary ammonia, a severe reduction of carbon dioxide tension in the alveolar air, an increase in the hydrogen-ion concentration of the blood, and an increase of three to five times in the amount of sodium bicarbonate required to alkalinize the urine, which was always highly acid. They were able to correct the acidosis in part or wholly by administration of sodium bicarbonate, preferably intravenously, or if this was not feasible, subcutaneously. They noted, but without pursuing the matter further at that time, "the continual drain of water from the tissues." However, they frankly admitted that the "acidosis may be entirely overcome, and yet death ensue as a result of it; it probably initiates many abnormal processes that we do not understand and that we have no way of overcoming." Their conclusion was that it was not the intermediary products of metabolism that were involved, "indeed, all proof of their presence is lacking. The condition depends on acidosis such as is found in cholera and a variety of other different diseases. The condition should not be, therefore, termed a food intoxication—it is not the presence of abnormal substances—it is the absence of substances that are very normal and very necessary to life."

Oscar Schloss of New York had also demonstrated acidosis in these so-called intoxicated children. Learning of Howland and Marriott's work, Schloss wrote to Howland saying he would defer his report until Howland and Marriott had published theirs. This he did. It was an act of courtesy and generosity from a younger to an older man which deserves great praise.

MacCallum and Voegtlin had shown that in the tetany following removal of the parathyroid glands the calcium in the blood serum was low: Howland and Marriott decided to see whether the calcium was also low in the tetany of infants. At the 1916 meeting of the American Pediatric Society their paper on "The Calcium Content of the Blood in Rachitis and Tetany" showed that in the former disease there was no more than a "very slight" reduction in calcium, but that in tetany the reduction was great during the active stage, returning to normal with recovery. For their biochemical determinations they devised a method applicable to one or two milliliters of serum, a significant step in the direction of microchemistry. They went on to treat the convulsions successfully by administering calcium. Here again, Howland's mind was the one which seized upon the opportunity.

There was a good deal of the magician about Marriott. Everything was easy. In the chemical laboratory Marriott was able in one way or another to meet Howland's every wish, often by the following morning. Howland pointed out the problem and Marriott developed the method to solve it, such as his colorimetric method for measuring the pH of blood serum. Their general outlook on life contrasted as much as their views on the entry of the United States into World War I. Marriott was what might be called a belligerent pacifist. Howland was vehemently pro-British and most outspoken in the belief that U.S. entry against Germany was not only necessary but right. Park could often hear their acrimonious discussions across the laboratory table.

When Marriott was offered the chairmanship of the Department of Pediatrics in St. Louis, Howland, believing that Marriott did not have sufficient clinical training to be a competent head of a clinical department, tried to keep him in Baltimore. Marriott's previous clinical experience before coming to Harriet Lane had been limited to two summers as the official physician in Yellowstone Park. He was fond of responding to the question of the commonest ailments he treated in Yellowstone Park—the answer: bear bites and geyser burns. It was unfortunate that Marriott and Howland had to separate, as they made a wonderful combination. Marriott had the imagination and the ingenuity, and Howland supplied the balance.

William McKim Marriott was born in Baltimore on March 5, 1885. He received his B.S. degree at the University of North Carolina in 1904. He taught biochemistry for several years and was awarded his M.D. degree by Cornell in 1910. That same year he went to Washington University in St. Louis as an instructor in biological chemistry. In 1914 he joined Howland at Johns Hopkins and became associate professor of pediatrics. In 1917 he returned to St. Louis as professor of pediatrics, a post he held until 1936. From 1923 until 1936 he was also dean of the Washington University School of Medicine. In 1936 he became dean and professor of research medicine at the University of California School of Medicine, but he died on November 11, 1936, shortly after reaching California.

The Rebirth of Parenteral Therapy

In 1832 Dr. O'Shaughnassy, a physician at Newcastle-upon-Tyne, sent to the editor of *Lancet* his famous report of the results of his examination of the blood in cholera, in which he found large loss of water, neutral salts, and free alkali, and accounted for these losses in the diarrheal stool. Thomas Latta, a physician in the town of Leith, near Edinburgh, who read his *Lancet* faithfully, at once set about applying these findings by injecting intravenously a solution containing sodium chloride and sodium bicarbonate. His first patient was an old woman severely ill with cholera. The dramatic outcome of this historic event is recorded in a report which he, too, sent to *Lancet*. After Latta's magnificent adventure, nothing more was done about replacement therapy until one hundred years later. Indeed, it was not until Marriott and Utheim directly measured the large reduction of the volume of blood in dehydrated infants that circulatory failure was recognized as the immediately dangerous event in infant diarrhea and it became clear that volume was the critical dimension of effective replacement therapy.

Dr. James Gamble awarded to Kenneth Blackfan the sobriquet of the Thomas Latta of our time. As Dr. Howland's perennial resident, Blackfan watched over his patients with a devoted solicitude. He became convinced that infants dehydrated by diarrheal disease needed more salt solution than could be provided by the subcutaneous infusions as used by Professor Garrod in St. Bartholomew's Hospital. Blackfan successfully argued his case and was permitted to try more vigorous replacement. The importance of adequate replacement of fluid loss was convincingly demonstrated by a dramatic reduction of mortality, which nowadays is sustained by continuous intravenous infusion. It is well to remember that important advances in medical science have been made and will continue to be made at the bedside by observant physicians. As demonstrated by the story of replacement therapy, critical judgment at the bedside may be the turning point of discovery.

Kenneth Blackfan began his medical career in 1905 as a country doctor. Eighteen years later he became Thomas Morgan Rotch Professor of Pediatrics at Harvard, and for a similar period carried his department forward with consummate skill and success. On graduating from high school in Cambridge, New York, he entered the Albany Medical School of Union University. During his third year, Richard Pearce came to the school as professor of pathology and bacteriology. Kenneth Blackfan responded to the enthusiasm of this fine instructor and student of disease and was permitted to work in Pearce's laboratory the following summer. A warm student-master friendship developed which ultimately determined Blackfan's future course in medicine. When Blackfan received his medical degree at the age of twenty-two, he returned to his hometown as a general practitioner. He always recalled those "horse and buggy" years with pleasure, but there were "disturbing visits" to nearby Dorset, just over the line in Vermont, where Richard Pearce spent his summers. Pearce encouraged Blackfan to seek a different career, and by 1909 he had persuaded the young country doctor to set out for Philadelphia, where Samuel Hamill and David Edsall found a place for him as resident in charge of a foundling hospital. Kenneth Blackfan thereupon became a pediatrician.

Two years later John Howland, then professor of pediatrics at Washington University, offered him a residency. This was a stroke of good fortune. It removed the adventurer from his lonely post in the foundling hospital, and after two years in St. Louis placed him in the group of young pediatricians who assembled around Howland in Baltimore. He became the most beloved member of this group, as the resident physician. None watched work under way in the laboratory with more eager interest, and he often found time to participate. For example, his work with Dandy on internal hydrocephalus has come to deserve that lofty adjective, "classic." As related, Blackfan's demonstration that dehydration is a much more dangerous feature of diarrheal disease than the state of acidosis shifted emphasis from alkali therapy to fluid replacement and produced the basis of the present effective treatment of this widespread scourge of infants.

When Kenneth Blackfan reached the age of thirty-seven, he was still a resident, having held this position for eleven years. As a result of this experience, he knew the existing body of knowledge in his chosen field; he knew its frontiers and he knew where the paths of progress lay. He was a superb diagnostician and a master of the hospital care of patients. In addition, his four years of country practice had taught him resourcefulness and had given him an understanding of the day-to-day realities of patient care. He was in all respects qualified for the diverse duties of departmental headship. His first commission came in the year 1920, when he was appointed professor of pediatrics at the University of Cincinnati. There he built up his department and guided it with outstanding success. Then in 1923 the fruits of eighteen years of education for leadership fell to Harvard.

James L. Gamble and "Gamblegrams"

At the 1918 meeting of the American Pediatric Society a paper of importance was presented by Kenneth D. Blackfan and James L. Gamble of Baltimore. This was their first appearance on an American Pediatric Society program. Gamble was not yet a member and was not present. The paper was on cholesterol metabolism of infants. The wording of their conclusions bears the Gamble imprint: "We feel that the consistently large negative balance found in these fairly normal and gaining infants while receiving the usual amount of cholesterol in their food is strong evidence in the direction of proving that cholesterol can be readily synthesized."

James Gamble never forgot the debt he owed to Howland, who gave "a young, ill-trained, would-be investigator a place in his fine new chemistry laboratory and sustained his courage by a kindly disregard of his first fumbling efforts." Recalling those days, Gamble stated:

This laboratory was the first one in this country for the study of disease in the clinic by quantitative methods of chemistry. It was the consummation of John Howland's clear vision of the value of such equipment in a university department. He brought a brilliant young biochemist from St. Louis to set it in motion. The ebullient McKim Marriott lost no time in doing this. We were all expected to make our own choice of features of disease to assail by approaches of our own devising so there was in his laboratory [Howland's] a happy lack of program and a delightful spirit of free adventure.

The establishment of the laboratory came opportunely at the beginning of the era of micromethods of measurement which greatly facilitated examination of biochemical events in patients. Clinical medicine was being given a large new armament and it was exciting to find that these methods which were being developed by Folin, Van Slyke and others made information we were after easy to come by.

It was indeed fortunate for the Johns Hopkins Department of Pediatrics that James Lawder Gamble began his meteoric research career in Baltimore.

He was born on July 18, 1883, in Millersburg, Bourbon County, Kentucky. His primary education began in the Millersburg Female College, an institution in which prepubertal boys were also enrolled. At the age of twelve, he was transferred to the Millersburg Military Institute, and when the time came to apply to college, he passed the entrance exams for Harvard without difficulty. However, because his parents believed that the Boston climate might be damaging to his health, he entered Stanford University in 1901 and enrolled in the premedical course. As stated by Loeb, Gamble "drifted" into medicine without any particular conscious motivation and with the natural assumption that he would devote his life to the practice of medicine. Gamble graduated from Stanford in 1906 with the assistance of an earthquake, which came in the spring of that year and eliminated the ordeal of final examinations. He entered Harvard medical school and graduated in 1910. He completed a two-year medical internship at Massachusetts General Hospital, followed by a six-month service at the Children's Hospital in Boston in 1913. He then went abroad to visit the famous European clinics. This represented a turning point in his career, for he became interested in the study of disease in man by the quantitative methods, cumbersome as they were at that time, of the biochemist and the physiologist. He worked in the laboratory of Otto Folin, where simple chemical procedures applicable to the study of metabolic processes in man were being developed. He then returned to Massachusetts General Hospital, where he began his career as an investigator in the small chemical laboratory there under Fritz Talbot. He later came under the influence of Professor L. J. Henderson, from whom he received further training in biological chemistry. His close contact with Henderson stimulated his interest in problems of electrolyte physiology.

In 1914 he heard about the first fulltime department of pediatrics at Johns Hopkins, with well-equipped laboratories for investigation. He accepted an invitation from Dr. Howland to come to Baltimore and arrived in January 1915. His entire teaching assignment consisted of two lectures a year on the food requirements of infants. The first of these lectures Dr. Gamble memorized so effectively and delivered with such fluency that to Dr. Howland's great merriment his material ran out in twenty-five minutes and he had to dismiss the class. Six months after his arrival in Baltimore, Gamble made the important decision to abandon a career in clinical medicine and to dedicate his life "to the study of disease by means of chemistry." He early developed the capacity to design simple experiments which yielded definitive answers.

After an absence during World War I, Gamble returned to Baltimore in 1919. By that time Dr. Howland had developed a deep interest in the treatment of epilepsy by the ketosis of starvation. Gamble went to work on this problem with two Canadian collaborators, Graham Ross and F. F. Tisdall. The design of the study was simple. Since there was no food intake or feces, the balance studies could be carried out by measurements on the daily urine collections and the blood plasma. The execution of the experiment was laborious and extended over a period of nearly two years. The analytical determinations were tedious, but rarely have data been subjected to more original deductive reasoning, according to Loeb. The results are best summarized in Gamble's own words:

One, the data display, in operation, the two adjustable components of the acid-base construction of urine (titrable acidity and ammonia production) which Henderson and Palmer described and which permit the removal of anion excess within the prescribed limits for urine acidity without expenditure of fixed base beyond the quantity which properly presents for removal. Two, they show the determining role of fixed base in sustaining the osmolar value of the body fluids because of the adjustability of the total cation-anion equality. Three, they show the relation of volume of the body fluids to fixed base content on the premise of preservation of the normal osmolar value with the corollary that, so long as the kidney is operating accurately, loss (or gain) of water and electrolytes will be parallel. On this basis the data were used to allocate losses of water from the body fluid compartments from measurements of outgo of intracellular and of extracellular base.

This study of fasting children begun in 1919 was finally published in 1923 and remains a classic work. Perhaps more significant than the contribution which these experiments made to the knowledge of electrolyte physiology was their influence on clinical research. At a time when most clinical investigation consisted of the recording of endless observations made on some new method, Gamble planned a crucial experiment to elucidate basic problems of function and applied chemical means to this end. In the words of Loeb,

These experiments constituted a pioneer approach to the interpretation of quantitative description in terms of the mechanisms involved. Meaning received the primary emphasis. The general design of the experiments devised by Gamble continues to be the pattern for most studies dealing with electrolyte and water metabolism today. Even the expression of data by simple graphic means, now known as "Gambelian diagrams" or "Gamblegrams," has been generally adopted and is a blessing for students, teachers and investigators alike.

At the May 1923 meeting of the American Pediatric Society, Gamble's last paper on work done in Baltimore entitled "On the Manner of Therapeutic Action on Tetany of Substances Producing Hydrochloric Acid" was presented. Also illustrated with the now famous Gamblegrams, it showed how calcium chloride, ammonium chloride, and hydrochloric acid alike produced a lowering of plasma bicarbonate with a simultaneous increase in chloride and a reduction of pH, increasing the ionization of serum calcium and thus inducing relief of tetany.

In 1922 Gamble returned to Boston as assistant professor of pediatrics. Finally, he was appointed professor in 1932. Gamble modestly pointed out that his work would not have been possible without Benjamin Kramer. "We had in our midst a versatile inventor of micromeasurements. The studies—of acid-base metabolism—would not have been possible without the methods of measuring sodium, potassium, calcium, and magnesium which Benjamin Kramer's ingenuity gave us." Howland was devoted to Gamble but never fully realized his potentialities until Gamble left for Boston and published the work on metabolism of starvation in children. Gamble told Park that Howland could not understand his decision not to take care of any patient in the Harriet Lane and definitely to abandon the idea of being a clinician. Howland believed that Gamble's chosen course meant failure—a man must head either for clinical medicine or for fundamental sciences; an intermediary position was totally impractical. After Gamble had gone to Boston, Howland made a determined effort to get him back, but failed.

The Conquest of Rickets

The key to the problem of rickets was to discover what prevented the deposition of calcium salts into the bone and bone-forming cartilage. In 1914 Marriott and Howland began to work on this problem. It was first necessary to be able to determine the concentration of the elements which compose the major part of the inorganic salts of bone, calcium, and phosphorus in the fluid from which the bones receive them, the blood. There were no techniques then available for the detection of these substances in the small amounts of blood that could be safely obtained from infants, so Marriott, Haessler and Howland devised methods, later superseded by better ones, which served the purpose. Marriott and Howland showed that in the active phase of the so-called idiopathic tetany of infancy the serum calcium was 5 to 7 mg/100 ml as opposed to a normal concentration of 10 to 11. In 1916 Marriott and Howland found the serum calcium concentration in cases of rickets without tetany to be normal or only slightly reduced.

In 1919 Kramer and Howland began a systematic study of rickets using the elegant micromethods devised by Kramer. They confirmed that in rickets the calcium of the serum may be reduced to a small extent, but even severe rickets with marked deformities and extensive radiographic changes usually showed only slight change in serum calcium concentration. They further discovered, coincidentally with Iverson and Lenstrup in Holland, that the concentration of serum inorganic phosphorus in uncomplicated rickets was without exception much lower than normal. In the seventy-two cases observed, the average concentration of inorganic phosphorus was 2.5 mg/100 ml, a reduction of more than 50 percent. In the same cases the average for calcium was 9.6 mg/100 ml, a reduction of approximately 5 percent.

Benjamin Kramer was one of the pediatricians with formal training in chemistry attracted to Howland's department because of the latter's interest in using chemical techniques for the investigation of disease. The importance of his contributions to these studies has not been sufficiently emphasized. Kramer successfully developed new micromethods for analysis of inorganic ions in serum, particularly calcium and magnesium, which were useful as diagnostic and research tools. Without these, their studies of rickets would not have been possible. Kramer left the Harriet Lane to become chief of pediatrics at the Jewish Hospital of Brooklyn and professor of pediatrics at the Long Island College of Medicine, which was subsequently taken over by the State University of New York. Kramer maintained interest in the application of chemistry to the diagnosis and study of disease, especially disorders of mineralization. He developed a pediatric research laboratory, which under the direct supervision of Albert E. Sobel further perfected microchemical methods. Sobel and Kramer published many studies of the calcification mechanism and of the biochemical behavior of lead in relation to calcium and phosphorus metabolism and vitamin D action.

An important chapter in the rickets story began when Dr. E. V. Mc-Collum set up his rat colony in the newly founded School of Hygiene and Public Health at Johns Hopkins in 1917. He and his associates, Nina Simmonds and Helen T. Parsons, were especially concerned with the defects of the diet which resulted in pellagra, since Dr. Joseph Goldberger had recently offered evidence that pellagra was a deficiency disease.

A decade earlier, while at the Wisconsin Agricultural Experiment Station, McCollum and Marguerite Davis had demonstrated the existence of vitamin A, the first fat-soluble vitamin to be discovered. They had also made great progress in determining the relative merits, from the nutritive standpoint, of the naturally occurring mixture of proteins in certain seeds and the shortcomings of the inorganic nutrients in the seeds of plants. In their study of the dietary deficiency of polished rice, they discovered that two classes of uncharacterized nutrients, one fat-soluble and the other water-soluble, were essential additives to the basic constituents of the diet. McCollum thus came to Baltimore with a fine background in nutrition research.

One afternoon in the autumn of 1918, John Howland asked McCollum whether anyone had ever produced experimental rickets in animals. McCollum replied that Miss Simmonds and he had produced a condition in young rats which they thought might be rickets and that they had such animals in the laboratory. They went to the laboratory, where Miss Simmonds exposed the skin over the thorax of one of the animals and revealed the "pigeon breast," Harrison's groove, and the wide costo-chondral junctions in the ribs which form the "rachitic rosary." Howland confirmed that the gross appearance of the thorax was similar to that seen in severe rickets among children. He asked McCollum how he had produced the condition. McCollum replied that he did not know what dietary factors were involved and could only tell him the composition and sources of the dietary ingredients. They were both aware that in order to discover the nature of the dietary defects which produced abnormalities in growing bones, as is the case in rickets, someone with expert knowledge of bone histology and bone pathology should examine and describe histologically the changes in bone structure produced by a wide variety of faulty diets. Howland agreed to invest in the necessary histological work, and so the cooperative project between the Department of Pediatrics in the School of Medicine and the Department of Biochemistry in the School of Hygiene began. Howland immediately sent a cable to Edwards A. Park, asking him to return to Baltimore. (Park was then in France in the Medical Corps of the Red Cross.) Pending his return, Dr. Paul G. Shipley was assigned to supervise the cutting, straining, and description of bone sections. Two technicians, Madeline Spencer and James Joy, worked in the Hunterian Building and were trained by Shipley in the techniques involved. They used thirty-day-old rats fed on a variety of diets which they predicted might lead to rachitic bone changes. When Dr. Park returned early in 1919, he and Dr. Shipley shared the pathological work.

Paul G. Shipley was a graduate of Yale University and received his M.D. degree from Yale in 1913. In that year he came to Baltimore to work in the Department of Anatomy under Dr. Mall. In 1917 he received an appointment in the Department of Pediatrics to work on the pathological studies of rickets. In 1926 he was made associate professor of pediatrics. His investigations were concerned chiefly with the problem of the calcification of bone, although he later became interested in lead poisoning and devised spectroscopic methods for the detection of lead in the body fluids. His report in 1932 was the first description of tick bite fever in Maryland.

Although rickets had been characterized as a definite disease by Glisson in 1660, little was known about it until Pommer in 1885 made extensive studies of the structure of rachitic bones. In 1890 Palm reported the results of geographic investigations and pointed out the beneficial effects of sunlight in the treatment of rickets. In 1904 Buchholz first called attention to the value of artificial light in the treatment of the disease, but the value of his work was overlooked, so that in 1918 the etiology of rickets was still a mystery.

Important clues to the etiology of rickets were provided by Mellanby, who in 1918 presented evidence that the disease was caused by a diet deficient in some accessory factor in nutrition. He demonstrated that certain fats (butterfat and, notably, cod liver oil) prevented the bone lesions caused by his experimental diets. He established a standard diet which regularly produced rickets in puppies, and using this technique, he tested many foods for their antirachitic value.

When the Hopkins group began to publish their results in 1921, they had completed studies of the effects of about three hundred experimental diets on hundreds of rats. They found that although the bones of young rats were highly responsive to dietary defects, the most significant factors for safeguarding normal bone growth were the ratio between the calcium and the phosphorus in the food and the kind of fat supplied. Low calcium and high phosphorus or low phosphorus and high calcium were disturbing to bone growth. The former relationship caused rickets complicated by tetany. However, with unfavorable ratios between calcium and phorphorus, rickets was not produced if the diet contained a small addition of cod liver oil or a large addition of butterfat. Kramer made numerous determinations of calcium and phosphorus in the rats and showed that the blood phosphate was low in the animals which showed rachitic lesions.

They further demonstrated that vitamin A was not related to rickets and concluded that a second fat-soluble vitamin, an antirachitic substance which they named vitamin D, existed. When small rats were restricted to one of their rickets-producing diets and were exposed to summer sunshine in Baltimore for five hours daily, they were completely protected against rickets. When kept out of the sunlight on the deficient diet, they developed severe acute rickets in twenty-one days. These observations on the effects of their experimental diets were in accord with the extensive clinical studies indicating that sunlight or artificial light containing ultraviolet rays would prevent or cure rickets in human subjects. The Hopkins group was able to produce, by dietary means, severe acute rickets in young rats in three weeks and to observe the healing process histologically under the guiding influence of the antirachitic substance, vitamin D. Thus, they developed a quantitative test for this vitamin based upon the extent of deposition of calcium salts in the line of provisional calcification in the long bones of small rats rendered rachitic by deficient diet. In 1922 this procedure was adopted as the pharmacopoeial method for standardizing vitamin D.

For McCollum, these cooperative studies with Dr. Park afforded the first opportunity to work with an expert in the special field of bone pathology. By pooling their expert knowledge in the two segments of biological science which they represented, they made discoveries which neither could have accomplished working alone. McCollum noted that discussion of any aspect of these investigations with Park never failed to stimulate constructive thought and to open vistas which had not before been evident.

Howland and his co-workers concluded that there must be a solubility product constant for calcium and phosphate ions which has a definite value at a given pH and temperature. When the calcium ion concentration is very low, no precipitation can occur. Likewise, when the phosphate ion concentration is very low, there is no precipitation because there is a definite physiological limit of increase of concentration for each ion in the serum. The calcium cannot increase indefinitely to compensate for a low phosphorus concentration and vice versa. Although the ionic concentration could not be measured, they did prove that the general principle held true clinically. They used as factors for a rough product the total concentration of calcium and phosphorus in the serum. If one multiplied the concentration of calcium by the inorganic phosphorus concentration, each expressed in mg/100 ml of serum, one obtained a product which in the normal child was between 50 and 60. When the product was below 30, rickets was invariably present. When it was above 40, either demonstrable healing was taking place or there had never been any rickets. With products between 30 and 40, rickets was usually present. The Ca-P product idea was really the brainchild of Benjamin Kramer.

At this juncture Marriott and Howland and later Kramer and Howland approached the subject of calcification experimentally. They made artificial serum with the same amount of sodium bicarbonate, magnesium, and sodium chloride contained in normal serum. They added varying amounts of calcium and phosphorus and kept the solutions at a constant temperature subjected to a variable carbon dioxide tension to give any desired pH. When precipitation occurred, they determined the composition of the precipitate. The solutions were made up with or without a colloid such as gelatin. In these experiments the pH of the solution varied between 7.35 and 7.45. The calcium concentration was not above the normal maximum and the inorganic phosphorus did not exceed 5.5 mg/100 ml, but the concentrations were altered so as to produce different Ca-P products. They kept the solutions at 37.5 degrees C. and determined the presence or absence of precipitation at the end of twenty-four to forty-eight hours. Precipitation could be brought about in a number of ways, such as increasing the pH by reducing the carbon dioxide tension, increasing the temperature, or altering the calcium and phosphorus concentrations: They found that the Ca-P product which determined precipitation in the artificial serum was about 40, strikingly close to that which they had arrived at from their clinical studies.

In a paper presented at the thirty-seventh meeting of the American Pediatric Society in May 1925, Shipley, Kramer and Howland confirmed Robison's observations that cartilage removed from rachitic rats and suspended in a solution of inorganic materials (especially phosphate and calcium) in concentrations corresponding to those present in the plasma of normal infants became calcified within a few hours, calcium being deposited in the provisional zone of cartilage. This effect could also be obtained when the bone was suspended in serum of normal infants but not of the rachitic ones. Kramer administered irradiated milk to eight rachitic infants and produced healing in every case. The chemical changes in the blood were the same as those in rachitic children following ingestion of cod liver oil or exposure to ultraviolet light or sunlight.

At the thirty-third meeting of the American Pediatric Society held in June 1921, John Howland's presidential address was on "Prolonged Intolerance to Carbohydrates," which he devoted mainly to a discussion of the celiac syndrome. This marked a major step toward an understanding of the disorder and outlined an effective plan of therapy that remained standard for many years. He said: "From a clinical experience it has been found that, of all the elements of the food, carbohydrate is the one which must be excluded; that with this greatly reduced the other elements are almost always well-digested even though the absorption of fat may not be so satisfactory as in health." Howland knew that wheat products were among the things at fault, but it was nearly thirty years before Dicke's observation narrowed the fault to gluten and afforded confirmation of Howland's keen clinical inferences.

Among the excellent pediatricians trained by Howland was Hugh W. Josephs, who remained in a senior post at Johns Hopkins after Howland's death. While he was on the Harriet Lane house staff, he developed an interest in diseases of the blood and became nationally known as a pediatric hematologist. One of his important contributions was the treatment of secondary anemia in infancy with iron and copper. This relationship had been shown in the experimental animal by a group of investigators at Wisconsin, but studies in Boston by Tracey Mallory and his group indicated that large amounts of copper produced hemochromatosis in experimental animals. Therefore, there was resistance to giving copper to patients for the treatment of anemia. It was later shown that the large doses of copper used by Mallory produced a secondary hemochromatosis because of excessive hemolysis and, subsequently, Joseph's findings were fully accepted. In his study published in the *Bulletin of The Johns Hopkins Hospital* in 1931, Josephs found that copper, when given in addition to iron, accelerated the rise in hemoglobin. Copper appeared to accelerate hemoglobin formation, but had no effect on reticulocytes.

Josephs, in collaboration with Graham Ross, described the first case of recurrent attacks of spontaneous hypoglycemia in a young black boy who came into the hospital repeatedly for vomiting and loss of consciousness. On some admissions he was given salt solution, but on others glucose was administered intraperitoneally. Josephs noted that when the patient was given glucose, he promptly regained consciousness. On the next admission, he was given orange juice by mouth, which produced a quick recovery. The diagnosis was confirmed by the finding of hypoglycemia during the attacks.

Josephs was also one of the pediatricians who had an early interest in sickle cell anemia. On October 26, 1928, he presented his findings on the clinical aspects of sickle cell anemia at a meeting of the Johns Hopkins Medical Research Club. He described the clinical findings in twelve cases of sickle cell anemia. Emphasis was placed on the joint symptoms and their similarity to rheumatic fever. Hepatomegaly was found in the majority of cases, and in one instance, cirrhosis of the liver.

Hugh Josephs remained an active and effective member of the Harriet Lane staff until his retirement in 1956. During this time, he produced many other interesting clinical investigative studies, mainly in the field of hematology.

Howland's Successor

Edwards Albert Park, whose association with the Department of Pediatrics began with the advent of John Howland, was chosen to carry forward this focus of pediatric excellence following the untimely death of his former chief.

Born in Gloversville, New York, in 1877, he was educated at Phillips Andover Academy and Yale University. He received his M.D. degree from the College of Physicians and Surgeons of Columbia University in 1903. He served a one-year internship at Roosevelt Hospital and a six-month residency at the New York Foundling Hospital. It was there that he met John Howland. Park then returned to the College of Physicians and Surgeons as an instructor in medicine and pediatrics. He also held the Proudfit Fellowship in medical research, and for a time an instructorship in pathology. He shared an office and worked with Dr. Theodore Janeway on blood pressure, his first venture in research. In 1912 Dr. Park was asked by Dr. Howland to come to Baltimore, an opportunity which he seized. Beforehand, however, he spent a year in Germany in the laboratory of the eminent pathologist M. B. Schmidt, at Marburg. Here he learned the marvels of bone growth and the manner of its disruption by disease, and for the rest of his life maintained a continuous devotion to this field of study. Park was ready for the study of rickets, which at that time was the most frequent disease of infancy. That cod liver oil could cure rickets was discovered some two hundred years before, and for generations students of the disease had been convinced of the preventive effect of sunlight. But at the turn of the century, "medicine became proudly scientific and the notion that oil from the liver of a cod fish could cure a human ailment received the disrespect it so obviously deserved." It would have to be proved in a scientifically acceptable fashion. This occurred rapidly following the discovery of Mellanby in England that rickets could be produced in animals by defective diets. This new experimental approach led at once to intensive study of the pathogenesis of rickets and, as recounted, the Baltimore team of Mc-Collum, Simmonds, Howland, Park, Kramer, and Shipley made many important contributions, culminating in 1923 in the discovery of vitamin D. From his position at the microscope, Dr. Park provided expert guidance for these classical experiments. "Rickets would have been demolished without assistance from Park but not with the elegance and ceremony which this grand old disease deserved and which his knowledge of the histopathology of bone provided."

In 1921, two years after his return from war service in France as a pediatrician in the civilian division of the American Red Cross, he accepted the chair of pediatrics at Yale. But in 1927 he returned to Baltimore as Dr. Howland's successor. He had found time with Grover Powers in New Haven to carry out experiments which beautifully illustrated the curative effect of sunlight on rickets. Park, in accepting the Kober Medal of the Association of American Physicians in a manner expected of such a modest person, gave the major credit for the work on rickets to Elmer McCollum.

Over the years Park continued to devote his talents to the study of the diseases affecting bone. He was one of the few investigators who correlated the histological changes in bone with clinical, biochemical, and radiological findings. Bone histology is particularly difficult because of the large volume of mineralized matrix which hampers microscopic study of bone structure. Dr. Park had the skill and patience to overcome these difficulties. He recognized the importance of correlating structure and radiographic changes so that bone x-rays could be properly interpreted. In addition to rickets, he studied scurvy, lead poisoning, and nutritional disturbances of bone growth. He described the early radiographic changes in scurvy and interpreted them in terms of the histology of the calcified cartilaginous plate at the metaphysis and of the diminished trabecular density of the bone cortex. He described the dense band at the metaphysis of the long bones in lead poisoning and showed that this was the result not only of the increased density of lead in the bones but of a disturbance in bone growth and remodeling. The trabecular structure of the bone was altered, leading to much more closely packed trabeculae at the growing ends of the bone. These studies led to observations of the effects of growth retardation on bone structure and elucidated the mechanism of the production of the so-called growth arrest lines in bone. He interested pediatricians and radiologists in the more careful examination of bone structure by demonstrating that the growth arrest lines persisted for many years, so that evidences of previous periods of growth arrest could be diagnosed by examination of x-rays of the long bones; in Park's own phrase, "the imprinting of nutritional disturbances on the growing bone."

Dr. Howland had used the general dispensary only for teaching, and did not permit the formation of specialty clinics. Park was convinced that the chronically ill child suffered most. Therefore, during his first year as chief of the Harriet Lane Home, in spite of great opposition, he started a series of disease-oriented clinics. Many of the doctors thought that these special clinics would weaken the dispensary, but Park relied on the resulting improvement in patient care to bring more children to the hospital. Indeed, he was right. News of the improvement in patient care traveled rapidly and brought an ever-increasing number of children with severe and unusual conditions to the clinic.

The following year Park decided that infants who were admitted to the infant ward, which was composed of the east and west side of the fourth floor of the Harriet Lane Home, should be separated according to whether their illness was infectious or noninfectious, and not according to the color of their skin. The wisdom of this decision was indisputable, and the first ward of the Johns Hopkins Hospital was integrated in 1928.

Park also built a strong Department of Social Service. The social workers not only interpreted the doctor's orders to the patient but they also visited the home and helped the patient carry out the doctor's recommendations. In short, the social workers were Park's solution to the present-day problem of medical compliance.

Park was an inspiring chief whose wisdom is amply documented by the succession of leaders in pediatrics who trained under him. He expressed his ideal of a pediatric clinic as follows:

It is a place where sick children get the best medical care available anywhere and well children obtain the best guidance of how to remain well; where teaching is accepted as an integral part of the day's work; where thought keeps overflowing into new channels of curiosity and takes practical form in study and experimentation; where the spirit which prevails is one of intense burning zeal for the truth, which means constantly to seek to learn more and to do better things; where the human side of things is never lost sight of or made subordinate to the rest; where there is a broad social outlook and a consciousness of obligations to the community, not only to the individual members but to the community as a whole, so that the clinic is accepted by general consent as a great directing influence.

During Park's tenure, excellence in research continued to flourish. His successor, Francis Schwentker, made many important contributions, perhaps the most notable being the production of "allergic encephalomyelitis" with myelin destruction in monkeys, induced by repeated injections of normal brain tissue. These important experiments had far-reaching human implications, including the paralytic sequelae of anti-rabies inoculations, the potential risks of immunization against poliomyelitis with anitgens obtained from the nervous system, as well as the important area of auto-immune disease.

Lawson Wilkins

Lawson Wilkins graduated from the Johns Hopkins Medical School in 1918 near the head of his class, but received his degree in absentia while in France as a member of the Johns Hopkins Hospital Unit in World War I. The Johns Hopkins medical students who had volunteered were given jobs as orderlies. One day they were summoned by the adjutant, who informed them that they had just been accorded M.D. degrees by the University and that they were now physicians. Having made this brief announcement he remarked, "Now go back to the work you are doing." Lawson was becoming an expert with the bedpan.

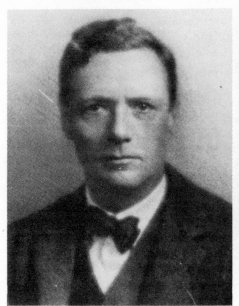

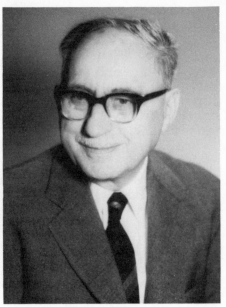

James Lawder Gamble
From Riesman's *History*

Benjamin Kramer
Courtesy of Dr. David Grob

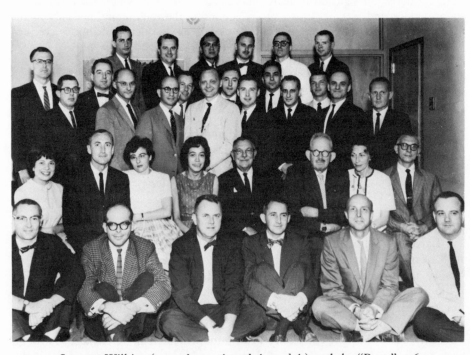

Lawson Wilkins (*second row, fourth from left*) and the "Boys," 1963
Courtesy of Dr. Claude Migeon

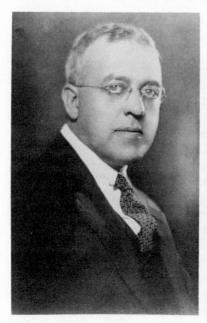

Paul G. Shipley
From the Archives Office, The Johns Hopkins Medical Institutions

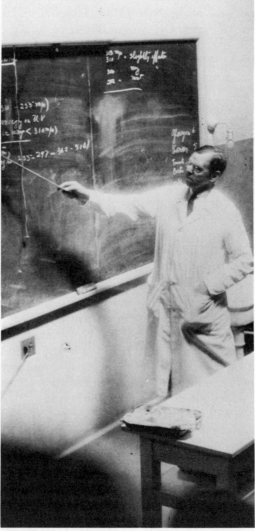

Edwards Albert Park
From the Archives Office, The Johns Hopkins Medical Institutions

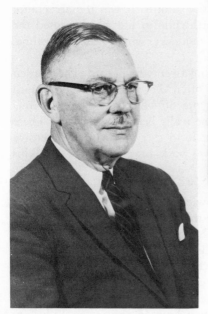

Lawson Wilkins
From the Archives Office, The Johns Hopkins Medical Institutions

At the expiration of the war, Wilkins obtained an internship in internal medicine at the New Haven Hospital under two of the ablest internists in the United States, Dr. George Blumer, a former pupil of Dr. Osler, and Dr. Wilder Tileston. He then accepted an internship in pediatrics at the Harriet Lane Home. He chose pediatrics because he thought it was the branch of medicine best attuned to the new biochemical and metabolic approach to disease at that time.

While an intern, Lawson started a special clinic for patients with congenital syphilis. He was impressed by the poor care these children were receiving, assigned as they were in haphazard fashion to a staff of interns lacking special knowledge of the disease or of the technical methods required; moreover, there was no follow-up system. Lawson organized their care and obtained a special social worker. The outcome was Howland's authorization of a special clinic for congential syphilis, the only specialty clinic in existence in pediatrics until 1927.

At the end of his internship at the Harriet Lane Home, Wilkins decided in favor of a life devoted to private practice. He made this decision because of his father. Wilkins, Senior, like his son, was tireless, alert to progress, open-minded to new ideas. He was probably the first physician in Baltimore to employ the clinical thermometer and to use diphtheria antitoxin. The elder Wilkins had always had an intense interest in his fellow human beings and their individual problems and could not conceive of complete satisfaction in life apart from the intimate contact with sick people which practice affords. It was the acceptance of his father's feeling for what was most worthwhile in life which caused the son to decline Howland's offer of an assistant residency, which was, at the time, the open gateway to an academic career.

Wilkins practiced pediatrics for the ensuing twenty-five years. The burden of work he carried was tremendous, and he often did not return home until eight, nine, or ten in the evening. Plenty of practitioners belong in academic medicine, and many men in academic medicine really belong in practice. There are, however, occasional supermen who are able to carry on a most extensive practice and to combine it with investigative work of great value. Wilkins belonged to this group of unusual men.

Very soon after he entered practice, his scientific studies began, and the subjects he chose concerned fundamental knowledge. His first paper, published with Benjamin Kramer in 1923, reported on the potassium content of human serum. In that same year he began work with Emmett Holt, Jr., on investigations of the calcium and phosphorus metabolism of rickets. In 1927 he undertook to cure rickets by an intramuscular injection of a cod liver oil derivative. Needing a biochemist, Wilkins obtained the cooperation of Charles Bills, who was at that time a postgraduate student under E. V. McCollum in the Johns Hopkins School of Hygiene. The interest which Lawson aroused in Bills concerning the nature of vitamin D was the immediate cause of the latter's entrance into steroid chemistry and not only determined the course of Bills's career but was also the starting point for his notable discoveries.

In the period between 1921 and 1927, Wilkins's studies took the form of reviews. These reviews were responses to requests from Louis Hamman and allowed Wilkins to become completely conversant with subjects of vital importance to him as a practicing pediatrician.

In the early 1930s Fritz Talbot of Boston sent Wilkins a child with epilepsy in the process of being treated with the ketogenic diet. Wilkins showed such interest in the treatment of epilepsy by means of the ketogenic diet that Park asked him to join Edward Bridge, who was then in charge of the epilepsy clinic at the Harriet Lane. As a result of his work with Bridge, Wilkins published a paper in 1937 on "Epilepsy in Childhood: I. A Statistical Study of Clinical Types; II. The Incidence of Remissions; III. Results with the Ketogenic Diet." This notable paper showed the care with which he kept his records and particularly the soundness with which he reached his conclusions. The detachment and common sense with which he approached his problems were particularly impressive. His work in the epilepsy clinic brought him into close contact with Park, and it was then that his potentiality in an academic atmosphere became apparent.

It was evident in 1935 that great advances were about to be made in endocrinology. Scientific knowledge had developed just enough to stimulate speculation. Falta had introduced the idea of multiple endocrine deficiencies, though his evidence was little more than guesswork. Under the leadership of men like Lewellys Barker of Johns Hopkins and Timme of New York, endocrinologists were making diagnoses of complex endocrine disturbances from little more than conjecture, and remarkable results from the administration of various hormone preparations by mouth were being reported. The practice of endocrinology was becoming very profitable. Wilkins, after reading Engelbach's book on endocrinology late one night, became so disgusted that he threw it across the room.

Children suffering from endocrine disturbances who came to the Harriet Lane Home outpatient department were being assigned at random to the doctors who were working there. There was no organization and no planned study. Park, recognizing the necessity of placing the management of children with endocrine problems on a sound basis, concluded that the only way in which this could be accomplished was to establish a special clinic devoted to the study of endocrinologic disorders. Anxious to place Wilkins at the head of some important section of the department, he offered Wilkins the directorship of the endocrine clinic. Wilkins replied by inquiring if Park wished to make him a charlatan. However, in spite of misgivings that the road led to moral depravity, Wilkins accepted the offer.

From 1935 to 1946, Wilkins continued to practice and at the same time to carry on his research and teaching in pediatric endocrinology. He was aided in his scientific work by a generous grant from the Commonwealth Fund, but this did not include salary, and he received none from the Johns Hopkins University.

At first he concentrated on the study of children suffering from thyroid deficiency, where he knew he was on solid ground. At the forty-ninth meeting of the American Pediatric Society in April 1937, Lawson Wilkins presented a classic study of growth, osseous development, and mental development in cretins and in dwarfs with special reference to thyroid therapy. His observations and conclusions have needed no significant revision in later years.

At the fiftieth meeting held in May 1938, Lawson Wilkins and his associates discussed creatine metabolism in hypothyroidism and dwarfism as influenced by thyroid therapy and pituitary extract containing the thyrotrophic hormone. Creatine output increased and the blood cholesterol fell in hypothyroid patients with thyroid therapy but not in other types of dwarfism. The latter did not respond to thyroid-stimulating hormone. These effects of thyroid medication in hypothyroidism appeared earlier and represented more delicate tests of thyroid response than increase in the metabolic rate. At the fifty-second meeting, May 1940, Wilkins discussed epiphyseal dysgenesis (stippled epiphyses), which he found to be a nearly constant phenomenon in hypothyroidism in early childhood and pathognomonic of the condition.

Later, J. J. VanWyk, M. M. Grumbach, T. H. Shepard II, and Wilkins reported the late results of treatment of sixteen thyrotoxic children with thiouracil drugs. Although four of the patients following initial improvement had eventually come to subtotal thyroidectomy, the rest had experienced sustained relief of symptoms, many of them for months and years after discontinuance of drug treatment. Persistent thyroid enlargement while under thiouracil treatment often responded dramatically to administration of desiccated thyroid gland.

Francis Schwentker, who succeeded Dr. Park in 1946, was able to offer Wilkins a "full-time" position in the department. This he accepted, even though it meant a considerable reduction in income. "He now had complete liberty, liberty to read, to study, to enter the laboratory and to think. In short his only compulsion was to do those things which he liked to do. No club behind, ahead nothing but carrots unlimited."

As the work on hypothyroidism waned, studies of the syndrome of sexual infantilism with ovarian agenesis and associated defects came into focus. Although these studies, like the thyroid work, brought no spectacular discoveries, they provided a great reservoir of knowledge, which became of inestimable value when the discoveries of sex-chromatin determination were announced in 1949 and the technique of sex-chromosome counting became available in 1959.

The pediatric endocrine clinic had inherited a large population of pseudohermaphroditic patients, particularly with the female pseudohermaphroditic-adrenocortical syndrome, who, in earlier years, had come to Johns Hopkins to Hugh Young's urology clinic for adrenocortical surgery. With the advent of the adrenocortical steroids and newer knowledge of the adrenal-pituitary axis, new hypotheses began to be tested in relation to the regulation of abnormal adrenocortical dysfunction. In the late 1940s and the early 1950s, this testing of new hypotheses became first a friendly rivalry and then a neck-and-neck race between the pediatric endocrine groups at Johns Hopkins and Massachusetts General Hospital. It was in December 1949 that testing in both institutions was first made of the effects of the newly synthesized adrenocortical hormone, cortisone, in the hyperadrenocortical female pseudohermaphrodite. The astoundingly successful therapeutic result was obtained by both. Lawson Wilkins and his group followed this contribution with intensive clinical and laboratory study of large numbers of affected infants and children, and these studies defined the rationale of the treatment and extended knowledge of the basic biochemistry of the syndrome and its subvarieties. As a result of these interests, Lawson Wilkins established the first psychohormonal research unit for the study of the psychology of hermaphroditism and related endocrine disorders. These studies, in which John Money was an important participant, increased fundamental knowledge of the process of psychosexual differentiation relative to genetic and hormonal variables and the sex of rearing.

Lawson Wilkins was a great leader, and his methodical approach, his superb record-keeping, and his broad knowledge of pediatrics allowed him to make many important contributions to pediatric endocrinology. He was not on a par with some others in terms of basic scientific contributions, but his influence was great and in every respect his name belongs on that list of famous offspring of the second generation of the Hopkins faculty.

One of his major contributions, in which he himself took great pride, was the training of the present generation of pediatric endocrinologists both in this country and abroad. The list of his pupils is long, and among them there are many who are now heads of departments of pediatrics or directors of pediatric endocrine clinics. Wilkins was very proud and fond of his fellows, whom he called "the boys," although a few "girls" belonged to the group. In the spring of 1963, only a few months before his death, Wilkins called all "the boys" and invited them to a scientific meeting in Baltimore. This was a momentous occasion and included the oldest boy, Walter Fleischman, who was Lawson's first associate in the endocrine clinic and who contributed most importantly to the thyroid work. After Lawson's death, "the boys" decided to have a reunion along with the second generation of fellows. Beginning in 1965, these meetings have taken place at Johns Hopkins every other year. By 1971 the group had become quite large, and a new type of administrative structure was needed for it. Thus, the Lawson Wilkins Pediatric Endocrine Society came into being. A constitution for the society was written, and Claude Migeon was elected founding president.

In 1942 Wilkins was promoted to associate professor and in 1957 to a full professorship. In 1953 he received the Borden Award of the American Academy of Pediatrics and in 1955 the Francis Amory Prize of the American Academy of Arts and Sciences.

Wilkins' studies were based on the most meticulous investigations of his patients, not on the literature, as is the case with so many others. For this reason, his work has a particular authority. The method which Lawson employed is that which von Pirquet used with such brilliance in his studies on allergy and on measles, the graphic method. All data collected were represented visually on running charts, which showed their qualitative, quantitative, and temporal relationships. They were accompanied by serial photographs of the patients themselves. The whole produces a statistical record, the significance of which is apparent at a glance.

Special clinics assigned to the study of particular diseases are the ultimate sources of knowledge concerning the outcome of disease. An endocrine clinic lends itself particularly to long-term study, for the patients are rare enough and, also, peculiar enough, to stand out clearly in the mind, and they tend to keep returning spontaneously because they continually require help. Moreover, in endocrinology, studies extending through the period of childhood into adult life and including the period of reproduction have a particular importance and, indeed, the question of longevity is involved. Wilkins' clinic has been distinguished by its long-term studies. In the systematic follow-up of his patients, the new data are entered on graphic charts which now in many instances cover years. These graphic charts are already a visual library of endocrinology. If the clinic is perpetuated indefinitely, these records will have the same importance in contributing to the knowledge of disease that biographies have in the formation of history.

Wilkins often stated that he would not have been deprived of his twenty-five years in practice for anything. It is interesting to speculate what influence this experience had on his final development and what would have happened had he committed himself to "full time" at the beginning. From the way in which Howland's clinic was organized in 1922, Wilkins would have undoubtedly been drawn into the vortex of biochemical research and become a biochemist in his own right. The direct approach to his problem via the test tube would then have become the primary motif. His experience in practice led him to approach the problems of his patients primarily as a physician, secondarily as a scientist. It enabled him to view his human subjects in totality and to move to the particular from the wide perspective of the general. The welfare of the patient was always the primary consideration.

Thus, Lawson Wilkins established a pediatric endocrine clinic at Hopkins which systematically applied laboratory methods to problems of hormonal imbalance in growing subjects. From observations carried out over long periods of time on individual subjects, there emerged important new knowledge of various deviations from the usual pattern of growth and of sex differentiation. Wilkins' volume *The Diagnosis and Treatment of Endocrine Disorders in Childhood and Adolescence* quickly became a standard text. Scholars came from all parts of the world to bring themselves up to date in this field, and Wilkins, a forceful and dramatic lecturer, was in constant demand as a speaker. Energetic, gregarious, outspoken, with a booming voice and enormous zest, he presented a vivid picture of the challenges and rewards of clinical investigation.

18 ❧ Johns Hopkins—Its Role in
Medical Education for Women

The entrance of women into the profession of medicine is an event of impor-
tance—not only to the medical profession, but to humanity and society, and it
will always have a place in human history.—Dr. William H. Welch: Memorial
for Dr. Elizabeth Blackwell, 1911

THE AMERICAN COLONIES, following closely the practices of their English
forebears, excluded women from the mainstream of medical education. A few
women were as educated in medicine as their male confreres: one of them, Dr.
Mary Jones, was convicted of witchcraft in the Massachusetts colony. In the
early nineteenth century a few women were educated under the apprentice
system, but the only "degree" a woman could receive at the time was a certificate entitled "Testimonial of Qualification to Practice the Obstetric Art." However, the United States, beginning in 1849 with Elizabeth Blackwell's graduation
from the Geneva College of Medicine in upstate New York, was the pioneer
in medical education for women.

That the Johns Hopkins University School of Medicine played a vital role
in this pioneering endeavor was largely the result of the efforts of four young
Baltimore women who were keenly interested in fostering opportunities for
women to obtain graduate education in various fields. The leader of the group
and the dominant personality was M. Cary Thomas, who because of her sex
had been rejected as a candidate for a Ph.D. degree at the Johns Hopkins
University. She studied abroad for her doctorate degree, became professor of
English and dean at Bryn Mawr College upon her return, and in 1893 was
made president of that institution. Her friend, Mary Elizabeth Garrett, had
inherited her father's fortune in 1884, and through M. Cary Thomas's influence
contributed to various educational enterprises, including the establishment in
1885 of the Bryn Mawr Preparatory School for Girls in Baltimore. The other
two young women were Mary Gwinn and Elizabeth King, and all four were
daughters of members of the original University Board of Trustees named by
Johns Hopkins.

Their opportunity to aid the cause of women in medicine came in 1888
when the Johns Hopkins Hospital was almost ready to open. In that year the
Baltimore and Ohio Railroad Company ceased paying dividends on its stock.
Since the income of the university was derived almost entirely from the stock
Johns Hopkins had owned in that company, it was clear that the university was

not in a position to finance the medical school in the near future. This was particularly disappointing because key members of the faculty had already been appointed, including Welch, Osler, Halsted, and Kelly.

On May 2, 1890, the Woman's Fund Committee was formed, its sole objective being to raise a sufficient sum of money to permit the School of Medicine to be established, and in return for the gift, to obtain a guarantee from the trustees that women would be admitted to the school on equal terms with men. Miss Garrett and her friends inspired women in other cities to accept the challenge, and fifteen regional committees were formed. Among the participants were Dr. Elizabeth Blackwell, Mrs. Julia Ward Howe, and Mrs. Benjamin Harrison, the First Lady, who was the head of the Washington Committee.

Within a few months $100,000, of which nearly half was contributed by Miss Garrett, was offered to the trustees. Initially there was strong opposition from the newly appointed faculty, but in the end they urged the trustees to accept the gift and the stipulations which went with it. The trustees promptly and unanimously voted to accept the gift with the proviso that the medical school would not open until a minimum of $500,000 was available. This proved to be a difficult task.

On Christmas Eve, 1892, Miss Garrett agreed to contribute the remaining amount ($306,977) in addition to her initial gift of $47,787. She did, however, impose an additional stipulation of higher scholastic standards of admission than had previously been contemplated by the trustees. Despite great anxiety over this new condition and rather tense negotiations, agreement was finally reached. On February 22, 1893, President Gilman officially announced that the Johns Hopkins University School of Medicine would open in October 1893, over four years after the first patient had been admitted to the Johns Hopkins Hospital.

This chapter relates the stories of four women graduates of Johns Hopkins who have made important contributions to medicine. Their experiences emphasize that the road to equality for women in medicine has been long and difficult. However, as we shall see, the trail has been blazed; women have become successful practitioners in both medicine and surgery, have made valuable contributions to medicine's scientific base, and have achieved the status of departmental heads.

Dorothy Reed

Edmund Wilson, of *New Yorker* fame, wrote a fascinating diary-notebook entitled *Upstate: Records and Recollections of Northern New York*. Wilson had an old family house—the Stone House—in Talcottville, a small community near Utica, New York. His delightful book covers the period 1950–1970, the chapters recounting his experiences with the people of that part of New York State and his family and friends. One of Wilson's favorite relatives, who summered with her mother in the Stone House, was "my pretty, dark cousin Dorothy whom I was always hoping to kiss." His portrait of Dorothy

Reed, later Dorothy Reed Mendenhall, a graduate of the class of 1900 of the Johns Hopkins Medical School, is a penetrating one.

Dorothy Reed was born into a family of superior social status. An intelligent and handsome young woman who possessed a very strong character, she had apparently intended to be a journalist, but was later diverted to medicine, influenced perhaps by physician relatives. In her own memoirs, she stated that her course of action was influenced by a need to "get into some work that interested me and be freed from having to live with my mother and do the sort of things she felt would be likely to make a good marriage." In the 1880s and 1890s medicine was still not considered an appropriate profession for women. But Dorothy Reed had enough tenacity, intelligence, and strength of character to accept the formidable challenge. It is of interest that after her graduation from medical school, while she was working in a hospital in New Jersey, a socialite relative regretfully declined, in view of Dorothy's position, to meet socially with her. This incident made Dorothy Reed feel for the first time what it meant to belong to a "minority." Her relatives, in all the years she was in Baltimore, always alluded to her as "being South for the winter."

Dorothy Reed's early education was at the hands of a tutor. Later she entered Smith College, of which her son was ultimately to become president. In the spring of 1893, when a sophomore, she was asked by one of her classmates, Bertha Bardeen, to look after her brother, who was coming from Harvard to see Bertha play tennis. It was while entertaining Charles Bardeen that she learned of the remarkable school of medicine being started in Baltimore to which he had been accepted and was to enter in the fall. Her interest aroused, she promptly wrote to Dean William H. Welch to inquire whether women were to be admitted, and eventually she entered the class of 1896. Charles R. Bardeen was a member of the first class at Hopkins and later became professor of anatomy and dean at the University of Wisconsin School of Medicine. His friendship with Dorothy Reed was a long one, as she went to live in Madison, Wisconsin, following her marriage to Charles Mendenhall.

From the time Dorothy Reed arrived at the medical school, she was frequently put in a position of having to defend her desire to become a physician. She had an unpleasant early experience with Dr. Osler, who tried to discourage her from becoming a medical student (although apparently she later became a favorite of his, and the admiration was mutual), and during her second year at Hopkins, she attended a lecture which, Dorothy said, "nearly sent me out of medicine." The lecture was given by an otolaryngologist on the diseases of the nasal passages.* He compared the cavernous tissues present in

* John Noland Mackenzie, clinical professor of laryngology and rhinology in the Johns Hopkins medical school and laryngologist to the Johns Hopkins Hospital. "The Physiological and Pathological Relations Between the Nose and the Sexual Apparatus of Man," Remarks made before the British Medical Association at its Montreal meeting, September 1897, *Johns Hopkins Hospital Bulletin* 9 (1898): 100. Mackenzie points out that the intimate relationship between the genital organs and those of the throat and neck seems to have attracted the special attention of the ancients, including Aristotle and Hippocrates. Mackenzie's attention was first attracted to investigation of the physiological and pathological relations between the nose and the genital organs by the case of a patient in London in 1879 who invariably

the nasal passages with the corpus spongiosum of the penis, and for the amusement of the male students he told many off-color stories. When he could not say things in English, he quoted Latin—and since Dorothy Reed had majored in Latin at Smith, she understood most of his quotations. When she later wrote of this incident nearly fifty years had passed, but according to Wilson, much that was said in that lecture was branded in her mind, and still "came up like a decomposing body from the bottom of a pool that is disturbed." Simon Flexner, who had presided at the lecture, afterwards apologized, but Dorothy decided that as long as she was in medicine, she would never object to anything that a fellow student or doctor did in her presence if he acted or spoke the same way to a man; but if he discriminated against her because she was a woman or was offensive in a way that he wouldn't be to a man, she would crack down on him herself or take it up with the authorities if he proved to be too much for her to handle. This position, which proved to be a viable one for a woman in medicine in the nineteenth century, apparently made life bearable for her, allowed her to make friends with some men who were not very pleasant persons but knew no better, and earned her the respect and friendship of many of her associates—although it didn't endear her to one or two she fell afoul of. As a result she developed an independence, even an arrogance, which she felt was foreign to her original nature. It was her belief that she was not such a nice person but a stronger one after Johns Hopkins.

An interesting sidelight of her medical school days at Hopkins are her comments, related by Wilson, about a fellow student, Gertrude Stein. Miss Stein was apparently as skillful at evading her course responsibilities as she had been at Radcliffe in her courses under William James. As she relates in her *Autobiography of Alice B. Toklas*, she had written on an examination paper: "Dear Professor James—I am so sorry but I really do not feel a bit like an examination paper in philosophy today." William James gave her an A and wrote: "Dear Miss Stein, I understand how you feel. I often feel that way myself." However, the doctors at Hopkins were not always so generous. According to Dorothy Reed, the professor of obstetrics did not think that Gertrude should receive a degree: "She could do nothing with her hands, was very untidy and careless in her technique and very irritating in her attitude of intellectual superiority which was marked even in her youth." The faculty decided to give her special consideration, however, probably on Dr. Mall's insistence, and he gave her a problem similar to one Florence Sabin had completed successfully in her fourth year. This involved the sectioning and reconstruction of a human embryo brain with the object of studying the development of the centers in the brain and the tracts leading from them. After working for several weeks on this preparation, Gertrude handed the results to Mall in the hope that she would receive credit for it in place of obstetrics, thus allowing her to graduate. Some days later Mall took the problem to Florence Sabin, saying:

---

suffered from coryza after sexual indulgence. Stimulated by this observation, he began the study of the subject, and five years later published the results of his investigations in an essay entitled "Irritation of the Sexual Apparatus as an Etiological Factor in the Production of Nasal Disease," in the *American Journal of the Medical Sciences* for April 1884.

"Either I am crazy or Miss Stein is. Will you see what you can make out of her work?" After studying the reconstruction carefully, Sabin concluded that Miss Stein must have embedded the cord when it was turned back under the embryo brain instead of extended from it. In no other way could the mysterious features of her reconstruction be explained. The model was eventually thrown into a wastebasket, and Miss Stein was refused her degree. In her book about Alice B. Toklas, Stein tells briefly of her student days in Baltimore and mentions a model of an embryo brain which she had made and which was of much service to the students.

Dorothy Reed's account of her life in Baltimore shows her readiness to protect and defend herself. She barely escaped rape and murder when the caretaker of the building in which she lodged came to her room and inquired whether he could be of any service to her. She produced a six-shooter (which, however, was not loaded) and locked the door. Half an hour later he had found an unprotected woman, and raped and murdered her.

In 1900 Dorothy Reed graduated fifth in a class of forty-three. In those days the twelve students with the highest grades were given internships. Dr. William Henry Welch explained to her that there was a "serious embarrassment" over the fact that both she and her fellow female student, Florence Sabin, were among the top twelve and both wanted to specialize in medicine. "There has never been more than one woman intern," he said. He asked her if she would take an internship in surgery or gynecology, but she declined. The morning after commencement she was given the position in medicine that she had earned. Soon afterwards she became very indignant when she received a "courteous" letter from Henry Christian, later professor of medicine at Harvard and physician-in-chief at Peter Bent Brigham Hospital, asking if she was quite certain that she wanted and was going to take her medical appointment, ending up by saying that if he couldn't have medicine under Dr. Osler, he would not stay in Baltimore.

After spending the summer in Boston studying pathology, she returned to Johns Hopkins to begin her internship, only to find that another controversy had developed about her appointment. Since two women had been appointed interns in medicine, one would have to be responsible for the white female ward and the other for the black ward. Dr. Henry M. Hurd, the hospital superintendent, thought it was impossible for a woman to serve the black males in Ward M. Dr. Sabin had apparently suggested that if only one internship could be awarded to a woman, the appointment should go to Dr. Reed; but Dr. Reed had no intention of assenting to any such disposition. She stated plainly that if either of them had to give up the internship, "I would be the one." But after all, Dr. Osler had given her the post and had congratulated her on it. Since Dr. Osler was away, she decided to speak personally to Dr. Hurd about the matter.

To my horror he said that he understood that it was I who wanted the colored wards. He had had experience with a similar woman physician ... who had a residentship at Hopkins before my day. He told me of her abnormal sex perversions. He said that of course he thought, and all my classmates and the medical staff would think the same thing—that only my desire to gratify sexual curiosity would allow me or any woman to take charge of a male ward.

When it came to Negroes, did I realize that the white nurses were always in danger on the male colored wards.... The male intern was all that kept them and the colored orderlies from insulting the nurses and women students—or more.... Finally, he said so much that my anger came to the rescue.

"Dr. Hurd," I replied, "I came to Baltimore to learn a profession.... I have spent six months as a clerk on the colored wards, male and female, surgical and medical. In that time ... I made most of the physical examinations.... As far as I know I gave satisfaction. Osler gave me the appointment and ... until he returns I shall be the intern of the colored wards and I shall do my best. If ... I find I cannot do my duties I shall tender my resignation to Dr. Osler."

Dr. Hurd's recollection of the conversation is not recorded, and Dorothy Reed's may be an exaggerated version written in retrospect. In any event, the path was obviously not an easy one for women in medicine in that generation. Dorothy Reed served her internship. In fact, although most interns at Hopkins left for the summer and let the fourth-year students take over the wards, she stayed until the last day. "Something Dr. Hurd had said of a woman being irresponsible and not to be trusted to see things through kept me at my post."

Dorothy Reed's major scientific contribution—a detailed description of what are now known as Reed-Sternberg cells—was made in 1902 while she was a fellow in Dr. Welch's Department of Pathology. There seems little doubt that the Reed-Sternberg cells were recognized by Greenfield as early as 1878. Their characteristics were next pointed out by Sternberg in 1898. Sternberg studied a series of cases of Hodgkin's disease combined with active tuberculosis, and only years later did he give up the idea that he was dealing with a peculiar form of tuberculosis. Therefore, one might argue that the greatest credit should go to Dorothy Reed, who described the cells even more accurately than did either of her predecessors and who clearly recognized that they were an essential part of the disease described by Hodgkin some seventy years earlier.

Dorothy Reed, reviewing surgical specimens and autopsy material considered to be Hodgkin's disease, found eight cases which closely resembled each other clinically and which had, she believed, a uniform histological picture. In her search for this material, she examined many specimens of true malignant disease, leukemia and tuberculosis, but in none of them did she find similar microscopic changes in the lymph nodes. Five of the cases in her series terminated fatally and three came to autopsy. In one case there was a generalized miliary tuberculosis, which from the history was apparently a terminal infection. No sign of tuberculosis was found in either of the other autopsy cases or in any of the extirpated glands, although careful search was made for tubercle bacilli.

The key contribution of Dorothy Reed's study was the description of the microscopic changes (Fig. 1). Since a diagnosis of Hodgkin's disease depends on the presence of these cells, the criteria for identifying them must be strict.

The studies of Florence Sabin on the development of the lymphatic glands proved of great value and assistance to her in the interpretation of her findings. A striking feature of her specimens were large giant cells, formed, she thought, from proliferating endothelial cells: transitions from epithelioid cells to large uninuclear cells, and from these to giant cells, in which one or more nuclei could be easily found. These giant cells were usually free in the interstices of the tissue but were occasionally seen on the reticulum, and with irregular protoplasmic processes. They occurred in great numbers in the large lymph sinuses of the node and occasionally appeared in the blood vessels. They varied from the size of two or three red blood corpuscles to cells twenty times larger. The smaller cells were usually round or somewhat polygonal; the larger cells were very irregular in shape. Cells having bizarre and irregular nuclei were found in the oldest growths. These giant cells, she concluded, were peculiar to this growth and were of great assistance in diagnosis.

Dorothy Reed summarized her study as follows: (1) We should limit the term Hodgkin's disease to designate a clinical and pathological entity, the main features of which are painless, progressive glandular enlargements, usually starting in the cervical region, without the blood changes of leukemia; (2) the growth presents a specific histological picture, not a simple hyperplasia, but changes suggesting a chronic inflammatory process; (3) the microscopical examination is sufficient for diagnosis; (4) eosinophiles are usually present in great numbers in such growths, but not invariably. Their presence strengthens the diagnosis; (5) the pathological agent is as yet undiscovered. Tuberculosis has no direct relation to the subject.

Dr. Reed also had talent as a medical illustrator, as evidenced by the accompanying illustrations.

Speculation continues as to the nature of the Reed-Sternberg cell. Immunoglobulin has been identified within these cells, suggesting that they might be neoplastic derivations of transformed lymphocytes. The increase in T-lymphocytes in the involved spleen in Hodgkin's disease has posed the question whether these T-lymphocytes represent a cell-mediated response against Reed-Sternberg cells or whether they represent precursor cells, the end stage of which may be Reed-Sternberg cells. However, others have suggested that Reed-Sternberg cells might instead be B-cells of histocytic origin.

After completing a year in pathology, Dr. Reed took a residency in pediatrics at the Foundling Hospital in New York (Dr. Edwards A. Park was an intern there in the same year.) In 1906 she married Charles Elwood Mendenhall, a physicist from Madison, Wisconsin, where she lived and raised her family. For the next nine years she retired from the medical profession to devote herself full-time to home and family. After her last son was born, Dr. Reed was offered a job lecturing and writing for the University of Wisconsin on nutrition, child care, and contagious diseases.

Dr. Reed's first child, a girl, died as a result of poor obstetrical care, from a condition that could have been prevented. After this tragedy, Dr. Reed was determined to improve obstetrical care in this country. In 1912 Congress created the U.S. Children's Bureau, and she worked through that bureau to help reduce the death rate of mothers and infants at childbirth. She found that the death rate in hospital cases far exceeded the rate in non-hospital cases, suggesting that women in childbirth were better off at home. Under the bureau's auspices, she went to Denmark, the country with the lowest maternal mortality rates, and learned that the midwife, who had been in charge of normal births for centuries, was trusted and respected. She was told that in the United States "you interfere—operate too much, we give nature a chance." Dr. Reed's report, published in 1929 and widely publicized, caused the revision of many delivery practices. Before her death in 1964, she also invented the "weighing and measuring test" which became nationally known as a guideline for identifying healthy babies, and carried out many other helpful works in the field of nutrition and child care. She looked upon her work in this area as a memorial to her only daughter.

At a time when women were shunned by the medical profession, Dorothy Reed Mendenhall had the strength of character and intellectual power to successfully complete her medical training, to make a significant contribution to the body of knowledge about disease, and to materially aid other women by her contributions to child and maternal welfare.

Helen Brooke Taussig

Helen Brooke Taussig is probably the best-known woman physician in the world. Clearly her fame rests, along with that of the late Dr. Alfred Blalock, on the development of the now famous blue-baby operation. Since 1945, the Blalock-Taussig procedure for the treatment of cyanotic congenital heart disease has saved the lives of more than twelve thousand children. However, Helen Taussig has done much more, making many basic contributions toward our understanding of the physiology of the heart and the circulatory abnormalities associated with congenital heart disease, as well as significant contributions to the study of rheumatic heart disease. Further, in 1962, she played an important role in pointing out the dangers of thalidomide and saved the American mother from the great tragedies which occurred in Europe and Great Britain.

The road to Helen Taussig's highly successful medical career was fraught with many frustrating and disappointing experiences, and it was only her drive and determination which allowed her to survive being female in a profession dominated by men. She grew up in a scholarly atmosphere in Cambridge, Massachusetts, where her father, Frank William Taussig, was a well-known economist and an adviser to President Woodrow Wilson. After attending the Cambridge School for Girls, Helen was admitted to Radcliffe College. She studied there for two years and then transferred to the University of California at Berkeley, where she received her A.B. degree in 1921. When she graduated, she considered a career in medicine, but her father suggested that public health was a more suitable occupation for a woman and advised her to apply to the Harvard School of Public Health, which opened in the fall of 1922. At that time President Lowell of Harvard was adamant against admitting women to the

Harvard medical school. When Dr. Taussig appeared for her interview, the dean of the School of Public Health told her that she would be permitted to study there but would not be granted permission to work for a degree. She recalls the conversation as follows: "Who is going to be such a fool as to spend two years studying medicine and two years more in public health and not get a degree?" she asked angrily. "No one, I hope," said the dean, to which she replied, "Dr. Rosen, I will not be the first to disappoint you."

Following these rebuffs, Dr. Taussig took a course in anatomy at Boston University, where she studied under Alexander Begg, dean and professor of anatomy. She recalls that Dr. Begg put a beef heart in her hand and told her that it would be worthwhile to become interested in one of the larger organs of the body as she went through medical school. She dissected the heart proficiently, and Dr. Begg, greatly impressed with her powers of observation and interpretation, advised her to apply to Johns Hopkins. All she would need, he said, was a good letter from Harvard. She obtained her Harvard letter from Dr. Walter Cannon, and as a result of this whole experience was clearly headed not only toward medicine but also toward cardiology.

She entered the Johns Hopkins School of Medicine in 1923 and received her M.D. degree four years later. She was elected to Alpha Omega Alpha, but lost out to Dr. Vivian Tappan when she applied for an internship in medicine. She became a pediatrician instead and received a fellowship in the medical cardiovascular division.

John Howland, who developed the first fulltime academic department of pediatrics, used the dispensary mainly for the teaching of students and house officers, being opposed, as we have seen, to the development of specialty clinics. Many thought that this arrangement provided inadequate care for children with chronic diseases. One such person was Howland's successor, Dr. Edwards A. Park, who believed that specialty clinics would not only lead to better care of the children but would also increase knowledge of disease. Thus, under his direction specialty clinics were organized, and Dr. Taussig, at a very young age and with little experience, was appointed physician-in-charge of the cardiac clinic of the Harriet Lane Home in 1930. This was one of the most perceptive appointments Dr. Park made.

Dr. Taussig's particular interest was the study and treatment of rheumatic fever. At that time the relation of streptococci to the pathogenesis of rheumatic fever was being studied actively, but her particular interest was more in the cardiological than in the bacteriological aspects of the disease. One of the early acquisitions in the heart clinic was a fluoroscope. Dr. Park told Helen that she should study each patient under the fluoroscope in different positions, as well as take x-rays and electrocardiograms. Dr. Mary Wilson's work had influenced Dr. Park a great deal, and he believed that viewing the patient under the fluoroscope in different positions might make it possible to differentiate early enlargement in rheumatic fever. He also insisted that one could not develop a pediatric cardiac clinic without studying congenital heart disease. Dr. Taussig accepted this latter assignment with little enthusiasm, as congenital heart disease did not at that time appear to have any pertinent research frontier.

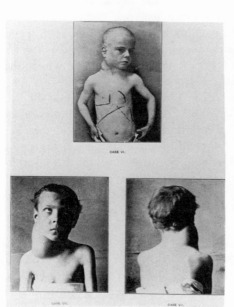

CASE VI.

CASE VII.   CASE VII.

Patients with Hodgkin's disease studied by
Dorothy Reed

Plate 5 from *Johns Hopkins Hosp. Reports*, vol.
10 (1902)

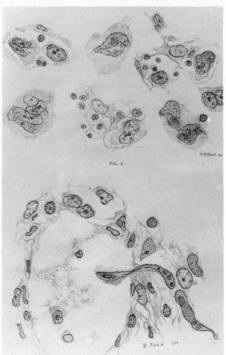

FIG. 4.

D. Reed

Fig. 1. Reed-Sternberg cells

The drawings of these histological sections were
made by Dorothy Reed.
Plate 7 from D. Reed, "On the Pathological
Changes in Hodgkin's Disease with Special
Reference to Its Relation to Tuberculosis," *Johns
Hopkins Hosp. Reports*, vol. 10 (1902)

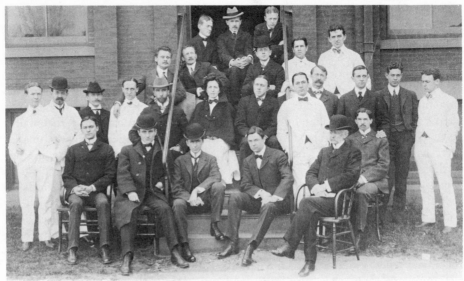

House officers of the Johns Hopkins Hospital, 1901

Dorothy Reed was a medical intern. The other female medical intern, Florence Sabin, is not in the
picture.
Courtesy of the Sophia Smith Collection, Smith College, Northampton, Mass.

234

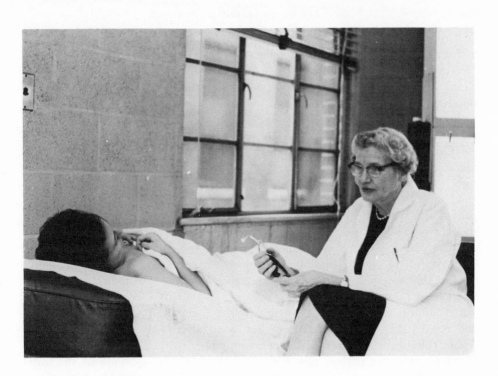

Helen Brooke Taussig
Courtesy of Dr. Helen Brooke Taussig

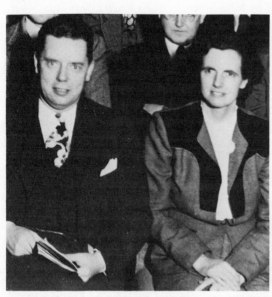

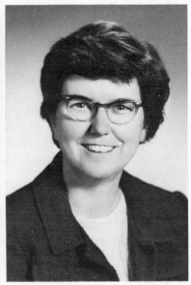

Philip S. Hench and Caroline Bedell Thomas
Courtesy of Dr. Caroline Bedell Thomas

Mary Ellen Avery
Courtesy of Dr. Mary Ellen Avery

In view of the embryonic status of the specialty clinics, there was no great enthusiasm on the part of the house staff to refer patients to the cardiac clinic. However, Dr. Taussig studied in meticulous detail every child who came to the clinic. She developed an enormous capacity for correlating data and understanding the functional circulatory changes brought about by various cardiac malformations. As a result of her work, she came to realize that most cyanotic babies showed enlargement of the right ventricle.

One day in 1933 she fluoroscoped a cyanotic infant and was impressed by the absence of any right ventricular shadow. She made the diagnosis of absent right ventricle; the electrocardiogram showed a left axis deviation. Another child was admitted a few weeks later who had a similar x-ray. When this patient was presented at ward rounds, the resident, Dr. John Washington, thought he had had put up the wrong film, but Dr. Taussig said: "No, that is not the wrong x-ray, it is another child with the same malformation." The similarity of the cardiac findings in these two patients crystallized in her mind the fact that specific malformations cause specific changes in the size and shape of the heart.

After this experience, the interest of the house staff increased, and more and more patients were referred to her. Soon afterwards, a patient was seen whose color became bluer and bluer and who finally died. The house staff wondered why the patient had died, since there was no evidence of the usual manifestations of heart failure. It was clear to Dr. Taussig that the patient had died of anoxemia and was found at postmortem to have extreme tetralogy of Fallot.

Dr. Taussig's next important observation was that some of these cyanotic patients got along reasonably well as long as their ductus arteriosus was open, but that they became more cyanotic and clinically much worse after the ductus closed. Thus, it gradually began to dawn on her that the basic problem was to re-establish flow to the lungs. At one of the Monday pathological conferences in 1939, Dr. MacCallum was trying to trace out the course of the circulation in a patient with pulmonary atresia. Finding this very difficult, he became somewhat mixed up in the process and then remarked that he still didn't know how this patient lived. Dr. Taussig spoke up and said that the circulation became incompatible with life and that is why we are studying such cases in this department rather than in Dr. Park's department. Since Dr. MacCallum had no great use for women in medicine anyway, one could have heard a pin drop at that point in the conference.

Dr. Taussig began to think of ways of trying to keep the ductus open. She searched the literature and considered such methods as nitrogen inhalation. Then she learned that Dr. Gross in Boston was tying off the ductus arteriosus in patients in whom it was the single persistent anomaly. It occurred to her that if one could close a ductus off, one could certainly put one in. Before Dr. Blalock's arrival in Baltimore (1941), Helen went to Boston to consult with Dr. Gross about the possibility of constructing a ductus arteriosus. He answered that it could be done, but he did not show the slightest interest in tackling the problem. Dr. Taussig told Gross that she was considering a move to Boston because of the illness of her father. After hearing her question and about her contemplated move, he advised her not to come where she would not be tolerated. "Stay where you are wanted," he said. It was fortunate for Hopkins that she decided to remain in Baltimore.

Before coming to Baltimore as surgeon-in-chief of the Johns Hopkins Hospital in 1941, Alfred Blalock had worked on various cardiac problems and had operated successfully on three patients with a patent ductus arteriosus. In addition, Blalock and Levy had studied the changes in pressure relations between the aorta and the pulmonary artery after an end-to-end anastomosis between the subclavian artery and a branch of the pulmonary artery. In the fall of 1942 the first operation at Hopkins for closure of the ductus arteriosus was successfully accomplished. At the end of the operation Dr. Taussig said to Dr. Blalock, "I stand in awe and admiration of your surgical skill, but the really great day will come when you build a ductus for a child who is dying of anoxemia and not when you tie off a ductus for a child who has a little too much blood going to the lungs." Dr. Blalock's reply was: "When that day comes, this will seem like child's play." Nevertheless, he had a receptive mind and took the problem to the laboratory.

As recounted by Ravitch, on a spring morning in 1943 Blalock asked the resident to accompany him to Harriet Lane for a consultation requested by Dr. Park. As the surgeons were leaving the ward after having seen the patient, Park asked Blalock whether he thought anything might be done for patients with coarctation of the aorta. Blalock's response was polite and noncommittal, but as he walked out of the Harriet Lane, he said to his resident, "I wonder how this could be approached in the laboratory." Some months later Dr. Park found on his desk a manuscript of a paper by Blalock and Park describing an operation for coarctation of the aorta in dogs, using the subclavian artery to bypass the constriction. In a later conversation, Blalock expressed to Park his concern about employing his coarctation operation in man, since so many of his dogs had become paraplegic when the aorta was cross-clamped during the procedure. As a result of the delay in trying this procedure on a patient with coarctation of the aorta, earlier operations were done by Crafoord in Sweden and Gross in Boston, both of whom employed excision of the coarctation and direct anastomosis. When Blalock discussed his studies on the operative relief of coarctation of the aorta in dogs at a Harriet Lane conference, Helen Taussig asked whether some operation could be devised to improve the pulmonary circulation in children with pulmonic stenosis. Blalock, of course, had the operative remedy at hand—the subclavian-pulmonary anastomosis performed in Nashville some years earlier in the attempt to produce pulmonary hypertension in the dog.

There is some divergence of opinion as to how the idea for the Blalock-Taussig operation came about. According to Dr. Taussig, in 1943 Blalock and Park were discussing the difficulties of cross-clamping the descending aorta. Dr. Park inquired: "Could you not use the carotid artery as a bypass? It is a long, straight artery and there are four vessels to the brain. Wouldn't it be possible to turn the carotid artery down and anastomose it to the aorta below the coarctation?" Whereupon Dr. Taussig spoke up and asked: "If you put the carotid artery into the descending aorta, couldn't you put the subclavian artery into the pulmonary artery?"

Dr. Blalock's version was put pithily in a letter of September 22, 1945: "I must say that if I made the statement to you that you could improve the condition of patients with aortic stenosis if you could find a means to allow more blood to reach the body, that I would be far from solving the practical problem." In 1965 Mark Ravitch wrote to Dr. Edwards A. Park about the matter. Dr. Park replied: "In my presence Dr. Taussig asked Blalock if he could not do something by operation to give patients with the tetralogy of Fallot adequate pulmonary circulation, on the grounds that such was what they required, but without suggesting how this could be done."

However the idea developed, Dr. Blalock invited Dr. Taussig to work on the problem with him in his laboratory. At this stage, the laboratory experiments were directed toward the production of pulmonary stenosis. Difficulty was encountered, as the ligatures around the pulmonary artery would cut through the arterial wall and the obstruction would not remain. A further difficulty was that even if stenosis was produced, it alone did not result in oxygen unsaturation of the arterial blood. Helen states that she suggested to Vivian Thomas, Dr. Blalock's technician, that he put a branch of the right pulmonary artery into the left auricle, thereby causing venous blood to be directed to the aorta. After the dogs had developed polycythemia, the proximal end of the subclavian artery could be anastomosed to the pulmonary artery to determine whether a reduction in the polycythemia would occur. Vivian Thomas did the first step the following day. That procedure alone did not make any difference in the red blood cell count, so he performed in addition a partial lobectomy of the right lung. This combination of operations resulted in some polycythemia, which appeared to be lessened by increasing the circulation to the other lung. These laboratory experiments were not entirely clear cut. Nevertheless, some two years after the suggestion that an operation to increase arterial blood flow to the lungs in patients with the tetralogy of Fallot might be developed, experiments had been done on some two hundred dogs.

It was decided to proceed with the operation of subclavian anastomosis to the pulmonary artery, to a significant degree on the basis of Dr. Taussig's strong conviction that it would help a cyanotic child. The early period was a trying one in terms of the technical problems of operating on very small and very ill children. However, Blalock's skill was equal to the task. The blue-baby operation soon became successful and brought deserved fame to both Alfred Blalock and Helen Taussig. Dr. Taussig reminisces that it did not take nearly as much courage to ask Blalock to do these operations as it did to recommend the first ductus operations in her patients, since the children with tetralogy had to live in an oxygen tent and were miserable, while the ductus patients were able to get along reasonably well.

After the first operation was carried out (November 29, 1944), Helen discovered that when cyanotic children became unconscious, as they frequently did from the anoxemia, morphine often had a dramatic effect. This was noted in patients who had received their pre-operative medication, and it was not clear at first whether the effect was caused by morphine or atropine. Later atropine was tried without effect. Everyone was reluctant to try morphine on an unconscious patient, but she pushed forward and showed that it was very helpful.

Dr. Taussig was promoted to associate professor of pediatrics on July 1, 1946, and became professor of pediatrics on July 1, 1959. She has received innumerable awards, including the Medal of Freedom, the highest civilian award that a U.S. President can bestow. In 1965 she was elected president of the American Heart Association, being both the first woman and the first pediatrician to hold that post, and in 1971 she was made a Master of the American College of Physicians. The American Heart Association has established the Helen B. Taussig lectureship, the first lecture presented in 1973. She was recently elected a member of the National Academy of Sciences and the American Philosophical Society, and has honorary degrees from more than twenty colleges and universities.

Dr. Taussig has remained very active in areas other than her primary love, pediatric cardiology, one of her most significant contributions being made in relation to the thalidomide problem. In 1961 one of the many foreign students whom she trained here provided the opportunity that permitted Dr. Taussig to play a key role in preventing a thalidomide disaster in the United States. This German student, Dr. Alois Beuren, told her in January 1962 about the incidence of a bizarre malformation—phocomelia—in certain newborn babies in Germany which it was thought might be due to thalidomide. Helen decided immediately to go to Germany and find out about this possible relation of phocomelia to thalidomide. She obtained the funds to do this, and by the time she had finished her tour of German medical centers, she was 90 percent convinced that thalidomide, a sleep-inducing drug widely utilized in pregnant women, was the cause of these cases of phocomelia. Lenz, a prominent German physician, had described the evidence against thalidomide at a medical meeting in Germany in October 1961. His report was published throughout Germany but was never mentioned in the American press. From Germany Dr. Taussig went to England, and was soon 99 percent convinced that thalidomide was the cause. On her return home she reported her findings at Johns Hopkins, and from the reception that she received there, she realized that the urgent danger should be more widely known. The American College of Physicians agreed to put an extra session on their already completed program so that Dr. Taussig could report her findings to this large group of physicians. She gave similar reports to the American Pediatric Society and wrote an editorial in the *New England Journal of Medicine*. These reports attracted the attention of Dr. Frances O. Kelsey of the Food and Drug Administration, who took steps to prevent the drug from being distributed for general use, thus averting a major catastrophe in the United States. By this effort Dr. Taussig not only saved many lives but also dramatized the need for more careful drug testing.

Caroline Bedell Thomas

In 1957 Caroline Bedell Thomas received the James D. Bruce Memorial Award in Preventive Medicine of the American College of Physicians. This award to Dr. Thomas was made for her original work on the sulfanilamide prophylaxis of hemolytic streptococcal infection to prevent recurrences of acute rheumatic fever. Her pioneering effort represented the first successful step in developing a specific preventive measure in the field of cardiovascular disease. The struggle to gain general acceptance of this simple measure was not a new experience in the field of clinical investigation.

The story begins in 1927 with the practical examination in bacteriology for first-year medical students at Johns Hopkins. Each student was given three test tubes containing "unknown" bacteria for identification. Caroline Thomas found that the first two organisms grew readily on a succession of appropriate media, but the third did not grow and did not take a characteristic stain. The anxiety typical of a medical student under such stress mounted. After a long, worried night of intense effort, her only positive result was that when stained with carbolfuchsin, instead of turning a rosy red as is characteristic of the tubercle bacillus, the preparation turned a pale lavender. When the deadline arrived, her answer was "tubercle bacillus." In fact, it turned out to be the causative organism of turtle tuberculosis, which stains atypically. This was her introduction to bacteriology.

During this period in her training, she was using a monocular microscope. By the end of the year she had developed piercing headaches and was at times seeing double. She consulted an internationally known ophthalmologist in Boston, who made a diagnosis of spherical torsion, for which he said there was no known cure. He told her that it would be advisable for her to withdraw from medical school. When Dr. Thomas returned to Baltimore in the fall, she spoke with Dean Alan Chesney in regard to withdrawing from school. The dean suggested that she see William H. Wilmer, the professor of Ophthalmology. This was a fortunate suggestion, as it turned out that her main problem was an extraocular muscle imbalance which could be corrected by prism exercises. Thus, she came very close to ending her career in medicine.

During the preceding summer she had met Ann Kuttner, who entered Dr. Thomas's own class as a second-year medical student at Johns Hopkins that fall. Dr. Kuttner had already received her Ph.D. degree from Columbia in 1922 under Hans Zinsser, and had done distinguished research for three years with Rufus Cole. While working with Dr. Cole at the Rockefeller Institute, she had been exposed to the work of Rebecca Lancefield, and thus Dr. Thomas for the first time heard about fundamental research on streptococcal infections. Her next contact with streptococcal infections came in 1929, when, as a fourth-year medical student, she made a study of the histories of all of the patients in the Harriet Lane Home who had had purpura hemorrhagica and those of a control group. The patients with purpura had had more episodes of streptococcal pharyngitis preceding their purpura than was found in the control group.

Her interest in bacteriological subjects continued during her internship and assistant residency in the Johns Hopkins Hospital, when she saw many cases of lobar pneumonia, meningococcus meningitis, and erysipelas, and treated them with specific antisera. Acute glomerulonephritis, a sequela of streptococcal infection, was also common among the ward population in those days.

In 1931, soon after Dr. Alvin Coburn had published his book *The Factor of Infection in the Rheumatic State,* Dr. Kuttner, who had also remained at Johns Hopkins and was Dr. Thomas's close friend, urged her to read it. In this book Coburn presented clinical evidence that beta hemolytic streptococcal infections preceded episodes of acute rheumatic fever.

While an assistant resident assigned to the heart station, Dr. Thomas was asked by Benjamin Baker to join him in a series of experiments on rabbits to see if a heat-killed culture of beta hemolytic streptococcus injected intrapericardially into rabbits sensitized to the same organism would result in cardiac lesions. The results showed that the hearts of the sensitized rabbits compared with those of the controls showed a marked nonspecific inflammatory reaction.

After two years of research in cardiovascular physiology, Dr. Thomas returned to the Department of Medicine. At the time it was unheard of for a woman to have a full-time appointment on the clinical faculty, and she did not receive one. When Edward Perkins Carter, who was in charge of the heart station, suggested that Dr. Thomas organize an adult cardiac clinic, Warfield T. Longcope, chairman of the Department of Medicine, approved. However, he warned that this clinic should not take any "interesting teaching cases" from the general dispensary, by which he meant patients with classical aortic insufficiency, mitral stenosis, and so on. Because of Dr. Thomas's fundamental interest in physiology, she concluded that the most interesting venture would be to study the earliest stages of disease and to investigate the physiological abnormalities that were occurring. She concentrated on four types of patients in the cardiac clinic: (1) young patients with a history of rheumatic fever but with minimal rheumatic heart disease; (2) patients with "early" essential hypertension; (3) patients with possible carotid sinus sensitivity; and (4) patients with heart block. Richard France was her associate, and the cardiac clinic they instituted met two mornings a week on the second floor of the Carnegie Building. They began to accept patients in September 1935, just one year before the advent of sulfanilamide. During that year, as they saw increasing numbers of young people whose health was severely threatened by the inroads of rheumatic fever, the questions constantly on their minds were: What can we do for these young patients? How can we interrupt the rheumatic cycle? It was in September 1936 that the possible answer came. Dr. Perrin H. Long had just returned from London, where he had seen the miraculous effects of sulfanilamide on beta hemolytic streptococcal infections being treated by Leonard Colebrook and his collaborators. Dr. Long reported this discovery one day at lunch and added the startling statement that when small doses of sulfanilamide were injected into the peritoneum of a mouse before it was inoculated with the beta hemolytic streptococcus, no infection ensued. While all of the other listeners were excited at the prospect of treating and curing usually fatal streptococcal infections such as meningitis, and serious ones such as mastoiditis, otitis media, pneumonia, and scarlet fever, Dr. Thomas's thoughts were entirely on her young rheumatic patients. Was it possible that by preventing the beta hemolytic streptococcal infections which preceded the rheumatic state, the disease cycle could be interrupted?

A later corridor conversation with Dr. Long resulted in the decision to give these patients a gram a day of sulfanilamide. This proved to be exactly the right dose. Dr. Thomas and her colleagues then began to test the double hypothesis: (1) that sulfanilamide would prevent beta hemolytic streptococcal infections in man as it did in the mouse, and (2) that in the absence of such streptococcal infections recrudescences of acute rheumatic fever would not appear. The next four years of study showed that the prophylactic use of sulfanilamide in patients susceptible to rheumatic fever was, indeed, highly successful. Not only did it prevent acute beta hemolytic streptococcal infections, but not a single major attack of acute rheumatic fever occurred in the treated group; in the untreated group, a number of major episodes took place.

However, Dr. Thomas's ingenious new discovery did not gain immediate and widespread acclaim. Dr. Longcope, influenced in all likelihood by Homer Swift, the authority on rheumatic fever at the Rockefeller Institute, did not accept the new results immediately. When shown a preliminary note to be published in 1937 outlining the first year's results, he said that it was too early to go into print and that the investigations should continue for at least five years before doing so. Whatever the connection may be, Dr. Thomas's application to the Johns Hopkins School of Medicine for a research grant of $500 to assist in the second year of this research was denied. But the cardiac clinic continued to operate even with no funds. Physicians and social workers alike were unpaid, and the sulfanilamide was supplied free of charge by the Winthrop Chemical Company.

Old ideas change slowly when new ones stand ready to take their place. In 1939, after three years of progress with sulfanilamide prophylaxis, Dr. Longcope one day told Dr. Thomas rather enthusiastically, while they were waiting for an Osler elevator, "Did you know that Dr. Homer Swift has found the cause of rheumatic fever?" This was the pleuropneumonia-like organism; its apparent relationship to rheumatic fever, work that was later disproved, had just been described in *Science* by Swift and Thomas McPherson Brown, a former resident in medicine. Previously, Dr. Homer Swift had treated a small number of patients with acute rheumatic fever with large doses of sulfanilamide and encountered toxic reactions. This in part may have explained his continuing opposition to the use of smaller doses of sulfanilamide as prophylaxis.

With the advent of World War II, the armed forces turned to a new sulfonamide derivative, sulfadiazine, to prevent beta hemolytic streptococcal infections in the large groups of young men living in close quarters in military barracks. Between December 1, 1943, and March 1, 1944, approximately 250,000 men in the United States Navy received a gram of sulfadiazine daily while an equal number served as controls. Commander Alvin F. Coburn, who had originally emphasized the importance of streptococcal infection in the development of rheumatic fever, directed this extensive program of mass prophylaxis, which was later extended to include more than 600,000 naval trainees. A well-documented review by Rosenberg and Hench of the results of sulfonamide prophylaxis of rheumatic fever both in civilian and military life summed up nine years of experience from 1936 to 1945 and left no doubt that an effective agent had been found which could be used on a mass scale to prevent rheumatic fever.

Because of her work on the prevention of rheumatic fever, Dr. Thomas was appointed as civilian consultant to the Surgeon General of the U.S. Army in 1944, and she wrote much of the army literature, which was intended for distribution to medical officers, on the subject of rheumatic fever. It was at this time that Philip S. Hench became familiar with her work, and he asked her to present it at a sectional meeting of the American College of Physicians in 1947. Dr. Hench fully appreciated the significance of her work, and it was undoubtedly through his initiative that Dr. Thomas later received the Bruce Award from the American College of Physicians.

Opposition to Dr. Thomas's conclusions continued, and on a program with Dr. Thomas as late as 1947, such an authority on rheumatic fever as T. Duckett Jones spoke about rheumatic fever as though there was still no means of preventing the attacks. He, like Dr. Homer Swift, had made a brief trial of the curative properties of sulfanilamide in acute rheumatic fever, but had given up the studies because the drug proved too toxic. Thus, he and Benjamin Massell were perhaps influential in steering the American Heart Association away from the use of sulfanilamide when that organization began to take interest in the prevention of rheumatic fever in the late 1940s and early 1950s. They recommended penicillin instead.

Dr. May Wilson, an American authority on rheumatic fever in childhood, did not believe during this period that there was any causal relationship between streptococcal infections and acute rheumatic fever. She took Dr. Thomas severely to task at a Chicago symposium from the point of view of the statistical validity of her studies. Later Hench encouraged Dr. Joseph Berkson, the statitician at the Mayo Clinic, to review Dr. Thomas's work in the light of this criticism. Dr. Berkson concluded that the work was entirely valid. In a letter to Dr. Thomas in 1952, Howard B. Sprague, chairman of the Scientific Council of the American Heart Association, said:

I believe you have a very good point about the matter of the prophylaxis of rheumatic fever with sulfa drugs. Actually the expense and the technical difficulties in the proper administration of prophylactic penicillin to school children are very real barriers to the use of this method, even though it may turn out to be more effective than sulfa prophylaxis. I agree with you that the technique of the use of the sulfa drugs should be defined for the medical profession. They appear to be somewhat more dangerous than is penicillin, but the risk must be very small.

Actually, the risk turned out to be much the same.

Over the ensuing years Dr. Thomas has continued to maintain an active career in clinical medicine and in clinical investigation in the Department of

Medicine. Medical students are fully aware of her prospective studies on the factors concerned in the development of coronary heart disease and hypertension in which they have been participants. Dr. Thomas, who was made a full professor of medicine in 1970, was one of the first women elected to the Association of American Physicians. Among her other honors are an honorary Doctor of Science degree from Smith College in 1955 and the Elizabeth Blackwell Citation from the New York Infirmary in 1958. Dr. Thomas is a Master of the American College of Physicians and a member of the American Society for Clinical Investigation and the American Physiological Society.

Mary Ellen Avery

For the third time the prestigious Thomas Morgan Rotch Professorship of Pediatrics at Harvard University is occupied by an individual who received a major portion of his or her training at Johns Hopkins. This post, which also carries with it the responsibility as physician-in-chief at the Children's Hospital Medical Center in Boston, is now held by Mary Ellen Avery, a 1952 graduate of Johns Hopkins. The first incumbent was Kenneth Blackfan, who served for many years as resident in pediatrics under Dr. John Howland in the pioneer days in Harriet Lane when the first fulltime academic department of pediatrics was being forged. Blackfan was succeeded by Charles Janeway, a 1934 graduate of Johns Hopkins whose father had been the first fulltime professor of medicine at Johns Hopkins.

Mary Ellen Avery, born in Camden, New Jersey, received her A.B. degree from Wheaton College (Mass.) in 1948 and her M.D. degree from Johns Hopkins in 1952. Following graduation from medical school, she received her intern and residency training in pediatrics at the Johns Hopkins Hospital.

She developed an early interest in problems of respiratory physiology in infancy and childhood, in general problems of the management of newborn infants, and in lung diseases, including tuberculosis. The year 1957 was eventful in terms of her research interest when, as a research fellow at Harvard, she began to study hyaline membrane disease. Dr. Avery and respiratory physiologist Dr. Jere Mead, with whom she was working at the Harvard School of Public Health, suggested that the pathogenesis of hyaline membrane disease might be related to a deficiency in lung surfactant. Hyaline membrane disease received its name because of the pink-staining coating found in the terminal air sacs of lungs of babies dying with respiratory distress. It outranks all other disorders, including complications of asphyxia, pulmonary hemorrhage, infections, and congenital malformations, as a cause of death in newborn infants. Although improved means of treatment and the development of pediatric intensive care has reduced the mortality rate, approximately ten thousand babies still die annually from this disease. In the affected babies, severe difficulty in breathing develops within a few minutes of birth. The premature newborn shows sternal and subcostal retractions, grunting, and whining, with rapid respiration. The immature lungs collapse almost completely each time the baby exhales rather than remaining partially expanded as is normally the case.

Two previous investigations led to Dr. Avery's conclusion that hyaline membrane disease might be due to a deficiency in lung surfactant. In 1955 Richard Pattle observed that alveoli are coated with a lipid and protein substance that somehow sustains lung bubbles, making them longer lived. Later John A. Clements, who worked at the U.S. Army Chemical Center at Edgewood and part time at Johns Hopkins, noted that this substance acts as a surfactant and affects the surface tension of the lungs. When the lung expands during inhalation, this surfactant increases the surface tension, thus enhancing the lung's recoil ability and elasticity. When the individual exhales, the surfactant produces a sharp decrease in surface tension, which prevents total collapse and allows the lung to remain somewhat aerated. When she became aware of these two findings, Dr. Avery recalled that infants dying of hyaline membrane disease had no air in their lungs at autopsy; thus the search began to find out if these babies had a surfactant deficiency. Using the Wilhelmy balance technique described by Clements, Avery and Mead found that at autopsy, infants weighing less than 1.1 kilogram at birth, as well as babies with atelectasis, lacked significant amounts of the substance needed to lower surface tensions, thus leading to the postulation that surfactant was a crucial factor in the pathogenesis of hyaline membrane diseases.

After returning to Hopkins, Dr. Avery, in collaboration with Dr. Sue Buckingham, discovered the source of lung surfactant. Dr. Buckingham noted that alveolar type II cells contained large osmiophilic inclusions or organelles that readily stained with osmic acid. Studies of the developing mouse lung revealed that surfactant was detectable at the same time that these osmiophilic inclusions appeared. In a subsequent study, radiolabeled precursors of the surfactant were injected. This material was found to localize in the type II cell, indicating that synthesis of surfactant took place in these special cells. These and further investigations on the lamb lung established the time of appearance of the pulmonary surfactant and paved the way for the important observation made by Liggins in New Zealand, that lambs born prematurely after maternal glucocorticoid administration were viable at a stage earlier than had been predicted. This led Avery and her co-workers to evaluate the role of glucocorticoid in the induction of the pulmonary surfactant. This work was done in collaboration with de Lemos, Shermeta, Knelson, and Kotas. Hydrocortisone given to one of twin fetal lambs during a one- to six-day period accelerated maturation of the lung. The effect was present in six lambs of more than one hundred days' gestation; but it was not demonstrated in one lamb injected after one hundred days. Infusion of the diluent without hydrocortisone did not affect lung maturation in the one lamb so treated. The lungs of the steroid-treated lambs were as much as one week more advanced in development than those of the twin control.

The discovery of the role of steroids in accelerating surfactant production may someday lead to a means of preventing hyaline membrane disease. At this time, however, the only way to reduce fatalities from the disease is by careful postnatal supportive treatment or by postponing the birth as long as possible.

During her days in Baltimore, Dr. Avery was concerned with other aspects of the control of breathing in the newborn, particularly with the initiation of breathing at birth. She and her collaborators wanted to know how the infant cleared lung liquid at birth. They described a syndrome, known as "transient tachypnea of the newborn," which they thought represented a delay in the clearing of lung liquid. This was a self-limited disorder presenting in the first days of life. Other studies on the control of breathing concerned cerebrospinal fluid, acid-base relationships, and carbon dioxide responsiveness of the newborn infant. During the 1960s, one of her major concerns was to emphasize the need to bring modern concepts of respiratory physiology to bear on the ventilatory problems seen in infants and to promote neonatal intensive care. She was the first to introduce the micromethodology for the measurement of blood gases in premature infants to the Johns Hopkins Hospital. Although she did not devise the technology, she was among the first to apply it in the management of such infants. She did much to promote the careful monitoring of these babies, and called the attention of the pediatric world to the probability that many infants were dying of too little oxygen because doctors were fearful of poisoning them with too much. At the time, there was a widespread fear that giving premature infants more than 40 percent oxygen would cause blindness due to retrolental fibroplasia. Her work in this respect was based on a retrospective review of autopsy protocols in association with Ella Oppenheimer and was published in 1960. This study was important in alerting pediatricians to the need for measuring the oxygen concentration in the blood if they were to provide appropriate ambient oxygen concentrations for premature infants. She clearly emphasized that it was the oxygen content of the blood which mattered, and that some infants might require 80 or 90 percent inspired oxygen to achieve normal arterial tensions.

In addition to her laboratory and clinical research contributions, Dr. Avery has written an excellent book entitled *The Lung and Its Disorders in the Newborn Infant*, first published in 1964 with two later editions, the most recent in 1974. She also co-authored, with Dr. Alexander Schaffer, a book called *Diseases of the Newborn*, published in 1971. She has also written many textbook chapters, largely motivated by the fact that her area of research is of recent development, is moving rapidly, and has obvious clinical implications. She has been very effective as well in building the bridge between physiology and bedside pediatrics. During her period in Baltimore, she worked closely with Dr. Richard Riley and Dr. Solbert Permutt, from whom she gained much background in pulmonary physiology. In 1973 she wrote an excellent review entitled "The Pulmonary Surfactant in Foetal and Neonatal Lungs."

In 1969 Dr. Avery became professor and chairman of the Department of Pediatrics of the faculty of medicine at McGill University, where she continued her excellent teaching and research programs. In 1974 she moved to Boston as Thomas Morgan Rotch Professor of Pediatrics at Harvard University. In her own words, "Perhaps the great challenge for the future will be to assess care and training programs. How that will best be done I do not know, but we need to restudy all facets of care and training. For example, perhaps a three year residency program is too long for a general pediatrician if the majority of problems can be handled by a family practitioner who has trained for as few as three months in the specialty. Complicated questions like that need to be evaluated anew."

As one reviews the careers of these important women in medicine, it is clear that during this last century the outlook for a career in medicine for women has gradually but constantly improved, so that today women are fully accepted as vital members of the medical scientific community. As illustrated by Dr. Avery's career, all avenues in the medical profession are now open to women.

19 ❧ Contributions of the Part-time Staff of The Johns Hopkins Hospital: Moore, King, and Gay

THE OUTPATIENT DEPARTMENT or Dispensary of the Johns Hopkins Hospital was organized in 1889 as follows, under William S. Halsted, chief of the dispensary: (1) Department of General Medicine, William Osler; (2) Department of Diseases of Children, William Osler and W. D. Booker; (3) Department of Nervous Diseases, William Osler and H. M. Thomas; (4) Department of General Surgery, W. S. Halsted, assisted by J. M. T. Finney; (5) Department of Genito-urinary Diseases, W. S. Halsted and James Brown; (6) Department of Gynecology, H. A. Kelly, assisted by Hunter Robb; (7) Department of Ophthalmology and Otology, S. Theobald and R. L. Randolph; (8) Department of Laryngology, John N. Mackenzie; (9) Department of Dermatology, R. B. Morison.

From the outset the hospital relied heavily upon a group of practitioners in Baltimore for the conduct of the Outpatient Department. Many of these men had obtained their special training abroad, as was the custom in those days. Some of them were given the privilege of admitting patients to the hospital, and this custom has continued to the present day. As the years have passed, the number of Baltimore practitioners working in the Dispensary has been great, and their total contribution both in teaching and in the care of patients has been outstanding. Furthermore, essentially all of the service rendered by this group has been without any monetary compensation from the hospital or the School of Medicine. Without their contributions, the hospital could not have grown successfully, nor would it have been possible to develop an effective teaching program for the students and the resident staff. This holds true today just as it did in the early days of the hospital and the medical school.

Over the years, many of these practicing physicians have engaged in clinical investigation. This essay will present the story of three such physicians—Joseph Earle Moore, John Theodore King, Jr., and Leslie N. Gay—who made important contributions to the development of medical knowledge as well as to the patient care and teaching responsibilities of the Department of Medicine.

Joseph Earle Moore and the Story of Medicine I

The Wassermann test for the diagnosis of syphilis was introduced into clinical practice in 1907. This immunological reaction, utilizing the phenomenon of complement fixation, has since been modified and simplified through the use of flocculation techniques. These various techniques, each carrying the name of the investigator who devised it, differ from each other only in minor technical details.

The antibody detected in syphilitic serums by nonspecific antigens is called "reagin" (because it reacts). In most normal human serum, the amount of reagin is so small as not to be detectible by standard serological tests as they are usually adjusted for sensitivity and specificity. However, reagin may increase in amount in the serum of nonsyphilitic persons during or after a number of acute infections with no etiological relationship to syphilis. In a few apparently normal persons enough reagin may be present in the serum to produce positive tests for syphilis with standard techniques. The tests in these cases are spoken of as biological false-positive (BFP) tests.

It became apparent for several reasons that BFP reactions were more frequent than had previously been believed. Beginning in 1938 a vast program of blood testing for syphilis was developed in the United States, and in many areas candidates for marriage and all pregnant women were required by law to have these tests, as were all armed services personnel at entrance into and again at separation from the military service. Thus, millions of Americans were subjected to this serological examination and new millions were tested annually. Mobilization of about 16 million young men in World War II resulted in epidemics of infectious disease (the exanthemas of childhood, viral respiratory infections, malaria, infectious hepatitis, and others) under conditions in which routine, often serial blood testing was possible in a manner not previously achieved in civilian medical practice. This combination of events provided new information regarding the comparative frequency of the BFP phenomenon, and it became clear that there were two types, acute and chronic. Acute reactions were characterized by the fact that they occurred during or shortly after a wide variety of unrelated nonsyphilitic infections and that they disappeared spontaneously within a few days, weeks, or at least less than six months after recovery from the illness. Chronic BFP reactions were marked by the absence of the known precipitating factors and by the persistence of reagin in the blood over many months or years, perhaps even for a lifetime, in many instances. When Dr. Joseph Earle Moore and his associates began their study of the chronic BFP phenomenon, it was only known that it occurred in patients with leprosy and had been reported in a few patients with discoid or systemic lupus erythematosus.

Until 1949, recognition of the BFP reaction was difficult. When a chronic BFP reaction was suspected, epidemiological investigation with serological testing and examination of familial and sexual contacts was necessary in order to verify the patient's statement of lack of exposure to the disease.

In a study of immunity in syphilis in 1939, Dr. Thomas B. Turner found that the serum of syphilitic animals or man contained an antibody that combined directly with virulent *Treponema pallidum*. But this phenomenon, indicating the presence in syphilitic serums of an antibody that destroyed *T. pallidum* organisms, was not then utilizable in any practical manner. Ten years later,

while working in Dr. Turner's laboratory, Robert Nelson studied the growth of
T. pallidum on artificial media. He was successful in maintaining the syphilitic
organisms alive, motile, and virulent for five to ten days on an artificial medium, largely free of tissue components. Nelson and Manfred Mayer next
mixed an emulsion of motile treponemes in this medium with syphilitic or
normal serum plus complement and observed the result directly under the
microscope. When the mixture consisted of normal serum plus treponemes plus
complement, the organisms remained motile and virulent. On the other hand, if
syphilitic serums were employed, the treponemes were immobilized and killed.
By appropriate absorption experiments, they demonstrated that the antibody
responsible for this phenomenon was distinct from reagin.

Moore and his co-workers quickly recognized that the treponemal immobilization test (TPI) might provide a clinically important tool for determining whether a positive standard serological test was due to syphilis or
represented a BFP reaction. Nelson and his associates soon demonstrated that
the "treponemal immobilization test" was negative in twelve acute BFP reactors, and soon afterwards that it was also negative in the chronic reactors. The
agreement between the clinical diagnosis and the results of the treponemal
immobilization test was remarkably close.

Thus, Moore now had the means of identifying the BFP reactors, and he
began a prospective clinical study to determine the nature of the chronic BFP
serological test for syphilis. In the initial studies of Moore and Mohr, the first
prerequisite for admission of a patient to the study was that he or she had been
routinely discovered to have a positive standard serological test for syphilis
(STS) known to have been present for at least one year, in the absence of any
history of infection with syphilis and of any physical evidence of the disease,
and that the spinal fluid was normal. In a group of 500 white private patients of
upper educational and socioeconomic levels, 40 percent of those who were
seropositive reactors were shown by means of negative TPI tests not to have
syphilis but instead to be chronic BFP reactors. Since there was some suggestion from available knowledge that these false positive tests might relate to
connective tissue disease, particular attention was paid to signs and symptoms
indicative of these diseases in the follow-up of these patients. Dr. Moore's first
report on the prospective study came in 1955. The series was composed of 148
chronic BFP reactors first discovered to have a positive standard STS in purely
routine fashion and who at the time regarded themselves as completely healthy.
At the time of the report these patients had been under clinical observation for
a minimum of one and a maximum of twenty years, with the average observation period being about six years. It became obvious that the chronic BFP
phenomenon was observed predominantly in females (70 percent). Further,
the data showed that in a few years after the appearance of the false-positive
test, 9 of 104 females in the series had developed verified systemic lupus
erythematosus. An episodic form of chronic illness, the manifestations of which
conform to those known to occur in systemic lupus erythematosus, had developed in 52 of the 148 patients in the series.

After Moore's death, this study was continued by Dr. Lawrence E. Shulman and Dr. A. McGehee Harvey. Further information verified the fact that females outnumbered males almost three to one, and follow-up studies showed that 7 percent of the females with a chronic BFP test ultimately developed systemic lupus erythematosus (SLE) and a large number had characteristic clinical features of SLE without any laboratory evidence considered diagnostic of the disease.

Of 192 subjects with a chronic BFP reported by Shulman and Harvey in 1964, auto-immune thyroiditis with hypothyroidism had developed in three. These authors had studied three other patients with auto-immune thyroiditis and a sustained false-positive test for syphilis. All six were females. Thus, the long-term follow-up of patients with a sustained BFP reaction has contributed important information to the problem of auto-immunization and auto-immune disease.

Dr. Joseph Earle Moore was born in Philadelphia on July 9, 1892, and died in Baltimore on December 6, 1957. His pre-medical education was obtained at the University of Kansas, where he also took the first two years of his medical training. He transferred to Johns Hopkins in 1914 and received his M.D. degree in 1916, after which he served for one year as a house officer in the Johns Hopkins Hospital. He then entered the army, attaining the rank of captain before his discharge. In France he came to the attention of Dr. Hugh H. Young, who was directing the venereal disease program of the American Expeditionary Forces. Thus began Moore's interest in the venereal diseases. When World War II ended, Dr. Moore returned to Baltimore and joined the Syphilis Division of the Department of Medicine. From that time forward, he was intimately associated with both the Johns Hopkins School of Medicine and Hospital.

The early years of the twentieth century saw some rapid breakthroughs in regard to syphilis with the discovery of the Wassermann test for diagnosis and the recognition of the *Treponema pallidum* as the causative organism. This was soon followed in 1910 by Ehrlich's discovery of salvarsan for the treatment of the disease. Up to that time at Johns Hopkins, patients with syphilis had been referred to the genito-urinary or the dermatology clinics, as was customary in other hospitals as well. However, through a grant from John D. Rockefeller, Jr., in 1914, a new clinic, designated Department L (for Lues), was organized. This clinic was the brainchild of George Walker, who was its first director. His principal assistant was Albert Keidel. In 1921 Keidel succeeded Walker as director of the clinic with J. Earle Moore, E. L. Zimmerman, and Harry M. Robinson as his principal assistants. Because of the interest that had developed in venereal disease control during and immediately after World War I, funds were attracted to this clinic and steps were taken in 1921 to develop research and teaching in syphilis on a fulltime basis within the Department of Medicine. Dr. Alan M. Chesney, then on the faculty of Washington University of St. Louis, was offered and accepted an appointment as associate professor of medicine, associate physician to the hospital, and co-director with Keidel of the syphilis clinic. Upon Keidel's retirement in 1929, J. E. Moore, who by that time had become one of the world's outstanding contributors to clinical syphilology, assumed the leadership of what was then called Medicine I. Under his leadership, the Johns Hopkins Medical Institutions were soon recognized as an outstanding world center for research in syphilis, as well as for postgraduate training in that field. Many young men on the faculty at Hopkins were able assistants to Moore in the activities of Medicine I, including Bowman J. Hood, Richard D. Hahn, Paul Padget, and Charles F. Mohr among others.

The first course in venereal disease control was offered in 1930 in conjunction with a similar one in tuberculosis control. The syphilis portion was under the direction of Dr. Thomas B. Turner. When Dr. Turner left to go to the International Health Division of the Rockefeller Foundation in 1932, Dr. H. Hanford Hopkins took charge. A short time later the interest in venereal disease control was hastened by the vigorous program instituted by Dr. Thomas Parran, then surgeon general of the U.S. Public Health Service. Dr. Moore proposed to the Public Health Service in 1936 that Johns Hopkins offer extended training in venereal disease control for public health officers and other physicians who had responsibility for municipal, state, or national programs. The Rockefeller Foundation was asked and agreed to assign Dr. Turner to Hopkins to develop these expanded training activities, which were undertaken by the School of Hygiene, the Hospital, and the School of Medicine. This venture was highly successful, and during the next ten years a succession of outstanding members of the U.S. Public Health Service, as well as a large number of health officers from all over the country, were sent to Johns Hopkins for this special training. This was perhaps the first experience of cooperation among the three Hopkins Medical Institutions in an academic activity. As a result, many excellent people were trained who later had distinguished careers in the U.S. Public Health Service and in the activities of the National Institutes of Health. This program continued into the World War II period.

One of the other outstanding features of Medicine I was the development of a family clinic, whereby an entire family in which a case of syphilis was suspected could be handled effectively. This clinic, which was conceived by J. Earle Moore, was under the immediate direction of Dr. Mary Stewart Goodwin, a Hopkins graduate and a member of the pediatric staff.

Medicine I was a model in many respects, but one particular aspect has not been sufficiently emphasized—namely, for the first time the study and treatment of a disease having such widespread effects in man was conducted by those who had basic training in general internal medicine, so that good medicine came first, the special interest in a single important disease being built on this sound foundation.

Dr. Moore's principal investigative efforts in the clinic were aimed at determining the best means of treating patients exhibiting the various manifestations of syphilitic infection, especially those with lesions of the nervous system. In 1933 he published his excellent monograph entitled "The Modern Treatment of Syphilis." It quickly became the authoritative text in the field, and went through a second edition. In 1943, when the efficacy of penicillin in the treatment of syphilis was discovered by Mahoney and his co-workers, Dr. Moore energetically worked on its effects in various types of syphilis and soon

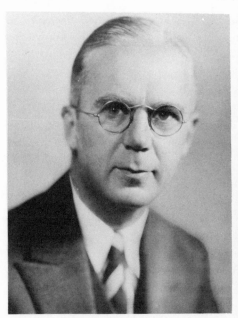

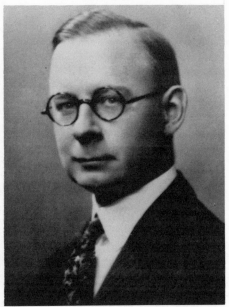

Joseph Earle Moore

From the Archives Office, The Johns Hopkins
Medical Institutions

Leslie N. Gay

From the Archives Office, The Johns Hopkins
Medical Institutions

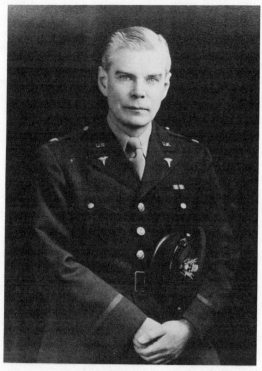

John Theodore King, Jr.

Courtesy of Dr. John T. King, Jr.

accumulated sufficient information to publish a new book entitled *Penicillin in Syphilis*. This volume appeared in 1946 and summarized all of the knowledge gained during World War II in the use of this new agent for the treatment of syphilis.

It was most impressive to see how, when the advent of penicillin suddenly changed the character of the syphilis clinic, Earle Moore developed a new interest based on his accumulated talents. With his vivid and fertile imagination, Dr. Moore immediately turned his attention to other problems in the area of chronic disease. He knew that the organization and the methods he had developed for long-term follow-up and study of a chronic disease such as syphilis could be ideally applied to some of these important problems. Out of this heritage came the medical genetics clinic and the Outpatient Center for Clinical Investigation, which are housed in the remodeled but hallowed halls of old Medicine I.

Discovery Through Clinical Observation: The Story of John Theodore King, Jr.

The time: the spring of 1927, during the course in physical diagnosis for the second-year students in the School of Medicine. The place: a small examining room in the Medicine III Clinic in the Carnegie Outpatient Building. The students had finished their examination of the patient and their findings were being reviewed by their instructor, Dr. John Theodore King. The patient was an elderly white man suffering from myocardial insufficiency. Examination of the heart revealed reduplication of the apex thrust that was clearly visible to the naked eye in this rather thin individual. This reduplication could be just as readily felt as seen. On auscultation at the apex, the heart sounds were barely audible. At the beginning of systole there was a soft sound and a soft murmur that were synchronous respectively with the two elements that formed the bifid systolic thrust. These unusual findings immediately aroused Dr. King's curiosity. To account for the obvious asynchrony of systolic ventricular activity, he suggested that the patient had a block of a branch of the bundle of His. A subsequent electrocardiogram verified this interpretation.

Unaware of any previous reports of the clinical diagnosis of bundle branch block, Dr. King decided to review the literature carefully and to look for similar signs in a large number of cardiac patients.

Accurate knowledge of bundle branch block came from experiments in dogs by Eppinger and Rothberger. They cut, respectively, the right, the left, and both branches of the bundle of His. Electrocardiographic studies in these experimental preparations paved the way for the recognition of bundle branch block in human beings. Dr. Edward P. Carter, who was for many years associate professor of medicine at Johns Hopkins in charge of the heart station, later amplified these observations by a study of the electrocardiograms in human cases. Eppinger and Rothberger made an observation of importance that had never been translated into clinical medicine: they noted a visible asynchronism in the ventricular contractions of the exposed hearts of their dogs immediately after section of one of the bundle branches. Dr. King reasoned that it should be possible to observe a similar asynchronism in the larger human heart in cases in which the apex thrust was sufficiently visible to be analyzed. With characteristic thoroughness, he analyzed the physical signs of all of the patients who had been studied electrocardiographically by Dr. Carter. He found that reduplication of the first sound was noted in six cases and a "canter rhythm" in two. The visible and palpable characteristics were not noted in sufficient detail to warrant any deduction as to the presence or absence of reduplication of the systolic thrust. King found that both Eppinger and Stoerk and Kauf were able to feel the reduplication of the apex thrust in bundle branch block, but the diagnosis in each case had already been made by the electrocardiogram. Cowan and Bramwell reported unfavorably on the possibility of clinical recognition of bundle branch block, concluding that there was no clinical sign of bundle branch block and only the electrocardiogram could establish the diagnosis. From his original observation and from the literature, Dr. King constructed the following hypothetical signs of bundle branch block:

Inspection: Reduplication of the systolic apex thrust (to be seen and to be checked by apex cardiogram).
Palpation: Reduplication of the apex thrust.
Auscultation:
a. Reduplication of S1 at the apex, or
b. Single S1 with asynchronous systolic murmur, or
c. Asynchronous systolic apical murmurs, or
d. Muffling of systolic sounds or murmurs to a mere sense of double movement.
Blood Pressure: Reduplication at the beginning of systole to be more significant in the presence of normal than of elevated pressure because of frequency of presystolic gallop in hypertension.

With this hypothetical picture in mind, Dr. King then examined one hundred consecutive patients with cardiac symptoms seen on the wards and in the dispensary of the Johns Hopkins Hospital. All patients were examined without any knowledge of the electrocardiographic findings. Immediately after the physical examination was completed, the diagnosis was written down, including a specific note as to whether or not the patient had bundle branch block. Six of the nine cases of bundle branch block were recognized from the physical signs elicited by Dr. King before confirmation by the electrocardiogram.

The results of this study were published in a paper entitled "The Clinical Recognition and Physical Signs of Bundle Branch Block," which appeared in the *American Heart Journal*. In an addendum to this paper, Dr. King noted that after the completion of his report he found a paper by Waldrop which had previously been overlooked because of its title. In this paper Waldrop mentioned a patient in whom he made the diagnosis of bundle branch block because of reduplication of the first and second sounds. He had not described the full clinical picture that Dr. King had worked out, but the diagnosis in Waldorp's patient was verified by electrocardiogram and at autopsy.

Thus, we see that an astute clinician, engaged in the daily process of teaching medical students, was able to make for the first time a clinical diagnosis of bundle branch block and to describe carefully the physical signs of this conduction abnormality in a simple, controlled clinical study.

John Theodore King, Jr., was born in Baltimore in 1889. He was descended from a long line of John Kings, but in 1844, the year in which his father was born, Theodore Frelinghausen of New Jersey, a man about whom his grandfather was very enthusiastic, was a candidate for Vice-President of the United States. This resulted in his son being named John Theodore King. Dr. King attended public schools until time for college preparation arrived. He then entered Boy's Latin School for three years of college preparatory work before entering Princeton University. Upon graduation, he entered the John Hopkins School of Medicine in 1910, receiving his M.D. degree in 1914. The following year he served his internship in medicine at Hopkins under the first fulltime professor of medicine, Dr. Theodore C. Janeway. He was one of the bright young physicians picked by Dr. Thayer as the assistant resident in charge of his private patients. This was a unique arrangement that had been provided for Dr. Thayer at the time he was offered the position as chief of medicine at Peter Bent Brigham Hospital. Thayer declined the invitation, and from then on he was permitted to have his own assistant resident, who helped in the care of his private patients. That a very distinguished group of physicians held that position is noted by Francis Rackemann in his biography of George Minot entitled *The Inquisitive Physician*:

Dr. William Sydney Thayer was Clinical Professor of Medicine at Johns Hopkins. He was a clinician of great ability, an excellent teacher and a charming person. He was the important consultant of medicine at Baltimore. He dressed immaculately —I can remember the black and white checked suit which fitted so well and the heavy rimmed pince-nez eye glasses on the end of a long black silk ribbon with which he used to twirl his glasses whenever he was thinking about something. Dr. Thayer was well known in Boston. Some of his family lived there. He was a great friend of Dr. Frederick C. Shattuck, his counterpart in Boston, and was very much like him, even to the flower in his buttonhole. One person who encouraged George [Minot] to go to Hopkins was Dr. Francis W. Peabody. He was four years older than George and since the Minots and the Peabodys knew each other as families so George had met Francis on numerous occasions. Francis had been a house pupil at the Massachusetts General Hospital and after that he had been one of the first to be invited to Baltimore to gain additional experience under Dr. Thayer. Dr. Reginald Fitz followed Peabody in 1911. After Fitz, Dr. Thayer had chosen Dr. Roy R. Snowden, a Hopkins graduate. These were outstanding young men and it was not surprising that Dr. Thayer should invite the next outstanding young man—Dr. George Minot—to follow them.

What more glowing endorsement could be made of John T. King as a young physician than to have received the honor of working as the resident for Dr. Thayer, in view of the star-studded lineage that had held this position.

In the years that have followed, Dr. King has been an outstanding medical consultant in Baltimore and has made many contributions to clinical science. He is a member of such important societies as the Interurban Clinical Club, the

Association of American Physicians, and the American Clinical and Climatological Association, of which he was president in 1950.

In the first edition of Dr. Helen Taussig's book *Congenital Malformations of the Heart*, she credits Dr. John T. King with being the one who publicized the clinical manifestations of coarctation of the aorta which led to its general recognition by clinicians. Dr. King had published a thorough study entitled "Stenosis of the Isthmus (Coarctation) of the Aorta and Its Diagnosis during Life" in the *Archives of Internal Medicine* (1926).

Shortly after King entered practice, he became interested in the study of basal metabolism and the method of determination which had recently been developed by Dr. Dubois of New York. King used Dubois's arrangement for the collection of CO_2 by weight in his laboratory setup in the Johns Hopkins Hospital. This was different from the other method then in use, which required the measurement of oxygen by volume to determine the basal metabolic rate. After several years of study, the CO_2 method was finally discontinued. Since it was not taken up by any of the manufacturers, the necessary apparatus was not available. However, as a result of these and other studies, Dr. King was elected to the American Society for Clinical Investigation. He maintained his interest in cardiovascular disease and in 1942 wrote, in collaboration with J. Creighton Bramwell, an excellent textbook of cardiology entitled *Principles and Practice of Cardiology*.

During World War I, Dr. King was assigned as a member of a small group to listen to chests and pick out cases of tuberculosis in soldiers before they went abroad. Because of his excellent training in physical diagnosis, he was able to identify a number of cases in this way. At this time, of course, x-rays of the chest were not generally available. The plates were made of glass, making widespread use very awkward. Later King was part of a notable group, organized by Francis Peabody of Boston, and including Dr. Joseph Pratt of Boston, Dr. Cyrus Sturgis, Dr. Leslie Gay, and Dr. Paul Clough, who took over a hotel with laboratory facilities in Lakewood, New Jersey, to study what was known as the "irritable heart" of soldiers, or "fatigue neurosis." It was not until later that the term "neurocirculatory asthenia" was suggested as a better designation for this condition.

During World War II, Dr. King was in charge of the medical service at the Walter Reed Hospital, where he and Aubrey Hampton described the frequent occurrence of pulmonary embolism with or without infarction of the lung in apparently healthy ambulatory individuals. These patients worked, had no cardiac disease, and gave no history of phlebitis. At times the onset was insidious and at others it closely simulated coronary occlusion, pneumonia, angina pectoris, or pericardial effusion. King and Hampton published a paper which pointed out that in cases of repeated pleurisy or pneumonia, especially if bilateral, pulmonary embolism should be suspected. This paper was instrumental in widening the horizon of physicians in the recognition of pulmonary embolism.

Dr. King has continued to practice medicine in Baltimore, and many patients, students, and house officers have benefited from his excellence as a clinician and as a teacher. He was honored in 1967 by being elected president of the John Hopkins Medical and Surgical Association.

A Remedy for Motion Sickness:
The Story of Leslie N. Gay

The history of Johns Hopkins is filled with examples of the recognition of an important need and the ability on the part of the departmental chairmen to select an individual capable of fulfilling that need. The development of the allergy clinic at the Johns Hopkins Hospital is a good example of this type of effective leadership.

Dr. Leslie N. Gay first came to Baltimore as a student in the John Hopkins Medical School in 1913. The year following his graduation he entered internship and residency training at Massachusetts General Hospital. When he returned to Baltimore in 1922, he worked under Dr. Evelyth Bridgman in the outpatient clinic and was asked to organize a group to teach physical diagnosis. His return to Baltimore coincided with a rapidly rising interest in the field of allergy in the United States. It was at this time that Dr. Warfield T. Longcope, Dr. Francis Rackemann of Boston, and Dr. Robert Cooke of New York organized the American Society for the Study of Hay Fever, Asthma and Allied Conditions, which subsequently merged with the Western Society and eventually became the American Academy of Allergy. One day Dr. Canby Robinson, who was serving on an interim basis as Professor of Medicine until the arrival of Dr. Warfield T. Longcope from New York, stopped Dr. Gay in the hall and said: "Gay, I want you to start an allergy clinic." Dr. Gay's prompt answer was: "I don't know anything about allergy." Robinson's reply: "Nobody else does."

This conversation was followed shortly by the birth of the allergy clinic in 1923. This was the third allergy clinic to be started in the United States. The first had been organized by Cooke in New York, and almost simultaneously Kessler had started another in Chicago.

The allergy clinic at Hopkins started in a small room next to the Main Admitting Office in the old Dispensary Building. Besides Dr. Gay, the only other worker was Dr. Nathan Herman. Soon, however, the clinic flourished, and they were joined by other young staff members who had developed an interest in the field. Their investigative work was primarily clinical in nature. They were the first to make an extensive clinical trial of ephedrine, which had been obtained from Dr. Reed, then pharmacologist-in-charge at the Peking Union Medical College. Gay and Herman published their studies of using ephedrine on one hundred patients with asthma in the *Bulletin of the Johns Hopkins Hospital*. They also began systematic surveys of pollen in the atmosphere in conjunction with the Department of Botany at the university. In 1929 and in 1930 these investigations represented pioneering observations in this area. The first studies of the effect of an air-conditioned environment on the patient with hay fever and asthma were carried out by Dr. Gay and his associates with equipment provided by the General Motors Corporation.

In association with Dr. Edmund Keeney, now director of the Scripps Clinic in La Jolla, California, long-acting epinephrine was developed for use in the patient suffering from chronic asthma. Just as one gives long-acting protamine zinc insulin, patients were given long-acting epinephrine, which saved them from the necessity of taking multiple doses of epinephrine each day. Epinephrine-in-oil was developed with the help of Eli Lilly, who was particularly interested in Johns Hopkins because of his relatives who lived in Baltimore. Hearing about this project of Dr. Gay and his colleagues, Mr. Lilly purchased $500 worth of dry powdered epinephrine from Parke-Davis. At that time Parke-Davis and Lilly had a "gentlemen's agreement" that neither would infringe upon the other's products. When Gay and Keeney were ready to publish their work, the results were turned over to the Parke-Davis Company at the request of Mr. Lilly, who said they would be the ones to manufacture the product.

The allergy clinic was the first to study the value and dangers of Isuprel. This drug, developed in Germany, was brought to the United States after World War II. Gay and his collaborators showed that Isuprel was dangerous as administered by the Germans, and that death was quite possible from overdose when it was given hypodermically. They showed that the safest method of administration was by mouth, using small sublingual tablets. Subsequently a spray was developed so that patients could use it more easily, but it was difficult to persuade them not to use this spray excessively.

The most exciting work done in the allergy clinic was a study of a number of drugs having antihistaminic action. In 1948 one of these drugs, compound 1694 (later known as Dramamine), manufactured by Searle, was found by accident to have a remarkable effect in preventing motion sickness. During an interview, a woman being treated for hives indicated that previously every time she rode a trolley car or got into an automobile she was incapacitated by severe motion sickness. She stated that since she had been taking the new drug, she had no further difficulty with motion sickness. Dr. Gay quickly perceived the importance of this observation and forgot entirely about the drug's antihistaminic effects. He was well aware of the serious problem that motion sickness had given troops crossing the oceans during World War II. He promptly gave the patient placebo capsules made up of sugar. She came back within two or three days, greatly disappointed that her motion sickness had returned.

With this pertinent observation and others to confirm it, the search was made for a means of testing this effect on a large scale. Dr. Gay got in touch with General Omar Bradley, who was then chief of staff of the army. General Bradley immediately called Dr. Gay to Washington because motion sickness had been a great hazard in the landing of troops in Normandy. Gay and Bradley met in October 1948, and on the twenty-seventh of November Dr. Gay and his associates sailed from New York on a troop ship for a twelve-day voyage to Bremerhaven. On board were fifteen hundred young, healthy soldiers. They were divided into groups in the best control fashion possible. The voyage was enlivened by severe North Atlantic storms, and sea sickness became a serious problem. The results of Gay's experiment were dramatic in that

Dramamine appeared to be successful not only in the prevention of sea sickness but also in relieving sea sickness after it had already developed. A man who had developed severe sea sickness while on placebo would be given Dramamine through a small syringe injected into his rectum. Within fifteen minutes he would ask for food and drink, which he had not been able to face for several days. On the previous trip of this ship at least fifty to one hundred soldiers had had to have intravenous fluids during the twelve-day passage, but on this voyage not a single man required such fluid replacement. The subsequent development of many other drugs capable of preventing motion sickness is a story well known to all, but many do not realize that it all began as an example of serendipity in research in the Allergy Clinic at the Johns Hopkins Hospital.

It was, indeed, an impressive evening for most of us present at the Johns Hopkins Medical Society meeting on February 14, 1949, when Dr. Leslie N. Gay and Dr. Paul E. Carliner presented their studies on the prevention and treatment of motion sickness. In the discussion of the presentation, Dr. Philip Bard pointed out that he had been close to this problem during World War II as a member of the National Research Council Committee on Motion Sickness. At that time the most effective preventive for motion sickness was hyoscine. He observed that the great contribution of Dr. Gay's work was showing the effectiveness of their drug on the treatment of people already sick. The full paper, "On the Prevention and Treatment of Motion Sickness," was published in the *Bulletin of the Johns Hopkins Hospital*. Later, additional work was done by Gay's group on the treatment of the nausea and vomiting of pregnancy with Dramamine.

Dr. Leslie Gay has been a very active and important member of the Department of Medicine since his return to Baltimore from Massachusetts General Hospital in 1922. He continued as the director of the allergy clinic until he reached retirement age in 1959, and has authored or co-authored almost seventy-five papers, most of them dealing with clinical subjects in the field of allergy. In 1946 he published a classic monograph, "The Diagnosis and Treatment of Bronchial Asthma." Dr. Gay is a past president of the American Academy of Allergy and in 1948 was awarded an honorary Doctor of Science degree from his alma mater, Lafayette College. He is now associate professor of medicine emeritus and still active in practice at the age of eighty-five.

Through the examples of J. Earle Moore, John T. King, and Leslie N. Gay, it is clear that the practicing physicians of Baltimore have contributed in many ways to the important activities of the Johns Hopkins Medical Institutions. And it is important to remember that they represent a large group of devoted physicians and surgeons, many of whom have made valuable original contributions to medical knowledge.

Joseph Erlanger

WHEN THE JOHNS HOPKINS School of Medicine opened in 1893, much had already been learned of the mechanics of the circulation by direct observation of and experiments on mammals. Instruments had been devised for exact measurement and direct recording of hemodynamic phenomena from the heart and various portions of the vascular tree. However, physiologists and physicians were aware that if such measurements could be made on the intact, unanesthetized animal and on man, much more could be learned about the normal circulation and its changes in various diseases.

As early as 1855 Vierordt had outlined a method of recording blood pressure by a counterbalancing pressure on the outside of a limb in man sufficient to obliterate the arterial pulse beneath. Many instruments had been constructed upon this principle, but none was entirely satisfactory. The best was that of Riva Rocci (1896), an instrument which Harvey Cushing brought back to this country after his study period in Europe.

An important contributor to cardiovascular physiology in the early days at Johns Hopkins was Joseph Erlanger, who later received the Nobel Prize for his work in neurophysiology. Both of his parents were immigrants who eventually settled in San Francisco, where he was born on January 5, 1874. In 1891 he enrolled in the "College of Chemistry" to prepare for the study of medicine. None of his forebears had ever followed a learned profession; he owed the idea of becoming a doctor to his elder sister—she had nicknamed him "Doc" because of his interest in lower forms of life. When the time came to choose a medical school, Erlanger was seriously considering the Cooper Medical School in his hometown until he heard from Walter Hewlett that the Johns Hopkins University had recently started a medical school which he believed would be "better than Harvard"—a strong recommendation indeed. Erlanger was admitted to Hopkins upon condition that he make up French during the summer vacation.

His knowledge of German proved helpful at Hopkins, for that was the period when many of the foremost American medical scientists were German trained. Because of the scarcity of textbooks in English, it was recommended that the students use Stohr's *Histologie*, Neumeister's *Physiologische Chemie*, Cohnheim's *Chemie der Eiweis Körper*, Hertwig's *Embryologie*, Spalteholtz's *Anatomische Atlas*, Ziegler's *Pathologische Anatomie*, Nothnagel and Rossbach's *Arzneimittellehre*, and Koenig's three-volume *Chirurgie*. Physiology was at that time strong in England, with Bayliss, Starling, Sherrington, Haldane, and others making important contributions. The recommended textbook in this subject was Michael Foster's. Foster, of course, was the teacher of Henry Newell Martin, the first professor of biology at Johns Hopkins.

Erlanger had had some research experience during his course in vertebrate embryology at Berkeley, but his first medical research effort was made during the summer vacation between his first and second years at Johns Hopkins. Unable to spend the vacation at home because of the cost of travel, he worked in the histological laboratory of Lewellys Barker on the locus in the spinal cord of the anterior horn cells that innervate a given voluntary muscle. Although Erlanger did not publish a paper on his work, Barker, in his book entitled *The Nervous System and Its Constituent Neurons*, mentioned Erlanger six times and reproduced three of his histological preparations, for which Erlanger received due credit.

Medical students in those days were stimulated to engage in research. Erlanger's first published research was "A Study of the Metabolism in Dogs with Shortened Small Intestines." The dogs used in the study were those which William S. Halsted and Franklin P. Mall had prepared in their search for reliable intestinal sutures. The object of their study was to determine the permissible length of intestine that could be excised surgically. Joseph H. Flint, a medical student who was working in Mall's laboratory, passed along the news that metabolic observations on these dogs were needed. Erlanger joined the study, which showed that there was a diminution in the absorption of fats.

Erlanger received his medical degree in 1899. After his year of internship in the Johns Hopkins Hospital, he was faced with the decision of whether to start practice or become a teacher and investigator. The only opportunity for the latter work was through a fellowship in pathology with William H. Welch, which he received for the year 1901, succeeding the two previous fellows, W. G. MacCallum and Eugene L. Opie. However, only a few days before the fellowship began, William H. Howell, professor of physiology, offered Erlanger an assistantship made available when George Dreyer, an assistant professor, resigned. Welch agreed to release Erlanger, and thus began Erlanger's career in physiology.

Physiology at that time was a three-man department, and Erlanger shared duties with the Instructor, P. M. Dawson, supervising the laboratory course for the medical students and preparing the demonstrations for Dr. Howell's lectures. The latter task was a tremendous responsibility, and two of his experiences are of interest. Dr. Howell wanted the class to see the capillary electrometer in action. This was a delicate instrument recently devised by English physiologists to record nerve action potentials. After several failures to make a capillary that was sufficiently sensitive for detection of the nerve action potentials, Erlanger succeeded in drawing one that recorded the action potential of the frog's heart, which was projected on the screen of the lecture room. The second experience related to the blood pressure machine, or sphygmomanometer. A Mosso instrument, which recorded the pulsation in the two first fingers of both hands, had just been imported from Italy. It was made of glass, and in preparing it for the demonstration, Erlanger broke it. Since the blood pressure demonstration was a must, he assembled a device of his own design with which the arterial pressure in the arm could be measured in man. Erlanger's instrument (1901) made it possible to determine the minimum (diastolic) and maximum (systolic) blood pressures with a high degree of accuracy. This apparatus combined features of the instruments devised earlier by Marey, von Recklinghausen, and Vierordt. It consisted of a pneumatic cuff, a Politzer bag, and a U-shaped manometer. A Ludwig Kymograph and tambour were used for recording. The interior of the tambour was in contact with the air column which transmitted the arterial pulse to the mercury manometer, and a writing stylus was attached to the tambour. Thus, the column of air, as it transmitted the arterial pulse to the mercury manometer, activated the tambour and stylus so that a graphic record was obtained. From his experiments on man as well as on an artificial circulatory model, Erlanger concluded that the maximum blood pressure corresponded to the point at which there was an abrupt increase in the amplitude of the oscillations of the arterial wall and that the minimum blood pressure was recorded at the point of maximum oscillation. Erlanger's contribution at this point in the development of blood pressure recording cleared much of the confusion, but his instrument was too cumbersome for clinical use. It was supplanted in 1905 when Korotkoff described the sounds heard over an artery at a point immediately below a compression cup. The point at which the sounds first appear has been universally accepted as the systolic pressure. However, the changes in the sounds that indicate diastolic pressure are more difficult to determine.

Erlanger spent the vacation period between his first and second years in the Department of Physiology in Germany. On his return to Baltimore he had an opportunity to make practical use of his sphygmomanometer in studies on a medical student with orthostatic albuminuria, Donald R. Hooker. Hooker, who later became the managing editor of the *American Journal of Physiology,* had already studied his malady from the chemical standpoint in collaboration with L. B. Mendel of Yale. Using Erlanger's instrument, they made plans to investigate it from the circulatory viewpoint. With Erlanger serving as the normal control, they used various procedures which were expected to alter the blood supply to the kidney, such as changes in posture. During these maneuvers, they followed the arterial and venous pressures as well as the blood flow in the arm and hand. The results of their studies were published in 1904 as a monograph in the *Johns Hopkins Hospital Reports,* their observations demonstrating that the output of albumin depended primarily on changes in pulse pressure rather than blood pressure.

In 1904 William Osler asked Erlanger to see a patient in the Johns Hopkins Hospital who exhibited the "Stokes-Adams syndrome," a condition characterized by a slow pulse and fainting spells. Erlanger's graphic records of the apex beat exhibited complete atrioventricular heart block. The patient had syphilis, and after he had undergone treatment his heartbeat gradually returned to normal, passing through all the stages of partial block in the process. The records were comparable to those obtained by Erlanger's medical students in the physiological laboratory by applying pressure on the atrioventricular junction of the turtle's heart. In the 1890s the German anatomist His had described the only conducting muscular connection between the atria and ventricles of the mammalian heart, the narrow atrioventricular bundle (AV bundle), and had shown that cutting that bundle resulted in permanent atrioventricular heart block. At that time at Johns Hopkins the anatomical phase of His's observations was being confirmed by Robert Retzer, who was working in Mall's anatomical laboratory. With this information available, Erlanger devised a clamp with which controlled pressure could be applied reversibly to the AV bundle of the dog's beating heart, permitting him to produce accurately all degrees of AV block.

During the summer of 1905 a medical student, Arthur D. Hirschfelder, collaborated with Erlanger in experiments designed to ascertain the relative action of the cardiac nerves, the inhibitors, and the accelerators during complete block (when the atria and ventricles were functioning independently of each other). It was Hirschfelder's first published work. Later, when Hirschfelder was professor of pharmacology at the University of Minnesota, he sent Erlanger his newly published *Textbook of Pharmacology*. To it was attached a card reading: "The harvest of the seed you planted in the summer of 1905."

During his fifth year in Baltimore, Erlanger was offered an associate professorship at Wisconsin at a salary of $2,500. He consulted Dr. Howell, who advised him to decline the offer, saying, "If they want you they will make a better offer." He was correct. The next year they offered Erlanger the professorship of physiology and physiological chemistry in the medical school, with a salary of $3,000. This offer he accepted. His work there and later at Washington University on the function of peripheral nerve fibers won him the Nobel Prize.

Theodore C. Janeway

One of the pioneers in the study of blood pressure in man was Theodore C. Janeway, the first full-time professor of medicine at Johns Hopkins. Before he came to Hopkins, Janeway also had the distinction of being the first to show that placing a ligature around a renal artery and temporarily compressing the blood flow resulted in elevation of blood pressure. Unfortunately, he did not follow up on this observation, and it remained for Goldblatt to devise a method of clamping the renal artery with partial interruption of blood flow, which could be maintained over a long period of time and thus produce a continuing hypertension.

The first paper in America that dealt specifically with blood pressure was the important presentation, at the twelfth meeting of the Association of American Physicians in 1897, by Abel and Crawford on the "Isolation of Chemically Pure Epinephrine." This was, however, experimental work. Richard C. Cabot of Boston made the first observations on human blood pressure reported to the Association of American Physicians in 1903 as part of a paper describing "Studies on the Action of Alcohol in Disease, Especially upon the Circulation."

This was a careful clinical study, using the Riva-Rocci sphygmomanometer and the original Oliver hemodynamometer in fifty-eight cases.

Janeway first presented his studies on blood pressure at the meeting of the Association of American Physicians, and then at the 1915 meeting he presented a very comprehensive paper entitled "Important Contributions to Clinical Medicine During the Past Thirty Years from the Study of Human Blood Pressure." Janeway's work began early in the century, and his first publication, entitled "The Clinical Study of Blood Pressure," appeared in 1904.

Chemical Transmission of Nerve Impulses

Elliott postulated in 1904 that some chemical was liberated at nerve terminals by the arrival of nerve impulses. In 1907 Dixon discovered the specific action of epinephrine, clearly stating that sympathetic nerves may produce their effects by liberation of epinephrine or a substance like it at their neural junctions. Until this time it was generally assumed that the waves of electrical potential accompanying impulses had force enough to leap across the resistance at nerve terminals, setting up new waves of excitation in the organs they supplied.

In 1906 William Henry Howell observed that when hearts were perfused with solutions free of potassium, stimulation of the vagus nerve was less effective, and that if the concentration of potassium ions was slightly increased in the perfusate, the vagus responded to subliminal stimulation. Two years later Howell and Duke published evidence that during vagal stimulation of the mammalian heart potassium was liberated into the perfusing solution. Howell interpreted these results, together with the well-known retarding action of excessive amounts of k-ions in the perfusing fluid on heart action, as evidence of indirect action of the vagus. The nerve impulses first liberated potassium from a bound, nondiffusible form in the heart tissue, and the free potassium ions then retarded the heart's action. It was later discovered that acetylcholine was the chief chemical liberated upon stimulation of the cardiac vagus nerves, but Howell, in experiments expressly planned for the purpose, was the first to produce substantial evidence showing that chemicals may be liberated at nerve terminals.

In retrospect, one must conclude that Dr. Howell's work was a significant contribution to the early development of the concept of chemical mediation of nerve action. It was also an important observation for the cardiac surgeon who makes effective use of the ability of potassium to produce temporary cardiac arrest.

William Sydney Thayer

William Sydney Thayer was born in Milton, Massachusetts, on June 23, 1864. He came from stock that represented the best of early New England character and grew up in an environment of scholarly interest of the highest type. Thayer graduated from Harvard College in 1885 and four years later received his medical degree from Harvard. The next two years he spent as a house officer at Massachusetts General Hospital in Boston. In November 1890 he came to Johns Hopkins as Osler's second assistant on the resident medical staff. In September 1891 he was appointed resident physician, a post he held for seven years. He then served as Osler's first assistant, with the rank of associate professor, until the time of Osler's resignation in 1905. He was appointed professor of clinical medicine in that year, and in 1918 he became chairman of the Department of Medicine in the Johns Hopkins University and physician-in-chief to the Johns Hopkins Hospital. He held these positions until 1921, when he voluntarily withdrew, believing that he should make way for a younger man. He maintained his connection with the hospital, sharing with his colleagues his great store of clinical knowledge.

During World War I he was appointed chief medical consultant of the United States Expeditionary Forces in France, with the rank of brigadier general. In 1927 he was elected president of the American Medical Association. For many years he was a member of the Harvard Board of Overseers, and he received many other honors, including an LL.D. degree from Edinburgh University (1927) and honorary membership in the Therapeutical Society of Moscow (1897), the Royal Society of Medicine of Budapest (1909), the Academy of Medicine of Paris (1918), the Royal Society of Medical and Natural Sciences of Brussels (1919), the Royal Society of Medicine, London (1923), and the Association of Physicians of Great Britain and Ireland (1925). He was also a member of the American Philosophical Society (1924) and a fellow of the American Academy of Arts and Sciences (1921). In 1927 a group of his friends established a fund in the university for an endowment to be known as the William Sydney Thayer and Susan Read Thayer Lectureship in Clinical Medicine. This was a unique token of appreciation of his achievements and a tribute to the memory of his wife, whose devotion to his interests had played such an important part in his life.

The preceding listing of facts about this outstanding clinician and scholar does not tell of the tremendous influence he had on American medicine and of the important contributions he made to medical science. The extent of his enormous role in American medicine was indicated by Simon Flexner, in his remarks at the dedication in 1934 of the new Thayer semi-private ward. Flexner's friendship with Thayer extended over a period of forty years, from the time they both arrived at the Johns Hopkins Hospital in the autumn of 1890, Thayer to go into the "house" under Dr. Osler and Flexner into the laboratory to study pathology under Dr. Welch. For seven years they were co-residents in the hospital. They met regularly at the head table in the old "officers' dining room" and were both influenced by the not infrequent presence at that table of that remarkable triumvirate—Welch, Osler, and Halsted. Others regularly present were Councilman, Abbott, Nuttall, Mall, Barker, and Frank Smith. The talk covered a wide range of topics, and there was much good-humored banter. Flexner remembered in detail his first meeting with Thayer. In 1887 the Ehrlich blood-staining technique had recently been published, and Dr. Welch had received from Ehrlich a small sheaf of student dissertations describing the method. These he turned over to Flexner, suggesting that he master the method and apply it to a case of leukemia in the hospital ward. To the modern student

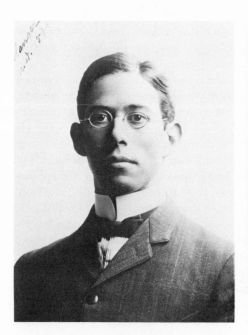

Joseph Erlanger
From the Archives Office, The Johns Hopkins
Medical Institutions

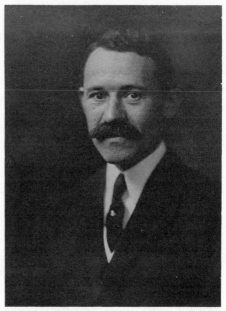

Theodore C. Janeway
From the Archives Office, The Johns Hopkins
Medical Institutions

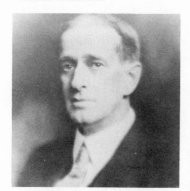

Edward Perkins Carter
From the Archives Office, The Johns
Hopkins Medical Institutions

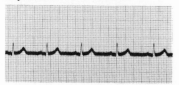

Fig. 1. Electrocardiogram taken
by Einthoven in 1902 before his
first publication

From Rijsmuseum Voor de Geschie-
denis der Natuurweten schaffen, P.
van der star. Courtesy of Richard S.
Ross.

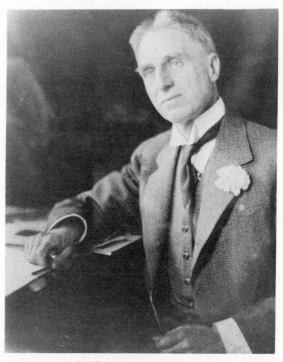

William Sydney Thayer
From the Archives Office, The Johns Hopkins Medical
Institutions

267

of clinical microscopy this may seem a rather insignificant event, but in those days it was pure adventure and exploration. To prepare the subtle, complex stains one had to acquire, by trial and error, great skill in executing the tricky film spreading and heating operations, and the differential staining and counting had to be carried out without example and wholly according to the sketchy printed descriptions. Flexner was persuaded to present his somewhat amateurish results at a meeting of the Johns Hopkins Hospital Medical Society. He relates how after the meeting an attractive young man with a pained countenance sought him out and asked where he had learned the blood technique. The young man was William S. Thayer, who had acquired expertise in the application of these new methods of study in his year abroad, either directly from Ehrlich himself or from one of his disciples. Thayer's experience with this new and exciting technique soon brought eager young doctors to the clinical laboratory to study under him, and in a short time it was being used widely throughout the country. (See the chapter on contributions to hematology.)

It is important to emphasize that during Thayer's year in Germany he had spent almost all of his time in pathology, which was the major attraction for him at that time, rather than in clinical medicine. He had studied diligently under Virchow, and if he attended any clinics or was attracted by any eminent clinical teachers, he made no reference to such study. He concentrated on strengthening his foundation in a branch of the natural sciences which was beginning to be called on more and more in an effort to discover the nature of disease.

As a young man, Thayer responded avidly to strong personalities among his teachers. The first of these was Reginald H. Fitz, professor of pathology at the Harvard Medical School in the days when pathology was a branch of clinical medicine. It was Fitz who first clearly described the syndrome of appendicitis. Although the clinical facilities in Boston surpassed the pathological, Thayer devoted himself to the laboratory and neglected the hospital wards. He was not projecting a future career, but was submitting to the compelling stimulus provided by Fitz, in whose activities pathology and practice were united. Medicine at that point represented to Thayer an opportunity to acquire methods of precision, and the pathological laboratory was the only available place in which to learn those methods that could be applied to the study of disease.

However, in 1890 an important event took place in Berlin, while Thayer was attending the Ninth International Medical Congress. The imposing Osler was pointed out to him: "a figure which stood out from all the rest. The alert figure with celtic features, drooping mustaches and small nervous hands; the physician-in-chief of the richly endowed, newly opened Johns Hopkins Hospital immediately arrested the young man's attention." How much of Osler was in that first glimpse, "of how little was I conscious at the moment. How little did I fancy that in three months I should be sitting at his table and that to him I should owe so large a part of the blessings of my life," Thayer wrote long afterwards. The life of Thayer the physician began at that point. He had again fallen under the dominance of a gifted man with a strong personality—this time a personality closely attuned to his own.

When Thayer arrived in Baltimore, two infectious diseases were rampant, malaria and typhoid fever. Thayer's studies in the clinical laboratory were directed toward malaria, for which his knowledge of Ehrlich's blood-staining technique especially qualified him. The discovery of the malarial parasite by Laveran, ten years earlier, had already been confirmed in America by Councilman and Osler. In Italy, strides were being made in the delineation and interpretation of this parasitic disease. Thayer's investigations with Hewetson fitted into and enlarged this expanding subject, and Thayer's *Lectures on Malarial Fevers*, superbly illustrated and published in 1897, carried the new knowledge throughout the English-speaking world. Soon such erroneous and confused diagnoses as "typhomalarial fever" were displaced, as laboratory diagnosis with the microscope supplemented clinical observation of patients.

Thayer made many interesting investigations of a clinical nature in relation to the cardiovascular system. His early studies of the physiological third heart sound, an auscultatory event he had discovered with Hirschfelder about the same time as Gibson of Edinburgh and some two years after Obrastzow of Kiev, were exemplary. Thayer was impressed with the accentuated third sound of mitral regurgitation. He pointed out that the third heart sound was loudest immediately after the subject assumed the recumbent posture—the so-called primo-decubitus position. He thought that this sound was due to "the sudden tensing of the mitral leaflet and perhaps the tricuspid value at the time of the first and most rapid phase of diastole."

Thayer also introduced the term "opening snap" for the characteristic sound heard in mitral stenosis, to correspond to the *"claquement d'ouverture* of the French." He was among the first to describe an epigastric venous hum with hepatic cirrhosis. With his pathologist colleague, William MacCallum, he bled dogs and studied the effects of anemia on the auscultatory findings in the heart, noting that these dogs developed an aortic diastolic murmur. Thayer was one of the early clinicians to employ blood cultures in the study of patients with fever and heart murmurs.

Thayer's early observations on bacterial endocarditis are also significant. In 1896 it was recognized that endocarditis and pericarditis were occasional complications of gonococcal infections, but the true nature of the process and their relation to the primary lesion were far from being settled. After Neisser's description of the gonococcus and the demonstration of satisfactory methods of culture by Bumm in 1885 and Wertheim in 1892, the various complications were studied with great care. Cases had been reported of ulcerative endocarditis with organisms resembling gonococci seen in the lesions by Gram's method (Winterberg, 1894).

Leyden carried the studies a step further when he stained gonococci on the heart valve in 1893, but blood cultures in his case were sterile. The first definite proof of the existence of a gonorrhoeal septicemia as well as of an ulcerative endocarditis due to the gonococcus was reported by Thayer and Blumer in 1896. The patient was a thirty-four-year-old widow who entered the Johns Hopkins Hospital on April 25, 1895. She had a history of "rheumatism" with polysynovitis. Three days before admission she felt tired and noted labial herpes. The day before admission she had a distinct chill. On examination she was febrile, had a pulse of 132 and a temperature of 102.2°F. There were signs of mitral valve disease with a loud first sound and a presystolic murmur. A slight leukocytosis was noted. The patient continued febrile and there was progressive enlargement of the spleen. On May 7 there was a presystolic thrill and a presystolic murmur followed by a snapping valvular first sound and a loud blowing systolic murmur transmitted into the axilla. She also developed a pericardial friction rub, and a faint diastolic murmur was heard along the left border of the sternum. The patient became progressively anemic, and numerous petechial spots were described.

On May 16 the patient died. An autopsy was performed by Dr. Simon Flexner, who found acute ulcerative endocarditis caused by the gonococcus, proven by cultures. The cocci presented the morphological features of gonococci and were obtained directly from the mitral valve. Blood cultures were positive for gonococci. Thayer felt certain that the organisms present in pure culture in the circulating blood and on the affected valve was the gonococcus of Neisser since (1) its form and arrangements were characteristic, (2) free cocci were frequently found crowded in the protoplasm of leukocytes in the thrombus on the valve, (3) the organism did not grow upon the ordinary media, (4) it grew readily upon a mixture of human blood and agar, and (5) it decolorized when heated and stained by Gram's method. (At this time Jesse Lazear, who was later to die of yellow fever in Cuba, was in charge of the bacteriological work in the laboratory of clinical microscopy.) Thus Thayer was the first to report a proven case of gonococcal endocarditis. His early work in this area culminated in the publication of a monograph, which appeared in the *Johns Hopkins Hospital Reports* in 1916. In 1930 he gave the prestigious Gibson Lectures in Edinburgh, which were titled "Bacterial or Infective Endocarditis." At that time the principle of treatment in this almost universally fatal disease was nil nocere. Thayer concluded that the widespread use of intravenous arsenicals and mercurials, and other so-called internal antiseptics, was irrational and dangerous. Following the appearance of the article by Capps, Thayer used arsenic in the form of cacodylate of sodium subcutaneously. "Used with care," he noted, "it is harmless." He had no idea as to whether it influenced the course of the disease. He concluded by saying that "at the present moment it is through scrupulous general care of the individual that the best results are to be obtained." These remarks of 1930 emphasize the tremendous advances in medicine that have been made in the past few decades.

Thayer rapidly became a vital force in medicine in the United States. In his delightful essays on the *Medical Education* of Jones, he states: "Twenty-five years have passed by. Great changes have taken place in medicine. Through the introduction of procedures, diagnostic and therapeutic, based on the application of the fundamental sciences, remarkable advances have been made in the art and science of medicine. Researches in no way inferior to those carried on in the laboratories of the fundamental sciences are being pursued by members of the clinical staff."

With this advance, Thayer detected a regrettable tendency, against which he warned: "A sound basis in the fundamental sciences, so desirable for the trained and scholarly physician, is in no way a shortcut to experience, practical and human, which always has been and always will be necessary to make a good diagnostician, a good doctor and a good clinical teacher." He deplored, therefore, that so large a proportion of American and foreign physicians were sadly lacking in the essential foundations of a training in clinical diagnostic methods, and he warned against a growing tendency to substitute laboratory reports for clinical observation. He spoke of such ancillary procedures as traps into which practitioners fall in too many instances and stressed that they could be liabilities as well as helps. He insisted that interest in bacteriological, sero-logical, and chemical tests was indispensable but that "the newer physical methods of exploration should not lead us to forget the necessity of prolonged and systematic training in ward and outpatient department, in pathological anatomy and in physical diagnosis."

Contributions to Electrocardiography

Students of bioelectrical phenomena had long known that in parts of the body where activity is evident, differences in electrical potential arise which result in the passage of so-called action currents from points of higher to points of lower potential. Waller showed that it is possible by connecting electrodes with the moist skin to collect these currents generated in the heart by means of an electrometer or a galvanometer. As the currents generated are extremely small, their detection is difficult, and clinical application seemed out of the question until the Dutch physiologist Einthoven adapted the string galvanom-eter for the purpose. Electric currents which are passed through a metal-coated fiber suspended in a magnetic field provoke a deflection of the fiber, which increases either with the strength of the current or the strength of the field. Einthoven passed the current from the heart through a microscopic thread (string) made of quartz or platinum, one to two microns in thickness, sus-pended in a very strong magnetic field. The movements of this thread were photographed through an illuminated slit on a rapidly moving film, and under a lens that magnified the thread and its movements several hundred times. The resulting photographic record yielded a curve known as the "electrocardio-gram" (Fig. 1). Einthoven accomplished this in 1903 and set up transmission lines to the hospital a mile and a half away so that he could take his records without moving patients who were critically ill.

In an article in Scientific American on July 22, 1911, describing heart diagnosis by electricity, it was stated that "this instrumental investigation serves not only for the discovery of disease but also for diagnosing its precise charac-ter. It is as yet too early to judge but many physiologists and physicians believe that it will prove to be a very valuable aid to the medical profession." At that time only three so-called heart stations were in operation in this country: at Presbyterian and Mount Sinai hospitals in New York and at the Johns Hopkins Hospital in Baltimore. As already described, Dr. George S. Bond played an important role in the introduction of electrocardiography into the Johns Hopkins Hospital. In later years Johns Hopkins was the scene of many contributions to our knowledge of the theoretical basis of electrocardiography, as well as to its clinical usefulness.

Edward Perkins Carter

Edward Perkins Carter was born in Williamstown, Massachusetts, on March 13, 1870, at which time his father was president of Williams College. Carter graduated from Williams and received his M.D. degree from the University of Pennsylvania in 1894. In that year he became a resident house officer at the Johns Hopkins Hospital and two years later a fellow in pathology. In 1898 he was the first resident physician in the newly opened Lakeside Hospital in Cleveland. In 1899 he studied in Vienna and then returned to practice in Cleveland. In 1912 he withdrew from private practice and spent the next two years at the University College Hospital Medical School in London. When the professional activities at Cleveland City Hospital were turned over to the faculty of Western Reserve Medical School, Carter returned to Cleveland as full-time chief of medicine at Cleveland City Hospital in 1914. In 1918 he came to Johns Hopkins as lecturer in medicine, holding successively appointments as associate professor (1924–1932) and adjunct professor of medicine (1932–1936). As a teacher he was at his best with a small group at the bedside.

His interest in research and the field of cardiovascular disease began early in his career. While still in practice he acquired a Mackenzie polygraph, with which he obtained records of the events of the heartbeat and pulse in patients in their homes. At Cleveland City Hospital he had the first electrocardiograph machine in that area: an old Cambridge instrument, which came over in the last shipment from England prior to World War I. He continued his observations upon the events of the cardiac cycle for many years, and his study of bundle branch block is still a classic. He was certainly among the first to recognize the high alveolar CO_2 content and unusual CO_2 tolerance of a patient with emphysema. After Carter assumed responsibility for the heart station or cardiographic laboratory at Hopkins in 1918, he produced several papers on the interpretation of the electrocardiogram. The most important was a study entitled "A Graphic Application of the Principle of the Equilateral Triangle for Determining the Direction of the Electrical Axis," published in the *Johns Hopkins Hospital Bulletin* in 1919 with Richter and Greene. Francis Dieuaide joined him soon after his arrival in Baltimore, and they carried out further studies in this same field.

William Hofmeyr Craib

It was in Carter's laboratory that much of the early work in cardiology at Johns Hopkins was done—notably that of William Hofmeyr Craib. Craib was educated at Gill College, Somerset East, South Africa. He was first in the colony matriculation examination, with exceptionally high marks in Greek. He received his B.A. degree with honors and was awarded the Jameson Scholarship for postgraduate study. After serving under General Botha in the Southwest African Campaign from 1914 to 1915, he went to France and served as trench mortar officer from 1916 to 1919 with the 29th Division. He was awarded the Military Cross and mentioned in dispatches. His degree in South Africa was awarded in pure mathematics, applied mathematics, and physics. After World War I he studied medicine at Cambridge and after clinical instruction in London graduated in 1923. After a year at Guy's hospital he received a Rockefeller Foundation research fellowship to work at the Johns Hopkins Hospital in Baltimore.

Upon his arrival at Hopkins he reported to Dr. Warfield T. Longcope, and having no official program in mind was assigned to the heart station under Dr. E. P. Carter, who suggested that he investigate the effort of thyroxine on the heart and blood vessels. Craib soon found that he was approaching clinical problems from an entirely new angle—seeing medicine for the first time as a science and not as a technique or craft. He has described his adventures with modesty and humor.

One day Craib was standing behind a group of students to whom Dr. Longcope was demonstrating a patient with a swollen abdomen and pitting edema. Dr. Longcope suddenly spotted Craib and said: "Ah, gentlemen; here is Dr. Craib straight from London, the very heart of electrocardiography. Let's ask him what he thinks." Turning to Craib he said, "Dr. Craib, according to the heart station report, this patient's electrical axis is fixed. Now, what does one conclude from that?" Craib was completely dumfounded. Electrical axes had never crossed his path at Guy's. His hands trembled and his palms grew damp. "Well, sir," he replied, "we're not very good on electrical axes at Guy's Hospital. But I would not be surprised if the right treatment might not be to loosen them up a bit—a powerful purgative such as a few drops of castor oil." It was a desperate effort in a desperate situation. Fortunately, Dr. Longcope tactfully went on teaching and Craib quietly retreated to find out what an electrical axis could possibly be. Back at the heart station he humbly inquired of the technician if she could enlighten him. She said to ask Dr. Carter when he came in, which he presently did. Carter seemed quite taken aback by the question. "But Craib," he said, "haven't you heard of Einthoven of Holland and Sir Thomas Lewis of London?" "Well, yes," Craib replied, "of Lewis certainly, but of Einthoven never. Didn't Lewis write a small book for students on the irregularities of the pulse?" "What a strange thing," said Carter, "the whole world hangs on every word that Lewis and Einthoven utter. Why, that large book lying there is Lewis' famous monograph on the subject of the electrical forces in the heart. Indeed, we call it our bible." By this time Craib was ready to sink into the floor and all he could say was: "Thank you sir, it seems there is a lot of reading for me to do. May I please borrow the book?" "Certainly," Carter said with a smile, "and I only hope you'll make more sense of it than I can."

As Craib began to read Lewis's book on the principles of interpretation of the electrocardiogram, he recognized that the explanation of the electrical phenomena described was not compatible with the theories of electricity taught him as incontrovertible dogma eleven years previously in Capetown, unless the electricity derived from living tissues was totally different from that encountered in inanimate matter. The explanation Lewis accepted was the "membrane theory" of Bernstein, according to which the electrocardiogram simply records a "wave of negativity" as the basis of the excitatory process and its tranmission. Craib, feeling it would be impertinent for him to tell Dr. Carter that Lewis's conclusions seemed completely untenable, decided therefore to study bioelectricity in his spare time. The next day he confided his doubts about the current theories of the electrocardiogram to Dr. E. Cowles Andrus. Andrus thought it a bit odd for someone to accuse a world authority such as Lewis of talking nonsense and that the chances, if not the certainties, were that Craib was wrong and Lewis right. "If you do produce something that makes it necessary for us all to think again and Lewis too—well, you'll certainly have put the cat among the pigeons in the world of muscle physiology." The next day Craib broached the subject with Dr. Carter, who happily said that if Craib was really keen to work on the fundamentals of bioelectrical phenomena with special reference to the electrocardiogram, he should by all means do so.

Lewis's statements about muscle electricity were based upon the theoretical electrical behavior of muscle strips. Craib, therefore, had to find muscle strips which could be suitably prepared, stimulated to activity, and kept alive long enough to record the electrical phenomena produced. Andrus suggested using the terrapin heart muscle. Craib cut a turtle heart into a number of strips, one to two inches long, and was delighted to find that each strip would beat on its own. Suspending the strips in physiological solution by a thread tied to each end and stimulating the strips at one end by means of a small electrical shock, he recorded a beat associated with a wave of excitation traveling from the stimulated end to the other. It soon became clear that Lewis' statements were not applicable to terrapin muscle heart strips, other experiments with frog skeletal and heart muscle showed that they, too, did not produce electricity in accordance with Lewis's theory. It then became necessary to produce a hypothesis that did explain the behavior of the muscle strips. The hypothetical field was worked out for Craib by Robert Canfield of the Department of Physics at the Johns Hopkins University. This stipulated that the electrical field around an intact heart should present characteristics typical of the summated effects of the large number of muscle strips that compose the heart. Craib then suspended a beating, intact, isolated heart at the center of a spherical bowl of physiological saline (a goldfish bowl) and measured the electrical field of potential set up around it during each contraction. The resulting measurements with the rough techniques available were so close to the theoretical forecast that he was now in a position to make a tentative statement to Dr. Carter. Since Craib's results were so revolutionary, they were reviewed in detail with Professor William H. Howell. Then Craib was sent by Dr. Carter to see Horatio B. Williams, professor of physiology at the College of Physicians and Surgeons in New York. Williams read over Craib's statement and then said to him: "It is difficult for me to say what I think. But before doing so, tell me who you are and what previous research you have done." "Well, sir," said Craib, "I'm not really anybody. I've never done any research until joining Dr. Carter's laboratory in

Baltimore." Williams replied, "But Craib, how can you then possibly be so impertinent as to speak of the world's greatest heart specialist and leader in electrocardiography in the way you do? Why, you actually suggest that the views he holds along with all of us don't make sense." Craib replied that he was not really criticizing Lewis, but simply wanted to know where his experiments were badly planned or where the interpretations and results were false. Williams then stated that there was no point in continuing the conversation. He wrote a letter to Dr. Carter warning him that publication of Dr. Craib's results might bring discredit on the laboratory. Carter, however, was determined that if Craib was to be condemned, at least the judgment would be a fair one. The next step was to submit the paper for presentation at the next meeting of the American Society for Clinical Investigation. Craib gave his paper, but unfortunately there was no discussion of it afterwards. However, Frank Wilson, the well-known cardiologist from Michigan, came up to him and spoke as follows: "Craib, may I say that I am the unhappiest man in America today. You see, I know you are right and that I have missed the bus. I have been working for years on the same problem. I have worked with Thomas Lewis, but I have reached the point of conviction that what you refer to as the negativity hypothesis is false and that currents around active muscle have points of entry and points of exit at the muscle surfaces. As I listened to you a full light dawned, and I felt it's kind of unfair that I should have got so close to the truth after years of thought only to be robbed at the post by someone who seems to have done only one experiment in his life. May I congratulate you on an excellent piece of work." Later Wilson, in his monograph on "Currents of Action and Injury," made generous acknowledgment of Craib's contribution. Wilson's support gave great encouragement to Dr. Carter and to Dr. Andrus, so that in spite of Williams's warning Craib was sent to Stockholm to read his paper at the International Physiological Congress in July 1926. The chairman of the session was Professor Einthoven of Leiden University, who was the doyen of electrocardiography. Craib gave his talk, showed his slides, and sat down. There was no discussion, and Einthoven, there and later, did not accept Craib's interpretation of his results.

Craib declined Carter's offer to continue work in Baltimore. Instead, he returned to England as medical registrar at Guy's Hospital and once more immersed himself in clinical medicine. But an opportunity eventually arose which brought him back to electrocardiography. This experience he has described in a memoir.

One day Sir Thomas Lewis called and asked Craib to show him his results. He ended up by attending dinner at Lewis's house. After dinner Craib tried an experiment on Lewis before telling him about his work. He asked Lewis why when he let go of a paper clip it fell to the table. Lewis said it was certainly due to the force of gravity. Craib then asked: "This force of gravity you talk of. Is this a fact or a theory?" "A fact, of course," said Lewis. Craib said: "The force of gravity you speak of is not a fact; it is a theory or hypothesis put forward to explain all sorts of observed phenomena." Craib then indicated that since they really did not speak the same language, it would be of no avail to discuss his theories with Lewis. Two weeks later he received another phone call from Lewis saying that he had changed his mind and thought he knew what Craib was getting at: "You are right about the force of gravity," he said. "It is a theory and not a fact." Craib spent a long period of time with Lewis talking about the electrical properties of matter. Lewis treated Craib with courtesy and patience, suggesting that he should really write up his work and asking that Craib let him see the manuscript in due course. Not long afterwards Lewis offered Craib a job in his laboratory under the aegis of the Medical Research Council at a salary of some £400 per annum.

Craib then set about to put his experimental work into a state fit for publication. He wrote thousands of words, which were carefully edited by Lewis, who was almost driven mad by Craib's colonial English. Craib has stated that he owes Sir Thomas an enormous debt of gratitude for his help in the writing of English and for his insistence on clear thinking and good literary style. The paper was entitled "A Study of the Electrical Field Surrounding Active Heart Muscle." Craib then studied the electrical fields of potential surrounding skeletal muscle, and his results were similar to those in cardiac muscle.

Sir Thomas suggested that the manuscript be referred to Professor E. D. Adrian for his comments. Adrian's reply soon came in a letter to Lewis condemning the work as unreliable, adding that he, Adrian, had tried to verify the results without success. He warned Lewis that discredit would be brought on the laboratory if such shoddy work were supported and encouraged. Lewis asked Craib if he could suggest a resolution to the problem. Craib pointed out that all of Adrian's work had been done using a capillary electrometer, recording the movements of a very fine column of mercury. His (Craib's) had been done with a string galvanometer and the Matthews oscillograph, both direct recording instruments. Adrian agreed to repeat Craib's experiment in his own laboratory. Adrian went into the darkroom where his experiments were conducted and soon called Craib in to look at the preparation he had set up. It was not exactly as Craib had described it, but Adrian thought that the difference was inconsequential. Craib, however, insisted that everything be arranged exactly according to his diagram. Craib then waited expectantly, hearing the sounds issuing from Adrian's laboratory as the excitation gadget, the falling of the photograph plate, and the swishing sound of an exposed plate being developed could be heard. This happened several times before Adrian finally emerged, walked quickly past, and said, "Craib, I'll publish your paper."

Receiving little encouragement in his efforts to study the complexities of bioelectrical phenomena, Craib returned to Africa in 1931. The following year he was appointed professor of medicine at the University of Witwatersrand, Johannesburg, a position he held for fourteen years. He was consultant physician to the South African forces during World War II, rising to the rank of colonel. In 1963 he was made an associate adviser to the Council for Scientific and Industrial Research and served on the Subcommittee for Medical Research. In 1965 he became vice-president on the council for Scientific and

Industrial Research and in 1972 a member of the Scientific Advisory Council of the Prime Minister.

Craib as a novice in research took a critical view of the "membrane theory" of Bernstein, and conceived the hypothesis that the excitatory process is due to the formation of electrical dipoles or doublets (Fig. 2). Despite the storm raised and the cool reception he received, Craib's conclusions have been abundantly confirmed, and form the basis of our present understanding of electrocardiography, including vectorcardiography.

E. Cowles Andrus

Another member of Dr. Carter's group was E. Cowles Andrus. While working for his master's degree at Oberlin College in 1916, Andrus had studied the effect of changes in the content of the perfusate upon the isolated terrapin's heart. When he came to Hopkins as a medical student in the autumn of 1917, he was excused from the course in histology on the basis of his work done at Oberlin. In recalling his first interview with Dr. Howell when he applied for work in the Department of Physiology, Andrus says: "Howell was gentle, quiet and relaxed and he put me quickly at my ease. I had started a project perfusing the heart of the terrapin and studying the effect of altering composition of the perfusate upon the rhythmic changes in 'tonus' of the atria. Dr. Howell listened to my report, encouraged me to continue, promised me a laboratory and introduced me to Charles D. Snyder under whose supervision I continued to work for the next two years." Although Snyder's investigations were in the area which would now be called "biophysics," he took a sympathetic interest in Andrus's experiments. Snyder was an outwardly shy person, but he had a dry sense of humor and a great capacity for friendship—Andrus considered his friendship to be one of the outstanding rewards of his medical school experience.

Andrus's comments on the Department of Physiology at that time are of interest:

The faculty consisted of only four individuals: Dr. Howell, Dr. Donald Hooker, Dr. Snyder and Helene Connet. As chairman, Dr. Howell was relatively inconspicuous because he was already engaged with activities connected with his appointment as Associate Director of the School of Hygiene and Public Health. His textbook was the student's vademecum, but his lectures, though based upon the book, were by no means simply excerpts from it. They included all the new advances in the field and captured the student's attention. Dr. Hooker lectured on the circulation and in the laboratory was engaged with studies on vasomotor control and the capillary and renal circulations. For those working in the Department there was a weekly journal club attended by staff and students where the results of work in progress in physiology as well as other departments were reported. At that time there were 90 students in each class in the medical school and the required course in physiology extended for three trimesters, from January of the first year to December of the second year. Laboratory exercises were conducted one afternoon weekly for two trimesters.

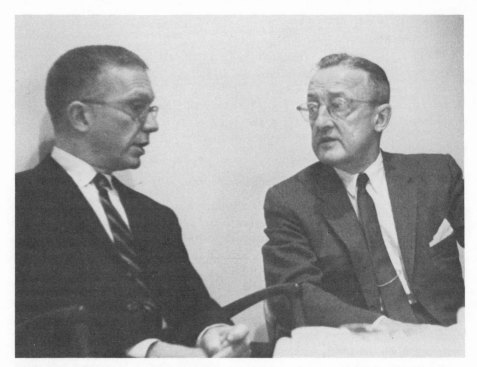

E. Cowles Andrus (*right*) and Richard S. Ross, dean of the School of Medicine

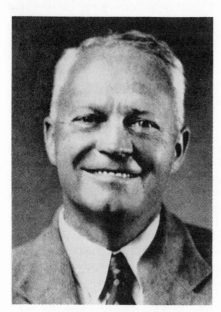

William Hofmeyr Craib

From G. E. Burch and N. P. DePasquale, *A History of Electrocardiography* (Chicago: Yearbook Medical Publishers, 1964). Reproduced with permission.

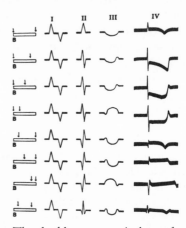

Fig. 2. The doublet concept in heart function

Craib compared (*Heart* 14 [1927]:71) the negativity hypothesis with the doublet hypothesis. The wave of excitation spreads from right to left along the muscle strip (B). The arrows indicate the site of electrode placement; the various curves to the right represent theoretic and recorded curves of variations in electric potential associated with stimulation of the muscle strip. Columns I, II, and III show electrocardiographic deflections expected: (I) according to the negativity hypothesis; (II) on the basis of doublets of short duration; (III) with doublets of prolonged duration and reversed polarity. Column IV shows the actual electrocardiogram.

278

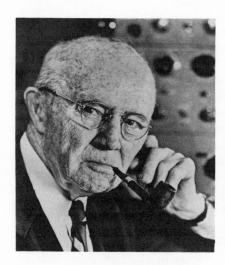

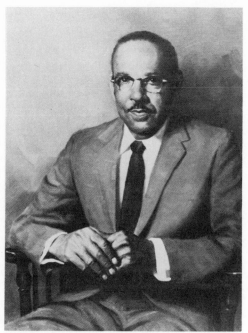

William B. Kouwenhoven

From *Modern Medicine*, copyright © 1967
by The New York Times Media Company,
Inc. Reproduced with permission.

Vivian Thomas

Courtesy of Vivian Thomas

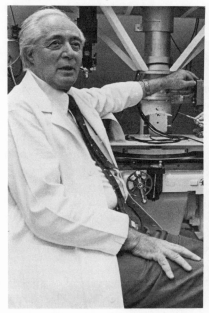

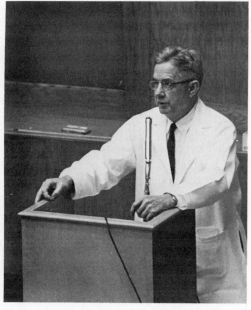

Richard J. Bing

Courtesy of Dr. Richard J. Bing

Alfred Blalock

From the Archives Office, The Johns Hopkins Medical
Institutions

Andrus and his brother, also a first-year medical student, were excused from the laboratory work in physiology as they had already had similar exercises while at Oberlin. Instead, they acted as laboratory assistants preparing the demonstrations for which their tuition, which had just been raised to $300 per year, was remitted. By far the most complicated experiment in the student laboratory course was the recording of blood pressure by cannulization of the carotid artery in the anesthetized dog. There were no exercises in neurophysiology beyond the simple nerve-muscle preparation and the demonstration of spinal reflexes in the frog. In comparison with present day methodology, the apparatus in the department was quite primitive, much of it having been put together by hand or otherwise fabricated by the investigator. Records of heartbeat, blood pressure or contraction of smooth or skeletal muscle were made by a paper-tipped stylus writing on a smoked paper; the smoking thereof and subsequent dipping in shellac for preservation was quite a messy process. "Gold-beater's skin" (calf peritoneal membrane) was a widely used material. For example, it was the basis of construction of the "Brodie bellows" for recording changes in air volume. Blood flow was measured by the "drip" method, or in the heart-lung preparation by a receptacle which was filled and emptied by dumping it at a given time interval. Action currents were recorded with a string galvanometer—Gasser and Erlanger did not introduce the cathode-ray tube until several years later, and amplification by electrical means was not then available. Electrical stimulation was accomplished with the induction coil, which was never free from after-discharge when an attempt was made to apply a single shock. Among the other special pieces of apparatus in the laboratory was a pump for perfusing the kidney with a cam so shaped that it delivered a pulsatile-like flow complete with dicrotic notch, an invention of Dr. Hooker's. Erlanger had devised two instruments: a clamp for producing heart block and a recording sphygmomanometer which was left in the laboratory when he moved to Wisconsin. Systolic pressure was recorded by the first pulse to come through as the cuff was deflated, and diastolic pressure was assumed to be that level at which the pulsations reached maximum amplitude. Snyder employed an impressive arrangement of thermocouple and mirror galvanometer for measuring the beat produced by cardiac muscle. Most ingenious was the Lucas pendulum devised by Keith Lucas of Cambridge, who was tragically killed during World War I. This consisted of a pendulum with switches arranged along an arc of 90° from horizontal to vertical, providing the means to deliver two stimuli at desired intervals. Although this sounds simple, each stimulus actually required four steps with separate switches: (1) to close the circuit to the tissue, (2) to allow current to flow into the inductorium, (3) to open the circuit, and (4) to "bread" the current in the inductorium. Thus a physiologist had to be a very "compleat" individual in those days.

After entering the clinical work of the third and fourth years of the medical school, Andrus transferred his activities to the heart station with Dr. Carter. He and Dr. Carter published a series of studies between 1921 and 1926 on the mechanism of cardiac rhythm. The membrane theory to explain the excitatory process in nerve and its application to other excitable tissues had been evolving since 1904. According to this theory, excitation involved alteration in permeability of the cell membrane and simultaneous depolarization. Nernst advanced the view that stimulation provokes a critical increase in the concentration of ions on either side of a semi-permeable membrane, and Lillie (1911) developed the concept that the process of conduction depends upon the excitation of adjacent areas by an action current developed at each excited point of the nerve. Keith Lucas and Adrian had described the phenomena associated with the "propagated disturbance" in the nerve, including the effects of blockade by pressure or narcosis. In 1921 Carter and Andrus, having demonstrated that an increase in pH of the perfusate increased heart rate and accelerated conduction and vice versa, advanced the theory that the rhythmic polarization and depolarization of the cell membrane, and therewith the potential difference so developed and discharged, was due to the gradient in hydrogen ion concentration across the cell boundary. They subsequently extended this concept to explain ectopic arrhythmias, assuming that local changes in hydrogen ion gradient increased local excitability. Subsequent studies confirmed the effects of the pH changes on cardiac rate and conduction, but their explanation turned out to be an oversimplification. The theory is fundamentally true but the responsible agent is potassium. They had apparently been dealing with a secondary effect of intra and extracellular pH upon the potassium flux.

In 1924, while Andrus was working in the laboratory of Sir Henry Dale in London, he demonstrated that the heart was more strikingly slowed by vagal stimulation in the presence of acidosis and showed greater acceleration with epinephrine in an alkaline medium. Furthermore, the heart rate and conduction were more rapid at any given pH when changes were effected by carbonic rather than by phosphoric acid. This indicated that carbon dioxide entered the cell and brought about a relative decrease in intracellular pH. There is now increasing evidence that this property of carbon dioxide is important in the presence of ischemia, resulting in intracellular acidosis. (Weisfeldt et al.) In the same year, while working in the laboratory of Sir Thomas Lewis in London, Andrus and Alan Drury demonstrated that acidosis and hypoxia caused the excitatory process in the dog's atrium to be conducted decrementally, slowing progressively as it spread. In 1924, while working at the Institute for Physiology in Vienna, Andrus showed that a single induction shock applied to the atrium of the turtle heart close to the end of the absolute refractory period was followed by a rapid "ectopic" rhythm, which persisted until interrupted by a second shock. That this was not due to a "circus movement" was proved by the fact that the sinus venosus continued to beat at its previous independent rate and rhythm.

In 1925, after Andrus returned to Baltimore, he worked with Dr. Carter on the refractory period of the normally beating dog's heart. For these studies it was necessary to drive the heart at a given rate and to introduce a stimulus after a controlled interval. With the assistance of Dr. Harold Wheeler of the Department of Physics, they designed a device which amplified the action current sufficiently to activate a magnet, which tripped a Lucas pendulum, making it possible to introduce a test shock at any given interval after a normal beat. With a special "balanced" induction coil they were also able to record from electrodes very close to the point of stimulation. Subsequently, they were able to insert a test shock at any desired interval following a normal beat and to follow that by a second shock at a controlled interval. They demonstrated for the first time that a single shock delivered to the body of the atrium soon after the end of the refractory period, while the vagus was stimulated, regularly provoked atrial fibrillation. Subsequently Padget and Andrus demonstrated that the refractory period of an early extrasystole was considerably shorter than that of a normal beat.

In 1940 Dr. Philip Hill and Andrus demonstrated that what was then called "angiotonin," now "angiotensin," provoked constriction of the coronary arteries in the perfused heart and conspicuously increased cardiac output in the heart-lung preparation. This was overlooked until 1960, when it was confirmed by Koch-Weser and others. Today augmented cardiac output is accepted as one of the contributing causes of sustained hypertension.

After a number of years in the heart station, Andrus entered practice in Baltimore, specializing in cardiology.

Heart Surgery—The Blalock-Taussig Operation

There is no more dramatic period in the history of medicine than the astronomical progress in cardiac surgery witnessed over the past twenty-five years. Up until that time surgeons regarded the matter of cardiac operations as did the British physician Stephen Paget, who wrote in 1896: "Surgery of the heart has probably reached the limit set by nature to all surgery. No new method and no new discovery can overcome the natural difficulties that attend a wound of the heart." Yet in a few short years the brilliant work of such pioneers as Alfred Blalock overcame many of these difficulties, and operations on the heart have become almost a matter of routine, with the saving of many hundreds of lives.

The event that triggered the spectacular advances in cardiovascular surgery was the famous blue-baby operation pioneered by Helen B. Taussig and Alfred Blalock of Johns Hopkins. The operation involved the creation of an artificial channel between the arteries of the lung and a branch of the aorta. The abnormality which they attempted to relieve was a curious combination of deformities of the heart known as the "tetralogy of Fallot." This congenitally linked abnormality was first noted by the famous British surgeon-anatomist William Hunter at the end of the eighteenth century, and was later described more completely by the French physician Étienne-Louis-Arthur Fallot. The syndrome consists of: (1) narrowing of the opening from the heart to the pulmonary arteries; and (2) a defect in the wall between the right and left ventricles which permits blood in one chamber to mix with that in the other. The functional result of this combination of defects is impaired circulation to the lungs, with the pumping of mixed venous and arterial blood from the ventricles into the general circulation without its passing through the pulmonary circulation. The clinical manifestations are cyanosis of the skin, due to lack of sufficient oxygenation of the blood; an increase in the number of circulating red blood cells by which means the body attempts to compensate for the lowered oxygen content; clubbing of the fingers; shortness of breath on mild exercise; and a noticeable tendency of the child with this defect to squat suddenly on the haunches after exertion. The solving of this important clinical problem was brought about by the diagnostic insight and skill of the pediatric heart specialist, Helen Taussig, and the surgical skill of Alfred Blalock. Taussig reasoned that the untoward effects of this cardiac anomaly were basically due to its interference with the flow of blood to the lungs. She noted that patients with a patent ductus arteriosis and tetralogy of Fallot did better than those with tetralogy of Fallot alone. The anticipated relief seemed attainable by an arterial anastomosis, which would increase the blood flow to the lungs. Blalock had been interested in the surgery of the blood vessels for many years, and was an expert in the techniques for anastomosing blood vessels. In his animal experimental work he had developed a method by which he could sever the subclavian artery which carries blood to the arm and shoulder and attach the business end of this artery to the side of the pulmonary artery beyond the point of constriction. This maneuver had the effect of shunting the mixed arterial and venous blood that came from the heart back into the lungs, thereby allowing it to accumulate its normal supply of oxygen. This maneuver was made possible since the ancillary or collateral circulation to the arm is sufficient to maintain adequate circulation in the upper limb even when the subclavian artery is cut. After practicing the necessary surgical procedures many times in the experimental animal, Blalock performed the first operation on a patient with tetralogy of Fallot in 1944. The success of this operation is now a matter of recorded surgical history. Hundreds of cases have been relieved of their symptoms with a mortality that was surprisingly low. Many of these cases survived long enough to have their pulmonic stenosis and ventricular septal defect corrected by open heart surgery.

Cardiovascular Physiologist—Richard Bing

The pioneering introduction by Blalock and Taussig of the blue-baby operation was a major turning point in cardiovascular surgery. However, the full potential of this development would not have been possible without the magnificent accomplishments of Richard J. Bing, who came to Johns Hopkins in 1943 to set up a diagnostic and clinical investigative laboratory in the Department of Surgery based on the newly developed technique of cardiac catheterization. Bing received a doctorate degree from the University of Munich as well as from the University of Bern. In 1935 he accepted a fellowship at the Carlsberg Institute in Copenhagen, where he worked with Alexis Carrel and Charles A. Lindbergh in their studies on whole organ perfusion. Later he continued these investigations at the Rockefeller Institute in New York. He joined the faculty of the College of Physicians and Surgeons (Columbia University) in 1939, and soon published his first independent research contribution linking hypertension to a breakdown of amino acids into pressor amines. The validity of his conclusions has not yet been proved, but there has been recent success in treatment based on preventing pressor amine release.

In organizing the cardiovascular research laboratory, Bing recognized the great potential of heart catheterization. He masterfully developed its use as a diagnostic tool in the study of patients with heart disease prior to operation, and also used it effectively as a tool for making quantitative physiological and biochemical measurements in patients with cardiovascular disease. His studies on the pathophysiology of the congenital malformations of the heart were published in a series of classic papers.

He perceived from the beginning that the catheter provided a means of investigating fundamental cardiac mechanisms in man, and he initiated some of the earliest studies of myocardial blood flow and myocardial oxygen consumption in man. He was the first to measure myocardial blood flow using nitrous oxide by a technique which he adapted from that devised by Kety and Schmidt for measuring cerebral blood flow. Dr. Frank Spencer, one of the many fine cardiac surgeons trained by Dr. Alfred Blalock, worked as a fellow for a year with Dr. Bing. In recalling that period recently (1974), Dr. Spencer stated: "I can hardly believe that twenty five years ago I was going over to Halsted 2 to persuade a man admitted to have his hernia fixed that he should also have his myocardial blood flow measured, but that is what we did." Many young men who trained under Bing subsequently established cardiovascular diagnostic laboratories of their own in other schools and hospitals.

In 1951 Bing became professor of clinical physiology at the University of Alabama, where he pursued his pioneering studies of myocardial metabolism. Subsequently he held appointments at Washington University and the Veterans Administration Hospital in St. Louis. In 1959 he went to Wayne State University as professor and chairman of the Department of Medicine. His administrative duties did not interfere with his work in the clinical laboratory, and he soon recognized another invaluable clinical tool—applying the principles of coincidence counting to the study of myocardial blood flow in man. Since 1969 Bing has been professor of medicine at the University of Southern California and director of intramural medicine and experimental cardiology at Huntington Memorial Hospital, where he continues active investigative work. In 1974 he received the Research Achievement Award of the American Heart Association.

Vivian Thomas

Vivian Thomas, who was Dr. Blalock's surgical technician and colleague in all of his studies on surgery of the cardiovascular system, wanted to be a physician when he registered to enter the Tennessee A and I, but the financial crash of 1929 obliterated those hopes. Instead he answered an advertisement for a laboratory helper at the Vanderbilt University School of Medicine, thereby solidifying his career pattern, as this was the start of his fruitful career with Dr. Alfred Blalock. Blalock soon recognized Thomas's unusual skills and taught him to carry out complex vascular and thoracic operations on his laboratory animals. Thomas soon became an outstanding surgical technical assistant and research associate. He contributed ideas to the work and kept beautifully detailed records.

When Dr. Blalock came to Johns Hopkins as chairman of the Department of Surgery in 1941, Thomas came with him and was placed in charge of the Hunterian laboratory. Here he played a vital role in training many of the young surgeons in the intricacies of experimental vascular surgery. During the first blue-baby operation on November 29, 1944, Thomas stood behind Blalock to offer helpful suggestions and advice. Fortunately, there is a record of Blalock's own evaluation of Vivian Thomas's role. In his NIH lecture at the dedication of the new wing of the clinical Center on September 3, 1963, Blalock indicated that he would place two nonphysicians on his list of major contributors to the field of cardiovascular surgery. One was Leon Schlossberg, a student of Max Broedel's who contributed so importantly with his outstanding illustrations; and the other was Vivian Thomas. Alex Haller, in a very delightful essay presented at the Halsted Society in 1974, told the following anecdote: While working with Glenn Morrow in the National Heart Institute in 1954, Haller was associated in the laboratory with another skillful technician, Alfred Casper, who had spent some time working with Vivian in Baltimore. While Haller was working on a dog, he got into troublesome bleeding from the pulmonary artery. He finally extricated himself successfully, and Casper expressed admiration at the way Haller had handled the situation. Feeling quite proud, Haller said, "Well, I was trained by Dr. Blalock." At that point he had completed only his surgical internship. A few weeks later they were again operating, and Haller got into even worse trouble. He literally did not know what to do. Fortunately Casper took over, placing clamps in appropriate positions, and the difficulty was successfully dealt with. Haller turned to Casper with great admiration at the end of the experiment: "I certainly appreciated the way you solved that problem. You used your hands beautifully." Casper looked him in the eye and with a little twinkle said: "I trained with Vivian." In 1969 a portrait of Vivian was presented to the Johns Hopkins Medical Institutions; a true token of his immeasurable contributions to the Hopkins Institution, to the Department of Surgery, and to mankind.

Cardiopulmonary Resuscitation

In 1973 William B. Kouwenhoven received the Albert and Mary Lasker Foundation Award for three important contributions to the care of patients with heart disease: (1) He and his colleagues confirmed the basic fact that an electric shock could reverse ventricular fibrillation of the heart; (2) they developed the devices for both open and closed chest defibrillation; and (3) they devised the technique of external cardiac massage. Dr. Kouwenhoven was an electrical engineer by training. He was professor of electrical engineering at Johns Hopkins from 1930 to 1938, and dean of the School of Engineering from 1938 to 1954. He became professor emeritus of electrical engineering in 1954, and in 1956 was appointed lecturer in surgery. In 1969 he received an honorary degree of Doctor of Medicine from Johns Hopkins, the first ever awarded by the university. Kouwenhoven's research illustrates the rewards of interdisciplinary cooperative research, and in addition portrays a dedicated, creative scientist who continued to make important contributions long after he had attained emeritus status.

In the 1920s the electric utility companies, concerned about the rising number of linemen killed by electric shock, began to support research on this problem. In 1926 Dr. L. W. Lieb, vice-president of Consolidated Edison of New York City, appealed to the Rockefeller Institute for help in reducing the high rate of electric fatalities. As a result of this appeal, five investigations were started, one of which was conducted by Professor William H. Howell of the School of Hygiene and Public Health at Johns Hopkins. Work on this project began under the supervision of William B. Kouwenhoven and Orthello R. Langworthy, who carried on extensive research on the damage caused by electric shock. Using rats as experimental animals, they studied the effects of DC and AC shock of high and low voltages as well as lightning discharges. Analysis of the problem in humans revealed that ventricular fibrillation occurred mainly from lower voltage shocks, while paralysis of respiration resulted from higher voltage. Donald Hooker, who was then associate professor of physiology at the Johns Hopkins School of Hygiene and Public Health, was successful in defibrillating a dog's heart but was unable to start it beating again. In 1930 Dr. Howell called attention to the work of Prevost and Batelly (1889), in which ventricular fibrillation was arrested in the animal heart by means of an electric countershock. He handed his group a reprint of the Prevost and Batelly paper and asked the simple question: "Is this true?" The answer quietly came back to him: "Yes." Soon after that Carl J. Wiggers of Case Western Reserve University in Cleveland attempted open chest defibrillation in the cases of ventricular fibrillation that occur occasionally in patients during a surgical operation. In 1947 Claude Beck, one of the surgeons working with Wiggers, reported the first successful open chest defibrillation in man with the electrodes applied directly to the surface of the heart. It was also found that with the heart exposed one could provide circulation of blood by squeezing the heart manually. Vivian Thomas of the Hopkins surgical laboratory built a number of open chest defibrillators, but obviously this method was not suitable in solving the problem of the electric industry.

World War II interrupted this research work on electric shock. After the war, Hooker had died and Langworthy had become involved with other problems. Kouwenhoven had moved to the Department of Surgery, then under the chairmanship of Dr. Alfred Blalock. In the early postwar period Dr. James Elam and Dr. Peter Safer perfected the mouth-to-mouth method of lung ventilation by expired air. It is an excellent method for oxygenation of the blood, but it does not produce any circulation.

Dr. William Milnor and Dr. Kouwenhoven began work on the development of a closed chest defibrillator in 1950, using at first capacitor discharges with electrodes on opposite sides of the chest. After some trials with this method, they discovered that a brief AC current of 20 amperes would defibrillate the heart successfully. Samuel Talbot, working on heart arrhythmias, asked them to demonstrate this method of defibrillating the canine heart. Under anesthesia ventricular defibrillation was induced, and thereafter normal rhythm was restored by a shock applied through electrodes attached to the sides of the dog's chest. However, since Talbot's experiments required strapping a vest studded with contact electrodes around the chest, no space was available for the defibrillating electrodes. They then found that the procedure was just as effective when one electrode was placed over the suprasternal notch and the other over the apex of the heart. Actually, such placements were superior to those previously employed, since the current then flowed longitudinally through the heart, allowing the intensity of the shock to be reduced by 50 percent. The Hopkins AC defibrillator was tested hundreds of times experimentally before being used on man on March 28, 1957.

Defibrillator tests had shown that there was a rise in blood pressure when a countershock was applied to the heart. It had also been reported that there was a slight rise in blood pressure when the mine safety electrodes were pressed on an animal's chest even before the countershock was applied. G. Guy Knickerbocker, who had joined Kouwenhoven's staff in July 1954, noticed this phenomenon and wondered whether manual compression of the thorax might be effective in producing some circulation of blood. Experiments were begun in which pressure was applied not only to the sternum but also on the sides of the chest. A number of animals suffered broken costal junctions and ribs, but the blood pressure rose to 40 percent of normal. This caused great excitement among the surgeons, particularly Dr. Henry T. Bahnson, who had recently joined the group. Further studies showed that a dog could be maintained viable for a period of ten minutes by the application of rhythmic pressure over the lower third of the sternum with a force of 80 to 100 pounds at the rate of 1 per second. On the night of February 15, 1958, Bahnson had the first opportunity to try this technique in a patient. He successfully resuscitated a two-year-old child whose heart was in ventricular fibrillation and reported to Dr. Kouwenhoven the following morning: "Bill, your theory works." In 1958 Dr. James Jude, a resident surgeon assigned to work with Dr. Kouwenhoven, applied external cardiac massage successfully to an obese woman in her forties who had developed ventricular fibrillation while undergoing anesthesia.

The Mine Safety Appliance Company's portable defibrillator was also developed during this program. In this device the electrodes which are placed on the skin of the chest to send the current through the heart are not connected to the charged condensers unless both are pressed on the chest with a force of at least 12 pounds. Thus accidental condenser discharges are avoided. This defibrillator has saved many lives and is part of the equipment of all modern hospitals. Now mouth-to-mouth artificial respiration provides oxygenated blood, and when it is accompanied by rhythmical pressure on the lower sternum there is sufficient pressure on the heart to circulate enough oxygenated blood to maintain life for an hour or more without resorting to thoracotomy.

21 ❧ Hematological Firsts at Hopkins

THE EVENTS DEPICTED in this essay illustrate an important principle: In the study of human disease seemingly minor details are often of vital importance. In the early days of the Johns Hopkins Hospital the clinicians who taught and directed the clinical services were meticulous in their attention to the intricacies of the history and physical examination. The examples described here show that such discipline in the observation and recording of facts can bear fruit in the laboratory as well. The individual who makes the first observation may not appreciate its full significance. Nevertheless, if the observation is accurate, if it is carefully documented and faithfully recorded, its significance will ultimately be recognized. Such observations are the keys which unlock the doors of knowledge. These keys are readily available to anyone of us who has the keenness to identify them and the initiative and curiosity to pursue them. Hopefully this essay will remind young men and women seeking perfection in the art and science of medicine today that success in medical research does not necessarily depend on the availability of complex equipment.

Several significant contributions to hematology were made by members of the original faculty of the Johns Hopkins School of Medicine before their arrival in Baltimore. Most notable were those by William Osler, William H. Welch, and William H. Howell.

William Osler and Blood Platelets

William Osler carried out important studies on the elements present in the circulating blood. These studies on the form and movement of the blood platelets were done with Edward Schafer in the physiological laboratory at University College in London, under Professor J. Burdon Sanderson. His observations were first presented in a communication by Professor Sanderson to the Royal Society of London on May 6, 1874, entitled "An Account of Certain Organisms Occurring in the Liquor Sanguinis" and were later published in the *Monthly Microscopic Journal* with one plate of nine figures. A considerable part of the communication described the changes in form which the "corpuscles" undergo when kept for some hours at the temperature of the body and examined in blood serum; but the "corpuscles" were described with figures and a true explanation given of the structure and formation of Schultze's granule masses.

Osler's observations were described in more detail in an article entitled "The Third Corpuscle of the Blood," which appeared in 1883:

In addition to the red and white corpuscles there are in the blood granular bodies of various size, from that of a red corpuscle to masses ten to twenty times as large. They were first described by Max Schultze and they may be called very appropriately, as I have been in the habit of doing for years, "Schultze's granule masses." In healthy adults they are not abundant as a rule, though exceptionally in persons in apparently good condition they abound.... The common opinion regarding them has been that they represent degenerated white blood corpuscles or a granular detritus resulting from their decay. I first showed that they were composed of distinct corpuscles, and that the masses did not preexist in the blood, but were formed at the moment of withdrawal by the aggregation of the corpuscles. At the edges of large groups, the disc-like corpuscles can be distinctly seen, and in the sulphate of soda solution such as used for mixing the blood in haemocytometer work, the corpuscular nature of the masses is quite clear. But what led me to this point was the fact of the impossibility of supposing that masses of the size of some of these could pass through the capillary—In the blood of the newborn rat they are most abundant, and the subcutaneous tissue was employed to investigate the condition of the masses within the vessels. It was then found that they do not preexist as aggregations in the blood, but are in the form of isolated corpuscles floating free with the other forms.

In a small artery or vein, there will be seen with the red and white cells small, pale corpuscles about $\frac{1}{4}$ the size of the red ones often in extraordinary numbers. A drop of blood from the tail of the same animal will show numerous granule masses, at the edges of which the corpuscles can be seen.—The corpuscles are discoid, pale, structureless and undergo peculiar alterations in shape elongating or presenting two or three fine hairlike extensions. They measure from $\frac{1}{8,000}$ to $\frac{1}{2,000}$ of an inch.

In this paper Osler also pointed out that until the previous year little or nothing new concerning these bodies had appeared. In that year Bizzozero of Turin published a paper in *Virchow's Archiv* which described these corpuscles again and advanced important views concerning their connection with the process of thrombosis and coagulation. Bizzozero's account of these corpuscles, which he called *blut plättchen* (blood plates), differed in no essential way from what Osler had already pointed out, and the figure of them in a small blood vessel is similar to that previously presented by Osler. However, the observation upon the connection of the corpuscles with thrombus formation was novel and important. Osler commented that the origin of these corpuscles remained a problem, but in his concluding remarks made the following statement:

First, there is in mammalian blood a third corpuscular element $\frac{1}{8}$ to $\frac{1}{2}$ the size of the red corpuscle. It can be clearly seen in the blood vessels of the living animal or in the vessels of freshly removed bits of tissue. It may be called appropriately the third corpuscle or "blood-plate" though the latter expression is not a very satisfactory one. Second, in blood withdrawn from the vessels these corpuscles aggregate together and form the well-known granule masses in which the corpuscles rapidly degenerate and lose their outlines. These masses, first described by Max Schultze should be known by his name. Third, there is evidence to show that the third corpuscle plays an important role in coagulation.

Although Osler wrote on many other aspects of hematology, including pernicious anemia with a description of the atrophy of the stomach, splenic anemia, and Laveran's organisms and their value in the diagnosis of malaria, his description of the blood platelets was undoubtedly his most important scientific contribution.

William H. Welch and Samuel J. Meltzer

During his six years in New York at Bellevue Hospital, Welch carried out only one experimental study in his pathological laboratory. From this single study, however, came a significant contribution to hematology.

The study was carried out with Samuel J. Meltzer, later a founder and the first president of the American Society for Clinical Investigation, who had asked Welch's permission to use his laboratory facilities. Meltzer had made several notable research contributions before emigrating to the United States from Germany, and after establishing himself in practice in New York, he became one of the original part-time members of the Rockefeller Institute and later a full-time member of that institute.

Meltzer suggested to Welch that they determine the effect on red corpuscles of shaking them with various substances presumed to be chemically inactive. For this work they needed some means of agitating the blood, and because of limited financial support, they borrowed a mechanical device for shaking bottles from Carl H. Schultz, a manufacturer of mineral waters. This machine, which could be kept in motion continually, was designed to allow several bottles, fastened parallel to one another, to be shaken to and fro longitudinally. There were 180 excursions per minute and the length of each excursion was 39 centimeters, resulting in a velocity of 1.17 meters per second. By shaking different bottles simultaneously under identical conditions, it was possible to investigate the action of different substances as well as the action of the same substance with various particle sizes.

With the naked eye they could see clearly the gradual change in the color of the blood, which became darker and darker, until at the end of seven hours it was absolutely black. Microscopically, no distinct change could be seen until the third hour. From that time on, there was progressive disappearance of the red blood corpuscles, the largest number of corpuscles disappearing rather suddenly between the fifth and sixth hours. Those which remained seemed to become paler, while the intervening fluid became less transparent. In the researchers' minds there was no doubt that the cause of this disappearance was mechanical. Although they searched diligently for red blood cell fragments and for shadows of the blood corpuscles, they did not discover either. They concluded that the destruction of the red blood corpuscles under the circumstances of their experiments was molecular and "tolerably" sudden. They observed that a certain "commotion of the hemoglobin" in the blood corpuscles appeared to precede their complete destruction, and that before their disappearance the red blood corpuscles lost some of their coloring matter: "It is perhaps only this loosening of the combination between hemoglobin and the stroma and not the expulsion of hemoglobin which is accomplished by the shaking. The complete separation of the hemoglobin from the corpuscle and its solution in the surrounding fluid occurs afterwards."

Almost three-quarters of a century later, exact measurement of the shearing stresses which rupture erythrocytes exposed to turbulent flow was made by Reuben Andres, Kenneth Zierler, and their associates. They found that mechanical destruction of erythrocytes was related to the kinetic energy per unit of time of the injection. By jet injection of a solution of sodium chloride *in vitro* into a pool of citrated human blood it was determined that hemolysis became detectable when the kinetic energy per second of injection reached 10,000 to 20,000 $g/cm^2/sec^{-3}$. It was still later before it was fully appreciated clinically that the shearing stress upon the red cells, stretching them within the circulation, causes them to lose membrane and eventually to be destroyed permanently.

A number of patients who have had Teflon prostheses or patches within their heart have developed mild to moderate hemolytic anemia. The peripheral blood characteristically shows spherocytes, burr cells, and schizocytes. The assumption is that increased turbulence of flow in the vicinity of the repair damages the red blood cells. This assumption is strengthened by the observation that patients who have undergone placement of aortic valve protheses are the group most likely to develop hemolysis. It has also been postulated that the anemia associated with a number of different disease states is produced by fragmentation of red cells within the circulation. Presumably the cells are damaged as they squeeze through small blood vessels occluded by fibrin or platelet plugs. The peculiarly shaped cells and cell fragments, as described above, are seen in the peripheral blood of such patients, and there may be marked hemosiderinurea. This has been labeled "microangiopathic hemolytic anemia," and may accompany malignant hypertension, eclampsia, the hemolytic-uremic syndrome in children, and rejection of renal homographs.

The first suggestion that mechanical deformation of red corpuscles by vascular lesions may result in anemia was made by Willys Monroe while he was working at the Marine Hospital in Baltimore. During this period he spent some time working in Dr. C. Lockard Conley's hematology division at Johns Hopkins. The suggestion was presented in a paper entitled "Intravascular Hemolysis—A Morphologic Study of Schizocytes in Thrombotic Purpura and Other Diseases," by Monroe and A. F. Strauss. In two cases of thrombotic thrombocytopenic purpura, they found appreciable numbers of erythrocyte fragments, which varied from barely visible granules taking a positive stain for hemoglobin to cells about half the diameter of a red cell. They postulated that these tiny cell fragments must have arisen by fragmentation of larger cells without loss of pigment. These small cells were first described by Ehrlich, who named them "schizocytes," or "split-cells." But their presence in tissue sections had been unrecorded until Monroe's observations. Monroe and Strauss noted that these schizocytes appeared most often at the site of vascular change, the highest output being from the coronary venous sinus. These studies led them to conclude that the study of erythrocyte fragmentation offered an important approach to the better understanding of many anemias. They pointed out Melt-zer's suggestion that erythrocytes were thrashed to pieces in whirls and rushes on the edges and corners of the circulation as the normal process of blood destruction. Ross, Robertson, and others showed by differential centrifugation that the only known normally occurring process of red cell destruction is fragmentation—a process which is accelerated in plethora and anemia.

Howell-Jolly Bodies

While at the University of Michigan, William Henry Howell published a comprehensive paper entitled "The Life-History of the Formed Elements of the Blood, Especially the Red Corpuscles." The major contribution in this paper was proof that the mature nucleated red corpuscles lose their nuclei by extru-sion, and not by absorption, in changing to the ordinary red corpuscle of the circulation. He observed the act of extrusion in part in living cells.

Howell also noted that severe and sudden bleeding (in cats) is followed by the appearance in the circulation of red corpuscles containing a large frag-ment of nuclear material. This fragment persists until the corpuscle disappears. He concluded that the greatly accelerated production of new corpuscles caused a too rapid extrusion of the nuclei, so that a portion remained entrapped in the corpuscle. This event was also described by Jolly, and hence these bodies have been designated as Howell-Jolly bodies.

Howell-Jolly bodies have been observed after splenectomy, in cases of splenic atrophy or congenital absence of the spleen, in hemolytic anemia, in pernicious anemia and sprue, and in thalassemia and leukemia. It is likely that they are produced by abnormal mitosis when single chromosomes become detached and fail to take part in the formation of the interphase nucleus.

Thayer Introduces Ehrlich's
Color Analysis at Johns Hopkins

Paul Ehrlich's researches in color analysis of the blood cells kindled a new interest in the study of leukemia. Among the first cases of leukemia studied in the United States with Ehrlich's new techniques were two at the Johns Hopkins Hospital in 1891. Both were described by Dr. Henry Toulmin at a meeting of the Johns Hopkins Medical Society on March 2, 1891, although the first case had previously been reported in the *Johns Hopkins Hospital Bulletin* in Janu-ary of that year.

The second patient was Mrs. Annie H., a black, thirty-one-year-old wash-erwoman who applied at the Dispensary on February 25, 1891, and was sent to the gynecological department for suspected "womb trouble." On transfer to the medical side, it was noted that over a period of two months she had lost fifty pounds in weight, had become pale in color, and had noted swelling of the abdomen. On examination there was marked enlargement of the spleen, and the mucous membranes were pale. The diagnosis of "splenic myelogenous leukemia" was made, and treatment with Fowler's solution was begun.

The follow-up to the first case was the report of a young boy who had entered the hospital with enlargement of the spleen. He, too, had "splenic myelogenous leukemia," and was treated with Fowler's solution and then sent home. On re-examination it was noted that his blood picture showed marked improvement.

The major discussant of this latter case was Dr. William S. Thayer. Thayer noted that beginning on November 2 he had had a chance to examine the blood with the new techniques developed by Ehrlich and had made careful counts of the blood corpuscles and estimated the percentage of hemoglobin as well. The patient had marked anemia, with a blood count of 3,430,000, on November 2, at which time the proportion of white to red blood cells was 1.0 to 18.8 and the hemoglobin was 51 percent. From this time on the patient had had no treatment, and when he was re-examined on January 29, the red corpuscles were 2,171,000 and the white corpuscles 714,000—a proportion of white to red of 1 to 3. The hemoglobin was 41 percent. On February 14, after the patient was again taking arsenic (Fowler's solution) in increasing doses, the white count had dropped to 33,000. On February 25 the white count was 9500. Thus, in less than three weeks after return to treatment, the excess in leukocytes had entirely disappeared.

Thayer then gave a résumé of the studies of Paul Ehrlich, first announced in 1877. In that year, while a medical student, Ehrlich described his careful researches made in the "color-analysis," as he called it, of the elements of the blood. He made use of dried cover-glass specimens, which were carefully prepared so as to have as thin a film of blood as possible and were "fixed" by heat. By studying the effect of various coloring matters, Ehrlich discovered that the protoplasm of certain leukocytes contained granules which had affinities for distinct classes of coloring matter, and that by using these coloring matters, cells which might otherwise be indistinguishable from one another could be differentiated. By these means, Ehrlich noted seven varieties of granulations in the blood of various animals. Of these, only three came into consideration in the study of human blood: (1) granules which had an affinity for eosin, (2) cells with basophilic granulation, and (3) the most common granulation in the blood, which was one stained by neither acid nor basic coloring matter alone but which takes on a stain when a fluid is used containing both. This is the so-called neutrophilic granulation, and occurs in the majority of leukocytes.

Thayer pointed out that in the splenic-myelogenous form of leukemia, one sees the greatest increase in white corpuscles under any conditions. The most characteristic feature of the blood is the appearance of a form of cell which is not normally seen. This cell is as large or larger than the large mononuclear variety in normal blood and morphologically similar to it, except that the protoplasm is filled with fine neutrophilic granules. These cells, called "myelocytes" by Ehrlich, appear to arise in the marrow. Other characteristic features in the blood are: (1) the enormous increase in colorless elements, (2) the increased number of eosinophiles, and (3) the presence of nucleated blood corpuscles.

In the case of leukemia under discussion, Thayer noted, the blood was typical of splenic myelogenous leukemia. Specimens were examined with different staining solutions: methylene blue; methylene green; dahlia; eosin and methylene blue; eosin, migrosin, and aurantin; and Ehrlich's triple stain of methylene green, acid fuchsin, and orange G. The myelocyte counts in this patient were as follows: on November 9—14.7 percent; on January 29—23.5 percent; on February 7—8.6 percent; on February 14—8.5 percent; on February 21—4 percent. The case under discussion was remarkable in many respects, and Thayer was not aware of any other case of undoubted leukemia where the excess in white corpuscles had fallen in so striking and critical a manner:

Just such a case as this demonstrates the value of these methods of study which we owe to Ehrlich. Though the physical examination of the patient at the present time might suggest most strongly a leukemia, the mere numerical estimate or, indeed, the examination of the fresh blood, might give us no hint that such a process had ever existed. The presence, however, of an appreciable percentage of typical myelocytes as revealed by these methods of contrast staining might put us upon the proper clue and lead us to anticipate or recognize the possibility of a future return of the leukemia.

Dr. Thayer had learned the techniques of study of the blood demonstrated by Ehrlich while studying in Europe for a year. When he returned to Baltimore, he stimulated much interest in these new techniques among the students and house officers. A number of new observations resulted, including that of the eosinophilia of trichinosis by Dr. Thomas R. Brown when he was a medical student.

It is of interest that Paul Ehrlich (1854–1915) was an indifferent student of medicine, occupying his time mainly with his experiments on dyestuffs and tissue staining. The results of his labors soon appeared in his improved methods of drying and fixing blood smears by heat; his triacid stain; his discovery of the mast cells and his detection of their granulations by basic aniline staining (1877); his division of the white blood corpuscles into neutrophilic, basophilic, and oxyphilic; his fuchsin stain for tubercle bacilli, based upon the discovery that they are acid-fast (1882); his sulphodiazobenzol test for bilirubin (1883); and his method of intravital staining (1886). He was a great pioneer in merging descriptive cellular pathology with experimental intracellular chemistry.

Auer Bodies

On April 25, 1903, a twenty-one-year-old youth was admitted to Dr. Osler's wards in the Johns Hopkins Hospital complaining of sore throat and nosebleed. On examination, both tonsils were seen to be markedly enlarged, almost meeting in the midline. The left showed an area of ulceration. The neck was swollen, due chiefly to enlarged glands. There were abundant purpuric lesions, and a general glandular enlargement was noted. Splenomegaly was also present. The patient was anemic, and on examination of the blood, the characteristic picture of what was thought to be lymphocytic leukemia was noted. (There is every reason to believe that the patient actually had myeloblastic leukemia.)

The patient was assigned to Dr. John Auer, a graduate of the Johns Hopkins School of Medicine and a house officer on Dr. Osler's service. Auer perceptively recognized structures which had not been previously described in this much-studied disease. In his own words:

In the cytoplasm of many of the large lymphocytes moderate numbers of indefinite granules were seen, so that these cells looked somewhat like myelocytes. In a few of the large lymphocytes the cytoplasm showed large refractile, rounded bodies; in others a refractile, rodlike body was present. In the nuclei of practically all the large lymphocytes a number of contractile, pulsating, clear areas were noticeable; in one instance pulsating structures were seen in the cytoplasm. These findings sum up the points to which I wish to call attention.

Auer's paper, which appeared in the *American Journal of Medical Sciences* in 1906, contained a number of freehand drawings of these peculiar intracellular structures.

From the available data Auer could not definitely state the significance of these bodies. However, he suggested the following possibilities regarding their nature: (1) artifacts, (2) cell constituents (large lymphocytes), or (3) parasites or fragments of parasites. It is interesting that Dr. McCrae considered the rods described in Auer's papers as identical with those noted by Dorothy Reed in a case of acute leukemia. Auer, however, believed that the structures described by Dorothy Reed differed in shape, size, and location from his "rods." Auer noted that the only parasite which so far had been found in human beings and which resembled his structures was the Leishmann-Donovan body (L-D). He believed that his leukemic granules closely resembled the form of the L-D body described and illustrated by Marchand and Ledingham, although he noted that nothing resembling a capsule was ever found enclosing his granules.

Auer bodies are rod-shaped peroxidase-positive structures in the cytoplasm which may be present in myeloblasts, myelocytes, or monocytes. They have been observed in as many as 25 percent of the cells in cases of leukemia. The nature and the significance of the Auer bodies have long been the subjects of investigation. From histochemical and electron micrograph studies, it seems reasonable to conclude that they are formed from azurophilic granules. Since the enzymatic content and structure of azurophilic granules conforms to that of lysosomes, the Auer body presumably represents an unusual form or abnormal development of lysosomes. It has been implied that they are present exclusively in myelogenous and in monocytic leukemia, but it remains to be proved that their formation is a phenomenon limited to leukemia. Although they are readily visible in Wright's stained preparations, a modification of the peroxidase stain facilitates their identification.

John Auer was born in Rochester, New York, on March 30, 1875. After receiving his M.S. degree at Michigan University in 1896, he entered the Johns Hopkins School of Medicine, graduating in 1902. After serving as a medical intern in Baltimore, he was a fellow and assistant at the Rockefeller Institute from 1903 to 1904. Then, after a year as instructor in physiology at Harvard, he returned to the Rockefeller Institute, where he held associate membership from 1908 to 1921. At that time he joined the faculty of St. Louis University as professor and director of the Department of Pharmacology, a position he held until his death. During World War II, he was a major in the Medical Reserve Corps, serving from 1917 to 1922. For five years he was secretary of the American Society of Pharmacology and Experimental Therapeutics, and was its president from 1924 to 1927.

During Auer's active research career at the Rockefeller Institute, his work was principally in the laboratory of Dr. Samuel J. Meltzer, whose daughter Clara he married in 1903. He was among the first to work on the phenomenon of anaphylaxis, publishing, with P. A. Lewis, a very important paper on the cause of acute anaphylactic death in guinea pigs in 1909. He also studied the motor phenomena of the gastrointestinal tract and conducted studies on sympathomimetic drugs, particularly epinephrine. One of his most important contributions was with Meltzer on the anesthetic properties of magnesium salts. They demonstrated that, in animals, this was a satisfactory way to control the increased muscular tone in tetanus. During his service in the Army Medical Corps during World War I, Auer treated a case of tetanus with intravenous injections of magnesium sulfate. Another outstanding contribution was his work with Meltzer on respiration by continuous intrapulmonary pressure without the aid of muscular action. This new method of applying anesthetics without movement of the chest wall was essential to the development of thoracic surgery.

While in St. Louis his major interest was teaching, and his well-known system of graphing and evaluating the composite result of a class experiment in pharmacology was greatly valued as a teaching method. During his period of internship at Johns Hopkins, he developed a deep appreciation of the human values in medicine, and these fundamental humanitarian beliefs he transferred effectively to his students in medicine and pharmacology throughout his career. He died in 1948.

William Lorenzo Moss

William Lorenzo Moss was born in Athens, Georgia, in 1876 and received the B.S. degree from the University of Georgia in 1901. He graduated from the Johns Hopkins School of Medicine in 1905 and the following year was a house officer at the Johns Hopkins Hospital. In 1907 he did postgraduate work at the University of Berlin, and from 1908 to 1910 he was instructor in medicine at Johns Hopkins and was placed in charge of the laboratory of the Phipps Tuberculosis Dispensary. From 1910 to 1914 he was an associate in medicine. He then left Johns Hopkins and held a variety of positions, first at the Institute for the Study of Malignant Diseases at Buffalo, New York, and later in preventive medicine and hygiene at Yale and at Harvard, being appointed assistant professor of bacteriology and immunology at Harvard from 1924 to 1929. From 1931 to 1934 he was professor of preventive medicine and dean of the University of Georgia School of Medicine.

Moss was well known for his interest in diseases of the blood and in tropical medicine. He was in charge of the Harvard Expedition to Peru in 1916 and was a member of the Scientific Expedition for the Study of Tropical Medicine in Central America in 1914. From 1928 to 1929 he was a member of the Crane–Field Museum Expedition to the Pacific, and he later participated in the Crane–Peabody Museum Expedition to New Guinea. He served overseas with the medical corps of the AEF during World War I, holding the rank of colonel.

It was during his period at Johns Hopkins (1909) that Moss made his observations on the iso-agglutinins and iso-hemolysins found in normal human blood which have such an important bearing on the occurrence of transfusion reactions. Before Moss's studies, numerous attempts had been made to establish some relation between the occurrence of iso-agglutinins and iso-hemolysins and various diseases, but the claims of various investigators who maintained that such relationships exist was not borne out by the accumulated evidence. Moss thought it likely that results of many observers were misleading because they were based upon the action of the sera investigated upon corpuscles from too small a number of individuals. It had been definitely established that a given serum may agglutinate or hemolyze the corpuscles of certain individuals but not of others, so that the results obtained in any series of cases would depend largely upon the corpuscles employed in the test. For this reason, in all of his studies the serum of each member of a series was tested against the corpuscles of every other member of the series, and the occurrence or absence of agglutination and hemolysis was noted.

In 1901 Landsteiner denied the specificity of the iso-agglutination reaction for diseases and pointed out that the phenomenon is also produced by the serum of healthy individuals. He attempted a classification of sera according to their iso-agglutinating action. His classification, which was generally accepted, was made up of three groups as follows: "In a number of cases (group A) the serum agglutinates the corpuscles of another group (B), not, however, those of group A; while the corpuscles A are agglutinated by the serum B. In the third group (C) the serum agglutinates the corpuscles of A and B." That this classification was imperfect was shown by Moss when he attempted to apply it to any series of twenty individuals in which he tested each serum against the corpuscles of every member of the series. Moss found that a classification that would cover all cases required a separation into four groups:

Group I: sera agglutinate no corpuscles. Corpuscles agglutinated by sera of groups 2, 3, and 4. Group II: sera agglutinate corpuscles of groups 1 and 3. Corpuscles agglutinated by sera of groups 3 and 4. Group III: sera agglutinate corpuscles of groups 1 and 2. Corpuscles agglutinated by sera of groups 2 and 4. Group IV: sera agglutinate corpuscles of groups 1, 2, and 3. Corpuscles agglutinated by no serum.

He found that the serum of members of any one group would not agglutinate or hemolyze the corpuscles of other members of the same group, but will agglutinate and may hemolyze the corpuscles of members of any other group

except those of Group IV. He indicated that this would have a practical application in the transfusion of blood from one individual to another. Moss's work
was carried out without his being aware that a similar classification had been
made a few years earlier by a Hungarian worker whose results had been published in a Hungarian journal not accessible to Moss. When this communication was called to his attention, Moss at once acknowledged its priority.

In 1914 Moss described a simple method for the indirect transfusion of
blood. The method consisted of two parts: (1) obtaining blood from the
donor, by means of an aspirating apparatus, and its defibrination by being
shaken in flasks with glass beads; (2) the introduction, intravenously, of the
defibrinated blood into the patient. He pointed out that he had used this
method for the past three years in about seventy-five cases and that it had
several obvious advantages over the direct method. It was much simpler in
execution and certain in operation. The amount of blood transfused was under
absolute control and could be measured exactly. He pointed out, however, that
one is using defibrinated instead of whole blood, which differs from the latter in
that it contains a large quantity of prefibrin ferment and has been deprived of
its fibrinogen. No instances of blood destruction in the recipient was observed
where homologous blood was used; that is, where the donor and donee belonged to the same group, as determined by the iso-agglutination reaction.

Moss's last contribution to the selection of donors for transfusion appears
to have been in 1917, when he published in the *Journal of the American
Medical Association* a simplified method for determining the iso-agglutinin
group in the selection of donors for blood transfusion. He points out that
during the past several years the procedure of blood transfusion by the indirect
method had become more popular because of the introduction of satisfactory
methods, but that there were still a sufficient number of "accidents" on record
to remind physicians that there was a real element of danger. While the technique of selecting donors of the same blood group was not difficult, it required
practice and was somewhat time consuming. Moss described in this paper a
simplified technique for the matching of blood for transfusion.

Cold Auto-agglutinin:
Its Discovery at Johns Hopkins

On the 19th of October, 1917, a young intern on the medical service at
the Johns Hopkins Hospital was examining the blood of a thirty-two-year-old
female just admitted with "bronchopneumonia." When the blood was drawn
into the diluting pipette, the red blood cells became agglutinated, clumps being
visible macroscopically as well as microscopically. The agglutinated cells could
not be broken up upon shaking, and an accurate count of them was impossible.

The intern, Ina M. Richter, was puzzled by this curious phenomenon, so
she sought help from a young instructor in clinical microscopy—Mildred Clark
Clough. Dr. Clough made a study of this unique phenomenon and characterized it with great thoroughness. The agglutination occurred only at tempera-

tures below 22 degrees C. and broke up if the preparation was heated to body temperature (Fig. 1). However, the agglutination returned again upon chilling the same preparation. The patient's serum produced similar agglutination of red blood cells from other individuals of the same blood group. However, when the patient's cells were washed free from serum, they behaved precisely the same as cells from other individuals and showed no tendency to agglutination, indicating that the phenomenon resided in the serum and was not a property of the cells. The active substance resembled ordinary agglutinin in many respects. It was active in high dilution (up to 1 in 500); it resisted heating to 60 degrees C. for half an hour but was destroyed at 65 degrees C.; it remained active when preserved in the icebox for several months; it was precipitated with the euglobulin fraction upon the addition of saturated ammonium sulfate solution. Further study showed that this agglutinin was distinct from the ordinary iso-agglutinins in the serum, since either could be removed from the serum, leaving the other intact. It was clear that this auto-agglutinin differed from ordinary agglutinins in several ways: (1) it was active only at low temperature, the agglutination breaking up on warming; (2) it was absorbed from the serum only at low temperature and was liberated from the cells on warming; (3) it was active on red blood cells from different species, including man, rabbit, guinea pig, hen, sheep, cat, and pig. A similar study of rouleaux formation was made in order to differentiate it more clearly from the activity of this auto-agglutinin. Unlike the auto-agglutinin, the rouleaux-forming substance was active only in concentrated serum. Its activity rapidly disappeared upon standing, and fresh cells were necessary for rouleaux formation. Although suggestive observations of a similar phenomenon had been reported, no clear identification of such a cold auto-agglutinin had been made previously.

The next question was whether or not this auto-agglutinin was related to the respiratory infection the patient had upon entry to the hospital. Although the titer of the agglutinin diminished as the patient recovered from the illness, it was still present. In spite of the fact that it became possible, when the patient became afebrile, to do a red count adequately without warming the serum above ordinary room temperature, the authors concluded that this phenomenon was not basically related to the respiratory infection, although it may have been enhanced by its occurrence. What threw them off the track was the discovery that a daughter of the patient showed a similar auto-agglutinin in her blood. It appeared to be somewhat feebler than that present in the mother's serum, but unfortunately the amount of blood they obtained was insufficient for further tests. There was no comment as to whether the daughter might have had a similar infection, which seems likely. Their conclusion, however, was that this peculiar auto-agglutinin was independent of the disease which the patient had, and was apparently hereditary.

The frequent development of cold auto-antibody in high concentration by patients suffering from viral (primary atypical) pneumonia or pneumonia due to mycoplasma was first conclusively demonstrated by Peterson, Ham, and Finland some thirty years later, in 1947.

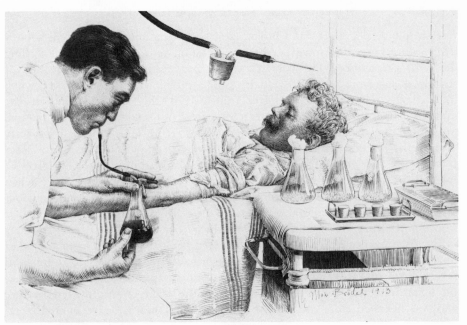

William Lorenzo Moss collecting blood from a donor for a transfusion

In this drawing by Max Broedel, the artist has depicted himself as the donor. The drawing appeared in an article by Moss on the indirect method of blood transfusion (*Am. J. Med. Sci.* 147 [1914]: 698).
Courtesy of Mrs. Ranice Crosby

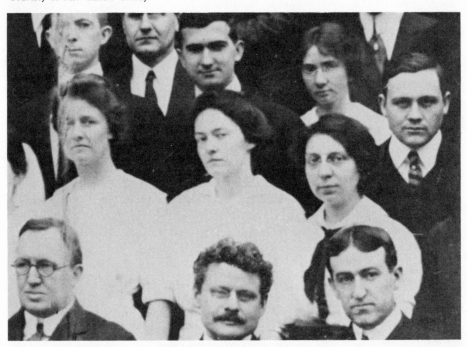

Mildred C. Clough (*center*)

From A. M. Chesney, *The Johns Hopkins Hospital and The Johns Hopkins University School of Medicine,* vol. 2, *1893–1905* (Baltimore: The Johns Hopkins University Press, 1958)

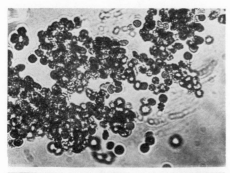
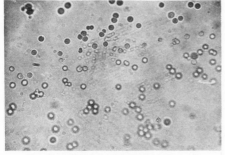

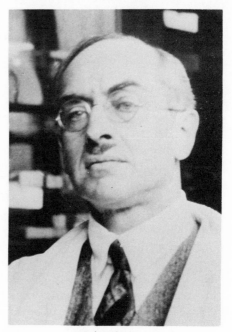

Fig. 1. Demonstration of the cold
auto-agglutinin

John Auer
Courtesy of Dr. Thomas Frawley

Top figure shows the auto-agglutination of the patient's cells by her own serum at room temperature. Bottom figure shows the same preparation after warming. The clumps are nearly, but not entirely, broken up.

From M. C. Clough and I. M. Richter, "A Study of an Auto-agglutinin Occurring in a Human Serum," *Johns Hopkins Hosp. Bull.* 29 (1918): 86, plate 16.

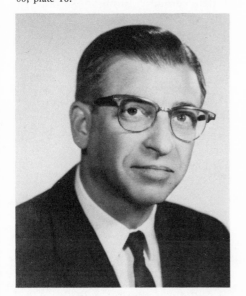

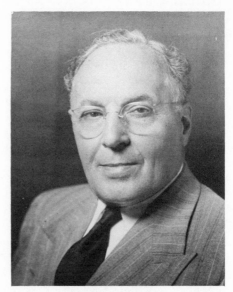

Irving J. Sherman
Courtesy of Dr. Irving J. Sherman

Verne Rheem Mason
Courtesy of Dr. Sherman Mellinkoff

Mildred Clark Clough was born September 14, 1888, in Newtonville, Massachusetts. She attended Wellesley College and received her M.D. degree from Johns Hopkins in 1914. She was an intern in medicine the following year and then served one year as assistant resident physician. After holding a Mary Putnam Jacobi Fellowship for one year, she became an instructor in clinical medicine at Johns Hopkins from 1916 to 1921. She married Paul W. Clough on September 5, 1916. From 1919 to 1922 she taught physiology at the Maryland State Teachers College and was physician in charge of the venereal disease clinic (women) of the Baltimore City Health Department from 1926 to 1932. She died on March 11, 1938.

Ina M. Richter was born on May 2, 1885, in San Francisco, California. She attended Bryn Mawr College and received her M.D. degree from Johns Hopkins Medical School in 1918. The following year she was a house officer in medicine at the Johns Hopkins Hospital. She received further training at the University of California Medical School, where she remained until 1926. She became a pediatrician and held a number of posts in the San Francisco area. She later served as a staff member of several hospitals in Santa Barbara, and was medical director of the La Loma Feliz School.

Sickle Cell Anemia: The First Molecular Disease

Johns Hopkins has been closely tied to the study of sickle cell anemia in general and in particular to the discovery that the disease is due to the genetically determined replacement of a single amino acid in a complex molecule. Sickle cell anemia was first described in 1910 by a Chicago physician, James B. Herrick, who two years later pointed out that coronary thrombosis could be recognized during life and need not end fatally.

The name, sickle cell anemia, was first coined by Dr. Verne R. Mason, while a member of the resident staff in medicine at Johns Hopkins, in an article which appeared in the *Journal of the American Medical Association* on October 14, 1922. His was apparently the fourth case of this disease to be described. In his discussion, Mason pointed out a number of facts which indicated that sickle cell anemia was a hereditary or congenital anomaly—an assumption supported by the history of disability in early life and by the occurrence of the disease only in Negroes.

Verne Rheem Mason, a native Californian, graduated from the Johns Hopkins Medical School in 1915 and remained on the staff of the Johns Hopkins Hospital and School of Medicine for the next six years as intern, resident, and instructor in medicine. In 1921 he returned to Los Angeles County Hospital, where for the next twelve years he had a major role in the instruction of the resident staff. When the University of Southern California School of Medicine opened in 1930, he was named professor of clinical medicine and contributed in many ways to the development of this school. He remained active in teaching and clinical investigation until his retirement in 1956. During World

War I, he served with Base Hospital No. 18, the Johns Hopkins unit in France, and in 1955 he became chairman of the Medical Advisory Board of the Howard Hughes Institute for Medical Research.

In 1923 John Huck, also at Johns Hopkins, presented evidence which strongly indicated that the sickling phenomenon was a property of the red blood cell itself, inherited by the individual according to the Mendelian Law.

Many are aware of Linus Pauling's epoch-making contributions to the study of sickle cell hemoglobin, but few are familiar with the interesting events which led Pauling to begin work in this area. The story began in Baltimore, when a Hopkins undergraduate, Irving J. Sherman, became interested in sickle cell anemia. As part of the work in an advanced genetics course, he undertook a study of the hereditary pattern in sickle cell anemia and sickle cell trait. This involved visiting the homes of families of patients with known sickle cell anemia in order to obtain blood tests on other members of the family. The standard technique for demonstrating the sickle cell at that time was the sealed, cover-slip wet preparation. Although Sherman pursued the study diligently, he was often disappointed by the unreliability of the test and curious as to why this preparation led to the sickling phenomenon.

The following year he entered the Johns Hopkins Medical School, and immediately approached Dr. Maxwell M. Wintrobe for permission to study the sickling phenomenon in his laboratory. His studies eventuated in the publication of a paper entitled "The Sickling Phenomenon, with Special Reference to the Differentiation of Sickle Cell Anemia from the Sickle Cell Trait." Sherman ultimately demonstrated that it was the reduction of oxygen tension which produced the sickling phenomenon, and that the blood of patients with sickle cell anemia would sickle at an oxygen tension considerably higher than that required to produce sickling in individuals with the sickle cell trait. This led to the demonstration that the venous blood of patients with sickle cell anemia contained a high percentage of sickled cell forms, whereas the venous blood of patients with sickle cell trait normally did not.

Many of his studies required periodic observations of the preparations for forty-eight hours, so that the experiments had to be started Friday evening or early Saturday morning, consuming many weekends and causing considerable loss of sleep. This was before the days of grants, and he had no technical personnel assisting him. Sherman does not recall the exact circumstances which led to the use of polarized light in examining the sickle cells, but he was quite excited by the birefringent effect, which he saw only in the sickled blood cell forms. He felt that this indicated a change in the physical state of the hemoglobin. Because this physical change occurred only with reduced oxygen tension and did not occur in normal blood cells, he concluded that the hemoglobin molecule itself was different. He discussed the problem with William Mansfield Clark, professor of physiological chemistry, who suggested that he try to differentiate the two hemoglobins either by crystallization or immunologically by guinea pig inoculation. Sherman extracted hemoglobin from normal individuals and from sickle cell patients, but had difficulty in crystallizing the preparations.

There was no cold room for his studies, and he had to use the roof of the hospital outside of the hematology laboratory during the cold winter weather. Passersby who saw him sitting in hat and coat on the roof of the hospital staring through a microscope from time to time must have thought that strange things were going on at the Hopkins. He also tried to sensitize guinea pigs to normal hemoglobin and to sickle cell hemoglobin in an attempt to differentiate the two.

Sherman was still working on these studies when he finished medical school in July 1940. He was forced to give them up, however, when he entered a surgical internship, for there were no nights or weekends off and essentially no free time during an internship in those days. In his final article he included his observations on the birefringent quality of sickled red blood cells in the hope that someone else would take up the problem and pursue it further.

Sherman had his early neurosurgical training with Dr. Walter Dandy at Johns Hopkins, and in June of 1943 he entered the army as a neurosurgeon. After World War II he completed his training at Montefiore Hospital under Dr. Houston H. Merritt, a Hopkins graduate, and Leo M. Davidoff. Subsequently he entered the practice of neurosurgery in Bridgeport, Connecticut, and has remained there since August 1947. He holds an appointment as clinical associate in neurosurgery at the Yale Medical School.

The second chapter in this fascinating story can be told best in the words of Dr. William B. Castle:

Linus Pauling and I were both members of a committee that eventuated in the publication of the book by Vannevar Bush, *Science, the Endless Frontier.* The committee met, among other places, in Denver, I think, in 1945. On the overnight train between Denver and Chicago, not long after leaving Denver, I had a conversation with Dr. Pauling about the molecular relation of antibody to antigen which was very informative to me. I then sketched a little bit of the work that Dr. Ham and I had been doing since 1940 on sickle cell disease and mentioned that, as stated by Dr. I. J. Sherman in 1940, when the cells were deoxygenated and sickled they showed birefringence in polarized light. This I stated meant to me some type of molecular alignment or orientation and ventured to suggest that it might be the kind of thing in which he would be interested. I am equally clear that I did not make the further generalization that it was orientation of the hemoglobin that might be doing this.

This event demonstrates unequivocally that on occasion, even if very rarely and inadvertently, committee meetings may lead to valuable results. In the following year, in collaboration with Dr. Harvey A. Itano, Dr. Pauling did find that sickle cell hemoglobin was the "kind of thing in which he would be interested," and in 1949 the epoch-making article entitled "Sickle Cell Anemia, A Molecular Disease," by Linus Pauling, Harvey A. Itano, S. J. Singer, and Ibert C. Wells appeared in *Science.* Their conclusions were based on the demonstration of an electrophoretically abnormal hemoglobin in the disorder. In a personal communication, Castle stated that he did not mention to Pauling the far more significant observations of Hahn and Gillespie in 1927, in which they made the following statement: "Sickle cell formation is a reversible phenomenon depending on the free or combined state of the hemoglobin of the susceptible corpuscles.

"The failure of corpuscles which have lost their hemoglobin to undergo sickle cell formation is consistent with our hypothesis relating the distortion to the hemoglobin—It is reasonable to suppose that sickle cells are formed in the body of an affected person wherever the oxygen tension and hydrogen ion concentration are such as to render the distorted form of the corpuscle stable." This is important in that it clearly implicates an abnormal behavior of hemoglobin, although not explicitly an abnormal hemoglobin.

Harvey and Janeway

On March 15, 1937, a thirty-six-year-old black chauffeur was admitted to the Johns Hopkins Hospital with acute follicular tonsillitis. Examination of the blood showed no anemia, the white blood cell count was 19,000 with 82 percent polymorphonuclear leukocytes, 3 percent juvenile cells, 10 percent lymphocytes, and 5 percent monocytes. The red blood cells were normal in size, shape, and hemoglobin content. The throat culture showed a pure growth of beta hemolytic streptococci. The patient was given 4.8 grams of sulfanilamide by mouth, and at the end of four hours the blood concentration was 10 milligrams per 100 milliliters. For the next two days the dose of sulfanilamide was 0.9 grams every four hours, the amount later being lowered to 0.6 grams every four hours. The throat infection cleared rapidly and the temperature and white blood cell count were normal on the third day of his hospital stay. On the fifth day of sulfanilamide medication, after two days without fever, a temperature of 102.6 developed. Believing this was due to the medication, it was promptly discontinued. The following day the patient complained of headache, was drowsy and weak and perspiring continuously. The mucous membranes were pale and icteric. Examination of the blood at that time revealed a red blood cell count of 1.57 million, with only 30 percent hemoglobin. There was a marked leukocytosis with 87,000 white blood cells of which 1 percent were myeloblasts, 20 percent juvenile cells, 53 percent polymorphonuclear leukocytes, 2 percent eosinophiles, 14 percent lymphocytes and 7 percent monocytes. The smear showed numerous nucleated red blood cells, polychromatophilia, and a reticulocyte count of 20 percent. The patient was given three 500-milliliter transfusions of citrated blood during the next forty-eight hours. The evidence of new blood formation as revealed by the reticulocytes and nucleated red blood cells gradually subsided. The striking leukocytosis fell slowly to a normal count, and mature cells soon replaced the young forms.

The following week a similar complication developed in a twenty-six-year-old black female who was being treated for acute tonsillitis with a peritonsillar abscess. The third patient who developed an acute hemolytic anemia while on sulfanilamide was a ten-month-old white female who had meningococcal meningitis.

These cases were reported in 1937 by A. McGehee Harvey and Charles

A. Janeway. The abruptness of onset of the hemolysis, its intensity, and the fact that it did not seem to be correlated with dosage distinguished this complication from the more slowly progressive anemias which had been observed to follow long, continued, and/or heavy dosage with sulfanilamide. In view of the later discovery of the role of glucose-6-phosphate dehydrogenase (G-6-PD) deficiency in this type of anemia, it is of interest that the first two patients reported were blacks. Harvey and Janeway pointed out the similarity between the sulfanilamide anemia and that produced by phenylhydrazine. Since this report, considerable progress has been made in understanding the nature of the hemolytic anemias caused by drugs or chemicals. Broadly speaking, there are two mechanisms: the first is direct interference with the metabolic processes of the erythrocyte by the drug or chemical; the second, which is relatively rare, is an immune one with the formation of antibodies against the drug, the erythrocytes being damaged as a result of drug-antibody interaction. In connection with the first mechanism, inherited erythrocyte G-6-PD deficiency is of paramount importance in explaining the unusual sensitivity of certain individuals to a wide range of drugs in dosages which hardly, if at all, affect normal people.

However, as more is learned, it is clear that the mechanisms are complex. A number of unstable hemoglobins are known to predispose to sulfonamide-induced hemolytic anemia, and two families with this disorder have been described by Dr. William Zinkham and his associates of the Department of Pediatrics at Johns Hopkins. Barton Childs, William Zinkham, and their collaborators also worked out the mode of genetic transmission of glucose-6-phosphate deficiency. They carried out a survey of randomly selected blacks to determine the frequency of primaquine-sensitive persons in this race. The method used was the glutathione sensitivity test. Relatives of reactors were examined by the same test to determine the distribution of sensitive persons within families. Affected relatives appeared in as many as three generations, suggesting genetic determination. They concluded that the most likely hypothesis for the mode of inheritance of a gene controlling this characteristic is that of sex linkage with incomplete dominance. Two Italian families containing individuals who had suffered hemolytic episodes following ingestion of fava beans were also examined by means of the glutathione stability test. The affected individuals were found to be reactors, as were some of their relatives, and the distribution of the characteristics within the families suggested that this syndrome, too, was associated with a sex-linked gene showing incomplete dominance and variable expression.

Later it was demonstrated that acetylphenylhydrazine is extremely toxic to enzyme-deficient cells and is used in the "Heinz-body development test" for primaquine sensitivity of Beutler, Dern, and Alving. It seems probable that the sulfanilamide drugs affect erythrocytes in a manner similar to the 8-aminoquinolines and that, when present, G-6-PD deficiency results in increased sensitivity to hemolysis by these drugs.

Charles Alderson Janeway was born in New York City on May 26, 1909, the son of Theodore C. Janeway, professor of medicine at Columbia and later

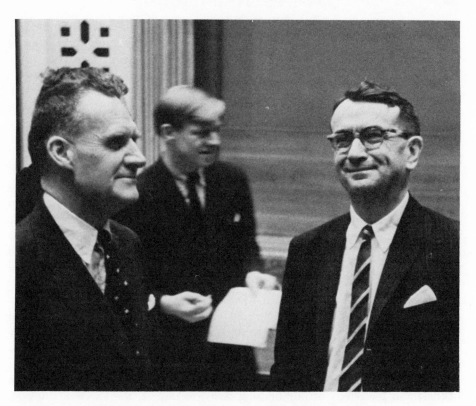

Charles A. Janeway (*left*) and A. McGehee Harvey
From the Archives Office, The Johns Hopkins Medical Institutions

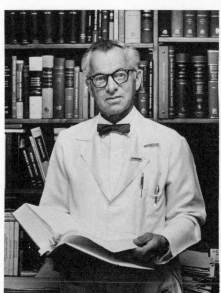

Maxwell M. Wintrobe
Courtesy of Dr. Maxwell M. Wintrobe

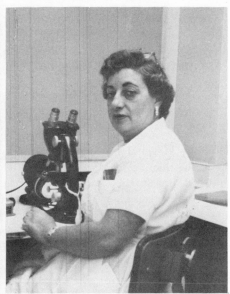

Regina Weistock
Courtesy of Regina Weistock

the first full-time professor of medicine at Johns Hopkins. His grandfather, Edward G. Janeway, was dean of Bellevue Medical College, the predecessor of New York University School of Medicine. After graduation from the Johns Hopkins Medical School in 1934, Janeway spent the next two years at Boston City Hospital, where he worked in the Thorndike Laboratory under an outstanding group including Minot, Castle, Keefer, and Weiss. The following year he returned to Baltimore as an assistant resident in medicine. In September 1939 he moved to the Department of Medicine at Peter Bent Brigham Hospital, which was at that time being reorganized by Soma Weiss. Janeway had charge of the Infectious Disease Division and the bacteriology laboratory. During World War II, Janeway worked with Professor Edwin J. Cohn of the Department of Physical Chemistry at Harvard, when Cohn was engaged in isolating the fractions of human plasma including albumin, gamma globulin, and a series of others. Janeway was given responsibility for the clinical trials of these first two products, albumin and gamma globulin. In late 1941 he was promoted from associate in medicine to assistant professor of pediatrics at Harvard, and moved his activities to the Children's Hospital.

In 1946 he succeeded Richard M. Smith as Thomas Morgan Rotch Professor of Pediatrics. During the ensuing years his conduct of that department was outstanding. His research interests in the years following his departure from Hopkins included the mode of action and clinical uses of the sulfonamides; the clinical effects and dosage of serum albumin and gamma globulin; the physiology of human plasma proteins; the dynamics of experimental serum sickness and the effects of immunosuppressive measures; the effects of measles, albumin and corticosteroids in nephrosis; and the delineation of the immunodeficiency diseases. He is a member of many important societies, including the American Society for Clinical Investigation, of which he was vice-president in 1952; the Association of American Physicians; the Society for Pediatric Research, of which he was president in 1954; and the American Pediatric Society, of which he was president in 1971. He is also a member of the Society of Scholars of the Johns Hopkins University.

Cryoglobulinemia

M.S.R., a fifty-six-year-old white housewife, was admitted to the Johns Hopkins Hospital on December 29, 1931, complaining of severe pain in the right shoulder, coldness of the hands and feet, and shortness of breath. In January 1931 sharp pain commenced in the right side of the neck. In August she began to complain of coldness and blanching of the hands and feet, which appeared suddenly and was aggravated by cold or dampness. In September nosebleeds commenced, recurring at weekly intervals. On examination in November 1931 she was thought to be suffering from Raynaud's disease. Bilateral thrombosis of the central veins of the retina was discovered. Later that month the patient had severe pain upon urination, followed by hematuria thought to be due to a renal stone. She was admitted to the neurosurgical service for cervical sympathectomy. Dr. Walter Dandy asked Dr. Henry M. Thomas, Jr., to see the patient in consultation. Thomas observed that she had hemorrhagic manifestations and asked Dr. Maxwell M. Wintrobe to see her.

After Dr. Wintrobe's clinical examination, he secured a sample of blood and prepared it for a hematocrit. The hematocrit tube was spun, and just as Wintrobe was ready to examine it he was called away from the laboratory. He placed the hematocrit in the refrigerator, which he sometimes did when he could not attend to the blood examination immediately. When he returned a short while later, he noticed that there was a large opaque layer above the packed red cells and the plasma was cloudy. He already knew that the patient had leukopenia and thrombocytopenia, but he was puzzled by the material present above the packed red cells. He stuck the hematocrit in his laboratory coat pocket and walked down to the wards to show it to Dr. Thomas. When he took the hematocrit out of his pocket, the material he had seen just a few minutes before had disappeared.

This led him to suspect that the patient had multiple myeloma, a diagnosis which was subsequently confirmed. Dr. Wintrobe, in collaboration with Dr. Mary E. Buell, made extensive studies of the blood in this unusual case and published a report in the *Bulletin of the Johns Hopkins Hospital* entitled "Hyperproteinemia Associated with Multiple Myeloma, with Report of a Case in which an Extraordinary Hyperproteinemia Was Associated with Thrombosis of the Retinal Veins and Symptoms Suggesting Raynaud's Disease." The summary of their article read as follows:

A patient who presented symptoms of coldness, blanching and a peculiar mottling of the extremities, as well as other signs of disturbed circulation, was found to have had in her blood a voluminous quantity of a substance which invariably was precipitated immediately on withdrawal of blood from the body. This material was found to be protein in nature. Autopsy proved that the patient suffered from multiple myeloma.

The chemical nature of this protein is discussed, and its relation to Bence-Jones protein considered. Among approximately 500 case reports of multiple myeloma, abnormality in the blood plasma has been found only in eight instances. Even in comparison to these cases, however, the case here reported seems to be unique.

It subsequently became obvious that this patient had the classical syndrome of cryoglobulinemia. This name for the protein precipitable in the cold-cryoglubulin was first introduced by Drs. A. B. Lerner and C. J. Watson in 1947.

Thalassemia Minor

In the April 20, 1940, issue of the *Journal of the American Medical Association*, there appeared an article entitled "A Familial Hemopoietic Disorder in Italian Adolescents and Adults: Resembling Mediterranean Disease (Thalassemia)," by M. M. Wintrobe, E. Matthews, R. Pollack and B. M. Dobyns of the Johns Hopkins Hospital. Shortly thereafter similar cases were reported in Boston. These cases represented the first instances of thalassemia minor described in this country. At the time, none of the American investigators were aware that similar cases had been described earlier by a Greek investigator, Caminopetros.

The sequence of events leading to the description of the cases at Hopkins emphasizes the value of an alert technician who functions as a member of the clinical team responsible for patient care. More than two years prior to the publication referred to above, a technician, Regina Weistock, noticed many stippled cells as well as target cells in the blood smear of a patient sent to the clinic for study. In view of the stippled cells, which suggested the possibility of lead poisoning, and slight icterus, she decided on her own initiative to do an osmotic fragility test, expecting it to show decreased resistance. However, the result was the opposite: the cells were more resistant than normal to decreasing concentrations of salt solution. When informed of these results, Dr. A. Murray Fisher had his patient return for a blood lead determination, which proved to be normal. Again the fragility showed that the cells did not break up until the concentration of salt was essentially zero and the same unusual cells were seen in the smear.

One month later another patient was seen whose blood on routine examination by Miss Weistock showed exactly the same changes. This patient had been referred to Dr. Fisher by Dr. Louis Krumrein, who had heard about the findings in the first patient. The lead level in the second patient was also normal. When Miss Weistock showed these results to Dr. Wintrobe, he suggested the possibility that there had been a mistake in the fragility tests. However, Miss Weistock herself was confident that she could not make a mistake four times in a row. They kept the results on these patients, both of whom were of Italian extraction, in mind, and saved the smears.

Two years later a patient with subacute Cooley's anemia was admitted to the hospital. Prior to this time, the blood of family members of a patient with Cooley's anemia either was not examined or the subtle changes present had been overlooked. In this case, however, Dr. Wintrobe had the other members of the family brought in for study of their blood. When Miss Weistock examined their smears, she immediately remembered the two patients who had shown similar findings two years before. These patients were recalled, and it became clear that all concerned had the same abnormalities, including the increased resistance to hemolysis. Dr. Wintrobe promptly recognized that they were dealing with the hematological abnormality associated with the thalassemia trait, and thus the paper was published describing what is known as "thalassemia minor." The carefully recorded observations by a competent technician and the prepared mind of a skillful hematologist turned the key which unlocked the enigma of this heritable disorder of hemoglobin synthesis.

Reggie Weistock is still a valued member of the Department of Medicine, having worked at the Johns Hopkins Hospital for forty-two years. She was born within sight of the hospital, at Fleet and Bond streets. She graduated from Western High School in 1928, studied at Goucher College for a year, and then began work in the family's wholesale paper and grocers' specialty business. During this period she attended the Johns Hopkins evening college, studying chemistry and other subjects in the School of Engineering. About a year later she was told by a family physician about careers open for medical technicians. She worked as a volunteer for nine months in the Baltimore City Health Department, during which time she continued to take night classes in chemistry, biology, and German at Hopkins. In 1931 she came to Hopkins with the idea of doing special course work in the School of Hygiene. At this time she saw Mr. Downey, assistant superintendent of the hospital, and was told that Dr. Wintrobe was looking for a volunteer to work in his laboratory. Thus began her training in hematology. It soon became obvious that she had unusual talent, and when the position as technician for the outpatient dispensary laboratory opened up six months later, on December 31, 1931, she was placed on the payroll for the first time as technician for the outpatient dispensary. When Dr. Wintrobe moved to Salt Lake City in 1943 she went to Utah with him. However, after only a short time, illness in her family necessitated her return to Baltimore, and since March 1943 she has continued to work as a senior technician at Johns Hopkins.

Although Maxwell Wintrobe has worked in several institutions and has more than any other single individual been responsible for the development of the excellent medical school at the University of Utah, he still considers Johns Hopkins as his "real school." He was born in Halifax, Nova Scotia, and moved to Winnipeg at the age of ten. He worked his way through school doing a variety of things, including giving violin lessons, teaching art, and helping to run a vinegar factory. He entered the University of Manitoba before his sixteenth birthday and although his goal was medicine, he decided not to major in science but to broaden his education by taking political economy and French as his major subjects. His graduation from medical school in 1926 coincided with Minot's discovery of liver therapy as a cure for pernicious anemia. Because he had seen many patients with pernicious anemia dying from the disease, this discovery made a great impression on young Wintrobe. On graduation he became a research fellow, with the task of trying to reproduce pernicious anemia experimentally. He worked in a small room in the basement of the medical school, where he trained himself in hematology. The following year (1927) he went to Tulane as an instructor, and since his "training" was in hematology he was advised to pursue this area. His attention was drawn to the virtually nonexistent knowledge of normal blood standards and the gross inaccuracy of the methods used in examination of the blood. He set out to work on this problem, and the Wintrobe hematocrit tube was soon devised. He remembers very well waking up in the middle of the night with the idea of the calculation of the indices of the red cells, which became a basic technique in modern hematology. Prior to Dr. Wintrobe's work, the blood values accepted as normal for the red cell count for men and women were based on the examination of two subjects in 1852 and 1854 by inaccurate and obsolete methods. Methods for the measurement of hemoglobin were also inaccurate. On this foundation the classification of anemias, which depended on the color index (a value determined by dividing hemoglobin expressed in percent by the red cell count multiplied by 2), was based. All anemias with a color index greater than 1 were primary and the "remainder" secondary. Little wonder that there was so much confusion and misunderstanding. The development of the hematocrit and reliable red cell indices made it possible for the first time to propose a sound morphological classification of the anemias.

At this time Dr. John Musser, his chief at Tulane, asked Wintrobe to help write the section on hematology in *Tice's System of Medicine*. The result was a classic hematology monograph based on Wintrobe's own work. This article proved extremely valuable, but its limited number of pages could not possibly hold all the information of importance which Dr. Wintrobe had accumulated. This, of course, ultimately led to Wintrobe's famous *Clinical Hematology*, which has gone through so many editions and is the bible in this field.

By a fortunate coincidence, Wintrobe then came to Johns Hopkins. Dr. Wintrobe wrote an article entitled "The Erythrocyte in Man" which was published in the journal, *Medicine*, in 1930. Dr. Alan M. Chesney, dean of the Johns Hopkins Medical School, was also the editor of this journal. Recognizing the talent of this young physician, who was recommended highly by Dr. Raymond Pearl of the School of Hygiene, whom Wintrobe had consulted in relation to the statistics involved in his studies on normal blood values, Chesney promptly invited him to join the staff at Johns Hopkins as his assistant in clinical microscopy. Those of us who were students at Johns Hopkins when Dr. Wintrobe took over the course in hematology had the good fortune to learn about the blood from this innovative hematologist who had so recently put the understanding and classification of the anemias on a firm base.

At Hopkins, Dr. Wintrobe continued to study the pathogenesis of pernicious anemia. He believed that to understand pernicious anemia one needed to fulfill "Koch's postulates," so he endeavored to reproduce the disease in an experimental animal. He knew that Ehrlich had described the early blood cells of the embryo and fetus as megaloblastic. He decided to study the blood of the embryo and fetus in humans whenever possible but more importantly in the animal. There was a large abattoir near the hospital where, from time to time, he could obtain eight or ten pig fetuses from a pregnant sow. He studied their blood and accumulated a great deal of data, not only on the appearance of the red cells, but also on their size and hemoglobin content, relating these to their gestational age. The full details of these studies were deposited in the Carnegie Laboratory in the Hunterian Building and a summary of the data was published in the *American Journal of Anatomy*.

The most interesting finding was that the younger the fetus, the more striking the macrocytosis, as if the fetus had the equivalent of pernicious anemia, as Ehrlich in a sense had implied. The changes in the blood of the fetus as it matured were similar to those seen in the blood of a patient with pernicious anemia who was being treated with liver extract. Wintrobe then thought that if he could study a newborn animal during the growth phase while the animal was on a diet lacking in extrinsic factor, perhaps he could reproduce pernicious anemia. He decided to start with an animal before it had received too much extrinsic factor in the diet and had stored too much anti-anemic principle for it to become depleted of this substance within a reasonable period of time. Working with three-week-old pigs presented several problems, among them feeding the animals. The diets were homogenized to resemble milk, and now arose the question of getting the food into the piglets; an artificial sow was being discussed. Fortunately, someone accidently spilled a batch of the milky diet on the floor, and the piglets quickly demonstrated that they knew exactly what to do with it. From these systematic studies on pigs came observations concerning the role played by various vitamins on blood formation and the effect of a deficiency of these vitamins on the blood and on the nervous system. Wintrobe showed that if given in large enough amounts, unautolysed yeast could produce a hematological response in pernicious anemia—an effect known to be due to folic acid.

Dr. Wintrobe then interested the Parke-Davis Company in providing support for his work on pigs. Johns Hopkins had never before accepted money from a pharmaceutical house. There was much ado about breaking tradition, but Parke-Davis agreed to terms which were so worded that no commercial advantage whatever accrued to the company.

In 1943 Wintrobe was invited to head the Department of Medicine in a new four-year medical school at the University of Utah. Dr. Isaiah Bowman, president of Hopkins at that time, pointed out to him that this represented an opportunity to pioneer in an area, without a medical school, about one-third the size of the United States. With additional urging from Alan Gregg of the Rockefeller Foundation, Wintrobe finally accepted the job. His outstanding contributions in the development of that medical school and his research, teaching, and writing have made him an important figure in American medicine. He richly deserves the honors he has received, which include election to the National Academy of Sciences and the Kober Medal Award of the Association of American Physicians.

22 ❧ Research at Johns Hopkins on the Thyroid Gland and Its Diseases

THE SPEEDS of essentially all of the basic cellular processes of the body are regulated by the thyroid gland, a small mass of pinkish tissue which weighs less than one ounce and is located just below the vocal cords. Disorders of the thyroid usually manifest themselves in one of two ways: the gland produces too much thyroxine and the metabolic rate increases (hyperthyroidism) or the gland produces an insufficient amount of this hormone, resulting in a metabolism which is below that necessary for normal function (hypothyroidism). When it develops rapidly, either condition may result in severe malfunction of both body and mind and may be associated with a disfiguring enlargement of the thyroid gland known as "goiter."

Goiter has been a well-known malady for centuries. Pliny the Elder, Vitruvius, and Juvenal commented upon the presence of goiter among the inhabitants of the Alps. (The term is derived from the Latin word *guttur*, meaning "throat.") In 1656 Thomas Wharton, an Englishman, proposed the name "thyroid," from the Greek word for "shield-shaped." A better understanding of the function of the thyroid came in 1883, when Swiss surgeons completely removed large goiters from a number of patients. Mechanical relief from pressure on the trachea and other organs caused by the large goiters was achieved, but within a few months all of the patients had developed severe thyroid insufficiency. Experiments removing the thyroid gland of animals in early life resulted in the symptoms associated with cretinism in man. Thus, it became known that the thyroid contains a substance essential for health and for normal growth and development. By the early 1890s physicians were treating patients with hypothyroidism by administering sheep's thyroid in the diet, and in 1896 the German chemist Baumann discovered that the thyroid contained iodine.

A number of physicians and surgeons at Johns Hopkins have played an important role in the development of our knowledge of the thyroid gland, and their contributions are the subject of this chapter.

The Operative Story of Goiter

In his classic monograph on the surgical management of goiter published in the *Johns Hopkins Hospital Reports* in 1920, William S. Halsted stated:

The extirpation of the thyroid gland for goiter typifies, perhaps better than any operation, the supreme triumph of the surgeon's art. A feat which today can be accomplished by any really competent operator without danger of mishap, which was conceived more than 1000 years ago, might appear an unlikely competitor for a place in surgery so exalted. There are operations today more delicate and, perhaps, more difficult, but they have followed naturally and easily in the paths made clear for them. But is there any operative problem propounded so long ago and attacked by so many which has cost so much thought and endeavor and so many lives before its ultimate solution was achieved?

At the time Halsted's interest developed in thyroid disease, two chief forms were recognized: the large colloid goiter, which often caused great disfigurement, distressing symptoms due to compression of the trachea, and insufficiency of thyroid secretion; and exophthalmic goiter, which was associated with symptoms of overactivity of the thyroid secretion and was accompanied frequently by exophthalmos. Both conditions often caused death and were a constant challenge to surgeons. The blood vessels in both conditions were so enlarged and numerous that hemorrhage during surgery was a serious hazard; so much so that eminent surgeons of the day declared that operations on the thyroid were not justified. Moreover, patients who survived the operation might gradually develop symptoms of hypothyroidism or those due to deprivation of the parathyroid glands. Halsted's operation, however, successfully avoided hemorrhage and protected the patient against removal of or injury to the parathyroid glands, and it was soon widely adopted.

Halsted became interested in studying the thyroid gland while working in Billroth's laboratory in Vienna in 1880. Wolfler, then an assistant to Billroth, was writing his classic monograph, *"Die Entwickelung und Bau des Tropfes,"* and occasionally went to Halsted's laboratory to study his sections of the salmon with reference to the development and structure of the thyroid gland in fish. Halsted did not recall, however, ever having seen an operation for goiter in Billroth's clinic, which he attended regularly.

Then in the autumn of 1887, at the suggestion of William H. Welch, Halsted began experiments on extirpation and transplantation of the thyroid in dogs, which resulted in the discovery, among other things, of the striking histological changes which signify hyperplasia and hyperactivity of this gland and which are similar to those found in Graves's disease. There is an interesting anecdote in relation to these experiments of Halsted. While he was doing this work in the Hunterian Laboratory, Victor Horsley from England was visiting Baltimore. Very excited about his results, Halsted showed all of his specimens to Horsley. It so happened that Horsley had already done similar experiments, and his work was at that time being processed for publication. However, being a courteous English gentleman, Horlsey did not mention this to Halsted for fear that it would hurt his feelings.

The remarkable discoveries by Gley (1891–1892) and Vassale and Generali (1896) of the vital importance of the parathyroid glandules also stimulated Halsted's interest in the surgery of the thyroid gland and suggested experiments in transplantation of these tiny epithelial bodies. From these experiments, the general law was developed that homografts of these glandules will not live and that for the successful transplantation of autografts a considerable deficiency must be created. Halsted made the startling observation that the life of a dog could be maintained by a particle of parathyroid tissue only one-quarter of a millimeter in diameter, the removal of which was followed by tetany.

In 1907, at Halsted's request, Herbert M. Evans made arterial injections of a dye to identify the location of all of the parathyroid glandules. As a result of careful anatomical studies by Evans and William G. MacCallum, and of Halsted's own surgical and experimental observations, the operative procedure for thyroid removal without damage to the parathyroids was developed. Although Halsted described the procedure on several occasions, he did so in such a fragmentary way that it did not attract much attention. Essential improvements in the operation over the twelve succeeding years, however, led to the publication of his classic monograph, admirably illustrated by Max Broedel, entitled "The Operative Story of Goitre: The Author's Operation." Thus, experiments undertaken primarily, so Halsted said, to determine the cause or causes of death after operations upon the thyroid glands, led to a better understanding of the surgical problems related to this important structure.

David Marine

While a student at the Johns Hopkins University School of Medicine, David Marine was inspired by Dr. Halsted to seek a career in research; his field of research, however, was chosen somewhat by happenstance. After graduation in 1905, he went to Cleveland for an internship in pathology. On his way from the train station to the hospital, he noticed that many of the dogs roaming the streets had large thyroid glands. When he arrived and was asked by his new chief what area of research he was interested in, he still had this on his mind and replied, "The thyroid." From then on he was a successful investigator of the physiology and pathology of the thyroid gland.

Marine conceived the idea that lack of iodine in the food and water supply might be the cause of the goiter in the dogs. By depriving experimental animals of dietary iodine, he produced goiters in them. Goiter prophylaxis by the addition of iodine to the diet had been tried as early as 1860, but the method fell into disuse and was forgotten after a decade of laboratory investigation. In 1916 Marine and Kimball prevented goiter in school children in Akron, Ohio, by this method. Marine urged that iodides be added to drinking water and table salt, but his proposals drew as much opposition as the addition of fluoride to the water supply to prevent dental caries did later. It took another ten years to convince the public that this simple measure would prevent endemic goiter.

Marine believed that endemic goiter can be produced solely by iodine lack. The normal functioning of the thyroid depends on the activity of the thyrotropic hormone of the anterior pituitary. The colloid material containing iodine is stored in the thyroid follicles, and the thyroid hormone is passed into the blood stream to maintain a normal metabolic rate. If the iodine supply is insufficient, this physiological concentration of thyroxine may not be maintained under increased need, as in puberty or during pregnancy.

In 1924 Marine advanced his theory known as the "Marine cycle." At a time of increased demand the thyrotropic hormone stimulates the cells which line the thyroid follicles, and as a result the individual cells increase in size (hypertrophy). Further action of thyrotropic hormone causes the individual cells to multiply by cell division so that the size and volume of the individual follicles are increased (hyperplasia). If an excess of iodine is made available, the enlarged follicles fill up with colloid. This excessive secretion ceases after a time, but the follicles are permanently enlarged in their resting state (involution). A continuation of this state leads to degeneration of the gland substance and the production of a simple colloid goiter.

Alan Mason Chesney

It had been postulated but not proven that goiter might be produced by an active goitrogen. This mechanism for the production of goiter (in contradistinction to the absence of iodine from the diet) was highlighted by a serendipitous observation made by Alan Mason Chesney in the autumn of 1927. During the course of his studies on experimental syphilis, Chesney noted that the rabbits in the colony were developing large goiters. The potential importance of this unexpected finding was recognized, and Warfield T. Longcope assigned Bruce Webster to search for the cause of the thyroid enlargement. Webster had arrived in Baltimore in July 1927 as a Jacques Loeb Fellow in Medicine and was working in the Division of Metabolism with Dr. George Harrop. Webster went to New York to confer with David Marine, at that time director of the laboratories at Montefiore Hospital. When he returned to Baltimore, he began an intensive study of these goitrous rabbits, which led to the publication of a series of papers on endemic goiter in rabbits. The first paper, published in the *Johns Hopkins Hospital Bulletin* in 1928, established that most of the rabbits in the colony developed goiter and that the event had no relationship to the syphilitic infection. The gross and microscopical appearance of the thyroid was that of a hyperplastic gland. The second paper, published simultaneously, demonstrated that heat production in the goitrous animals was 16.6 percent lower than in normal ones and that rabbits with the largest goiters showed the greatest depression in metabolic rate. The third of the series reported that when iodine was administered to the goitrous rabbits, there was a marked increase in metabolic rate, rapid emaciation, and in most instances death. The severity of the reaction bore a direct relationship to the extent of hyperplasia which existed before iodine was administered. Iodine tended to bring about involution of the hyperplastic thyroid gland, with a lowering of the alveolar epithelium. Areas of involution resembling colloid adenomata were observed. Both diffuse and localized areas of persistent hyperplasia were noted.

A subsequent paper by Webster and Chesney, entitled "Studies in the Etiology of Simple Goiter," which was published in the *American Journal of Pathology,* showed that the diet, which consisted almost exclusively of cabbage, appeared to be the major etiological factor, and that iodine administered orally completely protected the animal against the goiter-producing factor. This important discovery was substantiated by Marine and his co-workers and also by McCarrison in India. Since that time, small outbreaks of goiter have been reported in man in communities compelled by circumstances to exist mainly on cabbage. Later, in 1941, Thomas Henry Kennedy and Herbert Dudley Purves in New Zealand found that rape seed would also induce goiter.

Dr. Webster obtained a National Research Council fellowship and went to New York to study this problem further with David Marine. They published a paper in the *Journal of Experimental Medicine* on the occurrence of seasonal variations in the goiter of rabbits produced by feeding cabbage, presenting evidence that cabbage maturing in the spring and summer months has little goiter-producing power, while cabbage maturing in late autumn has much greater goiter-producing power. Other plants of the genus *Brassica* were also found to be goitrogens. Since these plants contain mustard oils, Marine and his co-workers (1932) were prompted to investigate the thyroidal actions of the isothiocyanates and their cyanide precursors. They demonstrated that acetonitrile and related compounds can produce thyroid hyperplasia and that the effect can be antagonized by iodine.

Bruce Peck Webster was born on November 1, 1901, at Lansdowne, Ontario, Canada. He received the M.D.C.M. degree from McGill University in 1925 and was awarded the Sutherland Gold Medal in Biochemistry. From 1927 to 1929 he served as assistant resident in medicine and Jacques Loeb Fellow at Hopkins. He became assistant professor of medicine at Cornell in 1932 and was promoted to clinical professor of medicine in 1964. He is a member of the American Society for Clinical Investigation. During World War II, he served with distinction and was awarded the Legion of Merit in 1945. He is a past president of the American Venereal Disease Association and the American Social Health Association. He has maintained a wide interest in internal medicine, with special attention to the venereal diseases.

Alan Mason Chesney was born on January 17, 1888, and died at the age of seventy-six on September 22, 1964. Almost his entire life was spent in close association with the Johns Hopkins University, the medical school, and the hospital. During these years his contributions, from professional, scientific, literary, and administrative standpoints, were outstanding.

Following his graduation from Baltimore City College, Alan Chesney attended the Johns Hopkins University, where he had a distinguished career in football and lacrosse. He graduated from the medical school with honors in 1912 in a class which contained such other notables as Ernest Goodpasture, Maurice Pincoffs, Mont Reid, and Lewis Weed. Following his internship and assistant residency in medicine at Johns Hopkins, he worked at the Rockefeller Institute for three years under Rufus Cole and O. T. Avery. With the entry of the United States into World War I in 1917, he was commissioned a first lieutenant in the Medical Corps, and at that time he married Cora Chambers. In 1919 he joined the faculty at Washington University in St. Louis as head of the Infectious Disease Division in the Department of Medicine, under Canby

Robinson. When Dr. Robinson took over the directorship of the Department of Medicine at Johns Hopkins, he brought Alan Chesney with him as associate professor to direct the newly created Syphilis Division. In preparation for this assignment, Chesney worked for a year with Wade Brown and Louise Pearce at the Rockefeller Institute, returning to Hopkins in 1922.

For the next ten years his energies were given primarily to the Syphilis Division, both in its clinical activities and in the experimental laboratory. His research during this period, related principally to immunity in syphilis, established him as an independent and imaginative investigator of infectious diseases. Among his major contributions were the demonstration of *Treponema pallidum* in blood, spinal fluid, and joint fluid of patients with early syphilis, and of the infectivity of virtually all organs of the rabbit in latent as well as early syphilis. Most important, however, was his long series of experiments covering a decade or more on the basic mechanisms of immunity in syphilis, which demonstrated the slow evolution of immunity in the experimental disease and established the fact that immunity persists long after elimination of the causative agent by specific treatment. His later contributions were in the study of the biological and therapeutic assay of penicillin in syphilis.

In 1927 Chesney became assistant dean of the School of Medicine, and in 1929 he succeeded Lewis Weed as dean, a post he held until his retirement in 1953. He saw the medical school weather the financial crisis of the Great Depression, following which there were the profound educational stresses incidental to World War II. After the war, he had the problem of adjusting administratively to the rapid expansion of research fostered by government support, which he did with good judgment and an acute sense of enduring rights and obligations of a free university. He was very active in the affairs of the Association of American Medical Colleges and served as its president in 1937. During this period, he wrote his three-volume history of the Johns Hopkins Hospital and the Johns Hopkins University School of Medicine from 1867 to 1914. The first volume was published in 1943, and the second and third in 1958 and 1963, respectively. Coincident with the fiftieth anniversary of the Johns Hopkins Hospital in 1939, he wrote and produced a one-act play entitled "The Flowering of an Idea," which conveyed in dramatic form the great vision of Mr. Hopkins and its practical realization.

A long list of honors came to Alan Chesney. As a result of his excellent research, he was elected to membership in the American Society for Clinical Investigation. In 1924 he became a member of the Association of American Physicians, and from 1923 to 1947 he served as editor of *Medicine*. He was president of the Medical and Chirurgical Faculty of Medicine in 1952, and from 1959 to 1961, president of the Johns Hopkins Medical and Surgical Association. He was awarded an honorary degree by the Johns Hopkins University in 1957.

One of his most inspiring actions was his fight against the antivivisectionists in 1950. This seemingly quiet academician became a vigorous defender of "the right," transforming himself at once into a practical ward politician and a civic leader. Public rallies were organized; faculty and students canvassed from door to door under his direction and on election day stood guard at the polls. The resulting avalanche of votes for this cause profoundly startled seasoned politicians, most of whom had sat carefully on the fence.

Few have served their university with such distinction as did Alan Chesney over a period of several decades.

Medical Thyroidectomy

Other Hopkins workers contributed importantly to the development of our knowledge about the thyroid, including the Mackenzies, the husband and wife team who worked in the School of Hygiene and Public Health, Curt P. Richter, Edwin B. Astwood, William F. Rienhoff, and John E. Howard.

As Cosmo G. Mackenzie has pointed out, all scientific discoveries have their roots in the past history of science and society. More often than not, however, they do not emerge in any clearly discernible or logical fashion from the previous body of scientific knowledge or from contemporary and direct attacks on related problems. Such was the case when he and his wife, Julia, uncovered within a period of a few months the goitrogenic activity of certain well-defined organic compounds: the sulfonamides, para-amino benzoic acid, and the thioureas. Their findings did not result from a direct study of the thyroid gland but, rather, from an effort to explain the amazing contradictions that existed in the symptoms produced by vitamin E deficiency in the rabbit and in the rat.

In 1931 Goettsch and Pappenheimer described a dietary deficiency disease in rabbits and guinea pigs characterized by dystrophy of the voluntary muscles. The animals' diet, which was composed of natural food, had been treated with an ethereal solution of ferric chloride in the hope of destroying vitamin E. However, potent samples of wheat germ oil, which had been shown to cure vitamin E deficiency in female rats, failed to cure the acute muscle degeneration described. This and other observations led to the conclusion that the acute degeneration of the voluntary muscles in these animals resulted from deficiency of a hitherto unknown fat-soluble factor, coupled, perhaps, with a concomitant deficiency in a new water-soluble factor. This was an exciting development, and Professor McCollum suggested that the Mackenzies investigate the nutritional factors responsible for this lethal disease. The Mackenzies soon recognized a species difference in the response to vitamin E deficiency, which they thought might be due to the synthesis of small amounts of vitamin E by the intestinal flora of the rat. They tested this hypothesis by administering a sulfonamide—sulfaguanidine—to their animals. This sulfonamide derivative, which had been synthesized by Professor E. K. Marshall, Jr., in 1940, was poorly absorbed in the intestinal tract and had been shown to reduce the concentration of coliform bacteria in the feces of mice. The Mackenzies tested the effect of the sulfaguanidine on weanling rats fed a purified diet containing all of the then-known vitamins except vitamin E. The control animals grew normally and were healthy in appearance. The animals fed sulfaguanidine, on the other hand, grew at a slower rate and after several weeks ceased to gain weight

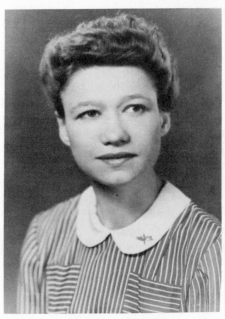

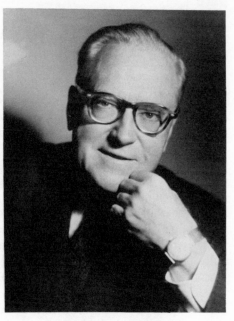

Julia B. Mackenzie
Courtesy of Julia B. Mackenzie

Bruce Peck Webster
Courtesy of Dr. Bruce Peck Webster

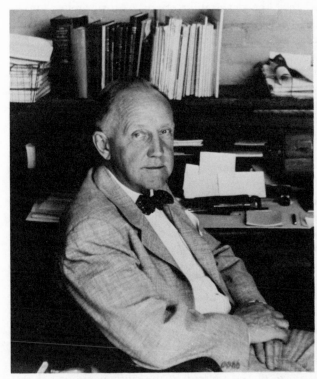

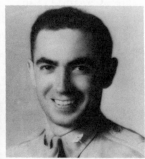

Cosmo G. Mackenzie
Courtesy of Dr. C. G. Mackenzie

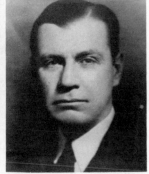

Alan Mason Chesney
From the Archives Office, The Johns Hopkins Medical Institutions

William F. Rienhoff, Jr.
Courtesy of Dr. Rienhoff, Jr.

and began to bleed from the eyes. A number of these animals were sacrificed and autopsies performed. Except for a loss of adipose tissue, the organs and tissues appeared to be grossly normal with one exception: in all of the animals fed sulfaguanidine, both lobes of the thyroid were greatly enlarged and hyperemic. These experiments were immediately repeated on weanling rats, with 10 percent yeast added to the sulfaguanidine diet. The results were startling. Although the yeast-supplemented animals grew at a normal rate and showed no sign of bleeding from the eyes, their thyroid glands were just as large and hyperemic as the glands of those who had received sulfaguanidine alone. The Mackenzies concluded that the sulfaguanidine produced a nutritional deficiency of unknown nature and, most important, an independent enlargement of the thyroid gland. Histological examination of the gland revealed changes resembling Graves's disease. The flat epithelial cells which normally line the follicles had been transformed into columnar cells of such height as to practically obliterate the lumen, which was essentially devoid of colloid. It was a spectacular display of a completely hyperplastic thyroid.

The investigators were faced with a choice: they could pursue the nutritional aspect of the problem and attempt to isolate and identify the factor in yeast which prevented the nutritional deficiency caused by sulfaguanidine, or they could investigate the mechanism of its action on the thyroid. Their decision to pursue the thyroid problem was based on a number of factors. In her years as a nurse, Julia had seen the devastating effects of toxic goiter and of myxedema. Cosmo recalled the winter of 1912, when his mother's sister, who was suffering from Graves's disease, had come to stay with them, and he had been scolded for calling attention to her loss of weight and the family "whispered" about her erratic behavior. Her cure by subtotal thyroidectomy left an indelible impression on him. Both of the Mackenzies had taken a special course in pathology given to students in the School of Hygiene by Professor Arnold Rich, who had stimulated their interest in the investigation of causes and mechanisms of human disease by his enthusiasm and penetrating analyses.

An additional factor in their decision was even simpler and perhaps more scientific. They were well aware of the work of Marine and his co-workers, who had noted that colloid goiter was common in both man and dogs in the Cleveland area, and who had correctly concluded that this was due to a deficiency of iodine in the water. They also knew from their course in nutrition that Alan Chesney and his colleagues had, in the late 1920s, discovered goiter in rabbits fed a diet consisting primarily of cabbage. This type of goiter was cured by iodine, but attempts to isolate the active goitrogenic factor had been very frustrating. The Mackenzies appreciated the significance of their observation of goitrogenic activity in a stable compound of known chemical structure. Their next step was to add more sodium iodide to the diet and also to inject it subcutaneously. This furnished no protection against the sulfaguanidine goiter. Thus their compound, sulfaguanidine, was unique among goitrogens in producing enlarged thyroids which could not be prevented by iodine. Indeed, the iodide actually increased the size of the thyroid in the sulfaguanidine-fed rats. On the basis of the study by D. D. Woods in 1940, which showed that para-amino benzoic acid inhibited the bacteriostatic action of sulfanilamide, they added the former compound to the experimental diet. It not only failed to prevent the action of sulfaguanidine on the thyroid, but when fed alone it exhibited goitrogenic activity in its own right, although to a lesser extent than sulfaguanidine. They now had two organic compounds of known chemical structure that exhibited goitrogenic activity.

Despite the administration of other sulfonamides to thousands of laboratory animals, there had never been any mention of an effect on the thyroid. The Mackenzies assumed, therefore, that sulfaguanidine was unique among the sulfa drugs and that its goitrogenic activity was related to the guanidine moiety of the molecule. Feeding guanidine and sulfanilic acid, both separately and together, however, did not produce any effect on the thyroid. Large doses of urea also provided negative results. It then occurred to them that the spatial relation between the sulfur and guanidine molecules might make sulfur derivatives and analogues of guanidine and urea worth examining. The first compound tested was thiourea, and its effect on the thyroid was dramatic, exceeding that of sulfaguanidine. Thus, three goitrogens had been discovered within a few weeks. They then proceeded to test sulfanilamide, sulfathiazole, sulfapyridine and sulfamethyldiazine on rats, and without exception each of them produced thyroid enlargement. Similar responses were obtained in mice and dogs. At the same time they tried a variety of thiourea derivatives, and all except acetylthiourea showed the typical thyroid response.

Histological examination of these glands by Dr. Arnold Rich led him to conclude that they were hyperthyroid. He recalled recently having seen sections of thyroid glands from rats fed phenylthiourea by Professor Curt Richter and Dr. Katherine Clisby of the Department of Psychiatry at Johns Hopkins. This compound is tasteless to some humans and has an extremely bitter taste to others, a difference that is genetically determined. Richter and Clisby were studying this compound in rats to see if they exhibited a similar taste discrimination. They found that the compound produced severe edema, and in those animals that survived, an enlargement of the thyroid. Thus, these workers had independently observed the effect of the thioureas on the thyroid. Rich pointed out that these glands, like those of the Mackenzies, showed an increase in the height of the epithelium and a depletion of colloid. His interpretation, as well as Richter's, was that this represented a compensatory response to a lowering of body temperature by the drug,—in other words, the apparent "hyperthyroidism" observed in the animals was the well-known reaction of the thyroid gland of rodents exposed to the cold.

This seemed unlikely to the Mackenzies, however. They attempted during the next few weeks to demonstrate a fall in body temperature in young rats fed thiourea and sulfaguanidine, but were unsuccessful. They believed the question could only be settled by measurement of the basal metabolic rate. By this time World War II had begun, there was already a shortage of metal, and the machine shop was so busy that no suitable measuring instrument could be constructed. Enthusiastic about the study, Dr. McCollum called the Carnegie Institute and asked if they might borrow the metabolic chamber originally used on rats by Francis G. Benedict in his classic studies on basal metabolism. The Carnegie officials graciously agreed to remove the apparatus from their museum, and it was with Benedict's copper chamber, with its water-sealed bellows, that the Mackenzies conclusively demonstrated that young rats fed sulfaguanidine or thiourea exhibited, after two weeks of goitrogen administration, a decline in oxygen consumption of 20 percent, as compared to control animals. Of a variety of compounds tested, only desiccated thyroid and thyroxine restored the basal metabolic rate to normal and completely abolished the hyperplastic appearance of the gland.

The next question was the mode of action. The Mackenzies showed that in thyroidectomized rats the drugs did not inhibit the action of thyroxine on the target tissues. Minute doses of the hormone restored the B.M.R. to normal levels. Therefore, they concluded that these drugs must block the synthesis of the thyroid hormone. Their next step was to demonstrate that in hypophysectomized animals the antithyroid drugs exerted no hyperplastic effect on the thyroid. Its appearance remained that of a resting gland. Finally, in normal animals the drugs produced histological changes in the pituitary that were typical of thyroidectomy. Their conclusions were that the sulfonamides and thioureas inhibited the synthesis of thyroxine and that this in turn lowered the basal metabolic rate. The normal feedback mechanism stimulated release of thyrotropic hormone, which in turn produced the spectacular hyperplasia without resulting in thyroxine synthesis.

Cosmo G. Mackenzie was born on May 22, 1907, in Baltimore. He received his A.B. degree from Johns Hopkins in 1932 and his Sc.D. in 1936. For the next two years he was a research associate in biochemistry at the School of Hygiene and Public Health at Johns Hopkins and for the four years after that assistant professor in biochemistry. He entered the Army Air Force in 1942 and was discharged in 1945. In the 16th Altitude Training Unit he showed production of the bends with exercise at low altitudes, measured the duration of useful consciousness at high altitudes, and demonstrated its prolongation by glucose ingestion. He also served as assistant director of the Physiology Section in the Research Division of the Air Surgeon's Office. After World War II he moved to Cornell University Medical College and worked with Professor Vincent du Vigneaud on the oxidation of methyl groups, the formation of one-carbon compounds, and their metabolic pathways. In 1950 he became professor of biochemistry and chairman of the department in the University of Colorado Medical School. Here, with Wilhelm Frisell, he studied the enzymology of one-carbon compounds and later with Julia Mackenzie the accumulation and metabolism of lipid in cultured mammalian cells. Dr. Mackenzie retired as chairman in 1973 and as professor in 1975, but he continues to work as professor emeritus in the medical school and the Webb-Waring Institute for Medical Research. He is a member of many distinguished societies, including the American Society of Biological Chemists and the American Institute of Nutrition.

Julia B. Mackenzie was born in Colorado Springs, Colorado, on April 5, 1911. She received her A.B. degree from Colorado College in 1932 and graduated from the Johns Hopkins Hospital School of Nursing in 1936. She received the Sc.D. degree from the Johns Hopkins University in 1939. From 1939 to 1944 she was first instructor of biochemistry in the School of Hygiene and Public Health, and then assistant professor. In 1947 she became research associate in biochemistry in the Department of Psychiatry at Cornell Medical School, where she demonstrated the antidystrophic activity of several new vitamin E derivatives. While an assistant professor of biochemistry in the Department of Pediatrics at the University of Colorado Medical School from 1951 to 1953, she elucidated the relationship between the erythrocyte fragility of premature infants and low blood levels of vitamin E. In 1954 she was named assistant professor of biochemistry at Colorado and was made full professor in 1967. In 1968 she was also appointed professor of anatomy. Her work for the last ten years has been in the field of cell culture, with particular reference to lipid metabolism. She is a member of the American Society of Biological Chemists, the American Institute of Nutrition, and Phi Beta Kappa.

The Mackenzies' studies on the goitrogenic activity of sulfaguanidine was first reported in *Science* in 1941. The fact that thiourea as well as a number of other sulfonamides possessed goitrogenic activity was outlined in an abstract in the *Federation Proceedings* in 1942. At the meeting of the Federated Societies held in Boston that spring, a verbal report was given of their results up to and including those obtained on the response of the thyroidectomized and drug-fed rats to thyroxine.

In the discussion which followed Julia Mackenzie's presentation, Dr. Edwin B. Astwood rose to say that he had obtained essentially the same results as the Mackenzies and advanced the same explanation for the mechanism of action of the sulfonamides and thioureas on the thyroid. The next week Watson Davis of Science Service urged the Mackenzies to say for national press release that possibly sulfonamides and probably thioureas could be used to treat toxic goiter in man. This they refused to do, partly because of the false hope that the cure of experimental muscular dystrophy with vitamin E had raised in patients with progressive muscular dystrophy and in their relatives. In addition, in the spring of 1942 the Mackenzies asked Dr. Perrin Long to try sulfonamides and thioureas in patients with toxic goiter. This was not feasible, Long said, because of the shortage of staff physicians as a result of the war.

It was Edwin B. Astwood who pursued the use of the thioureas in the clinical management of patients with hyperthyroidism. Astwood was at that time working at Peter Bent Brigham Hospital in Boston, but he had previously been a member of the Hopkins community. As a student at McGill, he had worked in the laboratory of Dr. J. B. Collip. He spent most of his fifth year of medicine as an intern and then tried to find a research position. Inexperience and lack of sponsorship frustrated these efforts, and the summer of 1935 approached with no research future in sight. A classmate and close friend was going to work for a year in surgical pathology at Johns Hopkins, and at the last minute Charles Geschickter said that Astwood might come. Astwood soon became disenchanted with looking down the microscope at tumors, and instead utilized the rat colony which had been set up to permit the assay of tumors for

sex hormones and gonadotropins. He had the good fortune to meet Curt Richter and Carl Hartmann, and he also spent time studying the literature on
endocrinology in the Welch Library. During his two years in Baltimore, he
studied in particular the endocrinology of mammary development in the rat,
and on the basis of this work and with Carl Hartmann's help, he obtained a
Rockefeller Fellowship—a real plum in those days, with a stipend of $1,800.
During the next two years, spent under F. L. Hisaw at the biological laboratory
at Harvard, he worked on the reproductive cycle of the rat and obtained his
Ph.D. degree.

He then accepted the challenge presented by Nicholas Eastman to establish an endocrinology research laboratory in the Department of Obstetrics.
With Eleanor Delfs and Georgeanna Seegar Jones, he initiated investigative
work along several lines. He and Dr. Jones published an improved method for
measuring pregnanediol in urine and with Dr. Delfs devised a method for the
determination of chorionic gonadotropin in blood. Meanwhile, by hypophysec-
tomizing rats—a rare skill in those days, one he had learned from Curt Richter
—Astwood showed that the corpus luteum of the rat is controlled by a third
gonadotropin, which he named "luteotropin."

After five years in the laboratory, he returned to clinical medicine when he
was offered a position by Dr. Soma Weiss, professor of medicine and chairman
of the department at Harvard and Peter Bent Brigham Hospital. It was just at
this time that the Mackenzies published their studies on sulfaguanidine and
Richter and Clisby published their work on phenylthiourea. Astwood's laboratory was involved in the elucidation of the interaction of the pituitary and its
hormones with the gonads, adrenals and thyroids, and thus technically and
methodologically it was uniquely prepared to investigate the mechanism of this
remarkable new phenomenon—goiter produced by pure chemical substances.
It was only a matter of weeks or at most a few months before Astwood
concluded that the mode of action was inhibition of the synthesis of thyroid
hormone—the goiter being compensatory and mediated by excessive secretion
of thyrotropin. Astwood was convinced that there was no goiter in the absence
of the pituitary, even if thyrotropin was given in replacement doses and the
action of thyroxine was not inhibited. Iodine reduced the goiter only slightly,
and most important of all, the goiter was prevented or cured when the rats were
given thyroxine. It could also be shown that the goitrous rats were hypothyroid.
Thus, he concluded that it was logical to try one of the active compounds in the
treatment of hyperthyroidism.

Later, in 1941, Soma Weiss suffered a subarachnoid hemorrhage and
died. The Department of Medicine at Brigham was left in the young but capable hands of Eugene Stead, Lewis Dexter, Charles Janeway, John Romano, and
Edwin Astwood. Each had responsibility for his field, with Stead as general
head and Janeway in charge of the students. In these circumstances Astwood
set out to try thiourea in hyperthyroid patients.

In those days, patients with Graves's disease were admitted to medicine
for two or three weeks and given iodine in preparation for a subtotal thyroidectomy. Astwood instead gave them one to two grams of thiourea a day. At first

the trials were discouraging. Finally, a new and severe case came along. No iodine had been given, and after thiourea was administered the patient's basal metabolic rate fell promptly. When thiourea was stopped, the patient relapsed; thiourea was given again with equal success. When the patient returned a month later, however, he was a sight to see. He was puffy and pale, and his eyes were nearly swollen shut. He had a croaky voice, and he moved slowly and with difficulty. He exuded a sickening, sweetish odor. At first Astwood, in his own words, "stupidly thought that this must be some horrible toxic effect of the drug." Several days later it dawned on him that this was acutely induced myxedema, which he was to see many times again. The substance responsible for the odor of patients taking thiourea, however, has never been elucidated. Astwood soon had other cases which confirmed the dramatic effect of thiourea, and the first clinical report was published in the *Journal of the American Medical Association* on May 8, 1943.

In the meantime many compounds had been tested for their goitrogenic effect. Thiouracil was found to be ten times more active than thiourea. This difference in potency did not carry over into man, thiourea actually being more active in man than thiouracil or the subsequently used propylthiouracil. In any event, Astwood's studies almost came to a halt when the seventh patient given thiouracil nearly died from agranulocytosis.

Concurrent with these studies on hyperthyroidism, observations were also being made on the effects of administering thyroid to patients with simple goiter. The effect of thyroid administration on the rats made goitrous with thiourea was so striking that this seemed an obvious thing to do. The predicted response was soon observed in many patients, but since the results were so expected and seemed so obvious, Astwood's group did not bother to publish it. When Monte Greer, who worked with Astwood, retrieved these data and obtained some additional information, a report was finally published in 1953, eleven years later. The medical storm and fury that this report stirred up, especially among surgeons, far exceeded in intensity that caused by the hyperthyroidism story. Astwood now believes that this discovery is of wider application and of greater importance than that of the antithyroid drugs.

William Francis Rienhoff, Jr.

On February 28, 1930, William F. Rienhoff, Jr., received the following letter from William Henry Welch:

Thank you very much for the reprint of your paper on the thyroid gland. I congratulate you heartily upon an extremely interesting, valuable and original contribution. You must have put a great deal of time, skill and energy into the work by the reconstruction method but it has been worthwhile. Your study would have delighted Dr. Mall and Dr. Halsted. You have brought out a number of new points. The comparison by your models between the normal thyroid and that of exophthalmic goiter is really fascinating.

With best wishes, I am,

Very sincerely yours William H. Welch

The contributions lauded in this letter from one of Johns Hopkins's original "greats" involved Rienhoff's study of the normal human thyroid and also of the gland in cases of diffuse goiter with hyperthyroidism from the standpoint not only of the individual follicles but also of the structure of the gland as a whole and of the various subdivisions or units into which the thyroid is divided. His reconstructions of normal and exophthalmic glands were made using the wax model methods previously employed by Dr. Franklin P. Mall. The study challenged a long-accepted statement by Wolfler. In 1883 Wolfler described rests of fetal cells between the follicles, which he thought persisted into adult life and later gave rise to tumors or neoplasms of the thyroid. Rienhoff set out to show this conclusion was inaccurate, as the methods available to Wolfler for study of the thyroid were inexact.

That the follicle of the thyroid represented the ultimate histological unit of the gland was generally accepted, but the manner in which the glandular mass is subdivided into larger regions composed of many follicles had not been described. In Reinhoff's study, not only did he use wax plate reconstruction to investigate a larger area of thyroid tissue than had been previously studied, but he also utilized the method of maceration and microdissection. Thus, he was able to visualize the spatial relationship of the individual follicles as well as the various regions, and in this way determine the presence of a true lobulation of the gland. The stained sections were continually referred to during the process of transferring the tracings of the photographs made of them to the wax plates. In order to include every epithelial cell, and thus detect the existence of any interacinar cell rests, either fetal or adult, serial sections of 10 and 20 microns in thickness were studied. No evidence of any interfollicular fetal cell rests or clusters of differentiated epithelium which were not a portion of the parenchyma was found. He noted many small follicles interspersed between the larger ones, and because of their small size, he suggested that they were not active at the time but represented a functional reserve. The noticeable reduction in number of these smaller follicles in the hyperthyroid gland confirmed this suggestion.

The wax reconstruction of the thyroid in exophthalmic goiter showed an enormous increase in the size of the follicles, and indentations in the wax models of these follicles bore witness to the papillomatous infoldings of the epithelium. The true external form of the follicle was brought out by the technique of maceration and dissection, while the internal shape or cast of the inside of the follicle was shown better by the wax models. By maceration and microdissection it was possible to demonstrate that the main mass of the thyroid gland is divided and subdivided into many connecting or annectant bars, bands, and plates of parenchyma, which in turn are composed of individual, discrete, and discontinuous follicles. There are no distinct and true lobules in the thyroid and it is incorrect to speak of it as a lobulated gland. These plates, bands, and bars of parenchyma are separated by clefts and spaces normally filled with tissue of mesenchymal origin, such as blood vessels, connective tissue, lymphatics, and nerves. They vary markedly in shape and size, the gland being irregularly broken up by the clefts and open spaces which form by their connections a fenestrated labyrinth in the gland mass. These bars, bands, and plates were always connected one with another, and no isolated regions of parenchyma completely surrounded by connective tissue were observed.

These astute and carefully executed studies designed to display the minute antomy of the normal thyroid and its changes in the course of exophthalmic goiter represented an unusual research accomplishment by a practicing surgeon. Rienhoff was awarded the Gold Medal Essay of the American Association for the Study of Goiter in the first year of its existence. The title of the first award essay presented at the meeting of the association in July 1930 was "A New Conception of Some Morbid Changes in Diseases of the Thyroid, Based on Experimental Studies of the Normal Gland and the Thyroid Gland in Exophthalmic Goiter."

William Francis Rienhoff, Jr., developed his interest in the thyroid during his association with Halsted. At that time patients operated on for exophthalmic goiter often had a postoperative thyroid crisis, with severe tachycardia and death. In 1923, after Plummer introduced iodine to control the symptoms of hyperthyroidism, Rienhoff began its use at Hopkins, and immediately the operative results improved. Rienhoff then became interested in the mechanism by which iodine caused these changes in the thyroid gland, and with Finney's permission did preoperative and postoperative biopsies on patients with exophthalmic goiter. Rienhoff had noticed during operations a striking difference in the gross appearance of the thyroid gland in patients with exophthalmic goiter treated with iodine in contrast to those who had not received it. The gland in the former patients was increased in size, seemed more resistant to the knife, and had more pronounced lobulations. The thyroid as a whole was less vascular in the iodine-treated patients. The most striking change noted, however, was the clear, lymphlike fluid which fairly dripped from the cut surface. This was assumed to be the colloid secretion of the gland. The gland in patients who had not received iodine was more vascular and on section gave the typical beefsteak appearance characteristic of Graves's disease. Rienhoff compared the histological changes in fifteen cases in which no iodine had been given with an equal number in which it had been used. The striking difference in the histological structure of the gland was at once apparent, but because of the varied histological picture that one may encounter in such cases, he felt it important to compare the histological structure of the same gland before and after the administration of iodine. The results of this study were published in a classic paper entitled "The Histological Changes Brought About in Cases of Exophthalmic Goiter by the Administration of Iodine." In each of the three typical cases of exophthalmic goiter, the basal metabolic rate was above 50. In each case under local anesthesia, the right upper pole of the thyroid gland was excised. The patient was then given Lugol's solution. Striking clinical improvement followed, and there was a precipitous drop in the basal metabolic rate. The gland was then removed at a later operation and examined. The most evident changes produced by iodine were an increase in the gross size and appearance of the thyroid gland and a decrease in the vascularity of the gland; a marked increase in the amount of colloid present; the presence of small tumefactions resembling beginning adenomata; and a change to a flat cuboidal epithelium. A comparison of this type of epithelium with the high columnar type present before the administration of iodine was striking. The papillomatous ingrowths of epithelium had been to a great extent mechanically flattened and uncurled by the increased intraacinar pressure as a result of the accumulation of colloid. For this reason the acini had become more normal in appearance, being regular in form and size, and the walls were smooth and even rather than irregular. Thus, Rienhoff demonstrated for the first time that in patients treated with iodine who have shown marked clinical improvement accompanied by a fall in the basal metabolic rate, there is a change in the histological structure of the gland from classical hyperplasia to a more colloid or less active state, approximating an inactive colloid goiter or a normal gland.

Another important contribution was the paper by Rienhoff and Dean Lewis entitled "Relation of Hyperthyroidism to Benign Tumors of the Thyroid Gland." This study of the involutional changes occurring in the thyroid glands of patients with exophthalmic goiter who were undergoing an iodine remission revealed striking similarities to the histological picture encountered in nodular goiter. It was shown that a clinically typical case of exophthalmic goiter associated with diffuse, smooth enlargement of the thyroid gland due to hypertrophy and hyperplasia of the parenchyma could give rise to a nodular goiter as a result of involutional changes in the thyroid concomitant with an artificial or spontaneous remission. These nodules or involutional bodies are not neoplasms but merely regressive sequelae of a previous hypertrophy and hyperplasia of the parenchyma. Their number and size depend on the number of remissions and the exacerbations in that gland.

Rienhoff also made many significant contributions to thoracic surgery. In July 1933, while operating on a three-year-old child with a fibrosarcoma of the lung, he introduced a new technical procedure. He opened the mediastinum transpleurally, isolating the intramediastinal branch of the right pulmonary artery, the upper and lower pulmonary veins, and the main bronchus. He ligated the three blood vessels separately, and after resecting the lung was able to close the stump of the right main bronchus by a single suture. He secured against air leak by oversewing the mediastinal pleura on the stump. Because the closure of the bronchus appeared safe, he did not drain the pleural cavity. The operation was a complete success, with no complications in the postoperative course. This technique removed the final bar to resection of the lung. Dissection of the hilar structures became the accepted technique for lobectomy and later made segmental resection possible. Rienhoff was also the first to emphasize that a concomitant thoracoplasty was unnecessary.

Rienhoff was born in Springfield, Missouri, on October 10, 1894. He graduated from Cornell University in 1915 and from the Johns Hopkins School of Medicine in 1919. Having stood academically in the first fourth in his class, he was awarded an internship in the Johns Hopkins Hospital. He began his intern year under the temporary chief, Hamman, but when Thayer returned from Europe, Rienhoff was assigned as his special intern. Following this year in medicine, Rienhoff transferred to surgery, serving as intern, assistant resident, and finally, from 1923 to 1925, as resident in surgery. He was Halsted's last resident.

After completing his surgical training under J. M. T. Finney, Rienhoff entered practice in Baltimore. Since that time he has been a member of the faculty of the Johns Hopkins School of Medicine, having advanced to the rank of professor. He is a member of all of the prominent surgical societies, including the American Surgical Association, Southern Surgical Association, and the German society Deutsche Gesellschaft für Chirugie (the first Hopkins member after Dr. Halsted). He is also a Foreign Fellow of the Royal College of Surgeons of London. In 1923 he married Frances Young, the daughter of Hugh Hampton Young, director of the Division of Urology. Two of his sons, William F. Rienhoff III and MacCallum Rienhoff, are graduates of the Johns Hopkins School of Medicine.

John Eager Howard

In 1889 Jonathan Hutchinson, an astute physician and surgeon, expressed his belief that all patients with thyrotoxicosis would have spontaneous remissions sooner or later and that subsequent relapse would not occur. Hutchinson's ideas were ingrained in Dr. John Eager Howard by his early clinical exposure to Dr. J. Howard Means and Dr. Warfield Longcope, who also felt that nearly all patients with thyrotoxicosis would have a spontaneous remission of their disease if given the time.

When in the 1940s, Astwood introduced the thiourea derivatives, he ushered in a new era in the management of thyrotoxicosis. Because of their capacity to inhibit proper utilization of iodine by the thyroid gland, these agents prevent chemical completion of the hormonal molecules and production of thyroid hormones is brought to a halt. The use of one of these blocking agents, became the first avenue of therapy even when some subsequent procedure such as surgery or radioiodine treatment was planned. It was soon found that after thyrotoxicosis had been controlled by such agents for six months to a year and the drug then withdrawn, there was recurrence of the disorder within a few months in about half the cases. This held true whether the drug was withdrawn gradually or abruptly and whether the patient had become distinctly hypothyroid during treatment or not. The most significant fact was that half of the patients did not have a relapse. It seemed likely to Dr. Howard that the blocking agents simply provided the time already alluded to, first by Hutchinson and later by Means and Longcope, for a true spontaneous remission to occur, and that after thiourea the remissions which persisted were in reality spontaneous and in no wise dependent on any specific activity of the drug. Based on this philosophy, Howard concluded that one approach to the therapy of thyrotoxicosis would be to control the disease, for a lifetime if need be, with a drug such as propylthiouracil until spontaneous remission occurred. Others had applied this method with success in a few patients for a number of years by lowering the dose of the drug when hypothyroidism occurred and raising it with the reappearance of hyperthyroidism. However, Howard found that he was unable to steer so nicely between Scylla and Charybdis and his patients seemed to fluctuate between the discomforts of too much or too little circulating thyroid hormones.

To overcome this dilemma, he decided to block completely production of the patient's own hormone with full thiourea dosage, and once this was achieved, to administer thyroid gradually to full replacement dosage, maintaining continuous administration of the blocking drug. This regimen kept the patient in a steady state of euthyroidism. It soon proved so successful in providing the status of well-being that many patients were reluctant to determine whether or not a spontaneous remission had occurred. Dr. Howard then faced the question of how would one determine this. The most obvious way was simply to withdraw the blocking agent and continue the thyroid hormone. If remission were not present, the combined quantity of endogenously made thyroid hormone and that which was given orally would soon produce clear signs of thyrotoxicosis. If the patient became aware of recurrence of symptoms, then one simply stopped thyroid therapy and reinstituted the program, just as when the patient was first seen. Using such a procedure, the proposed scheme of therapy could be carried out by a skilled clinician without resort to any laboratory procedures at all. However, to obtain a closer guide to the presence or absence of what Hutchinson called "a well-established recovery," Howard employed the following test: the blocking agent is withdrawn (administration of thyroid being continued) and five days later a radioiodine tracer test of uptake by the thyroid gland is performed. The theory is that if complete remission is present, there will be minimal uptake of iodine, just as if a healthy subject had been given full replacement doses of thyroid over an extended time. When the physician is convinced of the presence of a spontaneous remission, the thyroid blocking agent is withdrawn, but, an important feature of the regimen, full thyroid hormone replacement is continued. Should such replacement not be continued, the normal thyroid axis would be called into play, thyrotropin would again be released by the pituitary and the thyroid gland thus stimulated to produce the required amount of hormone. It seemed a better policy not to reawaken the axis, and simply to provide optimal thyroid hormone exogenously—a simple procedure of taking one pill each day. More important than any theoretical consideration was the success in his own patients. The presence or absence of exophthalmos accompanying the thyrotoxicosis has not affected choice in the use of regimen which has been discussed. In Howard's experience no patient has manifested progression of the ocular disorder since therapy started.

Jonas Stein Friedenwald

JONAS STEIN FRIEDENWALD was born in Baltimore on June 1, 1897. He was
the son of Harry Friedenwald, a distinguished ophthalmologist, scholar, and
historian, and the grandson of Aaron Friedenwald, whose name is prominent in
Maryland medical annals. Thus it was Jonas Friedenwald's rich heritage to be a
member of a proud and aristocratic Jewish family, fully dedicated to science
and scholarship, with a great sense of pride in the traditions of its people and
an impressive sense of personal honor and integrity. He received his education
at the Johns Hopkins University and was awarded the M.D. degree in 1920.
While serving for one year as a medical house officer, he met and married a
Hopkins nurse, Mary Louise Sherwin. Following this year in medicine, he
studied ophthalmic pathology under Dr. Frederick Verhoeff at Harvard, where
he received his M.A. degree.

From 1922 to 1923 he studied clinical ophthalmology under George E.
DeSchweinitz in Philadelphia, then he returned to Baltimore to begin the practice of ophthalmology with his father. On the surface his training might appear
to have been rather scanty for a career in either research or practice. However,
Jonas Friedenwald possessed an amazing brilliance and capacity for assimila-
tion. Not only was he a young man extraordinarily well trained for a career in
research and practice when he returned to Baltimore, but his accomplishments
were greatly enhanced by the tutelage which his talented father provided for
him in the field of ophthalmic surgery.

In 1923 he joined the pathology service at the Johns Hopkins Hospital
under Dr. William G. MacCallum and was placed in charge of ophthalmic
pathology. When the Wilmer Institute was founded in 1925, he became a
member of the clinical staff and was responsible for the pathology laboratory
and for instruction in ophthalmic pathology. He advanced rapidly through the
various academic grades, being appointed associate professor in 1931. Undoubtedly, he would have been appointed professor, but at that time only one
professorship was allowed in each department. One of the most impressive
tributes to this extraordinary man was that paid by Alan Woods. For thirty-two
years they were closely associated in the Wilmer Institute, and during the first
eight of those years, they worked side by side under the leadership of Dr.
William H. Wilmer. In 1933 Alan Woods was appointed chairman of the

department, a position which, he pointed out, could equally as well have been given on the basis of qualifications to Jonas Friedenwald. Woods, in fact, felt that Friedenwald was probably better qualified and would have filled the position with the greatest possible distinction. Woods also said that if failure to achieve this position was a personal disappointment to Friedenwald, he never showed it by work or by deed. During the twenty-two years of Woods's chairmanship, he proved a loyal friend, a faithful adviser, and a stimulating colleague.

During his career in the Wilmer Institute, Jonas Friedenwald inspired and trained innumerable young students, and was always at their disposal to talk about their pursuits and their goals. He could always be counted on to ferret out the basic problem and to solve the difficulties connected with it. Further, he carried on extensive basic scientific and clinical investigations, making impressive contributions in both areas. Because of his enormous fund of knowledge and experience, he was eagerly sought out by students, residents, clinicians, and investigators in a variety of fields at Johns Hopkins and throughout the country.

Friedenwald was at home in many areas of basic science. While his principal interest lay in pathology, he continually kept abreast of new developments in physics, mathematics, and chemistry. The latter interest is reflected in one of his most classic contributions. In 1929, at the Thirteenth International Congress of Ophthalmology in Amsterdam, Friedenwald gave the first report on his studies on the nature of glaucoma, in a presentation entitled "The Pathogenesis of Acute Glaucoma." In this paper he established, for the first time, the role of edema of the ciliary body in the pathogenesis of acute glaucoma and the regular association of ciliary edema, hemorrhagic, serous, and fibrinous extravasations with a rapid rise in ocular tension. As evaluated by Alan Woods, this study marked a milestone in his scientific career, since it initiated his entry into fundamental basic scientific investigation.

It later turned out that the changes in the ciliary body were the result, rather than the cause, of acute glaucoma, but this does not detract from the total impact of his contributions to the study of this disease. It was subsequently shown that acute congestive glaucoma is due to a pupillary block whereby aqueous humor cannot flow freely from the posterior chamber through the pupillary area because the iris is sufficiently in contact with the lens to cause an increased pressure in the posterior chamber, which then bows the periphery of the iris forward and brings it in contact with Schlemm's canal. There is an anatomical basis for this in that patients with this disease usually have a small corneal diameter and relatively shallow anterior chamber.

Continuing research in this field was destined to make Friedenwald internationally famous. The series of studies which followed began with an investigation of the mechanics of the circulation of the aqueous humor—the clear fluid which is constantly secreted into the anterior chamber of the eye through a complicated arrangement of channels and veins at the angle of the chamber. From here his studies proceeded to the formation of the aqueous; to the permeability of the ciliary body; to the dynamic factors which influence the secretion both of fluids and of colloids; to enzymatic oxidations and such various factors as ascorbic acid, epinephrine, cytocrome C, and cholinesterase, all of which play a role in mediating the passage of fluid across the ciliary-aqueous barrier. These studies were followed by one on Schlemm's canal and the factors which control and influence reabsorption of the fluid. These various studies formed the subject of his famous Proctor Award lecture in 1949 entitled "The Formation of the Intraocular Fluid." As pointed out by Dr. Thomas Maren in 1974, the original ideas expressed by Friedenwald in this lecture on bicarbonate formation in aqueous humor, its mechanism and relation to the treatment of glaucoma, have not only survived, but as a result of this man's intuitive genius, now constitute the basis for the understanding of the chemistry of aqueous humor secretion, the relations between ion transport and flow, and for the treatment of glaucoma with carbonic anhydrase inhibitors.

The basic concept put forth by Friedenwald in the Proctor lecture was that the ciliary process uses oxidative energy to separate protons and electrons at boundaries within cells. This produces an accumulation of hydrogen ions at one boundary and hydroxyl at the other. With the buffering of hydroxyl ions by carbon dioxide, bicarbonate is formed, balanced by sodium at the boundary, which he identified as the epithelial or secretory one. Others had postulated some of these ideas, but Friedenwald put them into perspective for an important secretory fluid which had previously never been considered in this light. As Maren emphasizes, this took imagination and courage, since the aqueous humor appeared at that time to be a neutral secretion. Friedenwald had no evidence that he was dealing with a fluid rich in sodium bicarbonate, although he recognized that other secretory organs do produce such a fluid. In the ensuing years an array of new investigations, many of which were encouraged by Friedenwald, clearly showed that his theoretical analysis was in fact correct. In chronological order these developments were: (1) finding bicarbonate excess in the posterior and anterior chambers of the rabbit eye; (2) demonstration of carbonic anhydrase in the ciliary process; (3) the development of powerful carbonic anhydrase inhibitors and the demonstration that these inhibitors (a) reduce the flow of aqueous fluid, (b) reduce pressure in the eye, (c) reduce the concentration of bicarbonate in the posterior aqueous of the rabbit eye and (d) control glaucoma in many patients. Just two years before he died, Friedenwald had the great satisfaction of reviewing in his modest way this extraordinary series of events, and in this last paper he showed, among other things, the relation between enzyme inhibition and physiological effect.

As so often occurs, recognition of the magnitude of his contribution came slowly, as there were certain gray areas about which there was reasonable controversy. Now these have been cleared up, and there can be no doubt that Jonas Friedenwald's contribution was fundamental to the understanding of the formation of aqueous humor and helped open the way for a more effective treatment of glaucoma.

At the time of his death in 1956, Jonas Friedenwald was still actively engaged in further investigations of this problem. He would be, as pointed out by Alan Woods, the first to admit that the complex problem of chronic glaucoma, which causes a high percentage of the world's blindness, is not yet solved; but through Friedenwald's effort, a long segment of the road toward this goal has been traversed. When the pathogenesis of chronic glaucoma is finally resolved, undoubtedly the solution will rest largely on the foundations laid down by Jonas Friedenwald.

Friedenwald's fertile mind addressed itself to many other problems in ophthalmology. In 1943 he became interested, as a part of the war effort, in wound healing. His investigations involved a technique for study of the mitotic activity during cell division, or cell division and regeneration of the corneal epithelium. During the war years almost all of the research facilities of the Wilmer Institute were devoted to the study of war gases, since one of the most important effects of the war gases of that era were on the eye. Friedenwald, a great humanitarian, was in charge of this investigation, much of which was classified. At the end of the war, however, seventeen of these studies were released and published in a single volume. War gases, fortunately, were never used, but swords can be turned into plowshares, and the information which came from Friedenwald's studies yielded basic data on the metabolism of the cornea and formed the basis for further studies on wound healing.

During the last decade of his life, Friedenwald's investigations were concerned more and more with enzymes and histochemistry. As indicated, whenever he became involved in any research endeavor, he acquired the basic knowledge necessary to occupy a position of leadership in that area. Characteristically, therefore, he developed an amazing knowledge of the phases of chemistry involved in these new projects, and as one distinguished professor in the medical school said: "This is a most phenomenal spectacle—an ophthalmologist is our foremost authority and most distinguished scholar in the field of histochemistry." Illustrative of this phase of his research career are the numerous papers concerned with the histochemical localization of cholinesterase in ocular tissues done in collaboration with George B. Koelle.

The ophthalmologist sees a particular type of exudate or hemorrhage in the retina either ophthalmoscopically or histologically, but the precise point in the vascular tree from which the exudation or hemorrhage arose usually escapes him. Even when he reconstructs in serial sections the neighborhood of a lesion, he can rarely be sure of the interrelationships. This question concerned Jonas Friedenwald, and he searched for suitable techniques with which he could visualize the blood vessel wall in preparations of whole unsectioned retina, believing that interesting relationships might emerge into view. In his Jackson Memorial Lecture, entitled "A New Approach to Some Problems of Retinal Vascular Disease," he describes how by good fortune a suitable technique became available and relates some of the fruits of its application. Friedenwald attempts to portray some of the excitement that he and his colleagues experienced during this study, which started as a routine systematic survey, not primarily directed toward retinal vascular disease. In the previous twenty years there had been a steady unfolding of techniques in the field of histochemistry—that is, techniques by which specific chemical components of the cells and tissues could be recognized in histological sections. The field had been given a more or less definitive pattern by the systematic studies of Wislocki and his colleagues at Harvard. They had applied these techniques to one tissue after another, but had not included the eye.

The first technique that Friedenwald chose was one for the demonstration of fixed carbohydrate that had recently been refined by Hotchkiss and Mc-Manus. The application of this technique to ocular tissues revealed many points of interest, particularly in the retina. The internal limiting membrane stained brilliantly, showing that this structure was a definite entity. Particularly striking in the retina was the fact that the endothelium of the whole vascular tree (arteries, capillaries, and veins) is surrounded by a brilliantly stained basement membrane. The presence of this vascular basement membrane can be recognized in other tissues; the existence of a capillary basement membrane in the kidney glomerulus is well known. Since the parenchyma of the retina normally contains no other structures that stain with this technique, it seemed possible that one might use it to obtain a view of the whole retinal vascular pattern in unsectioned flat preparations of the whole thickness of the retina. The modifications in the histological technique required to accomplish this purpose were worked out in Friedenwald's laboratory by Dr. Bernard Becker, and the applications of this technique in various pathological problems was pursued with Dr. Robert Day. Previously Dr. Friedenwald had reported that in the retinal lesions in diabetic retinopathy some of the small red spots observed ophthalmoscopically were not petechial hemorrhages, as they appear to be, but are actually small capillary aneurysms which could be recognized as such in serial sections.

Flat preparations of the diabetic retina showed great numbers of capillary aneurysms. These aneurysms always have both an afferent and an efferent connection and are therefore true aneurysmal dilatations, not endothelialized petechiae, which would be connected to the vascular tree by a single channel. Very commonly there is a cluster of exudates in the retina surrounding the aneurysms; thus, the majority of the exudates do seem to arise by leakage of plasma from the aneurysmal wall. Frequently there are also frank hemorrhages in the tissue adjacent to the aneurysms.

Friedenwald pointed out that in 1936 Kimmelstiel and Wilson described a form of intercapillary glomerular sclerosis which they believed to be characteristic of diabetic nephropathy. When kidney sections showing these lesions are stained for carbohydrate, the characteristic hyaline nodules stain intensely red, being similar in appearance to the thickened walls of the retinal capillary aneurysms. It was subsequently shown that the lesions in the kidney and the capillary aneurysms in the retina were in fact manifestations of the same vascular process which were found also in other areas.

Rich, Berthrong and Bennet discovered that renal lesions resembling those of the Kimmelstiel-Wilson nephropathy could be produced in the rabbit in a period of two to three weeks by the administration of 7.5 milligrams of cortisone daily. Friedenwald and Becker found that alloxan diabetes in rabbits predisposes these animals to the capillary lesion elicited by cortisone. On the basis of this and other evidence they speculated on the nature of the retinopathy. Friedenwald believed that the whole complex of symptoms, complications, and sequelae of diabetes might not be simply and directly related to the pancreatic dysfunction and the diminished insulin effect. In this respect, he was well ahead of his time.

Jonas Friedenwald's studies of various aspects of ophthalmic pathology are too numerous to catalogue in this chapter. These studies culminated in the *Atlas of Ophthalmic Pathology*, which was published by the American Academy of Ophthalmology and Otolaryngology and the Armed Forces Institute of Pathology. His continuing interest in mathematics and physics was constantly reflected not only in the directions of his scientific work, but also in practical day-by-day accomplishments. He served as chairman of the Committee on Tonometry and was largely responsible for the present standardization of tonometers and for many refinements and advances in their practical use. As early as 1924, he produced a new astigmatic chart and initiated explorations into the possible use of yellow-green light in ophthalmoscopy. These early investigations eventually culminated in the design of the famous Friedenwald slit-lamp ophthalmoscope in 1932.

Jonas Friedenwald, with his brilliant mind and wide range of interests, cultivated friendships with many important people, none of which was perhaps more important to him than that of Justice Felix Frankfurter's. When Jonas went to Boston to study, Frankfurter was then a member of the Harvard law faculty. Having known Friedenwald's father because of their common interest in Zionism, Frankfurter was introduced to young Jonas, who already had his medical degree and had, in addition, pursued basic mathematical studies at Columbia. Frankfurther learned that Jonas had previously come to the attention of the great Harvey Cushing, who quickly recognized the outstanding qualities of the budding young ophthalmologist. As a result, Cushing had asked him to make an eye examination of every patient in Cushing's neurosurgical ward at Peter Bent Brigham Hospital. Soon Frankfurter also learned that Jonas's talents far exceeded the boundaries of the medical sciences. In conversations with Frankfurter, Jonas probed deeply into the basic ideas of law and jurisprudence. They talked frequently, but Jonas kept after him for good reading matter. He wanted more than simple "fugitive talk." Frankfurter told him to read Holmes's *Common Law*, which is indeed rough going, not a book for the ordinary novice. Jonas not only read it but read it thoroughly, and Frankfurther remarked at the time: "This young doctor has asked me more embarrassing questions about some of Holmes's chapters than ever I was asked in dicussion about the book by colleagues of mine on the Harvard Law School faculty." And he emphasized that this was not a denigrating remark about the members of the Harvard law faculty.

The friendship with Frankfurter continued throughout Jonas's life and was marked by an exchange of letters which showed the depth and breadth of true scholarship. One incident is worth perpetuating. Frankfurter had always been troubled in trying to understand what is really meant by science. What constitutes science in any respectable use of the term? So he put the question to Jonas and received this answer, which is interrupted by Frankfurter's comments:

"Science is a social phenomenon. A scientific discovery does not become part of the body of science until it has been comprehended and confirmed by others. Even the most private scientific activity of the individual scientist must be based on the comprehension of what others have contributed. Consequently the language of science is as much a tool of scientific progress as any mechanical gadget which we use. If we allow that tool to be dulled, progress is slowed." (Frankfurter stated that it was almost impossible for him to imagine a more fruitful line of thinking than that statement opens up to the lawyer and judge, whose tools are words and nothing but words.) "This presents a continuing problem because the advance of knowledge results in the continuous change in the meaning of words." (A whole book on constitutional law could be written with that as the legend on the title page.) "When we succeed in inventing scientific words of enduring usefulness, we do so largely by naming the invariants we have discovered. In such case, the advancement of knowledge sharpens the denotation of our words and enriches their connotations. On the other hand, when we have not discovered the invariants and are forced to give names to evolving forms—such as sovereignty or senescence—" (think of combining, in one generalization, sovereignty and senescence!) "—progress of knowledge on social evolution may still enrich their connotations but unfortunately often shifts their denotations. If we ignore these shifts, we end up by talking incomprehensively, with rich connotations about an unspecified subject."

In another interesting conversation between the two, Friedenwald told Frankfurter a story that sheds light on his relaxed temper of mind. The justice had occasion to repeat to Friedenwald the cynicism of a friend about the medical profession. Friedenwald said that it reminded him of a minister who had come to see him recently suffering from eczema: "He had your friend's cynicism about the medical profession and said to me: 'After all these years of medical research I do not see why your profession has not found the cause of eczema.' I offered to bet him 10 to 1 that we would find the cause of eczema, before he found why the righteous suffered."

As pointed out by Abel Wolman, in spite of his broad and complex scientific interests and of the many contributions he made in his own country, he still had time to spread his abilities and interests abroad. Jonas Friedenwald was one of the prime movers in the establishment of a medical school in Israel. For twenty-five years he was at one time or another a member of the Board of Governors of the Hebrew University; of the Medical Reference Board, which had to do with developing the salient features of a medical school; of the development committee itself; chairman of the Subcommittee on Medical Education and of the Curriculum Committee; and in later years, a member of the Medical Advisory Board of the Hebrew University. The retinoscopy room of the Hadassah Hebrew University Medical Center in memory of Dr. Jonas Friedenwald is an indication of the tremendous gratitude of the faculty to him.

During his life Friedenwald received many honors, including the Research Medal of the American Medical Association in 1935; the Howe Medal of the American Ophthalmological Society in 1951, the first Proctor Award in 1949, as well as a host of other honors. He was an active member not only of the prestigious societies of ophthalmology, but also of the American Society for Clinical Investigation, an honor awarded to few in the field of ophthalmology. He also received the Donders Medal of the Dutch Ophthalmology Society in 1952. He was one of the editors of the *Archives of Ophthalmology* and the *Journal of Histochemistry and Cytochemistry*.

Curt Richter

Curt Richter was born and raised in Denver, Colorado. In his early years he worked in his father's structural steel and iron business, where he learned to run all of the machines. One of his main interests, when he was only five years old, was working at the forge—he had a real passion for beating hot iron into different shapes. After his father's death, in a hunting accident when Curt was eight years old, he spent six summers working on farms in northern Colorado, where he learned something that helped him all through his research career— patience. Early in his youth he developed a talent for measuring things, an aptitude he has carried on throughout his life. One occasion he remembers well: "My father and I had been out on a Sunday. When we returned he put two marks on a table and asked me to bisect the distance between them. I took one look and drew a line; I hit the exact center. That gave me a feeling that measuring things was something I had a talent for. Almost everything that I have done in research has involved some kind of measuring."

All through high school he was deeply involved in athletics—track, basketball, baseball, and skating. But he had no exposure to biology: "I can remember one time in high school, sort of degrading one of the boys I knew by saying, 'He takes biology.' I never had any formal training or experience in biology in the early years or, in fact, ever. When I graduated from high school, I followed a formula that had been left by my father. When I was quite young, he said we would go into business together and run his firm and that when I graduated from high school I would go to Dresden, Germany, to study engineering. He had a very high regard for German education." As soon as Curt graduated, he headed for Germany. He studied for three years at the engineering school in Dresden, which was the equivalent to the Massachusetts Institute of Technology in this country; and he had a wonderful time.

But then Richter's interests turned to other areas—he became absorbed with the opera, the theater, and literature—and before long he realized that he was somehow on the wrong track. When he returned from Germany after the first year and a half of World War I, he was certain he no longer wanted to be an engineer and went to Harvard to try his hand in a different field. Because of the years spent in Germany before and during the war, he decided to try international diplomacy, taking a course in this subject with Professor Wilson. The professor spent most of the class time quoting from Rudyard Kipling, and that ended Richter's interest.

He then tried economics, taking a course with Professor Taussig (Helen Taussig's father)—a special course with John Stuart Mill, David Ricardo, and Adam Smith. After about the fourth week in that course, he got a card from

Professor Taussig saying, "Mr. Richter, I don't think economics is your forte. I think you had better drop the course at once." He then gave up economics.

At that time he was also taking a course in the philosophy of nature, given by Professor Holt, which introduced him to psychoanalysis. The subject fascinated him, and he read almost everything that had been written by Freud and his disciples. Another course with Yerkes on animal behavior also interested him. He then had the good fortune to meet Professor Lawrence J. Henderson. "I don't know how we happened to get together, but he invited me very often to his home. We never talked about his studies on the blood, which I wouldn't have understood, but about general philosophy. What he had to say and the books he gave me to read had a great influence on me. I continued to visit frequently with him, almost up to the time of his death." After spending two years in the army during World War I, he decided to come to Johns Hopkins to work with John B. Watson, the behaviorist, who was then a member of the Department of Psychiatry.

He began to work with Watson in January 1919. His first morning on the job, Watson said to him: "I don't care what courses you take. As a matter of fact, you don't have to take any courses at all. All I care about is a good piece of research." That seemed like a wonderful plan to Richter, because he was a very poor classroom student. However, he did audit courses in anatomy and physiology, and studied neurology with Hal Thomas's father. He dissected a body in anatomy and did the laboratory experiments in physiology that he was interested in.

When I started with Watson, he assigned me a problem involving the study of learning in rats. I tried that for a little while, but it didn't interest me a bit. What did interest me was to see their activity erupt. The fact that they were active and why they were active excited my curiosity. This was my first experience with anything in biology; and it turned out to be a very lucky thing. Within two or three weeks after starting this research, I built cages myself which permitted the recording of the slightest movement of the rats. I found that they showed a very clear-cut, regular hour-and-a-half cycle. That further stimulated my interest, and opened the door to my continuing concern with periodic phenomena. At the same time, I found that rats, even when kept in constant darkness, still were inactive during the day and active in the night—showing the presence of an inherent diurnal clock. This was the first kindling of my studies on "biologic clocks." My early experience in the factory helped me a great deal in building my own apparatus and instruments, which I did consistently after that.

These studies, demonstrating the regular hour-and-a-half cycles and the inherent diurnal clock, were the basis of Richter's doctoral thesis. He has since published many papers on animal activity, and the subject is still one of his main research concerns.

Of his early education at Hopkins, Richter states:

The most important influence at that period was my relationship with Adolph Meyer, who was then director of the Phipps. John Watson only stayed at the Phipps for a year and a half after my arrival. He left for New York; I remained with Adolph Meyer. We became very close friends, and he had a great influence on my whole development. He had the same attitude that Watson had about the courses. He left it up to me as to what I did. He invited me to attend his staff rounds and to give some lectures. He also let me make records and work with patients. My education from that point on was largely through conversations. I saw a great deal of Professor William H. Howell, who helped me with my experiments, and I had many long talks with him. It was the same way with Dr. Herbert Spencer Jennings at the University. These were all chance encounters when we would meet in the library and talk for an hour or two. This did more for me than all the courses I could take. The same way with Professor John J. Abel; I spent many hours with him. He followed my experiments and was very helpful, as was Professor Andrews in the Biology Department at Homewood. Later on, influence of that kind came particularly from Elmer Mc-Collum of the School of Hygiene and Public Health. He took a great interest when I started my dietary self-selection studies. We were friends right up to the time of his death. I saw quite a good deal of W. G. MacCallum, mostly on an informal basis at the Maryland Club. Then there was Raymond Pearl, who was a close friend, and Dr. E. A. Park, who had a great influence on my work. I didn't see him much in the early years, but during the last twenty years, I visited with him regularly. I had many collaborators in the early days. Frank Ford and I published a number of papers; George Wislocki was a close friend, and we published a lot of papers together. Marion Hines, Sarah Tower, Carl Hartman, and Orthello Langworthy were co-workers, and I had a good many medical students who worked with me. I was lucky with having this freedom with Watson and with Adolph Meyer. I was lucky again when I went to the Institute for Advanced Studies in Princeton later on. When Oppenheimer greeted me, he asked me to sign the register at the institute. After this was done he said, 'Well, Curt, you've now fulfilled all of the obligations to the institute. You're on your own from now on.' Of course, the university at Hopkins, right from the beginning, gave me a very free hand. The fact is, I have never attended a single committee meeting.

Dr. Meyer turned over Watson's laboratory on the third floor of the Phipps to me, which he called the "psychobiology laboratory." This was a name he coined himself, and it has become widely used. My first studies were on spontaneous activity —what it is that makes an animal active and how can it be made more active or less active.

One part of this study dealt with the role played by the endocrine glands. Effects produced on spontaneous running activity in revolving drums by removal of the various endocrine glands was determined; likewise the effects of replacement therapy.

It was found that all of the endocrine glands have some influence in the control of activity, the hypophysis playing by far the most important part. The adrenals have a more important role in the wild Norway rats, who have such large adrenals; while the gonads definitely play the most important part in the domesticated rats, whose sex glands develop sooner.

The prefrontal cortex of the brain, the tip of the striatum, and particularly cortical area 9 in monkeys have an important part in the control of activity. After unilateral or bilateral removal of area 9, Dr. Marion Hines and Richter showed that monkeys become extremely active. With Hawkes and Langworthy, it was shown that removal of the frontal poles in rats and cats also results in greatly increased activity.

Over the years Richter has produced a great variety of periodic phenomena in animals by interferences with the endocrine glands or brain, by diet or by treatment with drugs. He has long been working on a collection of case histories of normal individuals and psychiatric patients who show various periodic disturbances. The main objective was to reproduce in animals cyclic changes found in man. One cycle produced by interference with the thyroid gland of rats, for example, very closely resembled the behavior of catatonic schizophrenics. Richter found that the twenty-four-hour and yearly cycles found in animals are definitely nonhomeostatic. They are independent of all external and internal disturbances, which, of course, makes these two cycles such reliable timing devices.

Another line of interest developed from Richter's fascination with the string galvanometer—an instrument which Dr. Meyer had purchased for Stanley Cobb, who had been in charge before Richter's arrival. Richter first used this instrument to study the psychogalvanic reflex:

I took my first record on Frank Ford, and it was really an amazing sight for both of us to see the changes that occurred with emotional stimulation. We used the string galvanometer for studies on the psychogalvanic reflexes of Phipps patients. Later on it was used to study electrical skin resistance, and extraordinary differences were found between various types of patients. Some patients had very active responses; many, none at all. After testing over thirty patients it became clear that most of the differences in galvanic responses depended on differences in the electrical resistance of the skin.

Richter then began to measure resistance of the skin in Phipps patients. This opened up a new field of research that has had the widest ramifications in the study of almost all functions of the body and personality. In a study of over three hundred Phipps patients and one hundred normals it was found that electrical skin resistance readings of patients extended far below the lowest levels of normals and far above the upper limits of normals; also that the skin resistance levels varied with the type of psychiatric illness.

Studies were then started to determine the physiological, neurological, and physical factors on which electrical skin resistance depends. For this study he used cats and monkeys, largely because of the porous nature of the pads of the feet and palmar surfaces of the hands. These studies lasted about ten years. New instruments, electrodes and techniques were designed to measure resistance of the skin on all parts of the body. Patients from almost all departments of the hospital, but mainly surgery and medicine, were used in the studies.

Areas of skin denervated by sympathectomy, peripheral nerve lesions, or spinal cord transections could be mapped to the sharpest borders; various types of peripheral vascular disease gave characteristic patterns; and areas of abnormal sweating could be accurately defined. Characteristic patterns were found in essential hypertension and various other specific clinical conditions. Of the greatest interest was the demonstration that areas of pain resulting from pressure on or irritation of nerves or referred from internal organs showed up very clearly in the electrical skin resistance patterns on the surface of the body.

One of Richter's first papers on this subject showed the great changes in skin resistance that occur during normal sleep. Later studies revealed that patients with various types of pathological sleep, particularly narcolepsy, have characteristic patterns. The skin resistance test was used for detecting the presence of lung tumors, particularly of the Pancoast type. He also showed Dr. John Bordley and Dr. George Hardy how the galvanic skin response in a simple conditioning process could be used for testing hearing in infants and children.

During World War II, Richter mapped peripheral nerve lesions on over six hundred soldiers in Walter Reed Hospital and on many patients who had had thoracoplasty operations. During the great attack in the 1940s on hyper-tension with surgical sympathectomy at all levels, Richter examined over two thousand patients at the Hopkins and at three other hospitals—in Boston, Ann Arbor, and Durham. Data obtained from these patients made it possible to construct a dermatome chart based on objective data rather than on results of sensory tests.

Another productive line of work came from an early study on alcohol initiated by Raymond Pearl. Richter found that when rats are given an 8 percent, 16 percent, or 24 percent solution of alcohol, they will reduce their intake of food by exactly the number of calories they are getting from the alcohol. This gave him the idea that animals have an inherent mechanism for regulating their dietary needs. When he heard about the control of the adrenals over salt metabolism, he decided to see what effect adrenalectomy would have on the appetite for salt. Sometimes within hours and certainly within a day after adrenalectomy, the animals began drinking large amounts of salt solution and kept themselves alive. These experiments showed that homeostasis for salt is maintained by (1) a physiological regulator (cortical secretion) and (2) a behavior regulator (voluntary intake of salt solution). These observations were then extended to many other instances of homeostasis, including the metab-olism of calcium by secretion from the parathyroid glands. Extensive studies were also made on dietary selections during pregnancy and lactation. Richter's paper with Lawson Wilkins on the greatly increased salt intake of a child with an adrenal tumor is one of the most interesting instances of self-selection in man.

When Richter first began reading about nutrition, he noted that most of the studies were made on whole diets or diets made up of a variety of foodstuffs including fats, proteins, carbohydrates, vitamins, and minerals. It seemed very difficult to draw any conclusions about the nutritive value of any one foodstuff. He and Dr. Emmett Holt decided to study diets consisting of a single food-stuff—a fat, protein or carbohydrate—to learn how long a rat of a standard age and weight could live on a single food, how active it could be, how much it would eat. Then a single mineral or a single vitamin was added for choice. For example, on dextrose alone rats survived thirty-six days on the average; when given access to a vitamin B_1 solution they lived twice as long—seventy-six days. Foods found in this way to have the best nutritive value were ultimately used in experiments in which rats were offered access to a variety of substances in separate containers. In one of the last experiments, they offered rats a choice of twenty purified foodstuffs in separate containers, including one fat, one protein, one carbohydrate, five mineral solutions, and six vitamin solutions. That the rats made good choices from this selection of purified foodstuffs was shown by the fact that they not only survived but grew, mated, and reproduced. But that their selections still lacked at least one nutritive substance was shown by the fact that none of the mothers succeeded in nursing the babies.

An outgrowth of these studies was an interest in the mechanism of taste. The studies on thiourea and its derivatives started with the observation that phenylthiourea (PTU), which had already been widely used in taste tests on human subjects, was highly toxic to rats. A small amount on the end of a toothpick sufficed to kill a rat. Field tests made to determine whether PTU could be used as a rat poison were negative. Rats could taste it. With the help of the DuPont Company, a search was made for thiourea compounds that had the same high toxicity as PTU but no taste. Hundreds of compounds were tested. Alpha-naphthyl thiourea, later called ANTU+, was found to be highly toxic with only the faintest taste. It had excellent results in the field and was finally used in a city-wide experimental rat-control campaign in Baltimore. The Office of Scientific Research and Development of the National Academy of Sciences financed this research on the development of a quick method of ridding a large city of rats in case the Axis powers (during World War II) started rat-borne germ warfare. After it was found that rats rarely leave their own block, the campaign was worked out on a block basis. Air-raid wardens for each block supervised the rat control campaign for their block. This operation involved the entire city, and over a million dead rats were recovered on the surface of the ground; large numbers had died in their burrows.

Much was learned in this way about the behavior of the wild Norway rat. Richter states:

Not long after our start on the Baltimore rat campaign and after we had trapped several hundred wild rats for laboratory studies, it became clear to me that the Norway rat offers a great opportunity for the study of the effects of domestication. With our trapping methods, thousands of wild rats became available to compare with domesticated rats. Studies were made of anatomy, physiology, pharmacology, reactions to drugs and behavior. Many differences in all categories were found. Some of the most interesting concerned the endocrine glands, particularly the adrenals, thyroids, pituitaries, and gonads.

With the wild rats Richter made a number of studies on stress and some incidental studies on the effect of the "sudden death reaction" of animals. Jars in which the animal was forced to swim continuously were designed to obtain a measure of fatigue and the effects of stress in domesticated and wild Norway rats. Jet pressure and water temperature were controlled. At 95 degrees F. and a 3-pound jet pressure, domesticated rats swam as long as forty to sixty hours, but wild rats (trapped from the streets) when placed in the jars violently examined the swimming jars from top to bottom for an avenue of escape.

When not finding one, they consistently died in eight to ten minutes. This sudden death was described as death by hopelessness, and was brought into relation with observations made by Walter Cannon on effects produced by bone pointing in wild natives in different parts of the world.

Another of Richter's interests was stimulated by John B. Watson, who was working on the grasp reflex of newborn infants. After Watson left Hopkins, Richter decided to investigate this reflex himself. With his interest in measuring, he decided to put the study on a quantitative basis. Watson had simply placed a pencil in the hand of the infant and then lifted it up suddenly, letting it hang. Richter worked out a set of parallel bars that small babies could grasp. Then he released them when they had their fingers around the bar. When they let go of the bar, they fell into a net. He obtained exact measurements of the "hanging time" of about one hundred babies and followed the development of the reflex with age. A parallel study was made on the grasp reflex of newborn rhesus monkeys. These studies were continued over long periods, with special interest in the changes that occurred from reflex to voluntary hanging; comparisons were made between action currents from forearm muscles. Studies were made of the "hanging times" in the earlier stages of voluntary hanging on children still in kindergarten up to the college period. A simple method was devised for determining what part of voluntary hanging depends on the grasp reflex—to what extent voluntary hanging depends on ability of the subject to release the grasp reflex. This study revealed interesting differences between individuals, particularly on patients with various types of psychiatric disease.

It was also found that bulbocapnine, a drug that elicits catelepsy in various animals, particularly in the rhesus monkeys, elicits the grasp reflex. The presence and strength of the reflex (hanging time) can be used to study the cataleptic effect produced by bulbocapnine. The grasp reflex was also used to measure effects produced on bulbocapnine catelepsy by various counteracting drugs. A study made with Dr. Marion Hines showed that removal of cortical area 6 in rhesus monkeys brings out the reflex.

Most of Richter's research has been concerned directly or indirectly with the nervous system, but some research in neurology was carried on more or less for its own sake: studies on the alligator brain with Dr. Charles Bagley; studies on decerebrate rigidity of the sloth with Dr. Leo Bartemeier; studies on the oculocardiac reflex of rabbits with Drs. Gillespie and Wang; electromyographic studies with Dr. Frank Ford on various types of spinal cord lesions; quill mechanism and motor cortex studies of the porcupine with Dr. Langworthy; conformation of the third ventricle with Dr. John Benjamin; comparison of Weigert-stained sections with unfixed unstained sections for study of myelin sheaths of the rat with C. Warner.

Over the years Richter worked out many different operations on the Norway rat—now over forty operations on the endocrine glands, almost all of the internal organs and the brain. These were all operations that were used in one of his experiments. The illustrations of these operations were prepared in collaboration with the medical artist P. D. Malone, one of Max Broedel's most talented students, now chief artist at the Lahey Clinic in Boston. These drawings, all made with the Broedel technique, are not only accurate in every detail but are beautiful to look at. They will be published soon in a book entitled *Experimental Surgery of the Rat*.

I think that covers in a very rough way the work that I have carried on. It may seem somewhat unrelated, but many of these studies overlapped in one way or another, so that they are not as independent as they might appear. A number of years ago, the first time I began to look at what I had done and the direction in which I was going, I found some consolation in a statement that was made by Magendie to Claude Bernard about his life: "Everyone compares himself to something more or less majestic in his own sphere, to Archimedes, Michelangelo, Galileo, Descartes, and so on. Louis XIV compared himself to the sun. I am much more humble; I compare myself to a scavenger. With my hook in my hand and my pack on my back I go about the domain of science picking up what I can find" (J. M. D. Olmsted: *Claude Bernard, Physiologist*, 1938).

The versatility of Curt Richter as an investigator is well described in the characterization by M. Brewster Smith, professor and chairman of the Department of Psychology of the University of Chicago, made when Richter was presented for the degree of Doctor of Science at that institution: "Distinguished researcher and teacher, whose persisting interests in the biological mechanisms of behavior led to simple, ingenious and elegant experiments and to multiple discoveries important to both psychology and biology."

Another remarkable tribute to his talents as an investigator was made to the author under rather unusual circumstances. During World War II, I met Sir McFarlane Burnet, the Nobel laureate from Australia, while he was making a consultant visit to the combat zone in New Guinea. When I told him I was from Johns Hopkins his eyes lighted up and he began to describe to me in glowing tones the very stimulating research scientist he had met in Baltimore— the scientist who had impressed him more than any other in his extensive visit to research laboratories in the United States because of his originality, ingenious approach to his experiments, and the breadth of his work—Curt Richter.

Curt Richter has received many honors in his long and distinguished career. He is a member of the National Academy of Sciences, the American Philosophical Society, and the American Academy of Arts and Sciences. He was awarded an honorary LL.D. degree in 1970 by the Johns Hopkins University. He has been honored with many distinguished lectureships, including that of the Harvey Society, The Gregory Society, Percival Bailey, and Samuel W. Hamilton. He holds the title of Professor Emeritus of Psychobiology and was honorary co-chairman (with E. A. Adolph) of the International Commission for the Study of Hunger and Thirst, Jerusalem, 1974.

George W. Thorn

A number of investigators at Johns Hopkins have contributed importantly to our knowledge of the adrenal glands and their function. In an earlier chapter mention was made of the communication of William Osler on "Six Cases of

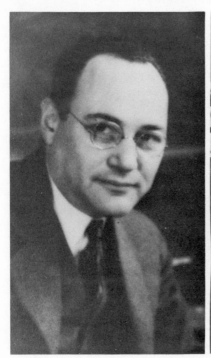

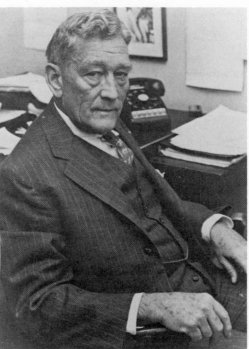

Jonas Friedenwald
Courtesy of the Library of the Wilmer
Institute

John Eager Howard
From *Johns Hopkins Med. J.* 131 (1972): 79

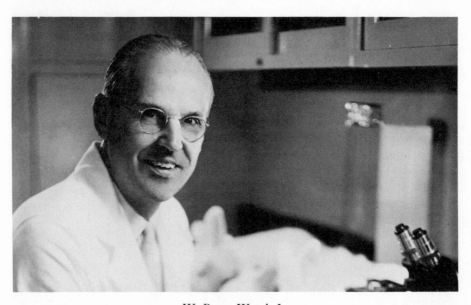

W. Barry Wood, Jr.

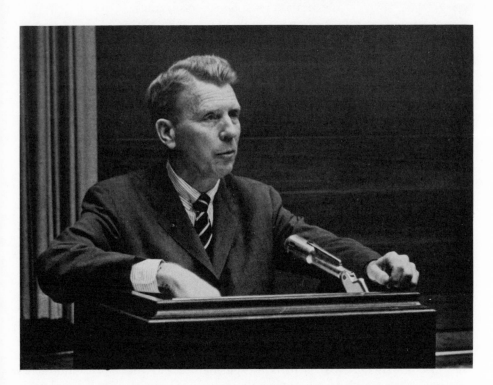

George W. Thorn
From the Archives Office, The Johns Hopkins Medical Institutions

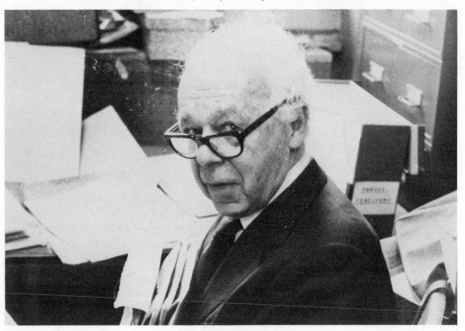

Curt P. Richter
Courtesy of Dr. Curt P. Richter

Addison's Disease, with a Report of a Case Greatly Benefited by the Use of the Suprarenal Extract." Particular credit must go to Osler for emphasizing the need in preparing the extract from fresh glands which are kept cold. He used hog adrenals, and years later it was demonstrated that this species has a much higher concentration of corticoids than do the arenals of grazing animals. Furthermore, Osler recommended extracting the glands with glycerin—also shown by Grollman, another Hopkins contributor, to be a particularly effective solvent for adrenal steroids. In the chapter on John Jacob Abel, an account was given of his isolation of epinephrine from the adrenal medulla.

Dr. George W. Thorn is another major Hopkins contributor to this field. A graduate of the University of Buffalo Medical School in 1929, Thorn became interested in studying the adrenal glands as an undergraduate student in the Department of Physiology. In November 1930 Hartman and Thorn published a method based on the maintenance of a normal growth curve in adrenalectomized rats as a standard assay for adrenal cortical extracts. They suggested that a unit of "cortin," injected twice daily, represented the quantity necessary for maintenance of normal growth in animals initially weighing 75 to 150 grams. With improved extracts, it was possible not only to maintain the lives of adrenalectomized animals indefinitely but to enable such animals to live an apparently healthy existence. Earlier Hartman and Brownell had described a simple process for the preparation of a concentrated cortical extract which contained less than 1:100,000 parts of epinephrine and could be administered intravenously as well as subcutaneously. In 1931 Hartman, Thorn, and their collaborators demonstrated the ability of this extract to maintain the health of patients with Addison's disease for a prolonged period. It was also shown effective in combating an acute adrenal crisis. Further clinical explorations by Hartman, Beck, and Thorn included studies on certain nervous and mental states, some of which improved under cortin therapy.

By 1936, Dr. Thorn had moved to Ohio State University as assistant professor of physiology and while there he demonstrated for the first time that the administration of a potent adrenal cortical extract could modify the renal excretion of electrolytes in normal subjects. In the fall of that year Thorn accepted a position at Johns Hopkins under his Rockefeller Foundation traveling fellowship to work with Dr. George Harrop in the Chemical Division of the Department of Medicine.

George Harrop's group was at that time particularly interested in the adrenal cortex. Harrop himself had developed an excellent technique for carrying out mineral balance studies on dogs. The standardization of the metabolic cages for the experimental animals, the technique for repeated bladder catheterizations, the well-controlled diets, and above all the skill of Dr. Harrop's laboratory associate, Harry Eisenberg, were important in laying the groundwork for future explorations in this field of medical research. In 1932 the classical studies of Loeb and of Harrop, Soffer, Ellsworth and Trescher demonstrated the beneficial effect of sodium salts in the treatment of patients with Addison's disease. Harrop's group also demonstrated the effect of adrenal extract on sodium and potassium balance in the adrenalectomized dog. In 1933

Kendall at the Mayo Clinic and Grollman at Hopkins obtained crystalline material from adrenal cortical extracts. This material appeared to possess cortical hormone-like activity.

In 1937, when Dr. Harrop accepted the post of medical director of E. R. Squibb and Company, Dr. Longcope asked George Thorn to head the Chemical Division. Thorn accepted and invited Dr. Lewis Engel, a young steroid chemist, to join him. Engel at that time was studying in Zurich, and his background knowledge in steroid chemistry was invaluable in their studies. When Engel arrived at Hopkins, he taught biochemistry to the third- and fourth-year medical students while they were assigned to the Department of Medicine. This was one of the first experiments of this kind to be carried out in an American medical school.

In 1937 Steiger and Reichstein announced the synthesis of desoxycorticosterone acetate (DCA), and in the following year Reichstein made available to Thorn a few milligrams of this newly synthesized adrenal hormone. Thorn clearly demonstrated at that time that while DCA administration was followed by a very striking retention of sodium and chloride, it did not correct the abnormality in carbohydrate metabolism characteristic of severe adrenal insufficiency. As long as the patients with adrenal sufficiency treated with DCA alone were able to eat normally, hypoglycemia was not a serious problem; but in the presence of acute stress or prolonged fasting, hypoglycemia developed rapidly.

The first instance of DCA-induced hypokalemic paralysis was reported in 1940 by Thorn and W. M. Firor. Severe paralysis involving the extensor muscles of the neck, hands, and feet occurred in a patient with Addison's disease given large quantities of DCA and supplementary saline and glucose solution in conjunction with a successful nephrectomy carried out for a tuberculous kidney. On two occasions in association with an abnormal lowering of serum potassium, this patient had the abrupt onset of severe flaccid paralysis, with complete recovery following reduction in DCA dosage and supplementary feeding of foods high in potassium.

Following the availability of 11-desoxycorticosterone, Dr. Francis Lukens referred to Thorn a patient with most of the clinical and laboratory findings of Addison's disease but with one notable exception—there was no hyperpigmentation. The serum sodium and chloride were low, blood urea nitrogen was elevated, and there were no abnormalities of the urine other than hypo-osmolality. The patient improved when large quantities of sodium chloride per day were administered, but the blood urea nitrogen remained elevated. Balance studies showed that this patient lost large quantities of sodium chloride in the urine despite a large daily dose of DCA, and it appeared that his renal tubular cells were refractory to salt-retaining adrenal hormone. He was also refractory to the renal effects of parathroid extract and antidiuretic hormone. This patient was followed for several years, and Dr. John Luetscher demonstrated a high level of "electrocortin" in the patient's urine—thus completing the presumptive diagnosis of adequate endogenous salt-retaining hormone but refractory end organ. This disorder was termed "salt-losing nephritis." Further studies on such patients helped to differentiate the pathophysiological changes in Addison's disease due to mineral hormone deficiency vis-à-vis those due to glucocorticoid deficiency.

One of the most practical things that came out of the availability of crystalline DCA was the development of long-term therapy by subcutaneous implantation of hormone tablets. Thorn and his collaborators first showed that carefully prepared tablets of crystalline DCA would maintain an adrenalectomized dog in excellent condition for periods of several months or more. From time to time, they removed the pellets, weighed them, and then replanted them. It was thus shown that over a prolonged period the amount of hormone was absorbed at a fairly constant rate. Therefore, it was possible to establish the number of pellets which when implanted would correspond to a given dose of hormone in oil injected subcutaneously once a day. The equivalence could be established by measurement of the electrolyte balance. If this could be maintained, then there was accurate physiological correspondence. These studies provided an excellent example of the manner in which experimental animal studies, especially those on dogs, have added so much to the improvement of medical care in man.

They then succeeded in applying this method to the treatment of patients with Addison's disease. It was found that a pellet of 125 to 150 milligrams of crystalline DCA could replace 0.5 milligrams of hormone in oil given as a single daily intramuscular injection. The patient could by this technique be provided with a continuous and effective source of hormone for periods of eight to twelve months. The small incision which was made at the time of implantation of the pellets served as a useful marker of any change in the patient's tendency toward hyperpigmentation. Later a technique of trochar insertion of the pellets eliminated the need for any operative procedure. Thorn's group noted that the pellets when removed for weighing were always surrounded by a neat capsule and could be "shelled out" like peas. It was clearly this fibrotic capsule which provided for the delayed absorption of the crystalline hormone. Now, of course, the use of DCA has been replaced almost entirely by the use of orally active, salt-retaining steroids such as 9-alphafluorohydrocortisone.

Thorn's notable studies of carbohydrate metabolism in Addison's disease while at Hopkins illustrate the importance of chance encounters in medicine. In 1940, as the result of a gift from Dr. E. C. Kendall of the Mayo Clinic of 85 milligrams of corticosterone and 33 mg of 19-dehydro corticosterone (Kendall's compound E-cortisone), he was able to compare in a patient with Addison's disease these two compounds, 11-desoxycorticosterone acetate and Wilson's adrenal cortical extract, under identical conditions. This represented the first time in which these 11, 17-oxysteroids had been tested in man.

The basis for Thorn's receipt of these very precious quantities of the two naturally derived corticosteroids was a long friendship with Kendall, which had begun in the summer of 1928. At that time Thorn, a third-year student of medicine, was serving as a camp physician on the shores of Lake Erie. One evening he was called to see Professor Kendall and his wife, who were desperately ill with high fever. In the succeeding decades their paths crossed many times, and Kendall had a continuing interest in Thorn's work. This led, of course, to his confidence in giving Thorn these corticoids, which had been isolated with such care and were available in such small quantities.

The results which Thorn obtained with a single injection of each of the substances provided clear insight into their pharmacological properties. Preliminary studies confirmed that patients with Addison's disease characteristically exhibit (1) a low normal overnight fasting blood glucose level, (2) striking hypoglycemia with continued fasting, (3) a decreased threshold for hypoglycemic symptoms, (4) a "flat" type of oral glucose curve, (5) absence of "rebound" in blood glucose curve following intravenously administered glucose, (6) decreased glycemic response to epinephrine, (7) abnormal increase in respiratory quotient following glucose administration, (8) high fasting (overnight) respiratory quotient, and (9) low basal metabolic rate. With the exception of its effect on the oral glucose curve, the abnormalities of carbohydrate metabolism were not significantly affected by 11-desoxycorticosterone administration. Treatment with large quantities of adrenal cortical extract (Wilson), cortisone-Kendall (33 milligrams) and corticosterone-Kendall (85 milligrams) were observed to (1) increase fasting blood glucose level; (2) decrease the standard respiratory quotient; (3) increase the blood glucose level and renal excretion of nitrogen and decrease the respiratory quotient following the standard intravenous glucose tolerance test, as compared to a similar test carried out under control conditions; (4) increase the threshold at which hypoglycemic symptoms appeared, and (5) increase the basal metabolic rate. These experiments in man supported the animal experiments of Long and his co-workers. They further suggested that the glucocorticoids increased the ability of the organism to form glucose and glycogen from nonglucose precursors and to impair the utilization of glucose, as indicated by the glycosuria which accompanied the administration of glucocorticoids and adrenal extract.

Thus the period 1940 to 1946 for the Addisonian patient was essentially one of treatment with 11-desoxycorticosterone acetate by intramuscular injection, subcutaneously implanted pellets, or sublingual administration, supplemented by adrenal cortical extract during periods of stress or crisis. Thorn's work while at Hopkins contributed to these important physiological and clinical developments.

In addition to his basic research work at Hopkins, Thorn also actively participated in the special clinical facility—Osler V—which had been designed by Dr. Warfield T. Longcope when the Osler Clinic Building was constructed in 1929. The establishment of such facilities was one of the important steps in the advancement of clinical investigation. Dr. Thorn gives the following account of the early use of this special ward:

My first contact with Osler V came in September 1936 when I joined George Harrop in the Clinical Division of the Department of Medicine. My responsibilities as a Rockefeller Fellow in Medicine included clinical responsibilities for patients on Osler V. At that time, as far as I can tell, John E. Howard and George Harrop were the two individuals who had admitting privileges. Then when George Harrop left in the summer of 1937, I took over his responsibilities for the operation of Osler V, the routine biochemistry laboratory [Mary Buell was the biochemist responsible for day-to-day supervision] and the research laboratories for our division. All of these and my office were located on Osler V and the 5th floor of the dispensary building.

Later when Lawson Wilkins began his clinical investigations on children with endocrine-metabolic disorders, we arranged for him to have admitting privileges on Osler V, since Harriet Lane could find no space for him! He was very appreciative of this and we all benefited from having his interesting patients and studies so near at hand.

The hospital made all of the beds on Osler V available to Thorn, Howard and Wilkins at no cost to the patients, but the hospital nursing service was not able to recruit nurses. This was a responsibility which fell on my shoulders and which was helped materially by the fact that George Koepf [research fellow] and his wife came from Buffalo. She was a graduate nurse and used to recruit from her friends at the Buffalo General Hospital. It appeared that many of the young women enjoyed a year at the Hopkins! Miss Nelson was our head nurse. She was also a trained dietician, but we had Betty Olsen [later Betty Hesser] as our dietician.

Early each fall Dr. Longcope would take me down to Winford Smith's office and we would negotiate for the academic year. This was always an interesting interview and I am certain without Dr. Longcope's strong and personal support the hospital would not have been nearly so generous.

The ward was closed in the summer. One year [1939] I took the whole unit to Saranac, where we studied electrolyte balance, adrenal function, etc. in patients with pulmonary tuberculosis.

Dr. Longcope made rounds once weekly on Osler V with us and always added a very important observation or raised a critical question. At one time or another we collaborated with other Hopkins departments. We had some of Helen Taussig's polycythemic cardiac patients in whom we administered DOCA to reduce their hematocrit in an attempt to improve their performance. As a consequence, Roger Lewis married one of these young women.

Palmer Howard was one of our first fellows and Kendall Emerson was one of the early residents coming from E. K. Marshall's department.

In summary—This was an extremely efficient and effective research unit, combining patient care, clinical investigation, student and house staff teaching, basic research in the biochemical laboratories and the great savings by having a joint relationship with the routine laboratory under Mary Buell.

In 1942 George Thorn became Hersey Professor of the Theory and Practice of Physic at Harvard Medical School and physician-in-chief at Peter Bent Brigham Hospital. His career since leaving Hopkins has seen not only the continuation of his productive work in the study of the adrenal gland and its diseases but also many other important endeavors in the field of endocrinology. He served with distinction as professor of medicine at Harvard until he became emeritus in 1972. For all of his outstanding work he has received many honors, including the presidency of the American Clinical and Climatological Association and of the Association of American Physicians, as well as of the Endocrine Society. He was elected to the Johns Hopkins Society of Scholars. He received the American Medical Association Gold Medal in 1932 and in 1939 and the Gordon Wilson Medal of the American Clinical and Climatological

Association in 1953. In 1955 he received the John Philips Memorial Award of the American College of Physicians, of which organization he is a Master. He is a Fellow of the American Academy of Arts and Sciences and editor-in-chief of the *Principles of Internal Medicine,* the textbook which was begun a number of years ago by Tinsley Harrison. He was further honored by Johns Hopkins by being invited to give the Thayer Lectures in 1967.

John Eager Howard

"Serendipity" is one of John Eager Howard's favorite words, not only because it is euphonious but because it has "hovered around my door due to an aberrant gene from my great-great-grandfather." In the Battle of Cowpens during the Revolutionary War, a retreat was ordered. General Howard preferred to charge, and a great victory was won—the first defeat of Tarleton's crack British regulars. When censured and told he might have been court-martialed, General Howard is said to have replied: "If we had been defeated, I would not be here." He received a Congressional Medal. This same ancestor caught his bride on the rebound, as it were. The record shows that she, of an ardent Tory family, would certainly have married Major André, had that gallant and charming soldier not been caught inveigling Benedict Arnold to become a traitor.

Howard was uncertain as an undergraduate about his career objectives. His banker father wanted him to join the family firm—or to join the ministry. Believing himself unsuited for either, he decided out of admiration for Dr. J. M. T. Finney and Dr. William S. Thayer to study medicine. Although exposure to Latin and Greek both at Hill and at Princeton hardly seemed appropriate preparation for medical school, in those days admissions committees were less concerned with brilliance in the physical sciences and stressed other factors indicating potential success as a practitioner. The Johns Hopkins University School of Medicine admissions committee made a perceptive choice when they accepted John Eager Howard.

Following graduation from Hopkins in 1928, Howard spent two years as a medical house officer at Massachusetts General Hospital. Then followed two years as an assistant resident and two years as a fellow in the Department of Medicine at Johns Hopkins. In 1934 he was appointed to his first faculty position at Hopkins as instructor in medicine and became a physician to the Johns Hopkins Hospital. For many years Dr. Howard directed the Division of Endocrinology and Metabolism of the Department of Medicine, and in 1960 he was promoted to a full professorship. In 1968 he assumed emeritus status, which has in no way slowed his pace. From 1957 to 1972 he was chief of medicine at Union Memorial Hospital.

The story of John Eager Howard's research contributions not only illustrates the meaning of serendipity but also demonstrates creative talent and ingenuity. In 1934, stimulated by Maurice Pincoffs, Halsey Barker and Howard reviewed the world's literature and attempted to construct a recognizable clinical syndrome in individuals having the rare tumor known as "pheochromocytoma," which induces periodic elevations in blood pressure. Because of this work, they were asked to see a patient in consultation who had recently had his appendix removed because of an episode of abdominal pain, although the appendix had not been inflamed. Hypertension developed abruptly after the operation and ran an unusually malignant course during the ensuing two months. Barker and Howard did not believe that a pheochromocytoma was present, but because of x-ray findings suspicious of an adrenal tumor, an abdominal exploration was performed. There was no tumor, but during the long operation, the intern holding the retractors became fatigued and loosened his hold, and a kidney came into full view. The surgeon noticed a curious yellow area and removed the kidney in the mistaken belief that it was cancerous. The patient's condition immediately improved and in a few weeks his blood pressure was normal. The lesion in the kidney proved to be an area to which the blood flow had been abruptly diminished. Thus, an extraordinary series of coincidences and "errors of both head and hand" led to the patient's cure.

It was not, however, until some fifteen years later that this strange clinical event yielded fruit of wider scientific moment. At that time a physician developed abdominal pain while driving his car and proceeded to the Johns Hopkins Hospital, where his normal appendix was removed. The surgeon sought other explanations for the pain but could find none. Two weeks later this physician again presented himself, this time with severe hypertension. After exhaustive tests, his physicians concluded that he had acute inflammation of the kidneys (hemorrhagic nephritis) and sent him home for a month of rest. During this period he became severely hypertensive and his vision failed, as did his heart, but his kidneys continued to function well. Since the patient's personal physician was ill, Dr. Howard was asked to see the patient. Howard could think of nothing more appropriate than to tell him about the patient he had seen fifteen years earlier; the physician in desperation immediately suggested that his kidney be removed. It required considerable persuasion before the urologist consented to perform the operation. It turned out to be rewarding, however, since exactly the same findings were present as in the first patient, and his blood pressure fell to normal.

It was Dr. Morgan Berthrong who provided the important clue from these two extraordinary cases. He discovered that in these two kidneys there were zones of tissue inadequately supplied with blood surrounding the zones of tissue completely dead, as the artery was occluded by a thrombus. In all the other kidney infarcts examined, the dead zones ended abruptly adjacent to perfectly healthy kidney. Thus, the presence of small areas of kidney inadequately supplied with arterial blood but not completely dead could result in severe hypertension.

This observation led Dr. Howard to tackle the problems of how one could detect such kidneys inadequately supplied with blood in whole or in part, and how such situations resulted in severe hypertension. These questions remain inadequately answered today, but serendipity again played a part in providing some diagnostic approaches to the identification of individuals with this rare but correctable form of high blood pressure. A third patient was seen who had recently developed hypertension and whose antecedent symptoms were almost identical to those of the two patients previously described. Aortography, a method of determining the status of abdominal arteries, had just been introduced, and by this technique, a narrowed artery to one kidney was visualized. Before operation, in the hope of disclosing some difference in the urine whereby patients with this type of hypertension might be identified, Dr. William W. Scott made urine collections from both kidneys simultaneously. Differences were found in the quantity of urine and in the concentration of two of the many urinary constituents studied. The patient's kidney was removed, and he also became normotensive. A year later, Edmund Yendt, a fellow in Dr. Howard's laboratory, called his attention to the studies of H. L. White on the changes in composition of urine following constriction of a renal artery in the dog. His findings were strikingly similar to those seen in the patient just described, and out of these observations came the well-known "Howard test," designed to determine the differential functional change in a kidney in which there is a lesion of this type causing hypertension.

Howard's research work on kidney stones is also fascinating. Whereas the disease of rickets used to be recognized exclusively in babies, in circumstances wherein the concentration of calcium or phosphorus is low in serum, a striking exception was found in uremia resulting from kidney insufficiency. In the uremic patient, rickets is almost invariably present, despite an elevated serum phosphorus and essentially normal calcium. Yendt found that the trouble lay in the uremic serum and not in the bones themselves. However, they were unable to determine what was in uremic serum that prevented deposition in the cartilage of calcium phosphate crystals. To find a possible inhibiting factor, another of Dr. Howard's fellows, William C. Thomas, Jr., put rachitic cartilages into normal urine. Despite an enormous concentration of calcium and phosphorus in the urine, the cartilage failed to calcify. It was, however, another example of sheer serendipity to find that urine from the first four patients who suffered from kidney stones did calcify the cartilage, although the calcium and phosphorus content of their urine was no higher than seen normally. It was soon learned that only an occasional urine specimen from patients who made stones caused rachitic cartilage to calcify. Suppose that the initial one or two such urine specimens had given no positive test? The matter would almost certainly have been dropped. As it was, the idea was pursued, and it was found that there is normally present in urine and in blood an inhibitor to calcification. This thesis has been pursued vigorously over the last five years by laboratories all over the world interested in calcification mechanisms in general, and to some extent by those working on kidney stones. Howard's group is still in the process of trying to clarify just what goes on—why one urine will cause calcification and another will not; but more important still, the basic crystallographic mechanisms involved in the formation of stones which will enlarge and become hard as opposed to the mechanisms for keeping crystals of any kind in a noncrystal, colloidal, or relatively fluid state.

The use of phosphate in the prevention of oxalate kidney stones came about in this way: Dr. William Boyce, a keen investigator of kidney stones who worked in Winston-Salem, where stones are plentiful, wanted to see whether phytic acid would chelate enough dietary calcium to prevent kidney stones. Though this notion seemed totally incorrect to Howard, a supply of phytic acid was given to thirty rural inhabitants of North Carolina who had more than five kidney stones a year for several years. Each was given the phytic acid and told to bring in a urine specimen once a month, at which time he would be given five dollars and a renewed supply of phytic acid. At the end of a year Dr. Boyce invited Howard to review the results, which were most dramatic. Twenty-eight of the thirty had just as many kidney stones as usual, but two had no stones and were utterly delighted. The urine of the two who had made no stones showed one striking difference from those who continued to make stones; namely, the phosphorus in their urine rose from the normal of 1,200 milligrams per day to 3 grams. Phytic acid is approximately 80 percent phosphorus. The incorrect conclusion was reached that the two who had made no stones were the only ones who could break down the phytic acid and absorb it. It was later learned that everyone can break down phytic acid with an enormous increase in urinary phosphorus. The two described were the only ones who had taken the phytic acid; the others had collected their money and thrown the phytic acid away. On the basis of the high urinary phosphorus of those two and the fact that Shorr's experiments with low phosphorus intake had created more kidney stones, stone formers were then put on phosphate therapy. This proved to be very successful in preventing oxalate stone formation.

In 1928 Fuller Albright came to Baltimore as an assistant resident in medicine because of a close friendship with Dr. Reed Ellsworth, one of Hopkins's most brilliant young investigators. John Howard met these two medical greats socially and began a lifelong friendship with them. Dr. Hugh Young was very fond of Ellsworth, who took Howard along when he examined the many extraordinary cases on Young's urological service. Ellsworth made some significant contributions to our knowledge of parathyroid function. At the annual Atlantic City meetings there were often violent polemics between Collip and Albright, sometimes almost resulting in fisticuffs. Albright insisted that the parathyroid's primary function was to make the kidney eliminate phosphorus, whereas Collip insisted that the primary function was on bone and its influence on calcium metabolism. Ellsworth proved Albright wrong when he and Futcher tied off the ureters so that no phosphorus could be excreted in the urine. In this preparation the injection of parathyroid hormone raised the serum calcium, and the typical skeletal lesions of osteitis fibrosa developed. In the test, which now goes by his name, Ellsworth injected parathyroid hormone intravenously and showed that within minutes phosphorus in the urine increases. The phosphaturia was even more dramatic in patients with hypoparathyroidism.

At the beginning of World War II, the armed forces predicted that the incidence of fractures among soldiers would be a serious problem. They requested, therefore, that the Office of Scientific Research and Development gather a research study group to see what could be done to expedite fracture union and prevent the development of kidney stones and urinary infection which followed prolonged immobilization. This task force, organized by Dr.

Howard Means and known as the "Macy Group," met three times a year to discuss the results of their studies. Howard was a member of the group and housed his human volunteers in the Osler V clinical research facility. Many interesting observations came out of Howard's studies. It was noted for the first time that negative nitrogen balance in injured persons is not affected by diet, provided the subjects are healthy. That is to say, there was tremendous loss of nitrogen in healthy persons after injury, but practically no loss in persons injured when debilitated. When the subjects were offered all of the salts of a normal diet but no food, these salts were completely rejected. Another important finding was that total intravenous feeding could be maintained for as long as fifty days and the nitrogen balance could be maintained by intraveous feeding just as well as by the feeding of steak and potatoes. These observations created great controversy at the meetings of the task force, and Ravdin, in particular, criticized them. It was later realized, however, that Howard's group had included potassium in the intravenous mixtures while the Philadelphia studies had not. And this was the crux of maintaining nitrogen balance during total intravenous feeding. As a result of such studies, potassium was first used as a therapeutic agent, both in the recovery period from diabetic acidosis and in severely potassium-depleted patients. There was at first strong criticism of these observations, too, and both Peters and Loeb doubted that the potassium-depleted person could retain potassium in far greater amounts than the relative proportion of phosphorus, sulfur, nitrogen, and other cellular ingredients retained. Nevertheless, this is now standard knowledge.

Thus, from the studies of Howard and others on the Macy committee, there came much new basic information on potassium metabolism as well as the successful use of intravenous feeding and data relating to protein metabolism in injury. Much of this original work has been overlooked by those contributing to these fields in later years.

During Howard's presentations before the Macy group on calcium homeostasis, it became evident to him that the bones must be a warehouse or storehouse for calcium from which the homeostatic mechanisms could either accept or provide calcium to the circulation to maintain the constant serum calcium concentration which had been demonstrated so beautifully years before by Hastings and McLean. Howard had pointed out that the amount of calcium needed for such homeostasis in times of greatest stress could be provided only from bone. Later, at a meeting of the Ciba Foundation in London, the idea was proposed that activity of bone cells governs such calcium homeostasis. It was suggested that these cells were protected by a membrane around the bone, and that it was this cellular activity which determined whether acceptance of calcium into the bone or provision of calcium from the bone to the external medium would ensue. When Dr. Park heard of this idea, he proceeded to demonstrate such a membrane histologically; these studies were published the following year in the *Journal of Clinical Endocrinology* but had previously been reported in an address before the College of Physicians of Philadelphia. This work was totally ignored until a year or two ago, when Neuman chemically proved the correctness of the view that there was a calcium pump in bone which, indeed, must be the mechanism whereby the homeostasis of calcium is maintained.

As a result of his outstanding research contributions, Dr. Howard has received many honors over the years. One of the most outstanding was the Passano Award in 1959. He is a member of all of the important medical societies; in 1961 he was president of the Endocrine Society and in 1973 president of the American Clinical and Climatological Association. In 1964 he received the Modern Medicine Award for distinguished achievement.

W. Barry Wood, Jr.

Careers are often determined by a chance event. Such was the case when W. Barry Wood, a chemistry major at Harvard College, unexpectedly met James Conant, then head of that department, one day in the hall. Conant inquired if Barry was enjoying himself and then took him to meet L. J. Henderson in the fatigue laboratory. Henderson suggested that Wood might study the leukocytosis produced by strenuous exercise, and thus began Wood's lifetime work with leukocytes. While an undergraduate, Wood made the interesting observation that the leukocyte count frequently doubled in short-distance runners, but then returned quickly to normal. With more sustained exertion and tension, as in football, however, the white blood cell count might increase by a factor of 3 or 4 and remain elevated for a matter of hours. He was obviously observing the mobilization of the marginal pool of intravascular leukocytes which followed brief bursts of intensive physical activity, plus the delivery of cells from the bone marrow pool when exertion was more prolonged. In 1932 there was no way to make this distinction, but in his published paper he recognized that storage pools must exist.

William Barry Wood, Jr., was born in Milton, Massachusetts, on May 4, 1910. During his years at Milton Academy, he had a superior academic record and also demonstrated exceptional ability as an all-around athlete, playing hockey, baseball, football, and tennis. It was not until his senior year that he took his first course in science, winning the senior science prize. At Harvard he won ten varsity letters, achieved national acclaim as an outstanding athlete, and graduated summa cum laude. The summer following his graduation, he married Mary Lee Hutchins, who became a graduate student at the Johns Hopkins School of Hygiene and Public Health when Woods entered the Johns Hopkins School of Medicine in 1932.

During his first year, he worked with Mansfield Clark, professor of physiological chemistry, and completed two pieces of investigation involving oxidation-reduction potentials. His interest in clinical investigation and clinical medicine received a tremendous surge during a clerkship spent at the Boston City Hospital, where he came in contact with Soma Weiss, William Castle, and Chester Keefer.

After medical school he was tempted to pursue a career in biochemistry, but by that time he had become fascinated with clinical investigation, so he entered residency training in medicine at the Johns Hopkins Hospital. In those days, assistant residents at Hopkins were encouraged to select a subspecialty area of interest to them. Barry's first choice was metabolism, but a senior resident had already chosen that area. Dr. Longcope suggested medical bacteriology. Barry visited Dr. Avery at the Rockefeller Institute, and after a stimulating interview, developed his lifelong interest in the pneumococcus. After finishing his residency training, he spent a year as National Research Council Fellow with Zinsser and Enders, then returned to Hopkins to begin his medical investigative career.

In 1942, just six years after receiving his M.D. degree, he was appointed head of the Department of Medicine at Washington University in St. Louis and physician-in-chief of Barnes Hospital. Here he made an impressive record, organized a fine department, and continued productive research in the laboratory. In 1955 he returned to Johns Hopkins as vice-president for medical affairs under a plan which permitted him to devote half time to research. Within a period of three years he gave up his administrative duties and accepted the chairmanship of the Department of Microbiology. Here he enjoyed the close association with students and research associates and co-authored what has become a standard textbook of microbiology.

His research work at Hopkins following his fellowship training, concerned the pathogenesis of pneumonia and the mechanism of recovery from pneumonia. His interest in the pneumococcus was reinforced by the stimulating conferences held on pneumococcal pneumonia by Arnold Rich. In St. Louis, Barry continued to work on the mechanism of recovery from pneumonia, recognizing the importance of surface phagocytosis.

During the early period in St. Louis, he again worked on leukocytes while studying the mechanism of fever. From then on, his investigative efforts, supported by his long-time associate Mary Ruth Smith and a steady stream of fellows, was primarily concerned with the pathogenesis of the febrile response. Beeson's discovery that granulocytic leukocytes are the chief source of endogenous pyrogen was confirmed, and much later evidence was obtained that macrophages can also produce endogenous pyrogen. This discovery was made independently by Elisha Atkins of Yale (a former associate of Wood's), and the two papers were published sequentially in the same journal.

Wood was the first to demonstrate that endogenous pyrogen injected directly into the carotid artery caused a more prompt and greater febrile response than did intravenous injection. This led to the hypothesis that endogenous pyrogen acts directly on the thermoregulatory centers in the hypothalamus. Subsequently, more precise proof of a direct action of pyrogen on the hypothalamus has become available (*J. Physiol.* 191 [1967]: 325. and *J. Neurophysiol.* 30 [1967]: 586).

Among Wood's distinctive contributions were the series of experiments in which he showed that rabbits made febrile by injections of endotoxin, viruses, antigens, and gram-positive organisms had circulating pyrogen which was quantitatively sufficient to explain their elevated temperatures. He showed for the first time that phagocytosis was an adequate stimulus for pyrogen release *in vitro* and that certain myxoviruses would also cause the same response. He clearly showed that blood leukocytes differed from exudate leukocytes in that the latter, but not the former, would liberate pyrogen spontaneously when suspended in saline. He did experiments on the metabolic basis of pyrogen production, showing the influence of various ions on the process. This work did not lead to any general conclusion, remaining as a series of phenomena devoid of an explanation. However, his work on the effect of metabolic inhibitors culminated in the demonstration that pyrogen was actually synthesized *de novo* by neutrophils from amino acid precursors. This work was published after his death, but his associates had given him the preliminary results and he knew that they would be successful.

During these final years of his research career, Wood did not neglect the pneumococcus. Two mechanisms of phagocytosis were known to participate in the destruction of pneumococci in the infected host: (1) his previously described surface phagocytosis, which operates in the pre-antibody phase of pneumococcal disease and may occur in the absence of opsonins of any kind; and (2) immune phagocytosis, which occurs late in the disease, when enough anticapsular antibody has accumulated to opsonize the encapsulated organisms. To these Dr. Wood and his associates now added a third mechanism that involves the participation of heat-labile opsonins. These heat-labile opsonins are immunologically polyspecific, and were shown to fix various components of complement, particularly C_3b, as the pneumococci were opsonized. Since C_3 reactive sites have been identified on the surfaces of granulocytes, the fixation of complement on the pneumococci was regarded as of probable importance in initiating phagocytosis. Furthermore, since these polyspecific, heat-labile opsonins are present in normal serum, it was suggested that they serve a significant function in early anti-pneumococcal defense.

Wood had an amazing capacity to budget his time. Throughout his career, for the most part, his mornings were dedicated to his administrative, patient, and teaching responsibilities and his afternoons to the laboratory; few things were permitted to interfere. He always found time to work, time to spend with his family, and time to keep physically trim by playing tennis.

He was a member of the Association of American Physicians, serving both as secretary and as president, and he was chosen to receive the Kober Medal of that association for 1971. In addition he was president of the Central Society for Clinical Investigation and of the American Society for Clinical Investigation. He was elected to the National Academy of Sciences and became a Master of the American College of Physicians. He was recognized as an outstanding medical statesman and served as adviser to many branches of the government, foundations, universities, medical societies, and many former students and associates.

Thus, Barry Wood excelled as a physician, as a teacher, as an investigator, and as an administrator. The Johns Hopkins Medical School appropriately memorialized him by naming the basic science building in his honor. A few years before his death, Barry Wood made the following statement:

While in high school I was certain that I'd become a teacher. In college I decided to become a doctor. In medical school I resolved to become both. Although this may sound a little like trying to have one's cake and eat it, too, it really isn't; for the doctor-teacher is an accepted hybrid of the medical profession—his unique opportunity lies in his daily contact with the students and in his chance to pursue research.

Medical students are an extraordinary group of people. Carefully selected and highly motivated, they become deeply absorbed in their exacting and fascinating work. To be associated with them in study and teaching is to be constantly subjected to a most potent kind of stimulus. As for medical research, it is difficult to conceive of a more gratifying form of human endeavor. In its modern scope it not only encompasses all of the natural sciences but of recent years it has begun to involve the social sciences as well. Its humanitarian possibilities are forever beckoning, sometimes at a distance and sometimes very close at hand.

As the final years of the first century of the School of Medicine come to a close, it is clear, when one views the career of some of the more recent members of the faculty, such as W. Barry Wood, Jr., that the strength and creative function of this school is stronger than ever, and that the heritage of excellence at Johns Hopkins is not just a tradition but a living symbol which constantly serves as a stimulus and driving force toward creative endeavor for all who are associated with the Johns Hopkins Medical Institutions.

IN HIS ADDRESS at the dedication of the Johns Hopkins Hospital in 1889, John Shaw Billings made the following comment: ". . . it is supposed that from this hospital will issue papers and reports giving accounts of advances in, and of new methods of acquiring knowledge, obtained in its wards and laboratories, and that thus all scientific men and all physicians shall share in the benefits of the work actually done within these walls." Such papers and reports did indeed pour forth from the hospital, and in the beginning the main vehicles of publication were the *Johns Hopkins Hospital Bulletin* and the *Johns Hopkins Hospital Reports*.

The Johns Hopkins Hospital Bulletin

The *Johns Hopkins Hospital Bulletin* was authorized by the hospital trustees in September 1889. A monthly publication with a subscription price of $1.00 per year, the *Bulletin* was to "contain announcements of courses of lectures, programs of clinical and pathological study, details of hospital and dispensary practice, abstracts of papers read and other proceedings of the medical society of the hospital, reports of lectures and all other matters of general interest in connection with the work of the hospital." Its original purpose, then, was to serve as a news bulletin, but as time went on more and more original communications appeared in the *Bulletin*, and as a result the *Bulletin* soon became a highly respected scientific periodical, doing much to carry the reputation of the hospital to other medical centers, notably in Europe.

From 1889 to 1924 the journal was supported entirely by the receipts from subscriptions and by a subsidy from the Hospital. Ownership was then transferred to the university, and its publication was aided by a subsidy from the DeLamar Fund of the School of Medicine. Its title was changed to *The Bulletin of the Johns Hopkins Hospital,* a new format was used, and a board of editors was appointed by the Advisory Board of the Medical Faculty.

Through the medium of the *Johns Hopkins Hospital Bulletin*, the various activities of the hospital and all of the important events were duly chronicled. Many of the investigations made in the various departments were brought to the attention of the medical world through this journal. It was a faithful mirror of the Johns Hopkins Hospital, and its establishment was one of the most important actions ever taken by the hospital.

The Johns Hopkins Hospital Reports

A month after authorizing the *Bulletin*, the hospital trustees authorized the publication of another Hopkins journal, the *Johns Hopkins Hospital Reports*. The purpose of this publication was to disseminate the results of scientific work carried out at the Hopkins. As noted, however, original work early on found its way into the *Bulletin*, and the *Reports* were used primarily for the publication of more lengthy articles, many of which were actually monographs.

When the Johns Hopkins University opened, and particularly after the inauguration of Welch's pathological laboratory, investigators had no suitable place for publication of their work in the United States. All of the existing medical journals in America were clinical journals, designed to serve practitioners and not adapted to the publication of basic scientific papers. This was understandable, since prior to that time there had not been sufficient research work done in this country to create the need for a scientific journal. To help solve the problem of lack of media for publication, President Gilman established under university auspices, but "open freely to contributions from every part of the country," special journals in subjects far enough developed to support such publications. In subjects where a university department was working almost alone, he encouraged the issuance of occasional volumes made up entirely of their own work, as in the case of H. Newell Martin's early studies on the isolated perfused heart.

When money was made available for inaugurating the *Johns Hopkins Hospital Reports* in 1889, Welch was authorized to devote the first volume to studies from his own laboratory. As Welch began editing the papers for this initial volume, he soon found himself struggling with a mass of detail. Illustrations were a real problem, as the plates necessary had rarely been used in the United States and therefore could best be prepared in Germany. This problem was solved, however, when Mall, who happened to be abroad, negotiated with a lithographer there for this work. Sometime after Welch began working on his pathological volume, Osler began to work on a volume of clinical reports. Osler's volume appeared in 1890, long before Welch's was ready for publication. Although Welch's volume was number 1, it was not finished until 1897, seven years after Volume 2 saw the light of day.

The *Reports* were to appear in individual numbers or "fasciculi," ten such numbers to a volume. For a time these volumes came out at fairly regular intervals, but since, as noted, the *Bulletin* began to publish more original investigations and doubtless also because the growth of specialty journals provided another outlet for such material, publication of the *Reports* became more infrequent and finally ceased in 1926.

Dr. Henry M. Hurd was the editor of both the *Bulletin* and the *Reports* from their inception until he relinquished the position in 1911. And he was an editor in every sense of the word. Any member of the staff who wandered into the superintendent's office late at night, when all was quiet, or on a Sunday afternoon, would find Dr. Hurd busily engaged in correcting galley proofs. Many of the articles were rather crude in their English construction, and had to be entirely recast by him. Under Hurd's editorship, these two Hopkins publications possessed a dignity and style rarely noted in medical periodicals of that time. The printing was good, the illustrations were excellent, and the text was remarkably free from typographical errors.

Hurd was born on May 3, 1843, at Union City, Branch County, Michigan. His father, a pioneer physician, settled in Michigan in 1834. Worn out by a laborious practice amid the hardships and privations of pioneer life in a malarious country, he died at the early age of thirty-nine, leaving a wife and three small boys. Hurd's mother remarried in 1848, and in 1854 the family moved to Galesburg, Illinois. In 1858 Hurd entered Knox College, where he spent two years. He subsequently devoted a year to teaching and general study, and in 1861 he entered the junior class at the University of Michigan, from which he graduated in 1863. He received his medical degree from Michigan in 1866 and spent the next year in New York in study and hospital work. He then moved to Chicago, where he was in general practice for two years. In 1870 he received the appointment of assistant physician to the Michigan Asylum for the Insane at Kalamazoo and entered that field of medicine in which he achieved distinction. Eight years later, he became assistant superintendent at the asylum, and on the opening of the Eastern Michigan Asylum at Pontiac in 1878 he was appointed its first superintendent, occupying that position for the next eleven years. It was during this period that his skill as an organizer, his broad cultural and literary attainments, and his effectiveness in the field of psychiatry became evident. He was active from the beginning with the Association of Medical Superintendents. During his period at the Michigan Asylum, he saw the treatment of the insane revolutionized by the abolition of restraint, the employment of the insane, the extension of the system of night nursing, the development of the "cottage plan," and the introduction of home comforts into the previously dull, unattractive institutional life. He was an ardent advocate of all of these progressive changes and was recognized as one of the outstanding psychiatrists of that period. In 1881 he visited Europe to study the treatment of the insane there, and his observations were the subject of a special communication to the joint boards of trustees of the Michigan asylums, published with the annual report of the Eastern Michigan Asylum for 1882. This and his other contributions to the literature, including numerous papers published in the *Journal of Insanity*, attracted widespread attention. A notable event was his presidential address in 1889 before the Alumni Association of the Medical Department of the University of Michigan, entitled "The Mental Hygiene of Physicians."

In June 1889 he was asked to take the post of superintendent of the new Johns Hopkins Hospital. The trustees of the Eastern Michigan Asylum at Pontiac were so concerned about losing him to Hopkins that one of the trustees came with Hurd when he visited Baltimore, hoping to persuade him to decline the offer. After he had met the Hopkins trustees and had visited the hospital, he turned to Hurd and said: "My object in coming with you was to see that you returned to Michigan, but I have changed my mind. If they offer you this position and you do not accept it, you will make the mistake of your life."

Thus, Hurd became, in June 1889, the first superintendent of the Johns

Hopkins Hospital, assuming his duties on August 1, at which time President Gilman, who had acted as director of the hospital since the preceding February, and Dr. John S. Billings, who had been medical adviser to the Board of Trustees for twelve years, terminated their connection with the hospital.

The Journal of Experimental Medicine

The problem of publication at Hopkins grew more difficult as Welch's laboratory expanded. Even though the *Johns Hopkins Bulletin* was intended for studies from the clinical departments, Welch's associates also used it as a means of getting their work into print.

One of the principal matters that came up for consideration by the Advisory Board in the autumn of 1895 was the establishment of a new medical journal. In 1893 the Advisory Board discussed a proposal to establish a new journal, to be called *Archives of the Medical Sciences* and to be edited by a committee under the chairmanship of Dr. Osler. This periodical was expected to publish results of investigations in any branch of medical science or art carried on at the Johns Hopkins University and Hospital, but for financial reasons the journal could not be started on the date proposed, January 1, 1894. At the Advisory Board meeting in the autumn of 1895, the matter again came up for discussion, and the available evidence indicates that it was Dr. Abel who revived the idea. He conferred with Dr. Welch, who immediately began to sound out several well-known American scientists to find out if they were interested. In a letter to Dr. Mall in 1895 Welch stated: "Abel is stirring up things for a new journal of high character for laboratory workers in this country in pathology, pharmacology and physiology. I think it may go through if we can secure Bowditch [Professor of Physiology at Harvard] and the important laboratory workers."

Abel provided an account of how the project got under way in an address given at the dinner of the Federation of the American Society of Experimental Biology on April 10, 1931 in Montreal:

I happened one day in the fall of 1895 to remark to President Gilman that we needed some sort of a journal in this country in which physiologists, pharmacologists, biochemists, pathologists and those engaged in research work in clinical medicine could publish their original researches. At that time, we had only open to us in this country purely chemical or medical journals as a medium for publication. The consequence was that most of us in that day sent our papers to foreign journals. A few days later I received a call from President Gilman who asked me to draw up a set of resolutions setting forth the needs for such a journal and to present them to the medical faculty of The Johns Hopkins University. We had a number of meetings and finally the Journal of Experimental Medicine, a journal of national scope published by D. Appleton and Company, made its first appearance in January 1896 with Dr. William H. Welch as its editor. The associate editors for physiology were Bowditch, Chittenden and Howell; for pharmacology, Abel, Cushny and H. D. Wood; for pathology, Adami, Councilman and Prudden; for medicine, Fitz, Osler and Pepper. Dr. Welch edited this journal most successfully and with meticulous care from 1896 to 1902, when it was taken over by the Rockefeller Institute for Medical Research.

Thus, the project finally succeeded, with Johns Hopkins agreeing to contribute $1,000 annually to the publication. It was the first American journal fully dedicated to the promulgation of basic scientific medical research studies.

The *Journal of Experimental Medicine*, as the new publication was called. was a radical experiment at that time. Many did not believe that America produced sufficient scientific work to fill its pages. In their eagerness to get the best work available from any source, the founders kept secret the fact that Johns Hopkins was contributing financial support. They wanted it to be a national journal and not to appear as a Johns Hopkins enterprise. A well-qualified board of associate editors was appointed from various universities to help evaluate the manuscripts and make recommendations to the editor. More important, these associate editors and their students were themselves asked to contribute papers, as were a group of fifty-six other scientists, who were designated "collaborators."

The journal was successful beyond all possible expectations. Medical research was then in a phase of rapid growth in this country, and American laboratories produced far more articles of high quality than anyone had foreseen. In 1897 the journal, which was printing six hundred pages a year and had at first been published irregularly, was definitely established on a bimonthly basis. Those who a short time before were afraid that there would be a lack of papers for even one periodical were looking frantically about for the development of another journal to help carry the growing load. Relief came when the *American Journal of Physiology,* sponsored by the American Society of Physiology under Bowditch's nominal and Porter's actual editorship, began publication in January 1898.

For Welch, however, the success of the journal brought with it penalties as well. At the end of the first six months, he wrote to Mall: "It will probably take me all summer to answer letters. The third number of the Journal will be a fat one and will be out this month." In apologizing to Herter for having to postpone the inclusion of a paper, Welch wrote in April 1897: "I have now waiting for publication enough articles to fill the next number which have been in my hands for from six months to a year. The writers are justly becoming impatient." Welch's greatest difficulties as an editor resulted from his attempt to take care of all of the details himself. His temperament did not permit him to accept assistance in this time-consuming work. He rarely consulted the associate editors, and shunning secretaries, he wrote all the voluminous correspondence in his own hand. He read every paper carefully. If he found it unacceptable, he returned it with a very kind note of rejection. If it required revision, he would often do the revision himself. Welch introduced the system of checking every bibliographic reference for which his excellent personal library sufficed and of giving references in a uniform style much like that used in the *Surgeon General's Catalogue* and the *Index Medicus*. After the papers were in proper form, Welch prepared the manuscript for the printer, read the proofs, arranged for illustrations, and laid out with his own hand the makeup of each issue. But gradually the volume of work got the best of Welch. He often failed to acknowledge the receipt of manuscripts. When many months had passed and their articles were not published, contributors began to request that the editor return their manuscripts. Still no reply. Dr. Henry M. Hurd, editor of the *Johns Hopkins Hospital Bulletin*, received many letters from some of the most prominent medical men in the country, begging him to rescue their manuscripts from Dr. Welch's study. As soon as Dr. Welch went off on one of his weekends, Dr. Hurd would go to his library, hunt among the many papers until he found the manuscripts he was looking for, and return them to the anxious authors.

One day when Hugh Young called on Dr. Welch and was admitted to his library, there was no place to sit down. The desk and everyone of the eight chairs were piled high with mail—most of it unopened. Dr. Welch apologized for the appearance of the room.

He explained that while I might think his study was in a state of disorder, he really had an excellent system. "On that armchair there I have the letters that have come during the past week; I hope to read these in the near future. On that chair, I have the letters that have come within the past month. On the other chairs are letters and magazines anywhere from six months to a year old which I hope to get to some time." As to the desk, he said that when it got too cluttered up he would open a newspaper and spread it over the letters and manuscripts and start afresh. I counted four such layers. There was one little corner of his desk pad which was vacant—just room enough to place a small sheet of note paper on which he wrote in his cramped handwriting.

I begged Dr. Welch to allow me to send him a dictaphone. I explained that anytime night or day, whenever he had a spare moment, he would be able to dictate his letters, that my stenographer would call the next morning for the cylinders and bring his typewritten letters back in the afternoon. He seemed greatly taken with the idea. I had my stenographer take the dictaphone to Dr. Welch and show him how to use it. The next day he returned and got a cylinder. I was anxiously awaiting to see what had been recorded. There was only one letter, which began: "Dr. Mr. Robinson, I wish to apologize for not writing sooner. I couldn't find time to— to— Young, I can't use this machine. Send your boy around to get it."

In 1901 Welch heard that Dr. Harold Ernst of Harvard was planning to start another periodical in the same general field as the *Journal of Experimental Medicine*. Ernst had founded the Boston Society of Medical Sciences in 1896 and had begun publishing its *Proceedings* in a small pamphlet, which he now wanted to convert into a national publication as the official organ of the newly organized American Association of Pathologists and Bacteriologists. The need for a special society for pathologists and bacteriologists and the fact that 1901 was the founding date of the Rockefeller Institute for Medical Research shows how rapidly medical science was progressing in the United States.

Welch tried to turn his journal over to Ernst, but when the Hopkins faculty discovered this, they pointed out that such a transfer was not permissible without the consent of the university. It was an awkward situation, settled by Welch's agreement to appoint an assistant editor. This, however, was never done. Welch got out several more issues, but after March 1902 the *Journal of Experimental Medicine* suddenly ceased to appear. No explanation was offered. Manuscripts continued to pour in, but not one was passed on to the printer. It appeared that Welch was limiting his activity as editor in an attempt to force the university's hand. In September 1902 he wrote to Herter: "I should be simply delighted if the Rockefeller Institute would take over the *Journal of Experimental Medicine*. The editorial burden weighs on me and I should be only too glad to part with it entirely. Or if that is not possible, to share it with you and Flexner." All of this was typical of Welch. During the early days of an important enterprise, he would be very active in it and even willing to do the day-to-day chores. But once the venture was well established, he was ready to relinquish his activities and let others take it over. He was persistent in this matter, and it was soon clear that the university would have to give up the journal. The Hopkins trustees agreed to turn the journal over to the Rockefeller Institute, and Flexner and Opie undertook its editorship.

Welch's habit of procrastination prevented him from completing even the necessary formalities. On December 24, 1903, Dr. L. Emmett Holt, the secretary of the institute, wrote somewhat frantically: "The executive committee . . . have received repeated inquiries and appeals from men who had sent articles to be published in the *Journal of Experimental Medicine* under the impression that the journal was already in the hands of the institute. As yet we have nothing to do with the conduct of the journal and we would like to know what response shall be made to such letters." Even after the institute secured legal possession of the journal in October 1904, Welch failed to turn over the manuscripts he had accumulated. Flexner finally had to make a special journey to Baltimore. When Flexner mentioned the object of his visit, Welch said he would send the manuscripts in a day or two; but Flexner was prepared. Welch succumbed to the pressure, and the repository of manuscripts scattered about his rooms were packed in a suitcase then and there.

The Journal of Biological Chemistry

The success of the *Journal of Experimental Medicine* and the rapid growth of biochemical research in the United States encouraged Abel to initiate steps for the foundation of still another publication—the *Journal of Biological Chemistry*. In the spring of 1903 he enlisted the aid of his friend Christian A. Herter, professor of pharmacology at Columbia University. Again it was at first doubtful whether a sufficient number of high-quality papers would be available. After numerous meetings and extensive correspondence between Abel and Herter, the first number of the journal appeared in 1905, with Abel and Herter as joint editors and A. N. Richards as associate editor. These three men were responsible for the immediate success of this journal.

It was decided that the format of the journal should closely resemble that of Hoppe-Seyler's *Zeitschrift für Physiologische Chemie* and that the subscription price should be so low that young workers could afford it. Financial deficits were foreseen as inevitable, and various means of meeting them were explored and discarded. A proposal from the secretary of the American Medical Association indicating the willingness of that organization to assume the financial burden, with the implication of participating in ownership, was not accepted because of the determination that the new journal should never enter into alliances outside the field of biochemistry, but should always be managed by and for biochemists, solely for the advancement of that science. Dr. Herter himself made up the deficits until his death five years later.

By the time scheduled for the publication of the first number in October 1905, five papers had accumulated and a list of 130 subscribers had been obtained. Osler was the first subscriber from Great Britain and Calmette the first from France. The first article was by Abel and Taveau on epinephrine; the second was by Reid Hunt on the action of thyroid on the toxicity of acetoni-trile. Its opening paragraph gives an idea of how far distant 1905 is in reality: "Speculation as to the function of the thyroid gland has taken two main directions; some supposed that these organs elaborate an internal secretion which is of itself necessary for certain processes of metabolism, while others think that their chief function is to neutralize poisonous substances originating in the body [enterotoxines] or introduced into it from without [iodine, for example]." The three subsequent issues brought Volume 1 to completion in June 1906. In it is to be found the first paper by Dakin published in this country; one by Treat Johnson and another by young E. V. McCollum on pyrimidines; four short papers by Herter on chemical byproducts of intestinal bacteria; and one by Jacques Loeb on the antagonism of magnesium and calcium ions. The subscription list more than doubled for the second volume, which was completed in January 1907. Waverly Press then became the printers of the *JBC*, their first scientific journal.

Upon the completion of Volume 6 in February 1909, Dr. Abel resigned his editorship to devote his energy to the formation of the American Society of Pharmacology and Therapeutics and to the initiation of its journal. Although he continued as a collaborating editor, his resignation really left Dr. Herter as sole editor until his untimely death in 1910. Herter's death involved not only the loss of a highly gifted leader but also the cessation of his financial support. Friends and relatives of Dr. and Mrs. Herter assembled a fund of $20,000 as a tribute to Herter's memory, which helped greatly in the future finances of the journal.

Christian Herter was an unusual man. His father was a successful architect in New York whose career was also cut short by death at the age of forty-four. Young Herter's home was a center of artistic rather than scientific culture. He received the equivalent of college training from private instruction under his father's guidance. From early boyhood his career goal was medicine, and he entered the College of Physicians and Surgeons at Columbia University in 1881, at the age of fifteen. He completed the course with distinction in three years and then served an internship at Bellevue Hospital. Herter's preceptor was William S. Halsted, then a demonstrator in anatomy. After his internship Herter studied pathology for a year in Baltimore under Welch, and then spent a year studying nervous and mental diseases in Zurich under Forel. He specialized in the latter field when he returned to America and began to practice in 1887. However, his interest soon turned to chemical problems, particularly those connected with pathological conditions. He equipped a laboratory in his own home for the study of his patients, then engaged a succession of well-trained chemists to work in his laboratory—the greater part of Dakin's career as a chemist was spent in Herter's laboratory—and with their help, trained himself in chemistry. Herter became competent enough in pathological chemistry to be made professor of that subject at Bellevue Medical College in 1898. His *Lectures on Chemical Pathology* was a unique book for its time. In 1903 he was appointed professor of pharmacology and therapeutics at Columbia. After spending a year in Europe with Paul Ehrlich and Hans Meyer, he discharged the duties of that position for six years before his death.

Herter's researches were designed not so much to advance a recognized medical discipline as to help his own understanding of medical problems which excited his special interest. He had little talent for organization, but the establishment in 1893 and the subsequent growth of his own laboratory was a unique venture in New York medicine. In 1901 he was one of the most influential of the six original trustees who organized the Rockefeller Institute. Herter also endowed two permanent lectureships, one at Johns Hopkins and the other at Bellevue, designed to acquaint medical students with the personalities of the creative investigators in the medical sciences.

It is of interest that in 1905 Abel's research went through a period of reorientation. During that period Jacques Loeb was engaged in systematic studies of the physiological action of ions. One of these studies dealt with the swelling of frog muscle caused by hydrochloric (HCL) and organic acids and indicated that organic acid was less effective than hydrochloric acid. Abel carried out similar experiments which suggested an apparent correlation between the degree of swelling and the diffusion constant of the acids. A brief account of this work was presented in 1907 at the first meeting of the American Society of Biological Chemists, a new society that owed its foundation primarily to Abel. It was he who took the initiative to call a meeting of biological chemists in New York on December 26, 1906. A few of the biochemists had expressed their reluctance to the organization of a new society, fearing that it might weaken the American Physiological Society and the American Chemical Society by the withdrawal of some of their respective members who were biochemists. However, these objections were removed by the well-considered remarks made by Abel at the New York meeting:

Scattered and divided forces cannot develop that coordination of effort that is desirable when many workers have one great interest in common. In such a case organization is beneficial. It encourages research; it furnishes the mechanism of confident criticism and helpful discussion; and lastly, the very fact that we feel impelled to organize willl make it evident to faculties of science and medicine and to scientific and medical societies that a great and growing department of research demands its fitting place in the general scheme of higher education.

Consistent with this viewpoint, Abel from his earliest days as professor of pharmacology at Johns Hopkins advocated independent chairs of biological chemistry. In 1908 he turned over responsibility for biological chemistry to Walter Jones, who was made the director of this new department.

Pharmacology and Experimental Therapeutics

By 1908 pharmacology had made sufficient progress in this country for Abel to assume the leadership in the foundation of the *Journal of Pharmacology and Experimental Therapeutics* and in the organization of the American Society for Pharmacology and Experimental Therapeutics. These projects he discussed at great length with his associates over the famous luncheon table in his department. Abel persuaded the Williams and Wilkins Company to publish the journal, which was incorporated in the name of Abel, Reid Hunt, and Carl Voegtlin. The first number appeared in June 1909, with Abel as editor. In the editorial announcement Abel expressed the opinion that "Every physician who has the best interest of his profession at heart feels that he must become familiar with the methods and principles and above all, with the actual objective results which are placed at his disposal by the sciences here represented." He quoted Paul Ehrlich's evaluation of the subjects: "There can be no doubt that the great fields of knowledge, pharmacology, toxicology and therapeutics, in their theoretical and practical aspects form the most important branches of medicine." During the sixty-six years of its existence, this journal has published numerous important investigations and since 1934 has been the official organ of the American Society for Pharmacology and Experimental Therapeutics. Abel was the first president of this society in 1908.

Abel's remarkable talent for oganization, rarely found in a man so dedicated to research, tremendously benefited experimental medicine.

Anatomical publications

Florence Sabin has described how a small group of men, returning to the United States from the study of medicine in Germany in the 1880s and finding no laboratories, equipment, or money for medical education, effectively organized to obtain all of these necessities. Within a decade laboratories were built and the more curious-minded of the students attracted to research. This led to numerous investigations of high quality, which created a pressing need for the formation of scientific societies and outlets for publication.

The Association of American Anatomists was founded in 1888. Although Joseph Leidy of Philadelphia was its distinguished first president, the society remained impotent until C. S. Minot and F. P. Mall became members. Mall had organized his department in Baltimore in 1893, but it was not until five years later that he and Minot joined the Anatomical Association. In one of his letters Mall stated, "Reform does not move rapidly unless there is someone behind it." This statement was never better illustrated than in this situation.

The first meeting of the association which Mall attended had a program including Mall's work on the origin of the lymphatics of the liver and the development of the diaphragm; Ross Harrison's, on the occurrence of tails in man; W. S. Miller's, on the lobules of the lung; M. Sudler's, on the structure of the gall bladder; and Broedel's halftones of the blood vessels of the kidney, together with papers by L. F. Barker, Pressman Keyes, and C. R. Bardeen, all from Mall's laboratory. Sabin points out that this program was like a breath of fresh air, "reminding one of the awakening of Rip van Winkle in a new era." There is sufficient documentation of Mall's role to demonstrate that he was always on the alert to find the good work which was being done in anatomy and to have it presented at the meetings of the Anatomical Association. As Dr. C. M. Jackson described it: "Modesty was Mall's most prominent personal trait, along with a Socratic propensity to ask searching questions. At the meetings of the American Association of Anatomists he was a great inspiration, but always 'behind the scenes.' He rarely appeared in the lecture room where the papers were being presented, and still more rarely, on the program. He spent most of his time chatting in the hall outside or at the demonstrations. Incidentally he was largely responsible for the emphasis on these demonstrations which constituted the most valuable and characteristic feature of our anatomical meetings."

Anatomy represented only one of many areas of medical science which were evolving at a rapid pace. It was becoming clear that still newer forms of medical publication were necessary. Instead of being diffuse in character, journals needed to be special, technical and national in scope. The first of the special journals to be formed in the United States was the *American Journal of Physiology* in 1898. For years this journal was edited on a sound scientific and financial basis by Dr. W. T. Porter of Harvard University. Subsequently, both this journal and the newer *Physiological Review* were run by Donald R. Hooker of the Johns Hopkins School of Hygiene and the Public Health. Dr. Hooker's editorship provided an impressive demonstration of the fact that an expert medical editor, with the aid of a skilled secretary and with the backing of an editorial committee, could publish a journal representing a scientific association on a sound financial basis without endowment or subsidies.

The first volume of the *American Journal of Anatomy* was published in 1901–02 due primarily to the efforts of Mall and Minot. Sabin points out that the initiation of anatomical publication in this country can be found in the correspondence between these two men. Minot's interests were primarily in embryology and he often discussed with Dr. Porter, the possibility of starting a journal of embryology. In a letter to Mall on March 21, 1900, Minot wrote: "In regard to the journal we need I have thought that a companion volume to Porter's *Journal of Physiology* would be the best plan. If my means permitted, I would have tried to start it, for Porter cordially approves. My idea has gone to and fro between a *Journal of Anatomy and Embryology* and of *Embryology and Cytology*." Mall's ideas were different, however. He believed that a general journal of anatomy should be considered first before any special journals were started; that such a journal should be national in character; that it should represent all of the fundamental problems of anatomy and should be of the widest possible scope and of the highest standards. He saw such a journal as an indispensable factor in demonstrating to the teachers and students of medicine the role of scientific anatomy in the development of medical science in this country. He foresaw what anatomy might mean not only for anatomical departments in medical schools but also for the other medical sciences with which its problems are related.

Mall's plan was as follows: To raise a sum of money, sufficient to guarantee prompt payment of the printer's bills, from those who might be interested in scientific publication in general; to use this fund as a trust and repay it from the income of the journal; to get the Anatomical Association to consider the journal as its own venture and include a subscription for it in the dues, thus getting an immediate personal circulation as well as the general circulation to libraries. Mall won Minot over to these plans and demonstrated the possibilities when Dr. Henry Knower of Mall's laboratory raised about a thousand dollars in Baltimore as a "guarantee fund." Minot then raised a similar sum in Boston, and finally Dr. George S. Huntington, professor of anatomy at the College of Physicians and Surgeons in New York collected a similar amount in that city. The fund finally reached a total of $5,000; the contributors were listed as founders of the *American Journal of Anatomy*, and their names published at the back of the first volume. Many of the contributors were not anatomists but physicians, surgeons, zoologists, and men interested in medical education, such as Gilman. Although many of those who contributed had doubts about the undertaking, they supported it on the basis of Mall's driving power and his skill in finance. The fund was held as a trust by Minot, Huntington, and Mall. The editors on the board of the journal were Lewellys F. Barker, Thomas Dwight, Simon H. Gage, G. Carl Huber, George S. Huntington, Franklin P. Mall, Charles S. Minot, George A. Piersol, and Henry Knower, who became the managing editor.

The first volume of the journal did not contain any published statement of its purpose, but the following letter was sent to possible subscribers:

We send herewith a notice of the new American Journal of Anatomy which we believe will be of the greatest service to anatomy in America, both by offering a medium for the publication of the best anatomical researches, and also of setting a higher standard of anatomical work and attainment. In order to put the journal upon a permanent footing it is necessary to have not less than 400 subscribers. We shall be very much gratified if your interest in the promotion of medical science induces you to become a subscriber.

The *American Journal of Anatomy* set aside a few pages for preliminary reports, short articles, critical notes on research and educational methods, and reviews. This material was soon issued as a separate publication known as the *Anatomical Record*. Both of these journals were a great success and provided an effective stimulus to research. They won immediate recognition both in this country and abroad as being a significant part of modern scientific medicine. Mall demonstrated that, besides being valuable to the scientist on the professional side, good scientific journals can be run on a sound financial basis. He directed the publication of the first seven volumes of the *American Journal of Anatomy* and the first volume of the *Anatomical Record* from Baltimore. In 1908, having other publication projects in mind, he turned both publications over to the Wistar Institute of Philadelphia.

Mall's first important undertaking in publishing was the ninth volume of the *Johns Hopkins Hospital Reports*, which was issued in tribute to Dr. William

H. Welch. Mall's best energies went into this volume, as a means of expressing his high regard for Dr. Welch. Mall's earlier days had been filled with anxiety about getting a start in scientific medicine in America; in a letter to Welch he said: "You made the opportunities here." Concerning the *Festschrift*, Welch wrote to Mall on May 13, 1900: "My first enthusiasm for this wonderful volume has not waned on closer acquaintance. I know that it would never have come into being except for you, and I cannot express my gratitude to you. In fact you were the incentive of so many of the contributions that my attitude to them is rather that of a grandfather than *in loco parentis*. You have been the greatest stimulus to scientific work on our faculty and have established the first real school of anatomy which this country has seen." A similar tribute to Mall was made by J. Whitridge Williams, who said: "The things which were unique in the early days of the Johns Hopkins Medical School were contributed by Mall, for without him we should have been just another good school."

Around 1912 Mall's plans matured for a new type of textbook in embryology, to which Minot was one of the outstanding contributors. This was the manual published in collaboration with Keibel. Although Mall planned it to be a start toward a publication called the *International Archives of Embryology*, the war effectually prevented this. The new archives became the *Contributions to Embryology*, published by the Carnegie Institution of Washington. Its development was Mall's last venture in publication, and not only represented the highest skill of the printer's art, being published on the finest paper and beautifully illustrated with lithographic plates, but also added to the highest scientific attainment in the field of anatomy.

Mall died in 1917, and two years later the ninth volume of the *Contributions to Embryology* was published as a tribute to him. Its foreword reads as follows: "The papers included in this volume have been contributed as a memorial by present and former members of the staff of the late Professor Franklin Paine Mall in recognition of his inspiring leadership and in response to the strong feeling of affection with which they had come to regard him. A volume of this nature had been under consideration to commemorate the approaching 25th anniversary of his occupancy of the Chair of Anatomy in The Johns Hopkins University." All of the contributors to this volume had been students of Mall's whom he had started in research, except for two foreign guests—Professor O. Van der Stricht of Ghent and Professor J. Duesberg of Liège. The advent of the war had brought these men to his laboratory, and both had contributed richly to Mall's pleasure and satisfaction. The memorial volume includes the exciting work of Sabin, E. R. and E. L. Clark, Margaret R. Lewis, Essick, L. H. Weed, George Corner, George L. Streeter, Warren H. Lewis, C. R. Bardeen, and Robert Bean. A very inspiring review of this volume appeared in the English journal *Nature* (*Nature* 106 [1920]:170).

American Journal of Hygiene

During the second academic year of the School of Hygiene and Public Health (1919–1920), The Society of Hygiene was established and a new publication was begun, the *American Journal of Hygiene*. Welch was the initiator of this new monthly journal. The first issue appeared in January 1921, with Welch as editor and Charles E. Simon as managing editor. Among the distinguished list of assistant editors, some of whom were on the faculties of other institutions, were Simon Flexner, Graham Lusk, George W. McCoy, M. J. Rosenau, F. F. Russell, Theobald Smith, E. R. Stitt, V. C. Vaughan, C. E. A. Winslow, Hans Zinsser, F. P. Gay, E. O. Jordan, and W. H. Park.

When Simon died in 1927, Roscoe R. Hyde became managing editor of the journal. By this time the editorial board was composed entirely of local faculty members, with Dr. Welch serving as honorary chairman. Beginning in 1938 but continuing in this format for only three years the journal was published in four sections devoted to: (1) epidemiology, biostatistics, and general topics; (2) bacteriology, immunology, and viruses; (3) protozoology and malariology; and (4) helminthology. In 1965 the name of the journal was changed to the *American Journal of Epidemiology*. Ownership of this journal has been in the Johns Hopkins University throughout its existence.

Journal of Urology

Within a year after the dedication of the Brady Urological Institute (1915), it was apparent that there was need of a journal for publication of papers by members of the urology staff. Dr. Young, after discussing the possibility of starting a special journal of urology with a number of prominent American urologists, made arrangements with the Williams and Wilkins Company of Baltimore to publish the *Journal of Urology*. The editors were John T. Geraghty, David M. Davis, Herman O. Mosenthal, and Hugh H. Young, editor-in-chief. The foreword in the first issue expressed the aims and ambitions of the editors:

Recent years have been very prolific in the production of splendid articles on the urinary tract, its adnexa and correlated subjects. Many of those from the Departments of Physiology, Pharmacology, Chemistry, Pathology and Bacteriology have been scattered through the various special journals on those subjects. The embryological and anatomical researches have likewise appeared in journals devoted to these fields. Medical articles on the kidney, adrenals, urine and so forth and the many diseases which are secondary are correlated, and surgical papers of a similar scope, have found lodgement in dozens of diversified journals all over the country.

The situation is such that one who is interested in all forms of research in this field, anxious to keep abreast with what the internists are doing along these lines and at the same time desirous of following the progress of surgical urology, is overwhelmed with the magnitude of the task and fails to discover much that is important. . . .

It is evident that some common meeting place is extremely desirable—some medium in which all types of papers upon the field of common interest may appear— Archives of Urology—historical, embryological, anatomical, biochemical, pharmacological, pathological, bacteriological, surgical and medical, experimental and clinical.

Such is what we hope to accomplish in the Journal of Urology and we bespeak for it the support and active assistance of all who come within the wide scope of its work.

The first issue appeared in February 1917 and contained 138 pages. This number, composed largely of experimental and research papers, gave evidence of the scientific character that the editors hoped to maintain in the *Journal of Urology*. When the second number appeared (April 1917), America had entered World War I and most of the editors had joined the AEF. Regardless of this interference, six numbers totaling 579 pages were issued in that year. In 1918, although many of the urologists were in France, the *Journal of Urology* had twenty-five original articles covering almost 500 pages.

At the annual meeting of the American Urological Association in 1920, it was proposed to publish a journal which would include the papers and discussions presented at the annual meetings. Realizing that it would be difficult to maintain the *Journal of Urology* if a second journal came into the field, Hugh Young proposed to the association that they take over the *Journal of Urology* without reservation and appoint a new board of editors. After accepting his offer a board of editors was chosen and Young was asked to continue as editor-in-chief. The other members of the editorial board were William F. Braasch, Henry G. Bugbee, Herman L. Kretschmer, and William C. Quinby. The arrangement provided that every member of the association was to be a subscriber to the *Journal of Urology*, and the financial status of the journal improved at once. In 1928 the twentieth volume was published. It included an accumulative index of the preceding ten years (which occupied 86 pages) and a very important series of papers. The two yearly volumes had grown to approximately 750 pages each. In 1934 Dr. William A. Frontz, who for seventeen years had been a very efficient editor, died and Dr. J. A. C. Colston assumed the position. For a number of years now Dr. Hugh Jewett has edited the journal.

The William H. Welch Library and The Institute of The History of Medicine

When John Shaw Billings, a medical biographer and one of the world's great bibliographers, drew up his plans for the Johns Hopkins Hospital, he curiously enough made only scant provisions for a library. His mind was evidently on larger things—on the general principles of organization and construction of a place where, as he expressed it, the students' knowledge was "not to be acquired from textbooks or lectures but from observation, experiment and personal experience." He doubtless recognized the close proximity of the surgeon general's library in Washington and also took it for granted that a small library would be established for books which were essential to the activity of that closely knit group of young men who first gathered in Baltimore.

THE EARLY MEDICAL LIBRARIES. With the opening of the Johns Hopkins Hospital on May 7, 1889, a medical library for the use of the resident and visiting staffs was established on the first floor, the north wing, of the Administration Building of the hospital. The collection of books during the first few years grew rapidly, largely because of the efforts of Dr. Henry M. Hurd. Within twenty years, the increase in the number of volumes caused the library to place a portion of its holdings in the basement of the building and to utilize an additional large room across the corridor from the original site. However, in spite of the efforts to provide for the growth of the library, the quarters in the Administration Building became increasingly congested. The overcrowding in the available rooms made effective use of the books impossible, but although the inadequacy of the library accommodations was apparent as early as 1915, for thirteen years thereafter the work of the library was carried on without interruption in these cramped quarters. To the general holdings of the hospital library, the following collections were added: the Morison Dermatological Collection (1897); the Howard A. Kelly Collection (1914); the Hugh H. Young Urological Collection (1917); the Henry J. Berkeley Collection of Psychiatry (1921); and the William Osler Collection (1921). At the end of the year 1928, the library contained over 31,000 bound volumes.

The library of the School of Medicine began with the purchase of a few volumes when the school was opened in 1893. This collection was initially housed in the old Physiology Building, where it remained until the opening of the new Hunterian Laboratory in 1914, when the library was moved to a series of rooms on the first floor of this new laboratory building. The library volumes consisted mainly of books and journals pertaining to anatomy, physiology, physiological chemistry and pharmacology. The general collection of the library was greatly strengthened by the addition of the Ahlfeld Teratological Collection, a gift to the university from Francis M. Jencks in 1905, and the Warrington Dispensary Collection, presented to the University by William A. Marburg in 1906. At the end of 1928 these library quarters had also become very overcrowded, containing more than 14,000 volumes.

When in 1916 the School of Hygiene and Public Health was established, a relatively large collection of medical journals and books was purchased as a working nucleus for its library. At first housed in the original building of the Johns Hopkins University, the library of the School of Hygiene was moved in 1925 to the new building adjacent to the medical school. In these quarters the library was satisfactorily accommodated, although by the end of 1928 it had grown to 11,000 volumes and included the valuable collection purchased for the school by Sir Arthur Newsholme, resident lecturer in public health administration from 1919 to 1921.

Thus various factors determining the growth of the Johns Hopkins Medical Institutions led to the formation and maintenance of these three distinct libraries. The hospital library, since it was founded before the medical school was opened, was logically the repository for clinical journals and books. The construction of the pre-clinical laboratories at a distance from the Administration Building of the hospital was the main reason for the establishment of a separate library for the basic science departments. Again, the library of the

School of Hygiene was initially necessitated by the housing of the school in buildings far removed from the hospital group.

So, for purely physical and chronological reasons, the three libraries were established separately, although the idea of a central medical library combining the collections of the hospital and medical school was generally accepted by the members of the Advisory Board of the Medical Faculty in the early years of the School of Medicine. The idea of centralization was discussed on many occasions, but in spite of the strong support given to it by Dr. Welch and Dr. Osler, no progress was made. After 1900 the movement began to gain further support and was especially promoted by Dr. Halsted. In 1918 Mr. George K. McGaw made the first of a series of gifts to the hospital in support of the library. Shortly before this and again in 1919, Dr. Halsted wrote to many of the alumni urging the idea of a central library and soliciting contributions of books. However, in spite of these stimuli, it was not until the period from 1922 to 1925 that the idea of combining the three separate collections began to take concrete form. Interest was developed not only in central housing but also in setting up an arrangement that would make the library more than just a well-run technical storehouse of medical literature. This important conception of the library was the initial phase of discussions which soon included the idea of an institute for the study of the history of medicine.

THE HISTORY OF MEDICINE. The footprints of Osler are seen in the early establishment of a Journal Club, which met every Thursday afternoon in the room set apart as a library to review and discuss articles from the contemporary literature relating to the day's work. Next came the formation of the Hospital Medical Society, which, according to the announcement in the first issue of the *Bulletin*, was to meet under the presidency of W. H. Welch on the first and third Monday of each month. For one of the early meetings of this society Dr. Billings brought from Washington forty-four carefully selected volumes, ranging from a fifteenth-century manuscript of Roger to the first edition of Jenner's *Inquiry*, to illustrate the discourse he gave on rare medical books. A surprising number of that early group showed an interest in medical history, and one finds in the Bulletin the following announcement: "The first meeting to organize the Johns Hopkins Hospital Historical Club was called to order by Dr. Osler in the hospital library Monday evening, November 10, 1890 at 8 o'clock. Thirty gentlemen present. Dr. Welch was elected President and Dr. Reese Secretary. Dr. Welch made brief introductory remarks to show the value of historical studies to the physician. He presented several histories of medicine and commented upon the merits of the various historians." Thus, the seeds were laid for what was ultimately to eventuate—the establishment of the Institute of the History of Medicine, with Dr. Welch as the first professor.

The Historical Society soon launched itself on a methodical survey of medical history that began bravely enough with a study of the Hippocratic writings. But the next year, in an effort to plumb the depths of Galen, the club nearly foundered, proving the wisdom of Garrison's advice that the beginner should back up into the subject rather than start out with its obscure origins.

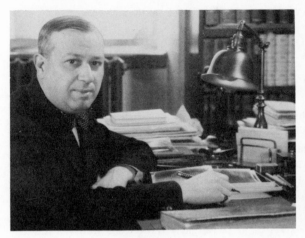

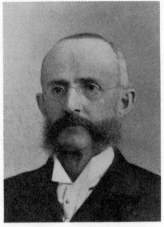

Henry E. Sigerist

From the Collection of the Institute of the History of Medicine, The Johns Hopkins School of Medicine

Henry Mills Hurd

The photograph was taken when Hurd came to Baltimore in 1889 as the first superintendent of the Johns Hopkins Hospital.
From *Johns Hopkins Hosp. Bull.* vol. 30 (1919), plate 42

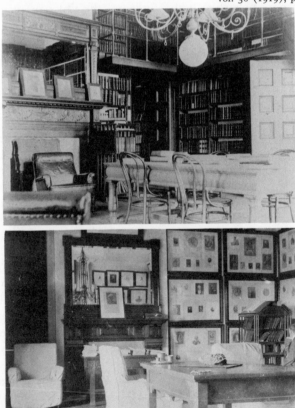

The original library (*top*) and the residents' reading room (*bottom*), Johns Hopkins Hospital, 1903

The library was then located in the present Board Room.
From the Archives Office, The Johns Hopkins Medical Institutions

The ambitious program was abandoned, the often delightful though desultory papers and essays that later characterized the monthly meetings being substituted for it.

Dr. Billings meantime had been coming over from Washington to deliver two courses of lectures—and prophetic were his chosen topics. One series was on the subject of hygiene, which after an interval of some thirty years bore fruit in the establishment of the new School of Hygiene and Public Health. The other course of lectures was on medical history, a subject which with the development later of the institute would have full opportunity to flourish under the care of the same person (Welch) who had said: "The study of the history of the various medical doctrines broadens a physician's view and liberalizes his conception of his profession."

Dr. Billings's afternoon exercises in those early days were slimly attended. Even with his rare gifts it was too heavy a historical meal for the undergraduate, and the members of the resident staff found themselves under so great a burden of bedside responsibility that their attendance was prevented. When Billings moved to Philadelphia on his retirement from the surgeon general's library, the formal lectures were brought to an end. They were replaced by something far more palatable to the students—the Oslerian method of slowly but surely arousing an historical appetite by the proper touch in each exercise upon the historical bearings of the subject under discussion, whatever it might be—an eponymic question asked, the original source books passed around, a paragraph read, a picture shown, or an incident related. In this way, by the process of repeated inoculations, many students who unquestionably would have sidestepped the formal course of lectures became unconsciously impregnated with something much more valuable to them in the long run than the acquirement of just a few more facts concerning diagnosis and treatment.

In spite of this early interest in the history of medicine, the general concept of an institute of medical history did not take on a definite character until the proposal for a medical library assumed final form in 1925. It was in October of that year that President Goodnow presented to Abraham Flexner, of the General Education Board of the Rockefeller Foundation, a detailed proposal for the establishment of a medical library at the Johns Hopkins University. In addition to the general thesis of the need of such a library in any educational community to promote an atmosphere of real scholarship, President Goodnow pointed out that the faculty of medicine had for many years appreciated the great opportunity existing in the field of medical bibliography —an opportunity to create in students and young teachers a cultural background of greatest service in making them familiar with the humanistic side of medicine. In his request for funds to establish a central library building he suggested that sufficient space be allotted in the building to house the proposed Institute of the History of Medicine. On February 1926 the General Education Board appropriated to the Johns Hopkins University the sum of $200,000 to serve as an endowment for a professorship of the history of medicine.

On November 1, 1926 Dr. Welch resigned as director of the School of Hygiene and Public Health to assume once more a position of leadership in the university—this time to inaugurate the newly created chair of the history of medicine. Later in November 1926 the General Education Board appropriated to the Johns Hopkins University the sum of $1 million toward the $1.5 million needed for the purchase of land and the construction and endowment of the central medical library. Subsequently, at a meeting in February 1927, the conditions of this appropriation were altered by the General Education Board so that the sum of $750,000 was made immediately available for the purchase of land and for construction and equipment of the library. In addition to this immediate grant, the General Education Board agreed to pay interest upon the sum of $250,000 provided the Johns Hopkins University raise $25,000 a year for the maintenance of the new library. In the event that the Johns Hopkins should capitalize its annual quota of $25,000, the General Education Board agreed to give to the university this sum of $250,000, provided that $500,000 for the endowment of the library be raised by the Johns Hopkins University before expiration of five years after completion of the building. In May 1928 the university received from an anonymous donor a gift of $500,000, thus enabling it to meet these conditions. In addition, the trustees of the hospital voted to continue their annual appropriations for library purposes and to turn this annual sum over to the central medical library for maintenance. A similar action was taken by the trustees of the Johns Hopkins University in regard to the annual appropriations for library purposes made in the School of Hygiene and Public Health and in the School of Medicine. These annual appropriations, amounting to $21,700, taken with the interest on the endowment of $750,000, provided the central medical library with an annual income approximating $60,000.

It was understood that the building should bear Dr. Welch's name, and so it was designated the William H. Welch Medical Library. Plans were developed for the building and ground was broken on November 29, 1927. On March 12, 1928, the cornerstone of the building was laid without ceremony but in the presence of a number of interested persons. The construction of the building occupied slightly more than a year, but on December 1, 1928, the assistant librarian and his staff were able to move into the building, although the removal of the books from the three constituent libraries was not undertaken until early in January 1929. The cost of the building and equipment was $625,000. The three institutions represented agreed that two representatives from each of the boards were to constitute a committee, with the professor of the history of medicine and the medical librarian as ex-officio members. During the academic year 1927–1928, the Medical Board of the hospital designated Dr. Warfield T. Longcope and Dr. J. Whitridge Williams; the Advisory Board of the Faculty of the School of Hygiene, Dr. Elmer V. McCollum and Dr. William W. Ford; and the Advisory Board of the Medical Faculty, Dr. William G. MacCallum and Dr. E. Kennerly Marshall, Jr.

In the spring of 1927 Welch departed for Europe to purchase books for the newly built medical library at Johns Hopkins. At that time Henry E. Sigerist had succeeded Karl Sudhoff as director of the Institute of the History of Medicine at Leipzig. On a visit to Leipzig Welch took Sigerist to Auerbach's

Keller, the place where Welch had had his eventful meeting many years before with John Shaw Billings. This meeting with Welch was the beginning of a sequence of events that brought Sigerist to America. In the autumn of 1931 Sigerist was invited to the United States for a lecture tour to begin at Hopkins. After he had spoken at Boston, Cushing promptly sent a telegram to Welch full of enthusiasm for Sigerist, who "has captivated everyone here by his modesty, learning, lively interest in everything and personal charm. I cannot imagine a more suitable person for the post or one more certain to develop it in the way you would desire." This was on November 30, 1931, and on Sunday, December 27, when Welch arrived in Minneapolis for a meeting of the History of Science Society, he recruited Sigerist as his successor to the chair of the history of medicine at Johns Hopkins.

Henry E. Sigerist, born in Paris in 1891 of Swiss parents, received his M.D. degree from the University of Zurich in 1917. In 1910–1911 he studied Oriental philology in Zurich and in London. Upon finishing his period of medical service in the Swiss Army he did postgraduate work with Sudhoff at Leipzig (1919), and in 1921 he joined the faculty at the University of Zurich as a medical historian. In 1925 he succeeded Dr. Karl Sudhoff as director of the Institute of the History of Medicine at Leipzig.

In spite of urging by all his teachers, Sigerist refused to specialize during his period of training in Germany. He delved as a young student into philology, history, science, and medicine. His was a truly comprehensive outlook. Languages, the humanities, and the sciences all fascinated him equally, and thus he remained a generalist. Ludwig Edelstein (at a memorial meeting held for Sigerist by the Johns Hopkins Medical History Club) commented that Sigerist's refusal to restrict himself to one particular field was the outcome of his innate curiosity. "Artless, unfeigned love of knowledge, as it was the stimulus of his research, also pervaded his writing, teaching and lecturing. It made every topic he happened to be concerned with come to life and unfailingly aroused and captivated the imagination as well as the interest of his audience." Sigerist commented himself on why he finally chose the history of medicine for his career: "Gradually I drifted into a field where I could combine all my interests, medical, philological, historical and sociological."

The study of the history of medicine at Hopkins now came under the influence and leadership of one who had the capacity to reconstruct past events from as universal a point of view as it is possible to achieve. In Sigerist's own words: "From the very beginning, I endeavored to correlate the history of medicine with the problems of our time." When Sigerist came on the scene, the history of medicine had recently passed the stage where it was just a hobby for interested physicians. Largely through Karl Sudhoff's efforts, it had been changed into a subject ranking as an academic pursuit in its own right. Sudhoff studied the history of medicine in order "to understand rather than to judge." Sigerist, however, "was intent on drawing lessons from his emphatic analysis of historical events and situations. He tried to orient himself in the life of the present by the insight that he had gained from the past." Edelstein also commented on another characteristic of Sigerist's scholarship: namely, the obligation he felt to take part in current events. Sigerist believed it important to bring his knowledge to bear upon the issues of his own time with courage and determination.

Sigerist's initial series of lectures at Hopkins before he was appointed to the professorship in the autumn of 1932 had been on the general subject of the evolution of medicine in its cultural aspects, with individual lectures devoted to the primitive conceptions of disease, the religious character of Oriental medicine, the philosophical attitude of the Greek physicians toward medicine, the bond of modern medicine, the cultural background of modern medicine, and the development of medicine during the nineteenth century. He also conducted a series of six seminars on the interpretation of medical texts. In addition to his outstanding contributions as a scholarly historian of medicine, Sigerist also had an important organizational role. He edited journals and founded series of books because he felt a strong urge to further medical history and to represent it in its many shades.

Chief among Sigerist's early accomplishments were the integration of the teaching of medical history with the program of the Hopkins Medical School, and the evolution of a journal—first as a section of The Johns Hopkins Hospital Bulletin (2 years) and for the next 7 years as an independent publication, the Bulletin of the Institute of the History of Medicine. In the teaching of medical history at Johns Hopkins, the Institute not only broadened the perspective of students, but no doubt inspired some to become medical historians—either by vocation or avocation. Meantime, the establishment of the journal was calculated to spread the gospel to the medical profession at large.

Well aware of a national mission, Sigerist was successful in bringing about a reorganization of the American Association of the History of Medicine. This body, largely made up of prominent physicians in Philadelphia, had already brought together individuals interested in medical history for pleasant annual meetings—a desirable first step in making men with common enthusiasms known to each other. The association was then organized on a national basis, using local groups as the constituent societies. Its very existence encouraged the formation of additional societies. In making the institute also available to the association as its official organ (1939), Sigerist provided the *sine qua non* for a real association, which was further provided with a constitution, officers, and annual meetings. To stimulate the interest of students, the Osler Medal was created and the Garrison Lectures were initiated. Through the *Bulletin*, and by means of questionnaire reports, Sigerist encouraged the teaching of medical history throughout the United States and Canada.

Only the passage of time will make it possible to put into perspective the influence of Sigerist as a historian. A contemporary evaluation is provided by the remarks made on one occasion by a distinguished group of medical historians and statesmen at a farewell dinner given for Dr. and Mrs. Sigerist on May 9, 1948. In his remarks at a meeting of the Johns Hopkins Medical History Club held after Sigerist's death (*Bull. Hist. Med.* 31 [1957]: 295), Owsei Temkin noted that philological analysis and cultural synthesis were the two main approaches of Sigerist to medical history. In Temkin's view, Sigerist considered it an important function as a medical historian to make the development of medicine understandable against the background of all factors that shape our civilization. The many interrelations between disease and civilization fascinated him and were studied at length in his *Civilization and Disease* of 1943. Temkin pointed out that the other two works in which he offered a synthesis of medicine were his *Introduction to Medicine,* known under the misleading English title of *Man and Medicine,* and the *Great Doctors.* Temkin believes that the latter was Sigerist's best book. Although it is a series of biographies, it does not concentrate on biographical detail but becomes a history of medicine in which the great doctors are points in its development. Yet as Temkin pointed out, the reader does not lose the feeling that he is dealing with men and not mere representations of abstract historical forces. Temkin concluded that *Great Doctors* shows Dr. Sigerist's mastery of his material, his instinct for avoiding factual historical mistakes and his great charm, which stimulated his audience.

Richard H. Shryock commented (at a farewell dinner given by Dr. and Mrs. Sigerist, May 9, 1948) on Sigerist's influence upon medical history in the United States:

For make no mistake, we are in the presence here of an historical phenomenon of continuing significance to this country. This phenomenon is what general historians term the transit of culture from Europe to America; in this case, the transit of the European—and particularly of the German—tradition in medical historiography to this side of the Atlantic. Similar transfers have taken place in other fields and in earlier periods, as when returning American students brought Scottish medicine here in 1760, French medicine in 1830, and German medicine in 1880. Rarely, however, has one man had such an impact on American scholarship or science as Sigerist has had on our medical history. One can think of partial parallels, as in the stimulus provided by his earlier compatriot, Agassiz, to certain natural sciences in this country, but the latter's influence was less unique. Sigerist found medical history here the avocation of a few prominent physicians; he leaves it a field in which there are not only a number of scholar-scientists who make it their vocation, but in which an increasing number realize the need for serious, continuous teaching, writing, and research. Sigerist would be the last to claim that he had accomplished this transformation alone; but when one recalls how many others who participated were directly or indirectly influenced by him, the primacy of his leadership becomes apparent.

In the words of Alan Gregg, Henry Sigerist

made us aware of the fact that medicine is the study and application of biology in a matrix that is at once historical, social, political, economic, and cultural. The practice of medicine is a part of sociology and a product of sociological factors. Sir Oliver Lodge once remarked that the last thing in the world that a deep sea fish could discover would be salt water. Henry Sigerist removed us, with the historian's landing net, from a circumambient present into the atmosphere of the past and thus discovered to us the nature of the new year in which we were swimming, floating, and betimes stagnating. He brought to American medicine the beginnings of what Josiah Royce declared was his idea of heaven—the knowledge of the significance of what you are doing.

Only experience can provide the alphabet with which to spell out the experiences of others. Santayana has warned us that he who ignores history is doomed to repeat it. Were you to ask me if anyone in the past fifteen years has been eager to make us Americans understand the richness and the power and the duty and the beauty and the meaning of scholarship and the potentialities of the universities I would think first of Henry Sigerist.

His scholarship appears to have been the natural consequence of an un-assuming industry and an amazing comprehension. Gregg tells the story of a dinner party at the home of Dr. Lewis H. Weed at which the conversation among a group of Johns Hopkins professors turned to the "hundred great books" used at St. Johns:

Stirred by a compelling mixture of sadism and masochism I suggested that we each tell how many of the hundred great books he had read. The high man said 32, the low 16. Then I pressed Sigerist for his score. With charmingly apologetic discomfort he admitted that he had read 94—adding that six of these he had not read in the original! This last embarrassed admission was never intended as a coup-de-grace to those who had not even considered that important detail—but quite gently it had, none the less, the effect of an urbane knockout....

I would name one other and vastly important imprint that Sigerist makes on American medicine—his relentless insistence that what we choose to do now with our present lives, is history in the making. To do this takes courage and a candor for which at times the general appetite flags, for to live *subspecie aeternitatis* is not always reassuring to those who live by current credos alone.

A long-time friend, Erwin H. Ackerknecht, interpreted Sigerist's period in America as follows:

Sigerist's migration to the United States in 1932 had a profound effect on his work....

Now he began to expound on the "crisis of medicine." In 1931 he began to put the "social environment" beside the natural one as a cause of disease. He dreamed of the "Asclepios politicos" and urged that the physicians should "keep pace with society." Sigerist always saw in medical history the bridge between the old humanities and the new science. To him the history of medicine was always both history *and* medicine; the medical historian always remained a physician who could contribute something to his profession. The environment of the United States, where most scholars place a high value on the social usefulness of their work, could only strengthen these tendencies. In his new sociological orientation he believed that he had found the ideal instrument for the realization of these goals....

Sigerist called his new orientation "sociology," but it had little in common with what is usually understood by this term in the writings of Durkheim, Max Weber, or Georg Simmel. The greater part of what he called "sociology" has been correctly defined by Milton Roemer as "the current patterns and problems of medical care in different countries," or social medicine. Sigerist collected a large amount of literature on his subject (which he called his "sociology collection") and studied conditions directly in the United States, Canada, Russia, South Africa, and India. The an-nouncement of a first course at Johns Hopkins on "The Social Aspects of Medicine" in 1934 marks the beginning of these activities which absorbed a great deal of his time and interest, and made him a public as well as a controversial figure....

Much of his sociology was and remained medical history, and is perhaps more precisely defined as "social history of medicine."

In view of the controversy over his many discussions and views on Soviet medicine, it is important to quote from the remarks that Sigerist made at his farewell dinner:

Whenever I had a chance, I enjoyed doing field work, in a number of European countries, in South Africa, Canada, India—all over the United States. And how could I have overlooked the Soviet Union, the country that was not talking about but practicing social medicine on one-sixth of the inhabitants of the earth? The studies I made during three summers in the USSR were perhaps the most inspiring of my whole career. Without the war I would have returned to that country every two or three years. I frankly admit that I was deeply impressed by all I saw, by the honest endeavor of an entire nation to bring health services to all the people irrespective of race, color, creed, sex, income: irrespective of whether the people lived in town or country. What we were talking about in America, the Russians were practicing as a matter of course.

After every trip I told my colleagues quite ingenuously what I had seen and thought. And it was a real shock to find that instead of being equally interested, many insulted me as being a Red or at any rate a poor fool who had been deceived. I knew better, suddenly the USSR became our most powerful ally, and there was in the United States an immediate and great demand for information on Soviet medicine. I was glad to be able to help in organizing the American Soviet Medical Society and in launching the American Review of Soviet Medicine. The Society and the Journal were started without any financial help. Those were difficult times when we worked feverishly day and night selecting articles from whatever journals happened to be available, translating them into Russian, editing them to make them pallatable to American readers, reviewing books, abstracting articles. The Society and the Journal were a huge success, and the membership and the number of advertisers increased steadily until the Russians had defeated the Germans on their front. Then all of a sudden American public opinion changed. But all of us who really know Soviet medicine will continue studying it no matter whether this is a popular venture or not, because we are convinced that the Soviet system of medical care is one that makes the best use of the present technology of medicine and brings the greatest number of services to the largest number of people.

Sigerist ended his remarks on a note of optimism:

There is no doubt that the world is in a turmoil today, as everyone who had some historical understanding expected it to be after the events of the last thirty-five years. We cannot spend years destroying material and cultural values, producing ever more powerful means of destruction, and then expect the world to be normal. Every shot that is fired anywhere in the world causes sorrow and hatred, and every new weapon that is forged causes suspicion and distrust. We cannot industrialize the world and expect to live as our ancestors did, and we cannot spread education and expect the colonial and semi-colonial people to accept political or economic servitude without rebellion. We happen to live in a period of transition, as there have been many times in the past before us, and in such a period conflicts, the clash of interests and ideas, are unavoidable. We are impatient because we would like to see the end of this period in our lifetime. We think we can all contribute to abbreviating it with goodwill, tolerance and an intelligent understanding of the process in the midst of which we find ourselves, which must lead to the acceptance of unavoidable changes in our way of life. As physicians we are the natural ambassadors of goodwill and as historians we have the duty to use our historical knowledge to help the people to understand the world in which they live and to help in creating an atmosphere of confidence. I have no doubt as to the ultimate outcome of the present historical process and I foresee a better world with more love, more beauty, more justice, more happiness and a better sense of value. We shall not live to see it but our children or their children will, and it must be our satisfaction to know that we have helped in preparing it.

To those who were exposed to the brilliance of his lectures and who later saw the enthusiasm with which he was received as he took up his duties at Hopkins in September 1932, his resignation from the medical faculty in 1947, in an "atmosphere of mutual disillusion and disenchantment," can only be viewed with sadness. It was an unfortunate event that this great medical historian found himself embroiled in the most controversial of contemporary issues, fired by prejudices deepened as a result of the war. And one can only look back at the comments of Dean Alan Chesney in a letter to President Bowman in 1942, while the controversy about Sigerist's attitudes toward Soviet medicine and communism were in their most bitter period. "Unfortunately Dr. Sigerist has made himself very unpopular with the rank and file of the medical profession because of his views on socialized medicine, and has caused a great deal of unfavorable comment, some of it unjustified in my opinion. He gives many persons the impression of being a propagandist rather than an objective historian in his pronouncements in the social field." However, Chesney, in reply to a letter from a physician in regard to Sigerist's activities, made the following comments: "The policy of this school has always been not to interfere with the expression of opinion by members of this faculty. For that reason I feel that it would be out of place for me as the executive officer of the school to make any comment upon Dr. Sigerist or his activities. If you feel impelled to take exception to statements made by Dr. Sigerist in public, it would seem to me advisable to make the protest directly to him, which in so doing you would give him an opportunity to state the bases upon which the statements were made."

In 1947 Sigerist retired to Pura, a village in the Italian part of Switzerland near Lugano, where he embarked on the writing of an eight-volume history of medicine. He died in 1957, his task still far from done.

25 ❦ The Story of Chemotherapy at Johns Hopkins: Perrin H. Long, Eleanor A. Bliss, and E. Kennerly Marshall, Jr.

Sulfanilamide Comes to Johns Hopkins: The Story of Perrin H. Long and Eleanor A. Bliss

CALVIN COOLIDGE, JR., son of the Thirtieth President of the United States, died of blood poisoning on July 7, 1924. A week before, he had developed what appeared to be a trivial blister on his right great toe while playing tennis. Two days later he noted a sharp pain in the groin, and Dr. John B. Deaver of Philadelphia was called in consultation. Soon the correct diagnosis was established—septicemia, or invasion of the blood stream by bacteria. An emergency operation was performed to establish drainage. All of the medical expertise of the country was brought to bear on the problem, but nothing could stem the relentless progress of the disease.

Some twelve years later the author of this chapter was sitting in the bacteriology laboratory on Osler VII, plating out cultures and talking to Dr. Perrin H. Long, who was working late that evening on his mice infected with streptococci. The phone rang. I answered it, and a woman's voice asked for Dr. Long. (Dr. Long had for the past few months been engaged in clinical studies with the new drug sulfanilamide, and was receiving calls from all over the country asking for advice about the use of the drug. He was also receiving a full quota of good-natured ribbing from his colleagues, who would call, announce themselves as some famous individual, and then give Dr. Long a dramatic but fictitious story about their problem.) When he answered the phone that evening, I heard him laugh and say, "You can't fool me this time. I know you are not Eleanor Roosevelt." Then he abruptly hung up the phone. Within a few seconds it rang again. This time when he answered it I heard him say in a very meek voice, "Yes, Mrs. Roosevelt, this is Dr. Long." The next day the newspaper headlines announced dramatically that the son of another president was ill, Franklin D. Roosevelt, Jr.; again, with blood stream invasion by streptococci. But this time the result was quite different, and later headlines signaled the news that the President's son had been cured by sulfanilamide. The beginning of a new era of "miracle drugs" was at hand.

In 1910, when Paul Ehrlich announced the discovery of salvarsan and its value in the treatment of syphilis, many believed that the control of all infectious diseases was within medicine's grasp. It was at this time that Ehrlich coined the word "chemotherapy," meaning chemicals used in the treatment of disease. Ehrlich's goal was the destruction of the specific disease-producing living agents within the body of the patient—that is, the synthesis of chemicals whose target would be the invading organisms, killing them without any harm to the tissues of the patient.

Shortly after Ehrlich's world-shaking discovery, World War I began, and little more was done to advance research in this direction between 1914 and 1920. After the war, some important advances were made in the chemotherapy of tropical diseases, as evidenced by the development of atabrin for the treatment of malaria and tryparsamide for the cure of African sleeping sickness. Attempts to control more common infections such as pneumonia and meningitis had not been successful, and there was widespread doubt that an effective treatment would ever be found. However, in 1932 a new group of chemical agents, which have since been called the "sulfonamide compounds," were tested for their effects upon streptococcal infections in mice. Successful results were first reported by Gerhard Domagk of Germany in 1935. The next six years witnessed a miraculous advance in the treatment of infectious diseases. The death rate from pneumonia was more than halved. Meningococcal meningitis, which formerly killed 40 percent of its victims, showed a decrease in death rate to 10 percent. Streptococcal bacteremia and meningitis, which had been almost universally fatal, were almost uniformly cured, and gonorrhea responded rapidly to the administration of sulfonamide drugs.

Although Gerhard Domagk did not publish his experimental studies of Prontosil until March 1935, reports of its clinical use began to appear in German medical journals in 1933, and French studies of a similar product were well under way by 1934. Most important was the demonstration by Jacques and Thérèse Tréfouël, François Nitti, and Daniel Bovet that the azo linkage was unnecessary and that the simple compound sulfanilamide was as effective as the dye (Prontosil) in the control of experimental streptococcal infections. It had been noted by Domagk and by others that Prontosil was ineffective *in vitro*. As Domagk put it, "It acts as a true chemotherapeutic agent only in the living body." The Tréfouëls, Nitti, and Bovet reasoned, then, that the dye must be altered in the body, presumably by breaking apart at the azo linkage. Professor Fourneau prepared sulfanilamide at their request, and as predicted it proved to be as effective a therapeutic agent as the dye. This brilliant discovery not only made things simpler but released the life-saving chemical from the restriction of use only under German patents.

Meanwhile, English workers were conducting studies with these new compounds. In the discussion following an address by Professor Hörlein of the I. G. Farbenindustrie (for which company Domagk worked) in October 1935, G. A. H. Buttle reported that he had found Prontosil effective in experimental streptococcal infections. By June 1936 Buttle, Gray, and Stephenson had worked with sulfanilamide and found evidence not only of its activity against a variety of streptococcal types in animals, but also that, unlike Prontosil, it suppressed the growth of these organisms *in vitro*. Then the Therapeutic Trials Committee of the Medical Research Council of Great Britain undertook a series of experiments. The results were published by the English scientists Leonard Colebrook and Meave Kenny on June 6, 1936. These authors described the effects of treatment with Prontosil on human puerperal infections, showing that the death rate was reduced by two-thirds. Their work stimulated enormous interest and activity in further study and testing of chemical compounds of the sulfanilamide type.

The pioneer American workers in sulfonamide therapy were Drs. Perrin H. Long and Eleanor A. Bliss of Johns Hopkins. Originally, they had been developing specific antisera for the treatment of streptococcal infections. Their work was well advanced when, in early 1936, after reading reports about Protosil in the German literature, they became interested in the sulfonamide compounds. In the summer of 1936, while attending a medical meeting in London, they heard Leonard Colebrook speak about his excellent results in treating "childbed fever" with Prontosil. They had the opportunity to talk to an associate of Dr. Colebrook's who, after developing septicemia by accidently infecting himself with streptococci, was treated successfully with Prontosil. This story convinced Long and Bliss of the value of the drug, and they immediately made arrangements to bring some of it back to Baltimore. Supplies were limited, but fortunately the Jackson Laboratory of Dupont and Company was able to provide them with sulfanilamide. Their immediate results in the treatment of experimental hemolytic streptococcal infections in mice seemed miraculous. Eight of the first ten mice treated survived, while all of the untreated controls died within twenty-four hours. When they found that large doses of sulfanilamide were not too toxic for mice, the decision was made to try the drug on patients.

An opportunity soon arrived when a seven-year-old child, severely ill with erysipelas, was admitted. Antitoxin had been given repeatedly without any improvement. Within twelve hours after the administration of Prontosil, the child's temperature was normal. The next patient treated was a woman dangerously ill with "childbed fever" whose temperature was 105°F. and who was having frequent chills. Sulfanilamide treatment was begun, and by the next morning her temperature was normal. Any skepticism about the drug was soon erased as patient after patient with streptococcal tonsillitis and pharyngitis, erysipelas, otitis media, and streptococcal bacteremia was promptly cured by its administration. By November 1936 Long and Bliss had accumulated enough experimental and clinical observations to warrant a report at the meeting of the Southern Medical Association held in Baltimore. This report was published in the *Journal of the American Medical Association* on January 2, 1937. From that time on, many new sulfonamide compounds became available.

Long and Bliss's clinical studies of the later additions to the sulfonamide family followed lines similar to their earlier studies, although after W. Harry Feinstone joined the group late in 1937, some pharmacological studies were undertaken. As we shall see later, most of the work in this area at Johns Hopkins was done by Professor E. Kennerly Marshall, Jr., and his group, who quickly laid the foundation for the science of chemotherapy. Long and Bliss

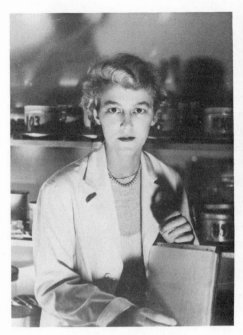

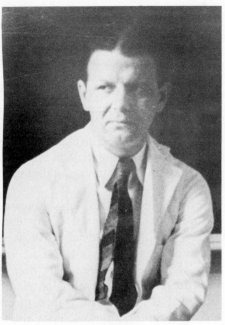

Eleanor A. Bliss

From *Harper's Bazaar*, 1949
Courtesy of Ms. Louise Dahl-Wolfe

Perrin H. Long

From the Archives Office, The Johns Hopkins
Medical Institutions

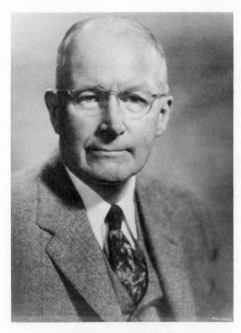

E. Kennerly Marshall, Jr.

From the Archives Office, The Johns Hopkins Medical Institutions

had a close association with them and profited immensely from Marshall's experience. Of the greatest importance was Marshall's method of determining the concentration of sulfonamides in body fluids. In the first published report of Long and Bliss, the lack of information on the absorption and excretion of sulfanilamide was noted. Dosage was aimed at attaining in the blood the 10 mg/100 ml concentration which had been found to be bacteriostatic *in vitro*. Thus, a daily administration of 1 gram per 10 kilograms of body weight was arrived at, the total amount being divided into four or six doses. It proved to be a shrewd guess, for when the assay method became available and the actual blood levels following various doses were known, the recommended dose for a concentration of 10 to 15 milligrams per 100 milliliters proved to be fairly accurate.

The mode of action of sulfonamide was a mystery for a while. Domagk had maintained that it was a true chemotherapeutic agent, specific in terms of Ehrlich's definition. However, further experience showed that this was not the case. Sulfonamides are not specific, nor are they protoplasmic poisons or bactericidal in the true sense. The bacteria in a patient given a sulfonamide are made to starve in the midst of plenty, since the sulfonamides interfere with their nutrition. The term coined to describe this condition was "bacteriostasis" —that is, the organisms cannot multiply, and thus fall easy victims to the natural defense mechanisms of the body, the white blood cells and the immune response. It was soon found by D. D. Woods, an English worker, that para-amino benzoic acid, a factor of the vitamin B complex with a chemical structure similar to sulfanilamide, was necessary for the growth of organisms. When a sufficient amount of sulfanilamide was present in either the artificial medium of a culture or in the body of an infected individual, the sulfonamide rather than the para-amino benzoic acid became fixed to the bacterial cell. This fixation blocked the utilization of para-amino benzoic acid by the parasites and they were literally starved to death.

During this very active period, Drs. Long and Bliss, as well as other members of the Johns Hopkins staff, made many important contributions to the development of this new, rapidly advancing field of chemotherapy.

Perrin Hamilton Long was born in Bryan, Ohio, on April 7, 1899. The descendant of a line of physicians who had practiced for many years in this small Ohio town, Long, after graduating from the local high school, entered the University of Michigan. His stay there was interrupted when he joined the American Field Service in 1917 to serve as an ambulance driver in France. In 1918 he was awarded the Croix de Guerre for bravery in action. After the war he returned to Michigan and married a fellow student, Elizabeth Griswold. In 1924 he went to Boston for three years, first as a fellow in the Thorndike Laboratory and then as an intern and resident on the Fourth Medical Service of Boston City Hospital. His chief there was Francis Peabody, for whom he developed a great admiration. After completion of his work in Boston, he spent several months at the Hygienic Institute in Freiburg, Germany, and then, in 1927, joined the staff of the Rockefeller Institute. Here, under the guidance of Simon Flexner and Peter Olitsky, he began his work in the field of infectious disease, concentrating on problems in virology. In 1929 he joined the faculty of the Johns Hopkins Medical School, of which he was a member for more than two decades. In 1940 Dr. Long was made professor and chairman of the Department of Preventive Medicine at Johns Hopkins.

In 1941 Dr. Long's academic pursuits were again interrupted, this time by the entry of the United States into World War II. Because of his in-depth knowledge of chemotherapy, he was one of a small group of consultants flown to Pearl Harbor to advise the government on the care of casualties immediately after the disaster of December 7, 1941. The following year he returned to active duty in the army and served in the African and Mediterranean theaters as a medical consultant. He retired from military service with the rank of colonel and was given the Legion of Merit. In recognition of service to the British, he received an honorary O.B.E. in 1945 and was elected to the Royal College of Physicians the following year. He was also awarded an honorary degree from the University of Algiers and later was made a Chevalier of the Legion of Honor.

After the war he returned to Johns Hopkins to continue his teaching and research, but in 1951 he departed for New York to assume the chairmanship of the Department of Medicine of the newly organized State University of New York, Downstate Medical Center, in Brooklyn. His new position ended his active period in the laboratory, but with unusual skill he turned his enormous energy to teaching and administration. He served in many consultant capacities, working with the National Research Council, the Veterans' Administration, the Public Health Service, and the U.S. Army. The latter service led to his promotion to the rank of brigadier general in the Reserves. In 1958 a laryngectomy for carcinoma curtailed his activities somewhat; his communication was limited to the use of an artificial larynx, impairing his effectiveness as a teacher He retired from academic life in 1961 but continued, however, to remain active, and edited several journals. He died suddenly of an acute coronary thrombosis on December 17, 1965.

Eleanor A. Bliss, the daughter of a professor of physics at the Johns Hopkins University, received her education at the Bryn Mawr School in Baltimore and at Bryn Mawr College in Pennsylvania. She received her Doctor of Science degree from the Johns Hopkins School of Hygiene and Public Health in 1925, writing her thesis on the "Anaerobic Spore-Bearing Bacteria in Baltimore Market Milk." For the next several years she worked with Dr. Harold L. Amoss on recurrent erysipelas, showing that it could be prevented by immunization with hemolytic streptococcal toxin.

In 1930 she joined in Perrin H. Long's study of the common cold and was delegated to make friends with fourteen chimpanzees—a hazardous occupation, as the chimps were not anxious to make friends with someone who pricked their fingers for daily blood counts. After Drs. Long and Bliss discovered that colds were "catching," the funds for this study ran out. Supported by a departmental fellowship, however, Dr. Bliss continued to work with Dr. Long on a variety of problems. In 1931 they identified the "minute" hemolytic streptococci which seemed to be particularly prevalent in the throats of patients with nephritis and rheumatic fever. By 1936 they were attempting to produce type-specific streptococcal antisera in some forty rabbits housed in the chimpanzee quarters atop the "old" Physiology Building when the sulfonamide era arrived. When Dr. Long became professor of preventive medicine, Dr. Bliss became a member of that department. In 1952 she was appointed dean of the Graduate School of Bryn Mawr College, from which position she retired in 1966.

One of her most cherished honors was to be invited by the French government, along with Perrin H. Long, E. Kennerly Marshall, Jr., and William Mansfield Clark, to attend the ceremonies connected with the fiftieth anniversary of Pasteur's death.

Eli Kennerly Marshall, Jr.:
Physiologist and Pharmacologist

In the fall of 1912 Eli Kennerly Marshall, Jr., a young instructor in Walter Jones's Department of Physiological Chemistry, went to an Italian market and bought some soybeans, from which he made the enzyme urease in order to study the decomposition of urea. Jones had stimulated Marshall's interest in methodology, and the young scientist promptly discovered a technique for the determination of urea in biological fluids. This was the first in a long series of major scientific contributions, most of which had important consequences for clinical medicine, by Abel's successor as chairman of the Department of Pharmacology and Howell's successor as chairman of the Department of Physiology.

Marshall was born in Charleston, South Carolina, in 1889. Some nineteen years later he stepped out of a train in Baltimore, walked to a rooming house on McCulloch Street, which was only a few minutes away from the Johns Hopkins Campus on Little Ross Street, and the following day enrolled for graduate work in chemistry. Thus began his career at Johns Hopkins which was to cover almost sixty years, with tremendous benefit to the Hopkins institutions.

Marshall received a good education at the College of Charleston, being the sole departmental student in chemistry there; but as Marin points out, Johns Hopkins was his real educational base. In 1911 his tutor, Associate Professor S. F. Acree, told Marshall that there was an opening in the medical school, in physiological chemistry under Dr. Walter Jones. Marshall applied for the job and was hired at a salary of $800 a year. The next summer he made the usual pilgrimage to Germany, working for a few months in Abderhalden's laboratory, where he began to learn about enzymes.

Marshall's work on urea brought him to the attention of Professor Abel, who was receptive to the idea of having Marshall join the Department of Pharmacology. Marshall had decided to do this principally on the advice of Jones, who told him that the horizons were greater in that discipline than in physiological chemistry. Abel encouraged Marshall to obtain his M.D. degree from Hopkins, which he did in 1917, but only with considerable difficulty; he took all of his preclinical work at the University of Minnesota during the summer months, since at that time a member of the Johns Hopkins faculty could not study in the school for credit. Marshall married a medical school classmate, Barry Carroll, during World War I, at which time he was assigned to the Chemical Warfare Service in Washington, D.C. While there, he recognized the talents of a young enlisted man who worked as a technician in his laboratory. He persuaded the young man to obtain his graduate degree at Johns Hopkins after the war. This Homer Smith did, in physiology, in the School of Hygiene, later becoming a distinguished renal physiologist and professor of physiology at New York University.

In Abel's department, Marshall's growth was rapid, due in no small part to the tutelage he received from Abel and the conversations around the famous lunch table, that "exclusive and unofficial Faculty Club of the Medical School" which was frequented by distinguished members of the faculty as well as visitors to the school. It was the intellectual center of the medical school in those days, even though the amenities consisted solely of tea, bread, and cold cuts served on an old wooden table with its feet in kerosene to ward off the cockroaches. Marshall's next move was in 1919 to the chair of pharmacology at Washington University in St. Louis, but his absence from Johns Hopkins was brief. He returned for good in 1921, succeeding William H. Howell as professor and director of the Department of Physiology.

Marshall's period in physiology was perhaps his greatest in terms of research contributions, and led to a scientific confrontation which as time passed was clearly resolved in Marshall's favor. The controversial area was the subject of a paper he published in the *Johns Hopkins Hospital Bulletin* entitled "The Mechanism of the Elimination of Phenosulphonphthalein—A Proof of Secretion by the Convoluted Tubules." In the concluding paragraph of this paper he made the following statement: "The problem which was presented in the introduction of this paper would then appear to be definitely settled, and satisfactory evidence would seem to exist that the processes which have been designated filtration, reabsorption and secretion are concerned in the formation of urine." As pointed out by Marin, only a careful reading of this paper can convey the excellence of the chemical and physiological techniques and the rigor and clarity of his thought. In terms of his views on secretion, Marshall had leaped some quarter century into the future. As one views the scene on the basis of present knowledge, it seems inconceivable that his ideas were so strongly opposed by such established leaders in the field as Arthur Cushny in Edinburgh and A. Newton Richards in Philadelphia. When he died in 1926, Cushny still had not accepted Marshall's idea of secretion; Richards did not finally relinquish opposition to it until about 1930. During this period of controversy, Marshall amassed an enormous amount of information in support of his views by studies on the comparative physiology of the kidney. One of his most notable contributions was the use of the aglomerular fish to cap his theory of secretion by the renal tubule.

Also during this period in physiology, Marshall made the first measurements of cardiac output in unanesthetized dogs, using the Fick principle, with analysis of the arteriovenous oxygen difference. The method he developed for man, using nitrous oxide and ethylene, remained standard until the advent of cardiac catheterization. These were classic studies which many physiologists had thought were impossible to accomplish.

In 1932 Marshall succeeded Abel as professor and director of the Department of Pharmacology and Experimental Therapeutics. His previous training and his career, which displayed the rationale of the pharmacologist as well as the chemist, physiologist, and physician, made him an ideal candidate to fill the shoes of the great Abel. Although it took some time before it was appreciated in the clinic, Marshall soon made another important physiological study. He demonstrated that in drug-induced respiratory depression, carbon dioxide alone is an inadequate stimulus to drive the respiratory center, and that anoxia plays a significant part. These findings clearly pointed to the hazards of administering oxygen under such circumstances. All are now familiar with the danger of carbon dioxide narcosis when oxygen is administered to patients with severe obstructive pulmonary disease and respiratory acidosis.

Three years after his advent as chairman of the Department of Pharmacology and Experimental Therapeutics, a complete reorientation of his research came about with the discovery of the sulfonamides. From that time on, his principal interest was chemotherapy. Marshall was quick to seize the opportunity to expand his knowledge, and within a year he had published a method for the determination of sulfanilamide. With the help of this new and powerful tool, he was able to map out its absorption, distribution, and excretion in animals and man. His work led to the establishment of rational dose schedules for these drugs, and he soon met the need for an intravenous sulfonamide with the introduction of sodium sulfapyridine. All of this work was original in both theory and practice, and Marshall stands in bold relief as a principal architect of the scientific age of chemotherapy.

Marshall also saw the necessity for a drug that would remain in the intestinal tract, and he prepared the poorly absorbed sulfaguanidine. According to Dudley, this preparation indirectly led to Marshall's playing a role in the outcome of World War II in the Pacific area. In 1942 the Japanese had managed to traverse the Owen-Stanley range in New Guinea and were on the verge of capturing Port Moresby, which would have led to the fall of Australia. Every Australian and American soldier that could be mustered was mobilized for service in that location to withstand the arrival of the Japanese. When the Japanese were on the outskirts of the city, a severe outbreak of dysentery occurred among the Allies. By good fortune, a sizable amount of sulfaguanidine was found in the medical supplies of the U.S. Army and flown to Port Moresby. This enabled the Australians and Americans to recover and to repel the Japanese attack.

However, World War II brought a prompt end to the work on sulfanilamide in Marshall's laboratory, and he assumed leadership of the important program to develop better means of treating malaria. He was principally responsible for the pharmacological studies on a national level and was director of an important research unit in his own laboratory, where he worked with unmitigated vigor during the entire war. This group worked on bird malaria, and by the closest attention to data obtained from the laboratory and from human volunteers, succeeded in defining the role of the four-amino and eight-amino quinolines in human malarias. There was a great controversy as to whether the quinolines should be given by a regimen calculated to maintain a constant blood level in the treatment of malaria. Marshall, who had introduced the concept of blood levels for the sulfonamides, demonstrated that this did not apply to the quinolines, which had a totally different pattern of distribution and mechanism of action. This indicated that he was a true scientist—flexible, realistic, and unfettered by traditional concepts. These characteristics also led him to be among the first to recognize that antibiotic management, too, could not be handled with the methods he had worked out for sulfanilamide.

Research was certainly the dominant theme of his career, but Marshall was also deeply devoted to the medical school. For thirty-five years he sat on the Advisory Board of the Johns Hopkins School of Medicine and fought for, among other things, improvements in the curriculum, free time for students, departmental autonomy, and high standards for faculty selection. He appreciated at an early stage the importance of clinical pharmacology, and before NIH grants became available, he established joint fellowships in medicine and pharmacology. Soon after World War II, in collaboration with Harvey in medicine, he helped to organize the Division of Clinical Pharmacology. As a tutor of young scientists, he was unsurpassed, instilling in them a rigorous sense of scientific discipline, integrity, and religious attention to controls.

Many honors came to him, although he was not what one would call an "organization man." His natural role was in the laboratory, where he was happiest. However, he was president of the American Society of Pharmacology and Experimental Therapeutics in 1942 and a member of the American Philosophical Society, the National Academy of Sciences and the Association of American Physicians. As Marin has pointed out, he was a bridge between the nineteenth and twentieth centuries for science, medicine, manners, the South, Maine, and Johns Hopkins.

A final anecdote: Back in 1926, when he was immersed in renal studies, he listened with only half an ear to his good friend Alan Chesney extol the virtues of Maine. Then he discovered in his reading that the goosefish was reported to have aglomerular kidneys. He recognized his opportunity to reinforce his thesis of renal tubular secretion, and when another friend, Warren H. Lewis, said that he was accustomed to eating goosefish steaks in Salisbury Cove, Maine, Marshall made immediate arrangements to spend the summer at the biological laboratory on Mt. Desert Island there, and he never missed a summer in Maine after that. The subsequent discovery that another aglomerular fish, known as the toadfish, was to be found in his own back yard in the Chesapeake Bay came far too late to alienate his affections for Maine.

Marshall is a distinguished example of the second generation of professors at Johns Hopkins. He had the unenviable task of succeeding not one but two of the remarkable and colorful members of the original faculty, but he soon demonstrated that he belonged in the same rank with such giants as Abel and Howell. He never departed from the tradition he inherited of absolute intellectual honesty and excellence in all his endeavors. He retired in 1955, but was active for many years as a visiting professor and as a consultant to the National Cancer Institute. He died in 1966.

26 ⚘ Discoveries at Johns Hopkins Related to the Nervous System and Its Diseases

Frank Rodolph Ford

DURING THE PAST few decades, studies of the process of nerve repair have led to a new theory of how the complex pathways of the central nervous system are formed in the embryo. For example, damage to the principal motor nerve of the face may result in a condition known as "crocodile tears." When the injured nerve regenerates, fibers that originally activated the salivary gland can go astray and connect themselves to the lachrymal gland of one eye. As a result situations calling for salivation induce weeping from that eye. Patients with this condition always wish to know whether normal function will return spontaneously, and if not, whether it can be restored by training and re-education. Formerly, neurologists agreed that the central nervous system was plastic enough to permit reconnection of any muscle's nerve to any other muscle with a good functional result, but in the past twenty-five years opinion has undergone a major change. The current view is that the connections required for normal coordination arise in embryonic development according to a biochemically determined plan that precisely connects the various nerve endings in the body to their corresponding points in the nerve centers of the brain and spinal cord. Although these higher centers in the brain may be capable of extensive learning, the lower centers in the brain stem and the spinal cord are implastic. Thus, the disordered connections set up by the random regeneration of injured nerves cannot be corrected by re-education.

One of the important milestones in the emergence of new ideas about the functional plasticity of the nervous system was the sharp challenge to the old concept presented in 1938 by the work of Frank R. Ford and Barnes Woodhall. In describing their extensive clinical experience with functional disorders following the regeneration of nerves, they concluded that these abnormalities persist in most affected patients for years without any apparent improvement. Their excellent report cast serious doubt upon the then-accepted methods of therapy and the theory that rationalized them.

In that same year Roger Sperry began his important investigations, the aim of which was to find out if functional plasticity was a property of the higher brain centers only or whether it extended to the lowest levels of the spinal cord. He switched the nerve connections between opposing muscles in the hind limb of rats in such a way as to reverse the movement at the ankle joint. Much to his surprise, the anticipated adjustment never occurred. The rats seemed unable to correct the reversal of motor coordination produced by the operation. When they tried to lift the affected foot it pulled downward; when they tried to rise on the ball of the foot, their toes swung up and they fell back on their heels. All efforts at re-education had little or no effect on the rat's motor system. These experiments were expanded to include sensory function and were done in other animals, including monkeys. Years of testing and observation failed to achieve any generalized positive correction in the action of cross-innervated muscles. Sperry found that while in most cases humans can learn to control transplanted muscles, they can do so only in simple, slow voluntary movement, the control of complex, rapid, and reflex movements is limited at best, and is subject to relapse under conditions of fatigue, shock, or surprise. Humans do seem, however, to have a greater capacity for adjustment than the subhuman primates. Such re-education as does occur must, therefore, be due to the greater development of higher learning centers in the human brain. Contrary to earlier opinion, it does not reflect an intrinsic plasticity of nerve networks in general.

The careful clinical studies of Ford and Woodhall were recognized by Sperry as an important contribution in unseating the theory of peripheral nerve plasticity. Since the organization of the lower nerve centers and the peripheral nerve circuit in higher animals seems to take place only in the early plastic stages of growth, it is now clear that injury to them later on cannot be repaired by any amount of re-education and training.

Many more examples of Ford's powers of observation and evaluation might be cited. Among the most notable: In 1936 he assessed the importance of vestibular reflexes on the basis of neurologic findings in patients subjected to section of the vestibular nerve by Dr. Dandy for relief of Ménière's disease; he predicted the troubles that would, and did, follow bilateral section of this nerve. In 1937 he considered perceptual disorders associated with lesions of the inter-hemispheric commissure, the corpus callosum. Geschwind in 1965 acknowledged the paper by Trescher and Ford as important in "the disconnection syndrome." Discussed in that paper was removal of a third ventricle cyst, in which there was section of the posterior half of the corpus callosum resulting in alexia in the left visual field.

Frank Rodolph Ford was born in Baltimore on October 21, 1892. His early schooling was in Baltimore, but the family later moved to Virginia, where he successively attended a local Virginia school and studied under a private tutor. He finished his schooling at the Boys Latin School in Baltimore and then entered the Johns Hopkins University. After graduation from the Johns Hopkins Medical School in 1920, he served as a house officer in psychiatry under Dr. Adolph Meyer. Dr. Ford soon realized that his interest and capabilities did not fit well with the life of a psychiatrist. He found neuroanatomy and neuropathology, which he had a good taste of in Dr. Meyers laboratory, much more stimulating.

As a result of this experience, he migrated temporarily to New York, where he received his training in clinical neurology at Bellevue Hospital under the colorful Foster Kennedy. There is one anecdote of his experience there that helps to characterize Dr. Ford. He observed that the various neurological consultants who made daily rounds had what to him was a rather annoying habit. Only the first consultant who saw the patient would leave a detailed note; those who examined the patient later simply concurred with the original impression. In order to glean all of the knowledge that might ensue from having the independent views of several expert neurologists, Dr. Ford simply removed each consultation note from the chart, replacing them only at the time of the patient's discharge.

On his return to Baltimore, Frank Ford became a house officer in neurology, at that time a subdepartment of the Department of Medicine, and quickly became known as a master of clinical neurology. He had an unusual ability to arrive at the most suitable answer to a neurological problem with an apparent minimum of effort. It was often said by his colleagues that they would prefer to have the "Judge's" opinion, after he had simply walked past the door of a patient's room, than that of most any other consultant after the performance of a lengthy and complex examination. One of Ford's most important functions was to serve as the clinical neurologist for the neurosurgeon, Walter E. Dandy. It proved to be a fruitful association, both in the cataloguing for investigative purposes of the important clinical material which passed through the neurosurgical service and also from the viewpoint of student and house officer instruction.

As pointed out by Arthur B. King, one of Frank Ford's students, neurology at that time (the mid 1930s) had little student appeal. Neuroanatomy was presented in a rather confused manner; physiology was in a state of flux; pathology ignored the field entirely and the current textbooks of neurology were unimaginatively written. But he says:

Suddenly in the third year of medical school, we students were exposed to a man who was a chain smoker, appeared in ruffled clothing, spoke with a slight lisp, had a pixie-like twinkle in his eyes and so great an economy of movement that he appeared almost constantly bored. Miraculously, however, he made the elucidation of clinical neurological problems simple, readily understandable and enjoyable. While he pointed out to the students their lack of understanding of the anatomy and physiology of the central nervous system, he quickly imparted his belief to them that there was hope for improvement. In fact he indicated a little attention to detail might even make them good diagnosticians. It didn't take long for us to learn that the "game of medicine" for Dr. Ford was to locate and define the pathologic process. Care and treatment of the patient were not for him but were like the plague, to be rid of as soon as possible.

Among the famous conferences in the history of the Johns Hopkins Medical Institutions are the Saturday morning sessions on Neuro-ophthalmology held by Dr. Frank B. Walsh and religiously attended by Dr. Frank Ford. Frank Walsh's description of these conferences summarizes Dr. Ford's personality and approach very well:

His pattern after arrival never varied. He would walk across the lecture room, deposit his hat on the radiator cover, and go to his front row seat on the aisle. There he was available for quiet greetings or questioning, and completely relaxed, he proceeded to take a long cigar from a pocket, light it, and await the appearance of the first patient. Immediately he gave complete attention to the history as presented and in many instances he already had observed significant abnormalities as the patient walked or was wheeled into the room. All became aware that the chronology of symptoms and signs registered almost automatically in his mind. His memory of cases, names and writings was phenomenal. It was my practice first to obtain audience participation and carefully to avoid obtaining Dr. Ford's comments until all others had finished their discussion. When I asked Dr. Ford to evaluate the situation his answer was directed to me in a low voice and only those close to him could hear his remarks. I would summarize what he had said. This exercise became completely routine. In his discussion, Dr. Ford always placed his comments into one of three categories: first, when he was completely sure of the principal diagnosis he stated this in few words; second, when several possibilities existed, he gave an appropriate explanation of each; third, when the diagnosis was completely obscure, he prefaced his observations by "I do not know." This self discipline was a prominent feature of Dr . Ford's personality. When the diagnosis was certain, that is category one, he would willingly indicate the reasons leading to that conclusion. One soon learned that to argue against his unqualified diagnosis was utterly without merit. When the diagnosis fell into category two or category three, Dr. Ford was at his best as a teacher and it was then that his subtle humor often lightened the occasion.

Among Dr. Ford's hobbies was clay modeling. This artistic diversion complemented his wife Louel's fascination with paintings. Dr. Ford shaped human figures, at least a thousand, each of which displayed his complete knowledge of anatomy. These figures depicted strength or weakness, wore a smile, a snear, a grimace, an expression of triumph or despair. His collection was arranged in groups, each group based on some story taken from the Old Testament. Those select few who had the opportunity to be shown these works were treated to a commentary about what each situation portrayed in these models, often in grim detail.

In spite of the fact that Dr. Ford was adverse to travel, attended no national meetings, and did not feel compelled to publish papers at frequent intervals, he was, nevertheless, widely recognized in the broad field of neurology. He developed an intense interest in pediatric neurology as well as in the neurological problems of adults, and being very systematic, he accumulated an enormous wealth of neurological material in patients of all ages for later study. By 1937 he was able to complete his classic book on diseases of the nervous system in infancy, childhood and adolescence. This monograph proved so popular and the amount of new material so great that as soon as he completed one edition he would begin the revision for the next. This text went through five editions, the final, sixth revision being sent to the publisher shortly before his last illness. Translation of editions four and five into Italian, Spanish, and Polish gives testimony to its great value, and more will be said later of its significance.

Ford was the first neurologist to develop a logical approach to the clinical disorders of the developing nervous system. In 1895 Bernard Sachs of New York wrote a textbook entitled *A Treatise on the Nervous Diseases of Children for Physicians and Students.* After that time there was no additional effort to display this difficult area of neurology for the student until Frank Ford's textbook appeared in 1937. Ford's monumental work was soon recognized as the classic presentation of developmental neurology. It was a one-man production, and represented in essence a clinical research accomplishment of the highest order. The following preface appeared in the first edition:

The diseases of the nervous system of infancy and childhood constitute a very difficult field which belongs to both the neurologist and the pediatrician but which has not been cultivated intensively by either. The neurology of childhood is still in an early stage of development as contrasted with that of adult life, and even the common neurological disorders of this period are, to a great extent, obscure. I have attempted, therefore, to bring together and to analyze all available information about these conditions in the hope that I may be able to clarify the situation to some extent. I have tried first of all to develop a classification based primarily upon etiology, with due emphasis upon clinical features rather than a purely anatomical classification as is customary.

This is a very modest appraisal in view of the fact that he was the first to present this difficult field in a logical fashion. In summarizing Dr. Ford's contributions in this field, Guy McKhann said: "I should have realized earlier, that Dr. Ford was the greatest expert in the clinical aspects of developmental neurology there has ever been. Further, I doubt that his level of expertise will ever be achieved again."

Philip Bard

To those familiar with the national pastime of baseball, the trio of Evans, Tinker, and Chance, that immortal double-play combination, represents the apex of excellence. The first three professors of physiology in the Johns Hopkins University School of Medicine represent an analogous degree of excellence in that important field of medical science. Henry Newell Martin, William Henry Howell, and Eli Kennerly Marshall, Jr., were giants in terms of their creative endeavors in the world of physiology. The odds would have been great against anyone who wagered that equal stature would be attained by the fourth incumbent in that chair when he arrived in Baltimore in 1933 at the age of thirty-four, having published only three papers dealing with his own independent investigations. However, over the ensuing thirty-one years as Professor of Physiology, Philip Bard lived up in every respect to the high standards of excellence that his predecessors had established in biology and physiology. There is no better confirmation of his right to stand in the ranks of his predecessors than the tribute paid to him at a dinner held in his honor prior to his official retirement in 1964: "Retiring and modest in his person, absolute in devotion to scholarly endeavor, enjoying to the full the pleasures of the free academic life, he has over these years brought distinction to our faculty, inspiration to our students, leadership to our university, and a happy, good fellowship to his colleagues."

Philip Bard was born in 1898 in Ventura County, California. He attended the Thacher School, founded in 1889 by Mr. Sherman Day Thacher of Yale College, in Ventura County. It was Thacher who put the idea of becoming a doctor into Bard's head. He frequently reminisced about Bard's uncle, Dr. Cephas L. Bard, who had served as an army surgeon at the end of the Civil War, after receiving his M.D. degree at Jefferson Medical College. He came to California shortly after his brother had arrived there and became a pioneer physician in Ventura County and later president of the California Medical Society. After Philip Bard expressed an interest in the study of medicine, his brother, Dick, sent him a copy of the then-current 1914 edition of Dr. William H. Howell's textbook of physiology. Bard vividly recalls the experiments of Walter B. Cannon on gastrointestinal motility described in that book. What a remarkable sequel, that he should later earn his Ph.D. in Cannon's laboratory at Harvard and then become one of Howell's successors in that chain of physiological giants at Johns Hopkins!

After his return from service in World War I, Dr. Bard consulted Walter C. Alvarez, then a practitioner in San Francisco. Alvarez told him about his own period in Walter Cannon's laboratory and how the experience had shaped his career interest in the gastrointestinal tract. He also told Bard about Bayliss's *Principles of General Physiology*, thus introducing him to the second of the great classics in that field. At Princeton, of course, Bard came under the influence of Edwin Grant Conklin, that incomparable embryologist and cytologist; and even more important in terms of influence on his future career, the great physiologist, E. Newton Harvey, with whom he spent an additional year at Princeton as a graduate student.

After Princeton, Bard went to Boston to study with Cannon. He soon became interested in an area of research which, with one or more variations, was to form the continuing theme of his scientific career. In searching for those conditions which induce vigorous sympatho-adrenal medullary activity, Cannon recalled previous experiments on dogs and cats in which an animal surviving decortication displayed anger on slight provocation. Cannon had done a series of acute experiments in which the cerebral cortices were disconnected from the brain stem. These cats exhibited a remarkable group of findings which Cannon termed "sham rage." Bard was encouraged to determine the locus of the central mechanism essential for this activity which so closely resembled the behavior during rage of a normal animal. Bard succeeded in showing that the region necessary for "sham rage" was located in the caudal half of the hypothalamus. He concluded that the hypothalamus is not an "autonomic center" but a part of the brain which contains neural mechanisms necessary for complex patterns of behavior, such as display of emotion and defense against heat or cold. These experiments represent the initiation of his life-long interest in the physiology of the nervous system.

In 1928 Bard returned to Princeton as an assistant professor in the Department of Biology, and had three very pleasant years continuing his research and conducting the course previously given by E. Newton Harvey, who was then a research professor. In 1931 he returned to Cannon's department as an assistant professor in physiology. Here he had ample facilities for research, and most important of all, an opportunity to collaborate with David Rioch, who had just come from Johns Hopkins to Harvard in the Department of Anatomy under George Wislocki. They studied the behavioral capacities and deficiencies of four cats from which Bard had removed all cerebral cortex and different amounts of the rest of the forebrain. At the same time Bard explored the basic neural control of two groups of postural reactions, absent or very deficient in decorticate animals. He found that they depend on the sensory-motor cortex and remain unimpaired when the remainder of the cortex is removed.

In March 1933 Bard received an invitation from President Joseph S. Ames of the Johns Hopkins University to become professor and director of the Department of Physiology. This post had become vacant as a result of the transfer of E. K. Marshall, Jr., to the Department of Pharmacology on Dr. Abel's retirement. At that time there were only three staff members in the physiology department—Charles D. Snyder, Chalmers L. Gemmill, and Evelyn Howard. Bard recruited Chandler Brooks, his first Ph.D. student at Princeton, as an instructor, and also a fourth-year student, Clinton Woolsey, who gave up an appointment in surgery to join the department as an assistant. Both of these men ultimately became directors of important physiological enterprises and achieved eminent success in the field of physiology. Over the years Dr. Bard recruited many other outstanding physiologists, including Elwood Henneman, professor of physiology at Harvard, and Bard's successor at Johns Hopkins, Vernon Mountcastle, who has continued without interruption basic work in neurophysiology of the highest quality.

By the time he arrived in Baltimore, Bard had become adept at intra-cranial surgical procedures in cats, dogs and monkeys. He points out that there were so many important problems which seemed approachable by these techniques that he failed to learn the elements of electrophysiology, which subsequently advanced knowledge of the nervous system far beyond other approaches. In 1936 Woolsey and Bard realized that the technique they were using, that of cortical ablation, in determining the control of the placing and hopping reactions by the precentral and postcentral gyri of the monkey's cortex had reached the limits of valuability. At that time Wade Marshall set up a cathode ray oscillograph with appropriate amplifiers in the physiology laboratory, and the three investigators began to study the question of whether evoked potentials would throw further light on the cortical representation of somatic sensibility. This study resulted in the first systematic mapping of the primate postcentral gyrus by this pioneer technique. Woolsey applied this method widely, and many of Bard's pupils who subsequently entered the laboratory learned to use it in analysis of several central sensory systems. Bard himself, while he encouraged work in these directions, went back to his old-fashioned ablation technique for further experimental adventures.

With Woolsey and Brooks, Bard carried out an extensive comparative study of the cortical control of the postural reactions, showing their increasing corticalization in phylogeny and their loss following discrete local lesions of the somatotopically related portions of the sensory and motor cortices. As pointed out by Mountcastle, these studies represent the limit to which the methods of surgical ablation and clinical examination could be pushed in the elucidation of cortical function, and they culminated in Bard's Harvey Lecture of 1938. Subsequent studies were made of hypothalamic function in regulating sexual behavior and the reproductive cycle, in governing the pituitary gland and its target organs, in regulation of body temperature, and in the production of fever.

In his student teaching Bard gave of himself in a very personal way. His course contained a minimum number of lectures and emphasized individual initiative, free time for scholarly endeavor, and small group laboratory exercises. These laboratory sessions were not aimed at the repetition of experiments, the results of which were already known. He used them to bring teacher and student into direct exchange around a naturally occurring problem designed to enhance the student's powers of observation and reasoning and to teach him to evaluate evidence in a critical way. In addition, he instituted a more lively program of postdoctoral training than had existed previously in the basic science departments at Johns Hopkins.

Bard, of course, has received many honors and has contributed in many ways, not only to Hopkins, but outside of his home environment as well. He was president of the American Physiological Society from 1942 to 1945 and then served for many years as a member of its Board of Publication Trustees. His laboratory program was interrupted for four years in the mid-1950's, when he served as dean of the medical faculty. Since his retirement, he has remained an active investigator in the laboratory of physiology. He is a member of the National Academy of Sciences and the American Philosophical Society.

Poliomyelitis Research

There is nothing more thrilling in the research history of the Johns Hopkins Medical Institutions than the studies of Howard A. Howe and David Bodian on problems relating to poliomyelitis. Howe began working on poliomyelitis in 1936 in the Department of Anatomy, under a grant from the President's Birthday Ball Committee. He and his associates, Robert Ecke and Talmadge Peele, developed a laboratory capability for work on experimental poliomyelitis in rhesus monkeys and demonstrated that poliovirus could spread along known nerve fiber pathways in the brain. In 1938 their grant ended, but the Commonwealth Fund offered to support research in this area for a two-year period. Also in that year, Dr. David Bodian joined Howard Howe's group as a research fellow—a momentous event for the future of poliomyelitis.

Dr. Bodian came to Hopkins after serving as a National Research Council Fellow at the University of Michigan with Professor Elizabeth Crosby, the distinguished neuroanatomist. He received his Ph.D. degree at the University of Chicago in 1934 and went on to take an M.D. in 1937, and his extraordinary ability was quickly recognized by C. Judson Herrick, the outstanding neurologist of that period. Within two years after Bodian joined Howe, they had done a number of experimental neuroanatomical and pathological studies in monkeys and chimpanzees that established them as one of the important poliomye-litis research teams in the country.

Their early research efforts were concerned with an analysis of the inter-action of poliovirus and the nervous system, of the mode of spread of virus in nerve fibers, of the route of entry of virus into the nervous system, and of the conditions which might produce refractoriness of nerve cells to infection with the virus. For example, in 1939 they demonstrated the preferential nerve fiber pathways of poliovirus in the brain and the existence of susceptible and refrac-tory centers of viral multiplication. In 1941 evidence was found for intra-neuronal multiplication of poliovirus and its spread within axons. In the same year they determined the rate of poliovirus spread in peripheral nerve axons in retrograde direction, and first demonstrated that chimpanzees could be infected with poliovirus by feeding, without involvement of the olfactory bulbs. They also demonstrated that, contrary to widely held belief, the olfactory bulb was not the major route of poliovirus entry in man. Importantly they found that nonparalytic cases of poliomyelitis could have as severe pathological involve-ment as paralytic cases, the difference being that in nonparalytic cases the destroyed motorneurons in the spinal cord were too separated to involve a single functional muscle group sufficiently to result in a noticeable loss of motor power. These early studies were put together in a classic volume, *Neural Mechanisms in Poliomyelitis,* published by the Commonwealth Fund of New York in 1942. Some of the original papers were published in the *Bulletin of The Johns Hopkins Hospital.*

A very important event took place in 1941 when Dr. Kenneth Maxcy applied to the new National Foundation for Infantile Paralysis for a long-term grant. Maxcy had graduated from the Johns Hopkins Medical School in 1915 in the same class as Dr. Thomas Rivers, the foundation's scientific adviser. In 1917 they had both been assistant residents on Dr. Howland's service in pedi-atrics. After World War I Maxcy joined the U.S. Public Health Service and gained an international reputation because of his work on murine typhus. In 1929 while he was investigating an outbreak of the disease in the South, he came to the conclusion that the reservoir of the disease would probably be found in rats and mice and was probably spread to the human population by means of fleas or mice, reaching these conclusions from the epidemiological data. This work paved the way for Hans Zinsser, who, while investigating an outbreak of typhus in Mexico, showed that the red flea was responsible for the spread of this separate variety of typhus. As a result of his classical work, Maxcy was elected to the National Academy of Sciences.

In 1929 Maxcy left the Public Health Service and became a professor of preventive medicine at the University of Virginia. Then, after serving at the University of Minnesota for a period in 1938 he joined the School of Hygiene and Public Health at Johns Hopkins as professor of epidemiology. Maxcy believed that if the polio problem was ever to be solved, it would be necessary to construct a broad program to study not only the spread of the virus in the human body but its distribution in a community as well. He hoped to establish a permanent research center at the School of Hygiene and Public Health that would devote itself to the study of polio and other viruses. He wanted to bring together a nucleus of research workers in various disciplines such as pathology, anatomy, virology, and epidemiology and later to add additional workers from such fields as biochemistry and physics. In order to do this he recognized that he would need funds not only to establish the center but also to give security to the workers for a period of at least five years. Prior to 1941, research grants were made on a year-to-year basis and were very modest. Thus, it was a tremendous venture for Maxcy to approach the National Foundation and ask for a long-term grant.

The foundation fortunately agreed to Maxcy's proposal, but it took a number of months to work out a final arrangement. Basil O'Connor, the director of the foundation, recognized that such an agreement would probably serve as a model for other long-term grants, and he wanted to see that all of the details were worked out properly. In return for a grant of $300,000 for a period of five years, the Johns Hopkins University agreed to establish a research center in the School of Hygiene and Public Health which would devote itself to the study of poliomyelitis. The foundation accepted the fact that all research undertaken by the center was to be determined solely by the director of the center and his associates.

The success of Maxcy's plan was assured when he obtained the services of Howard A. Howe and David Bodian, who had done such creditable work on neuroanatomy in relation to poliomyelitis. Dr. Weed, director of the Department of Anatomy, accepted the transfer of Dr. Howe from the medical school to the School of Hygiene. Dr. Bodian, who had left the medical school in 1942 to accept a position as assistant professor of anatomy at Western Reserve, returned late in 1942 to join Dr. Maxcy's group in the School of Hygiene.

To help the work of this group, the Johns Hopkins Medical School assigned to Dr. Maxcy laboratory space in the new Hunterian Laboratory Building. With new and larger facilities, an expanded program could be developed which was capable of studying monkeys in numbers sufficient to enable quantitative analysis.

Another stroke of good fortune came to the group when in 1942 David Bodian met Isabel Morgan (later Isabel M. Mountain) at Woods Hole. Daughter of the first American-born Nobel laureate, Thomas Hunt Morgan, she received her Ph.D. degree in bacteriology under Stuart Mudd at the University of Pennsylvania. She then went to the Rockefeller Institute to work with Dr. Peter Olitsky on immunological studies of encephalitis viruses. Bodian persuaded her to come to Baltimore to carry out similar studies on experimental poliovirus infections; she had begun work with poliovirus at the institute in 1941. When she arrived in Baltimore in 1944, the group embarked on a program in which studies of the epidemiological, immunological and pathological aspects of poliomyelitis were closely intertwined. Morgan's first project was to find out whether she could induce resistance to an intracerebral inoculation. She also wanted to see whether a correlation between antibody and resistance could be established. She inactivated a strain of poliovirus with formalin, and by giving monkeys multiple intramuscular inoculations of this inactivated virus, she finally induced resistance to intracerebral inoculation of live poliomyelitis virus in her animals. She discovered that such immunity resulted when monkeys had achieved a titer of 1 to 3,000 of antibody in the serum. Moreover, there was a good correlation between the degree of resistance and the level of antibody.

In 1949 the group made the important discovery that there were only three major immunological poliovirus types, and that all were genetically stable, as contrasted with influenza virus. The National Foundation later created a large typing program in four laboratories in order to be certain that there were no other virus types, such as one might see in such bacterial classes as the pneumococcus and the streptococcus. This was absolutely vital if there was ultimately to be a successful vaccine. However, it was the study of Bodian, Howe, and Morgan which was the first to show that there were three major immunological virus types and that their specific antibodies were present in equal amounts in human gamma globulin—very basic information along the road to the successful development of a poliomyelitis vaccine. In spite of the debacle of the Park-Brodie and Kolmer vaccines of 1935, when numbers of children contracted poliomyelitis because the vaccines contained live virus, Howard A. Howe, as a result of the progress that had been made with the establishment of the three immunological types, was enthusiastic about the possibility of a vaccine being developed.

By 1951 Isabel Morgan had demonstrated beyond any doubt that she could immunize rhesus monkeys with formalin-inactivated viruses of all three basic immunological types to a degree that made it impossible to infect such animals with poliomyelitis by the most sensitive route. At that time, however, most virologists still believed that it was not possible to immunize against poliomyelitis with a formalin-inactivated virus. Isabel Morgan converted these "doubting virologists," which was quite an accomplishment. In 1950 Howard Howe extended Morgan's original observations by immunizing chimpanzees and monkeys with both formalin-inactivated vaccines and live virus vaccines against all three types of polio. He soon discovered that while those animals which received formalin-inactivated vaccine could not be prevented from having an alimentary infection and putting out virus in their stools, they nevertheless resisted paralysis upon intracerebral and oral challenge. Most important were his observations that the antibody responses to all three poliovirus types were within satisfactory limits, and that adjuvants were able to stimulate antibody responses to small amounts of formalin-treated material. He believed that his results made it feasible to try formalized material on children. About a year later he inoculated a few mentally defective children in a Maryland home with formalin-inactivated vaccine and showed that the children did develop antibodies against all three polio types. This work was very important but since the material was made of monkey cord, the danger of an allergic encephalomyelitis was an unacceptable risk for large-scale immunization programs.

As pointed out, David Bodian, while testing the polyvalent characteristics of poliovirus antibody in gamma globulin, discovered that it contained antibody

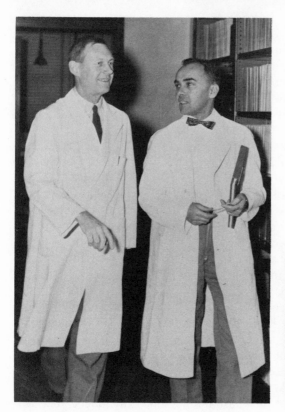

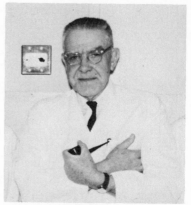

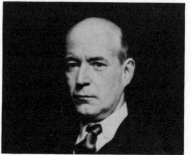

Howard A. Howe (*left*) and David Bodian
Courtesy of Dr. David Bodian

Frank Rodolph Ford
From the Archives Office, The Johns Hopkins Medical Institutions

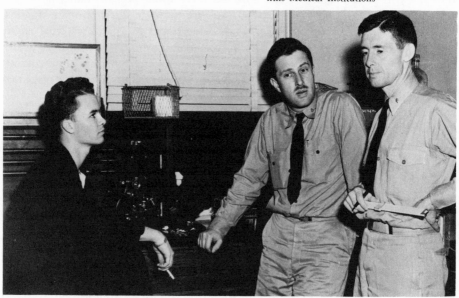

Joseph L. Lilienthal, Jr. (*center*) and Richard Riley (*right*)
From the Archives Office, The Johns Hopkins Medical Institutions

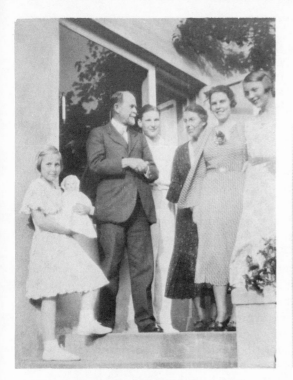

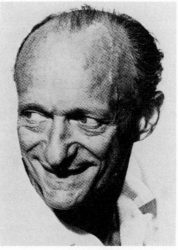

Isabel Morgan (*second from right*)

This picture shows Isabel Morgan with her father, Thomas Hunt Morgan (*second from left*), and her mother (*third from right*). The Morgans were visiting friends in Oslo on their way to Stockholm, where Dr. Thomas Morgan received the Nobel Prize for Physiology and Medicine. Courtesy of Dr. Isabel Morgan Mountain

Stephen W. Kuffler

Courtesy of Dr. Stephen W. Kuffler

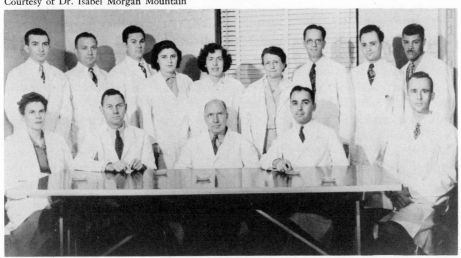

Poliomyelitis research group

Seated (*left to right*): Isabel M. Morgan, Howard A. Howe, Kenneth Maxcy, David Bodian, C. Schwerdt; standing (*left to right*): W. M. O'Leary, W. D. McClaskey, W. Bender, J. Pausch, P. Heaton, Mrs. Cleary, V. Talbert, J. Lazuick, and T. Greene
Courtesy of Dr. David Bodian

in equal titer to all three known types of poliovirus. Gamma globulin was also shown to be successful in the prevention of measles, and Joseph Stokes, Jr. demonstrated that even a small amount of gamma globulin would give protection against infectious hepatitis. As a result, Dr. William Hammon set up a field trial of the effectiveness of pooled gamma globulin in preventing poliomyelitis.

By 1951 virologists had found other things that made vaccine a distinct possibility. Not only had Isabel Morgan shown that formalin-inactivated polio virus could be used for immunization purposes, but John Enders and his group had demonstrated that the virus would multiply in nonnervous tissue in culture, an observation which won his group the Nobel Prize. Also, the immunological typing program carried out by the National Foundation had by this time reached the conclusion that there were only three major immunological types of poliovirus. However, it was still not known whether poliovirus reached the central nervous system by way of peripheral nerves or the blood stream. If it traveled by the nerves, most scientists were resigned to the fact that protection could only be achieved by a high antibody titer. If, however, it traveled by way of the blood stream, then the titer of antibody could be much smaller. The field trial conducted by Dr. William Hammon in September 1951 at Provo, Utah, showed that gamma globulin, even though only a small amount of antibody was present, would protect against paralytic poliomyelitis. The importance of this observation was immediately understood by Dr. David Bodian at Johns Hopkins and Dr. Dorothy Horstmann at Yale. Given the validity of these findings, they concluded that poliovirus travels from its portal-of-entry to the central nervous system by means of the bloodstream, and they both began the search for evidence of viremia. Cynomologous monkeys and chimpanzees were fed poliovirus, and after several days blood specimens were collected and tested for the presence of poliovirus. They quickly discovered virus in the blood between the time of feeding and the development of the paralysis. Previous investigators had missed this viremia because they took the blood specimens too late in the course of the disease, that is, after the development of the paralysis. As soon as these investigators found the viremia in animals, they searched for it in early human cases, and soon discovered viremia in abortive cases of poliomyelitis. In 1951 Bodian and his co-workers demonstrated that low levels of passive antibody were capable of preventing poliomyelitis in monkeys infected intramuscularly or orally with paralytic doses of virus. The same was true of the viremic phase of poliovirus infection in monkeys. In 1953 these workers showed a correlation between the occurrence of viremia and subsequent paralytic infection in chimpanzees.

In 1956 Bodian did important work in establishing the pathological criteria to be used in the monkey safety test for the approval of polio vaccines. At an early stage in the safety testing of commercially produced Salk vaccine, a certain batch passed by Parke-Davis was sent to the NIH for further testing. The Division of Biological Control informed the Vaccine Advisory Committee that this particular batch of vaccine was causing poliomyelitis in monkeys. Dr. Bodian and Dr. Rivers hurried to the NIH so that Dr. Bodian could examine the sections of the spinal cords in monkeys, since he was the recognized expert in the pathology of poliomyelitis infection. Dr. Bodian soon discovered that the so-called poliomyelitis lesions were, in fact, old dengue-virus lesions. The monkeys, who came from the Philippines, apparently had been infected with dengue virus and had recovered. This story does not reflect poorly on the Division of Biological Control: the people were first rate, but at that time there were almost no neuroanatomists who had had experience in the histopathology of poliomyelitis. Subsequently, Dr. Bodian and others trained many people to be experts in this field so that they could man the necessary positions in the laboratories of the pharmaceutical firms where the clinical and histopathological problems of poliomyelitis arose during safety testing.

These most important studies by the poliomyelitis group at Johns Hopkins and the successful cultivation of poliovirus in tissue culture by Enders and his co-workers resolved the pessimism of the early 1940s and created a sound foundation for the development of both types of poliomyelitis vaccine. Thus, Hopkins contributed greatly to the conquering of this most distressing disease —paralytic poliomyelitis. The studies continued, of course, and in 1956 the group determined the sites of poliovirus multiplication in tissues of chimpanzees after virus feeding. In 1960 they demonstrated that low levels of passive serum antibody are capable of limiting poliovirus excretion from the throat but much higher antibody levels are required before fecal virus excretion is affected. In 1964 Bodian made the first electron microscopic study of the poliovirus-infected motorneuron with demonstration of the cytoplasmic effect of virus and of viral aggregates in cytoplasm.

Dr. Bodian, who was made professor and director of the Department of Anatomy in 1957, has continued his outstanding contributions to Johns Hopkins. He became emeritus at the end of the 1974–1975 academic year.

Dr. Howe graduated from Yale University in 1925 and from the Johns Hopkins University Medical School in 1929. He became an assistant in anatomy after his graduation and was promoted to the grade of associate in anatomy, a position he held from 1940 to 1942. In that year he was made associate professor of epidemiology and became adjunct professor in 1947. He assumed emeritus status in 1961.

Stephen W. Kuffler

Members of the faculty of the Johns Hopkins School of Medicine have made many important contributions to the neurological sciences. Perhaps no other, however, has done more with less facilities than Stephen W. Kuffler. Kuffler was born on August 24, 1913, in Hungary. He received his medical degree from the University of Vienna in 1937. After only one year as an assistant in medicine and pathology in Vienna, he migrated to Australia, where he met John C. Eccles, the director of the Kanematsu Institute of Pathology at the Sydney Hospital, and who later became a Nobel laureate. During the next seven years Stephen Kuffler spent a profitable period on important studies of the end-plate potential in the function of the myoneural junction, which clearly demonstrated his talents in basic science.

During this time he also met the author who was attached to the Johns Hopkins 118th General Hospital stationed in Sydney during World War II (1942). Kuffler and I became close friends, and together we made a number of studies on nerve injuries in the military population. After the war I became director of the Department of Medicine at Hopkins, and with the help of Detlev Bronk, I made it possible for Kuffler to come to this country to work in the laboratory of Ralph W. Gerard in Chicago. When the Division of Biomedical Engineering was established in the Department of Medicine, under the directorship of Samuel W. Talbot, I brought the availability of this brilliant young neurophysiologist to the attention of Alan Woods and Philip Bard. Kuffler was successfully recruited for an appointment as an assistant professor in ophthalmology at the then princely salary of $4,500.

Upon his arrival in Baltimore, Kuffler was housed in the Wilmer Institute basement, which at that time was dark, cluttered up, and the occasional home of Sam Talbot, who was engaged in transferring his activities to the Department of Medicine. Stephen Kuffler wasted no time in developing an amazing research unit, which finally grew to a cadre of ten talented young men. With Talbot's help he begged, borrowed, and constructed equipment to carry out his neurophysiological studies. The services of a young electronics engineer by the name of Robert Bosler were obtained. He was relatively untrained at that time but had a natural talent and an instinctive ability to solve problems of instrumentation. Eminently successful, he worked with Kuffler throughout the Hopkins years and still is the major contributor to the technical aspects of Kuffler's department at Harvard.

First Kuffler resumed the work on neuromuscular transmission he had begun in Australia, bringing it to a satisfactory conclusion in 1948 by accumulating rigorous evidence in favor of chemical rather than electrical transmission at the neuromuscular junction.

As director of the neurophysiological laboratory in the Department of Ophthalmology, Kuffler's interest then turned to an analysis of retinal function in the cat. As a result of Talbot's excellence in optics, a multibeam ophthalmoscope was designed, which took several years to construct. (The description of this important instrument was eventually published in 1953.) This ophthalmoscope enabled Kuffler and his group to stimulate the retina precisely with various patterns of light while the investigator could look at the fundus of the eye and himself observe the stimuli. This tremendous advance was coupled with another—a new method of recording from individual ganglion cells without opening up the eye. Thus they had developed the techniques of working with precision on a practically intact visual system.

In 1948 Carlton C. Hunt came to work in human neuropharmacology with the author. It was felt that he would profit greatly by spending his first year with Stephen Kuffler, and as a result of this, he never returned to the Department of Medicine, later becoming an outstanding professor of physiology. With Kuffler he began an investigation of muscle spindles, their sensory and motor innervation, and their role in maintaining posture. In collaboration with Hunt and an Englishman named Quilliam, the motor innervation of the muscle spindles was unequivocally established as was the manner in which they operate. As a result of this work, the study of muscle spindles, feedback control, and postural mechanisms became a flourishing area of neurophysiology. In 1949 Gilbert Ling, a young Chinese scientist who had developed the first intracellular microelectrode, came to Kuffler's laboratory and concentrated on studies of the cell membrane, producing some very stimulating hypotheses on the nature of membrane potentials. He later became a professor at the University of Pennsylvania.

By 1952 the first phase of Kuffler's studies on the visual system was essentially completed. He attributes the success of these experiments to the relatively simple innovations they had introduced. The first was to use the natural media of the intact eye and the second was to ask what seemed a deceptively simple question: What is the best way of influencing the cells in the visual system to fire impulses? The answer was quite clear that the receptive field of each ganglion cell on the retinal surface was concentric, with a central portion working in the opposite way from the peripheral portion around it. For example, a small spot of light may excite a ganglion cell if placed precisely into the center of its receptive field; but if the same spot of light was moved in any direction within one or two millimeters, the response of the same cell would be the opposite—it would be inhibited. On the other hand, if the entire receptive field was stimulated by covering it with light, the responses tended to be weak. Although these results might appear paradoxical, they became central for understanding the neural organization of the retina and provided a successful model for a neurological interpretation of many aspects of perception of contrast and of pattern vision.

When Carlton Hunt left the laboratory, Miles Vaughan Williams of Oxford came for two years. With Kuffler he published a series of papers entitled "The Small Nerve System in the Frog" and provided a clear demonstration of the existence of specific "tonic" or "slow" muscle fibers, a distinct entity which had a separate innervation as well as a reflex regulation. The parallel effort of dividing the work in the laboratory between the visual system and other neurophysiological problems continued throughout Kuffler's stay at the Wilmer Institute.

Another important line of work was initiated in 1954, when Carlos Eyzaguirre, after a period in the Department of Medicine, went to work in Kuffler's laboratory. He and Kuffler studied a rather primitive stretch receptor from crustacean preparations and worked out the sequence of events that intervened between the application of external energy and the initiation of impulses. This new preparation proved an important one, as it was applicable to many other systems and eventually led them into neurochemical studies and the establishment of a new transmittor substance, gamma-amino butyric acid. Eyzaguirre eventually became head of the Department of Physiology at the University of Utah.

Perhaps the most exceptional work started at the Wilmer Institute was that of Torsten Wiesel and David Hubel. Wiesel came in 1955 from the Karolinska Institute in Stockholm, and Hubel joined Kuffler in 1958, after finishing his residency in neurology at Johns Hopkins. They pursued the analysis of receptive fields started by Kuffler, and carried the work right into the visual cortex. In their hands the receptive field studies proved a powerful tool, and as a result we now have a much better idea of how our nervous system processes information. Their work related directly to many fundamental questions, such as the initial development of connections in higher centers and how these can be influenced by the environment, particularly in the early period of life.

At the Wilmer, obligations for administration and teaching were minimal, informal, and therefore enjoyable. The productivity was greatly enhanced by the youthfulness of the group and the great number of bright young men who came to the laboratory for training and experience. It is amazing how many of the young men who came in the years between 1947 and 1959 are now heads of departments of physiology, or have become internationally known as physiologists or cell biologists. In addition to Hunt, Qulliam, Ling, Vaughan Williams, and Eyzaguirre, there were Wolfgang Trautwein, Otto Hutter, Kenneth Brown, Susumu Hagiwara, David Ottoson, Horace Barlow, Charles Edwards, Josef Dudel, Taro Furukawa, David Potter, and Edwin Furshpan.

Not only was there an excellent tradition of scholarship in Kuffler's group, but there was also great devotion to the work, which was pursued with considerable gusto and at times frivolity. For example, together with other young and not-so-young investigators, they formed the "Know Nothing Club," which used to meet for drinks, a good meal, and a lecture afterwards. If time grew short and the spirits too high and strong, they left out the last portion of the program, namely, science. The principal source of this esprit-de-corps undoubtedly rested in Stephen Kuffler.

With the great influx of excellent young talent from all parts of the globe, Kuffler's laboratory expanded into several rooms, and a new neurochemistry laboratory was added. Nevertheless, by 1958 Kuffler had accumulated so much young talent that there was insufficient space for him in the Wilmer; so the choice had to be faced whether to disperse or stick together. There were enough bright people to form a new department. This was recognized by Harvard Medical School, particularly by Otto Krayer, the chairman of the Department of Pharmacology. Thus, Kuffler states, "with a certain amount of reluctance about ten of us left Wilmer Institute in 1959 to migrate north to Harvard Medical School." Within a short period Harvard took the unusual step of creating a Department of Neurobiology and six full professorships for Kuffler's group, which has made outstanding contributions since that time.

Kuffler's scientific work has had a strong impact on several areas of the neurological sciences, and his experimental studies have repeatedly opened up new fields of research. In recognition of his many contributions, honors have flowed steadily to him. He is a member of the National Academy of Sciences and a Foreign Member of The Royal Society, the Royal Danish Academy of Sciences, and the Austrian Academy of Sciences. He has given many prestigious lectureships, including among others the Harvey Lecture, the Ferrier Lecture, the Silliman Memorial Lecture, and the Sherrington Lecture. He received the Proctor Award in Ophthalmology and the Dixon Prize in Medicine from the University of Pittsburgh. In 1971 he was the recipient of the prestigious Passano Award and in 1972 the Louisa Gross Horwitz Prize in Biology from Columbia University. For a time he held the titles of Robert Winthrop Professor of Neurobiology and Chairman of the Department of Neurobiology at Harvard Medical School. In 1974 he was made the John Franklin Enders University Professor. He holds the honorary degrees of Doctor of Medicine from the University of Bern, and Doctor of Science from Yale University, Washington University, and the University of London.

Myasthenia Gravis and the Thymus Gland

In closing this series of vignettes describing the many faces of research in the Johns Hopkins Hospital and the Johns Hopkins School of Medicine, I would like to describe the work of my colleagues, Richard Masland and Joseph Lilienthal, and myself on the disease known as myasthenia gravis and its relationship to the thymus gland. The term "myasthenia gravis" comes from the Greek *mys* (muscle), *asthenia* (weakness), and from the Latin *gravis* (heavy). Thus it implies a marked or severe muscle weakness. An English physician, Thomas Willis, first described the chief symptoms of asthenia of voluntary muscle with recovery after rest. In speaking of "the palsy" in his London *Practice of Physick*, he said the following:

There is another kind of this disease depending on the scarcity and fewness of the spirits; in which the motion fails wholly in no Part or Member, yet it is performed weakly only, or depravidly by any—Those who being troubled with a scarcity of spirit will force them as much as they may to local motions, are able at first rising in the morning to walk, move their arms this way or that, or to lift up a weight with strength, but before noon the stores of the spirit which influence the muscles being almost spent, they are scarcely able to move hand or foot. I have now a prudent and honest woman in cure, who for many years has been obnoxious to this kind of bastard palsy, not only in the limb but likewise in her tongue; this person for some time speaks freely and readily enough, but after long, hasty, or laborious speaking presently she becomes mute as a fish, and cannot bring forth a word, nay, and does not recover the use of her voice until after an hour or two.

This was an isolated observation, and it was over two hundred years before this syndrome was again referred to in the medical literature. However, in the past hundred years it has intrigued many scientific investigators.

In 1932 Lazar Remen of Munster, Germany, first demonstrated the effect of neostigmine on a patient with myasthenia gravis. In 1935, while an intern on the medical wards of the Johns Hopkins Hospital, I took care of two patients with myasthenia gravis, the first in this hospital to receive treatment with neostigmine. My interest in this disease was kindled by this experience, and it deepened a few months later when I heard Dr. Walter B. Cannon lecture on the new evidence relating to the chemical transmission of nerve impulses. Dr. Richard Whitehill, a fellow house officer, and I demonstrated the value of neostigmine as a specific diagnostic test in patients with myasthenia gravis. We also confirmed the fact that quinine produced an increase in the muscular weakness in patients with myasthenia gravis.

In the spring of my second year as assistant resident in medicine, Sir Henry Dale came to Baltimore to give a series of lectures. Dale had recently won the Nobel Prize for his brilliant work in demonstrating the relationship of acetylcholine to transmission of the nerve impulse across the neuromuscular junction. I was fortunate enough to be able to make arrangements to spend the next two years working in Sir Henry Dale's laboratory in London—the first year under a fellowship of the American College of Physicians and the second year with support from the Rockefeller Foundation.

After arriving in Dale's laboratory in September 1937, my first effort was to study the mechanism of action of quinine on neuromuscular function, using the technique which had been developed in that laboratory. These studies revealed that quinine has a number of actions on skeletal muscle. Most important, it abolished the response of the normal mammalian muscle to injected acetylcholine, a phenomenon that proved to be due largely to the curariform action of quinine, which was demonstrated for the first time in these experiments. This finding was of great interest, since quinine increased the degree of muscular weakness in the patient with myasthenia gravis, and Jolly, many years before, had pointed out the analogy between curare poisoning and the fatigability of the muscles in patients with myasthenia gravis. Curare, of course, is the generic name for various South American arrow poisons, and it has a long and romantic history. It has been employed for centuries by the Indians of the Amazon River for killing wild animals used for food. It produces death from muscle paralysis, the key feature of which is the type of fatigability seen in myasthenia gravis.

Since my long-term objective was to learn more about the basic nature of myasthenia gravis, much of my time in Sir Henry Dale's laboratory was spent in trying to adapt the special techniques which they had devised for their animal experiments to the study of neuromuscular function in man. This was a difficult step. In the first place, one had to be certain that the motor nerve to the muscle from which one is recording the muscle action potential has received a supramaximal stimulation but not one sufficiently strong to induce repetitive discharge of the nerve. Secondly, one must have a quantitative way of recording the action potential of the whole muscle in man. The electric current that must be applied to the nerve is strong, and in addition to the pain which may be induced, a stimulus artifact is usually produced which interferes with the visualization of the action potential—the stumbling block for those who had attempted to do this unsuccessfully in the past.

A second step was to apply the pharmacologic agents to be studied, including acetylcholine, as close to the muscle as possible in order to duplicate to the fullest extent in man the "close arterial injection" that had been so successful in providing evidence that acetylcholine was the normal transmittor substance. Brown, Dale, and Feldberg developed the technique of "close arterial injection," which permitted rapid injection of acetylcholine directly into a single muscle. The resulting contraction of the muscle closely simulated that resulting from a maximal motor nerve stimulus. This quick response of the muscle was abolished by curare even more readily than its response to a nerve impulse, and a small amount of the anticholinesterase drug eserine changed the simple twitch produced by a single motor nerve stimulus into a repetitive response—an evanescent tetanus.

With partial curarization in the experimental animal, two processes were demonstrated to take place at the neuromuscular junction following the passage of a single nerve impulse—a brief period during which the response to a second or test stimulus to the nerve was enhanced or facilitated and a longer period during which it was profoundly depressed. This depression was thought to be due to the inability of the acetylcholine released and replaced at its normal rate to excite all of the muscle fibers in the presence of the partial neuromuscular block produced by curare. When a tetanus was applied to the nerve, the response to a test stimulus to the nerve at varying intervals thereafter was greatly potentiated.

Thus, the methods which I was trying to develop for studies in man would have to be sufficiently quantitative to reproduce these events seen in the normal and partially curarized animal if one hoped to elucidate the nature of the defect in neuromuscular function in myasthenia gravis. The following key findings in the experimental animal are among those that we successfully reproduced in the experiments in man: (1) the response to acetylcholine excitation and the late depression of neuromuscular function produced by acetycholine; (2) the conversion of the single response of the muscle to nerve stimulation to an evanescent tetanus by eserine or neostigmine; (3) the phenomenon of facilitation and depression in the partially curarized animal; and (4) the post-tetanic facilitation seen in the partially curarized animal.

In 1939, working in collaboration with Dr. Richard L. Masland at the University of Pennsylvania, we successfully overcame the difficulties in obtaining satisfactory electromyograms in relation to maximal nerve stimuli in man. Electrodes for recording the muscle action potential were fixed to the skin. The stimulating electrode was pressed firmly over the ulnar nerve, just below the elbow. The action potential being observed by means of the cathode ray oscillograph, the strength of the nerve stimulus was gradually increased until the muscle action potential reached a maximum size. Subjects were then partially curarized, and the time course of the response to paired stimuli at varying intervals was entirely suitable for studying the physiology and pharmacology of neuromuscular transmission in man.

Our next step was to study the electromyogram in patients with myasthenia gravis. It was soon discovered that the response of the myasthenic muscle to a single maximum motor nerve volley excited a reduced number of muscle fibers. The second of the two responses to nerve impulses at varying intervals was further reduced, as in the partially curarized individual. When the nerve was stimulated with a series of electrical impulses, in other words a tetanus, the resulting muscle action potential showed a progressive decline in voltage. Neostigmine abolished the abnormalities in the electromyogram in myasthenia gravis, and the abnormalities were increased by the administration of a small dose of quinine.

Studies done at Johns Hopkins in 1941 with Dr. Joseph Lilienthal, Jr., while we were both members of the resident staff, showed that when injected into the brachial artery, the neostigmine produced a prolonged paresis of the injected extremity, during which a muscle action potential evoked by supra-maximal stimulation of the ulnar nerve was followed by repetitive activity. This was undoubtedly due to the persistence of acetylcholine released from the nerve ending. The initial response to a single stimulus was not altered from the normal, showing that this neuromuscular block caused by neostigmine was different from that produced by partial curarization. These experiments fur-nished clear evidence that one could observe the state of neuromuscular trans-mission in man as accurately as one can determine the status of a patient with diabetes mellitus by estimation of the blood glucose. They indicated a striking similarity in the neuromuscular block in the patient with myasthenia gravis to that produced by curare in the experimental animal.

The studies carried out between 1939 and 1941 strongly suggested that a curare-like action was responsible for the neuromuscular block. It seemed logi-cal that such a substance might be present in serum, and we turned our atten-tion to the thymus gland as the possible source for such a substance. It had been known for some time that abnormalities in the thymus gland were present in a large percentage of patients with myasthenia gravis and that a number of these patients had a tumor of the thymus. The possibility that there might be a curare-like substance in serum released from the thymus was enhanced by the occasional observation of neonatal myasthenia. Infants born of a myasthenic mother occasionally have a characteristic difficulty in feeding due to weakness of the circumoral and other muscles, a weakness which is relieved by the administration of neostigmine. This neonatal myasthenia persists for only a few weeks, then spontaneously disappears and has no tendency to return at a later age. The explanation suggested to us by this was that a curare-like substance capable of crossing the placental membrane was present in the mother's serum.

When Dr. Alfred Blalock became professor of surgery at Johns Hopkins, Joseph Lilienthal and I approached him with the proposition that we determine the effect of total removal of the thymus in a series of well-studied patients with myasthenia gravis. The literature at that time contained several reports of surgical removal of a thymic tumor with what appeared to be a beneficial influence on the course of the myasthenia gravis. In none of these cases was an effort made to search for and remove all thymic tissue. The fifth such operation had been carried out in 1939 by Dr. Blalock, a cystic tumor being removed from the thymic region. No other thymic tissue was visualized, although the search of the anterior mediastinum was not a thorough one. Thus, Dr. Lilien-thal and I, in the belief that our experimental evidence at that point justified such an experiment, proposed to Dr. Blalock that he systematically remove all of the thymic tissue from a series of patients with myasthenia gravis. Dr. Frank Ford, who had followed our work carefully, agreed with our proposal, and his stature and influence were helpful in persuading Dr. Blalock to undertake this approach.

Three principal methods of study were employed in estimating the effect of thymectomy in our patients: (1) a careful study was made of the degree of clinical fatigability without medication and after a given dosage of neostigmine; (2) quantitative studies of the response to nerve stimulation of the type already described were carried out and the effect of neostigmine on this response to nerve stimulation was also carefully recorded; and (3) the general course of the disease and the total need of the patient for neostigmine were carefully recorded.

These studies were reported for the first time in an article entitled "The Treatment of Myasthenia Gravis by Removal of the Thymus Gland—Preliminary Report," published in the *Journal of the American Medical Association* in 1941. For the first few months after the operation, several of the patients showed progressive improvement in strength and no longer required neostigmine therapy. Five months after the operative procedure, electromyographic studies demonstrated that (1) a larger number of muscle fibers responded to maximal motor nerve stimulus, and (2) there was greater efficiency in the transmission of pairs and trains of maximal motor nerve stimuli across the neuromuscular junction. In addition, the intra-arterial injection of neostigmine, in contrast to its effect before thymectomy, now produced (1) repetitive response to a single stimulus and (2) normal local paresis and a depression of neuromuscular function in two of the patients. These studies indicated that in certain individuals the thymus played an important role in the pathogenesis of myasthenia gravis. Although there was no absolute proof that the improvement was related to thymectomy, subsequent experience indicates that this was the case. This was the first time that objective evidence of an effect of the thymus in man had been demonstrated.

Joseph Leo Lilienthal, Jr., was born in New York City on November 1, 1911. After graduation from Phillips Exeter Academy in 1929, he entered Yale University and received his B.S. degree in 1932. He graduated with the class of 1937 from the Johns Hopkins School of Medicine and on June 25, 1937, married Katherine Arnstein. He made an outstanding record as a medical house officer at Presbyterian Hospital in New York City, and then returned to Baltimore as an assistant resident physician. He served as chief resident on the Osler service in 1941–1942. The following four years he served with distinction as an officer in the Naval Medical Corps at the School of Aviation Medicine in Pensacola. He was a lieutenant commander at the time of his discharge in 1946. After the war he returned to Baltimore as associate professor of medicine in charge of the Physiological Division, and his outstanding record as a physiologist, teacher, and clinician led in 1950 to his appointment as professor of environmental medicine in the School of Hygiene. He reorganized this department, which had formerly been the Department of Physiology under Dr. William H. Howell, broadening the scope of its activity toward the study of man and the influences of his complex environment upon physiological function. He created a unique and effective relationship between the Schools of Hygiene and Medicine which was very fruitful, and could never have been accomplished without his stimulating personality and outstanding ability as a scientist and administrator. His amazing drive, intellectual capacity, and loyalty made it possible for him to remain at the same time an outstanding contributor to the teaching and patient care program of the Department of Medicine.

As an investigator, he clearly demonstrated the breadth of his intellect by making fundamental contributions in both basic physiology and clinical medicine. One of his earliest interests, which has already been described, was the physiology and pharmacology of neuromuscular function in man. He later showed versatility by bridging the gap to lower mammals by his important studies on the constituents of muscle, the effects of alpha-tocopherol phosphate, the action of decamethonium, the origin of fibrillary potentials in denervated muscles, and his final work on the effect of stretch on metabolism of skeletal muscle. One of his most important collaborators during this period was Dr. Kenneth Zierler.

During his period in the navy, his interest in the field of respiratory physiology and diseases of the lungs began. These basic studies on the relations of oxygen, carbon dioxide, and hemoglobin in the blood of man and on the determination of the physiologically effective pressures of oxygen and carbon dioxide in alveolar air under various experimental conditions had far-reaching practical significance in their application to the study of disease in man.

Lilienthal gave generously of his time in support of governmental activities, serving as consultant to the Office of Naval Research, the Department of the Army, the National Science Foundation, and the National Institute of Health. At the National Research Council he served on the Committee on Naval Aviation and also on the Committee on Naval Medical Research. His distinction as a scientist led to his election to the American Society for Clinical Investigation, the American Physiological Society, and the Association of American Physicians. His premature death in 1955 was a great loss to the Johns Hopkins Medical Institutions.

References

PREFACE

Billings, J. S. "The Plans and Purposes of The Johns Hopkins Hospital." In *The Johns Hopkins Hospital. Addresses at the Opening of the Hospital*. Baltimore: Privately printed. 1889.

Comroe, J. H., Jr. "What's Locked Up." *Am. Rev. Resp. Dis.* 110 (1974): 111.

Comroe, J. H., Jr., and Dripps, R. D. "Ben Franklin and Open Heart Surgery." *Circ. Res.* 35 (1974): 661.

Gregg, A. "Dr. Welch's Influence on Medical Education." *Bull. Johns Hopkins Hosp.* 87 (1950): 28 (Suppl.).

Shannon, J. A. NIH: "Present and Potential Contribution to Application of Biomedical Knowledge." In *Research in the Service of Man: Biomedical Knowledge, Development and Use*. U.S. Senate, 90th Congress, 1st Session, Document No. 55, 1967, pp. 72–85.

Technology in Retrospect and Critical Events in Science. Prepared for the National Science Foundation by Illinois Institute of Technology Research Institute under Contract NSF-C535, December 15, 1968.

1. A CENTURY OF CLINICAL SCIENCE AT JOHNS HOPKINS:

CONTRIBUTIONS TO MEDICINE BY STUDENTS, HOUSE OFFICERS,

AND FACULTY

Billings, J. S. "The Plans and Purposes of The Johns Hopkins Hospital." In *Johns Hopkins Hospital: Addresses at the Opening of the Hospital*. Baltimore: Privately printed, 1889.

Blalock, A. "The Nature of Discovery." *Ann. Surg.* 144 (1956): 289.

Bronowski, J. "The Creative Process." *Sci. Amer.* 199 (1958): 59.

French, John C. *A History of the University Founded by Johns Hopkins*, p. 82. Baltimore: Johns Hopkins University Press, 1946.

Gregg, Alan. "Dr. Welch's Influence on Medical Education." *Bull. Johns Hopkins Hosp.* 87 (1950): 87 (Suppl.).

Huxley, Leonard. *Life and Letters of T. H. Huxley*. Vol. 1, pp. 465–467. London: Macmillan and Co., 1900.

Osler, W. "Looking Back." *Johns Hopkins Hosp. Bull.* 25 (1914): 354.

Thoms, Herbert. *Classical Contributions to Obstetrics and Gynecology*, p. xiii. Springfield, Ill.: Charles C Thomas, 1935.

2. PIONEERS IN UROLOGY: JAMES R. BROWN AND HOWARD A. KELLY

Brown, J. "Catheterization of the Male Ureters. A Preliminary Report." *Johns Hopkins Hosp. Bull.* 4 (1893): 73.

Brown, James. "Catheterization of the Male Ureters." *Johns Hopkins Hosp. Bull.* 6 (1895): 12.

Brown, James. "Obituary." *Johns Hopkins Hosp. Bull.* 6 (1895): 95.

Burnam, Curtis F. "Howard Atwood Kelly." *Bull. Johns Hopkins Hosp.* 73 (1943): 1.

Chesney, A. *The Johns Hopkins Hospital and the Johns Hopkins University School of Medicine: A Chronicle*. Vol. 1, 1867–1893. Baltimore: Johns Hopkins University Press, 1943.

Cordell, E. F. *The Medical Annals of Maryland: 1799–1899*, p. 334. Baltimore: Williams & Wilkins Co., 1903.

Cullen, T. S. "Dr. Howard A. Kelly." *Johns Hopkins Hosp. Bull.* 30 (1919): 287.

———. "Dr. Howard Kelly, the Last of the Johns Hopkins Hospital's Big Four." *Johns Hopkins Alumni Magazine*. 31 (1943), March and June, pp. 35 and 106.

Kelly, H. A. "The Examination of the Female Bladder and the Catheterization of the Ureters under Direct Inspection." *Johns Hopkins Hosp. Bull.* 4 (1893): 101.

———. "The Direct Examination of the Female Bladder with Elevated Pelvis—The Catheterization of the Ureters under Direct Inspection, with and without Elevation of the Pelvis." *Am. J. Obstet. Gynecol.* 29 (1894) 1.

———. "Testimonial Dinner to H. A. Kelly." *Bull. Johns Hopkins Hosp.* 53 (1933): 74.

Kelly, H. A., and Burrage, W. *Dictionary of American Medical Biography*, p. 153. New York: D. Appleton & Co., 1920.

TeLinde, R. W. "Howard Atwood Kelly." *Am. J. Obstet. Gynecol.* 68 (1954): 1203.

Young, H. H. *A Surgeon's Autobiography*, p. 76. New York: Harcourt, Brace & Co., 1940.

Young, H. H., and Davis, D. M. *Practice of Urology.* Vol. 1, p. 245. Philadelphia: W. B. Saunders Co., 1926.

3. MEDICAL STUDENTS ON THE MARCH: BROWN, MAC CALLUM, AND OPIE

Ashford, Bailey. *A Soldier in Science*, p. 42. New York: William Morrow and Co., 1934.

Barron, M. "The Relation of the Islets of Langerhans to Diabetes with Special Reference to Cases of Pancreatic Lithiasis." *Surg. Gynecol. Obstet.* 31 (1920): 437.

Brown, Jeannie Albert. *Dr. Tom Brown, Memories.* New York: Richard R. Smith, 1949.

Brown, T. R. "Studies on Trichinosis." *Johns Hopkins Hosp. Bull.* 8 (1897): 79.

———. "Studies on Trichinosis, with Special Reference to the Increase of the Eosinophile Cells in the Blood and Muscle, and Origin of These Cells and Their Diagnostic Importance." *J. Exp. Med.* 3 (1898): 315.

———. "The Blood in Certain Cutaneous, Nervous and Miscellaneous Diseases, with Remarks upon the Origin and Significance of the Eosinophiles." *Md. State Med. J.*, July 1902, p. 303.

Chesney, A. M. *The Johns Hopkins Hospital and the Johns Hopkins University School of Medicine, A Chronicle.* Vol. 2, *1893–1905*, p. 4. Baltimore: Johns Hopkins University Press, 1958.

Flexner, Simon. "William George MacCallum." *Science* 99 (1944): 290.

Forbus, Wiley D. "William George MacCallum (1874–1944)." *J. Pathol.* 56 (1944): 603.

Hirsch, James G. "Eugene L. Opie (1873–1971)." *Trans. Assoc. Am. Physicians* 84 (1971): 31.

Longcope, W. T. "William G. MacCallum (1874–1944)." *Trans. Assoc. Am. Physicians* 58 (1944): 28.

———. "William George MacCallum (1874–1944)." *Bull. Hist. Med.* 18 (1945): 207.

MacCallum, W. G. "On the Pathology of Haematozoan Infections in Birds." *Johns Hopkins Hosp. Bull.* 8 (1897): 51.

———. "On the Haematozoan Infections of Birds." *Johns Hopkins Hosp. Bull.* 8 (1897): 235.

———. "Notes on the Pathological Changes in the Organs of Birds Infected with Haemocytozoa." *J. Exp. Med.* 3 (1898): 103.

———. "On the Haematozoan Infections of Birds." *J. Exp. Med.* 3 (1898): 117.

———. "On the Haematozoan Infection of Birds." *Johns Hopkins Hosp. Bull.* 9 (1898): 18.

———. "On the Production of Specific Cytolytic Sera for Thyroid and Parathyroid, with Observations on the Physiology and Pathology of the Parathyroid Gland, especially in its Relation to Exophthalmic Goitre." *Trans. Assoc. Am. Physicians* 18 (1903): 35.

———. "On the Relation of the Islands of Langerhans to Glycosuria." *Johns Hopkins Hosp. Bull.* 20 (1909): 265.

MacCallum, W. G. and Voegtlin, C. "II. Relation of Tetany to Calcium Metabolism." *Johns Hopkins Hosp. Bull.* 18 (1908): 244.

———. "On the Relation of the Parathyroid to Calcium Metabolism and the Nature of Tetany." *Johns Hopkins Hosp. Bull.* 19 (1908): 91.

———. "On the Relation of Tetany to the Parathyroid Glands and to Calcium Metabolism." *J. Exp. Med.* 11 (1909): 118.

Opie, Eugene L. "On the Haemocytozoa of Birds." *Johns Hopkins Hosp. Bull.* 8 (1897): 52.

———. "On the Haemocytozoa of Birds." *J. Exp. Med.* 3 (1898): 79.

———. "On the Relation of the Chronic Interstitial Pancreatitis to the Islands of Langerhans and to Diabetes Mellitus." *J. Exp. Med.* 5 (1900): 419.

———. Special issue of *Archives of Pathology* dedicated to Eugene L. Opie, vol. 34 (1942).

Rich, Arnold R. "Dr. William George MacCallum (1874–1944)." *Johns Hopkins Hosp. Bull.* 75 (1944): 73.

4. TWO MYCOSES FIRST DESCRIBED AT JOHNS HOPKINS

Bechet, P. E. "An Outline of the Achievements of American Dermatology Arranged in Chronological Order." *Bull. Hist. Med.* 19 (1946): 291.

Chesney, A. M. *The Johns Hopkins Hospital and the Johns Hopkins University School of Medicine, A Chronicle.* Vol. 2, p. 342. Baltimore: Johns Hopkins University Press, 1958.

Cordell, E. F. *Medical Annals of Baltimore (1799–1899),* p. 410. Baltimore: Williams & Wilkins Co., 1903.

Garrison, F. H. *An Introduction to the History of Medicine,* p. 649. Philadelphia: W. B. Saunders Co., 1929.

Gilchrist, T. C. "Blastomycosis—Description of the First Case. Preliminary Report Read Before American Dermatological Association, May 1894." In Duhring, *Textbook of Cutaneous Medicine.* Vol. 1, p. 157. 1895.

———. "A Case of Blastomycetic Dermatitis in Man." *Johns Hopkins Hosp. Reports,* 1 (1896): 269.

———. "Two Rare Cases of Diseases of the Skin." *Johns Hopkins Hosp. Bull.* 7 (1896): 138.

———. "A Bacteriological and Microscopical Study of Over Three Hundred Vesicular and Pustular Lesions of the Skin, with a Research upon the Etiology of Acne Vulgaris." *Trans. Amer. Dermat. Assoc.,* 1899, p. 87.

———. A Bacteriological and Microscopical Study of Over Three Hundred Vesicular and Pustular Lesions of the Skin, with a Research upon the Etiology of Acne Vulgaris." *Johns Hopkins Hosp. Reports* 9 (1900): 409.

———. "Some Experimental Observations on the Histopathology of Urticaria Factitia." *J. Cutan. Dis.* 23 (1908): 122.

Gilchrist, T. C., and Stokes, W. R. "The Presence of an Oidium in the Tissues of a Case of Pseudo-lupus Vulgaris." *Johns Hopkins Hosp. Bull.* 7 (1896): 129.

Kelly, H. A., and Burrage, W. C. *Dictionary of American Medical Biography,* p. 1081. New York and London: D. Appleton & Co., 1928.

Robinson, H. M., Sr. "A Short History of Dermatology as It Progressed in Baltimore." *Bull. School Med. Univ. Maryland* 37 (1952): 9.

Schenck, B. R. "On Refractory Subcutaneous Abscesses Caused by a Fungus Possibly Related to the Sporotricha." *Johns Hopkins Hosp. Bull.* 9 (1898): 286.

5. TEACHER AND DISTINGUISHED PUPIL:
WILLIAM HENRY WELCH AND GEORGE HOYT WHIPPLE

Charache, P., Bayless, T. M., Shelly, W. M., and Hendrix, T. R. "Atypical Bacteria in Whipple's Disease." *Trans. Assoc. Am. Physicians* 79 (1966): 399.

Chesney, A. M. *The Johns Hopkins Hospital and the Johns Hopkins University School of Medicine.* 3 vols. Baltimore: Johns Hopkins University Press, 1943, 1958, and 1963.

Flexner, A. "William Henry Welch." *Bull. Johns Hopkins Hosp.* 87 (1950): 39.

Flexner, S., and Flexner, J. T. *William Henry Welch and the Heroic Age of American Medicine.* New York: Viking Press, 1941.

Hendrix, T. R., and Yardley, J. H. "Whipple's Disease." In *Modern Trends in Gastroenterology—4,* p. 229. Ed. W. I. Card and B. Creamer. London: Butterworth & Co., 1970.

Minot, G. R., and Murphy, W. P. "Observations on Patients with Pernicious Anemia Partaking of a Special Diet." *Trans. Assoc. Am. Physicians* 41 (1926): 72.

Riedman, S. R., and Gustafson, E. T. *Portraits of Nobel Laureates in Medicine and Physiology,* p. 171. London, New York, and Toronto: Abelard-Schuman, 1964.

Turner, T. B. *Heritage of Excellence: The Johns Hopkins Medical Institutions 1914–1947* Baltimore: Johns Hopkins University Press, 1974.

Welch, W. H., and Nuttall, G. H. F. "A Gas-Producing Bacillus [Bacillus Aerogenes Capsulatus, Nov. Spec.] Capable of Rapid Development in the Blood-Vessels After Death." *Johns Hopkins Hosp. Bull.* 3 (1892): 81.

Welch, W. H. "Observations Concerning the Bacillus Aerogenes Capsulatus." *J. Exp. Med.* 1 (1896): 5.

Whipple, G. H. "A Hitherto Undescribed Disease Characterized by Deposits of Fat and Fatty Acids in the Intestinal and Mesenteric Lymphatic Tissues." *Johns Hopkins Hosp. Bull.* 18 (1907): 382.

Wintrobe, M. M. "Anemia, Serendipity and Science." *J.A.M.A.* 210 (1969): 318.

Yardley, J. H., and Fleming, W. H., II. "Whipple's Disease, a Note Regarding PAS-Positive Granules in the Original Case." *Bull. Johns Hopkins Hosp.* 109 (1961): 76.

Yardley, J. H. and Hendrix, T. R. "Combined Electron and Light Microscopy in Whipple's Disease: Demonstration of 'Bacillary Bodies' in the Intestine." *Bull. Johns Hopkins Hosp.* 109 (1961): 80.

6. PHARMACOLOGY'S GIANT: JOHN JACOB ABEL

Abel, J. J. "On a Simple Method of Preparing Epinephrine and Its Compounds." *Johns Hopkins Hosp. Bull.* 13 (1902): 29.
Abel, J. J., and Crawford, A. C. "On the Blood-Pressure-Raising Constituent of the Suprarenal Capsule." *Trans. Assoc. Am. Physicians* 12 (1897): 461.
Abel, J. J.; Rowntree, L. G.; and Turner, B. B. "On the Removal of Diffusible Substances from the Circulating Blood by Means of Dialysis." *Trans. Assoc. Am. Physicians* 28 (1913): 51.
———. "On the Removal of Diffusible Substances from the Blood of Living Animals by Dialysis." *J. Pharmacol. Exp. Ther.* 5 (1913): 51.
———. "Plasma Removal and Return of Corpuscles [Plasmaphaeresis]." First Paper. *J. Pharmacol. Exp. Ther.* 5 (1914): 625.
"Dr. John T. Geraghty." Baltimore *Sun*, August 18, 1924, p. 16.
Edmunds, C. W. "Presentation of the Kober Medal to John J. Abel." *Trans. Assoc. Am. Physicians* 49 (1934): 5.
Geraghty, J. T., and Rowntree, L. G. "The Value and Limitations of Functional Renal Tests." *J.A.M.A.* 61 (1913): 939.
Keith, W. M., and Hench, P. S. "Leonard George Rowntree, 1883–1959." *Trans. Assoc. Am. Physicians* 73 (1960): 29.
Lamson, Paul D. "John Jacob Abel, A Portrait." *Bull. Johns Hopkins Hosp.* 68 (1941): 119.
Marshall, E. K., Jr. "John Jacob Abel, 1857–1938." *Trans. Assoc. Am. Physicians* 54 (1939): 7.
———. "John Jacob Abel—Decade 1913–1923." *Bull. Johns Hopkins Hosp.* 101 (1957): 311.
———. "Abel the Prophet." In *John Jacob Abel, Investigator, Teacher, Prophet*, p. 6. Baltimore: Williams & Wilkins Co., 1957.
Rowntree, L. G., and Geraghty, J. T. "An Experimental and Chemical Study of the Functional Activity of the Kidneys by Means of Phenolsulphonephthalein." *J. Pharmacol. Exp. Ther.* 1 (1910): 579.
Voegtlin, Carl. "John Jacob Abel, 1857–1938." *J. Pharmacol. Exp. Ther.* 67 (1939): 373.
Young, Hugh H. *A Surgeon's Autobiography*, p. 92. New York: Harcourt Brace & World, Inc., 1940.

7. NEUROSURGICAL GENIUS: WALTER EDWARD DANDY

Barr, J. S. " 'Sciatica' Caused by Intervertebral-Disc Lesions." *J. Bone Joint Dis.* 17 (1937): 323.
Barr, J. S.; Hampton, A. O.; and Mixter, W. J. "Pain Low in the Back and Sciatica: Due to Lesions of the Intervertebral Discs." *J.A.M.A.* 109 (1937): 1265.
Blalock, A. "Walter Edward Dandy (1886–1946)." *Surgery* 19 (1946): 577.
Campbell, E. "Walter E. Dandy—Surgeon, 1886–1946." *J. Neurosurgery* 8 (1951): 249.
Dandy, W. E. "Fluoroscopy of the Cerebral Ventricles." *Bull. Johns Hopkins Hosp.* 30 (1916): 29.
———. "Ventriculography Following the Injection of Air into the Cerebral Ventricles." *Ann. Surg.* 68 (1918): 5.
———. "Loose Cartilage from Intervertebral Disc Simulating Tumor of the Spinal Cord." *Arch. Surg.* 19 (1929): 660.
Dandy, W. E., and Blackfan, K. D. "An Experimental and Clinical Study of Internal Hydrocephelus." *J.A.M.A.* 61 (1913): 2216.
Dandy, W. E., and Goetsch, E. "The Blood Supply of the Pituitary Body." *Am. J. Anat.* 11 (1910): 137.
Fairman, D. "Evolution of Neurosurgery Through Walter E. Dandy's Work." *Surgery* 19 (1946): 587.
Goldthwait, J. E. "The Lumbosacral Articulation: An Explanation of Many Cases of 'Lumbago,' 'Sciatica' and Paraplegia." *Boston Med. Surg. J.* 164 (1911): 365.
Middleton, G. S., and Teacher, J. H. "Injury of the Spinal Cord Due to Rupture of an Intervertebral Disc During Muscular Effort." *Glasgow Med. J.* 76 (1911): 1.
Mixter, W. J., and Barr, J. S. "Rupture of the Intervertebral Disc with Involvement of the Spinal Canal." *N. Engl. J. Med.* 211 (1934): 210.

Oppenheimer, H., and Krause, F. *"Ueber einklemmung bzw. strangulation der cauda equina." Deutsche Med. Wchnschr.* 35 (1909): 697.
Wolfe, Thomas. Biography from *Concise Dictionary of American Biography*, p. 1242. New York: Charles Scribner's Sons, 1964.

8. EARLY CONTRIBUTIONS TO THE SURGERY OF CANCER:

WILLIAM S. HALSTED, HUGH H. YOUNG, AND JOHN G. CLARK

Baumgartner, A. *"Maladies de la mamelle." Nouveau Traite de chirurgie, Le Dentu-Delbet* 32 (1913): 270.
Bloodgood, J. C. "Operations on 459 Cases of Hernia in the John Hopkins Hospital from June, 1889 to January, 1899." *Johns Hopkins Hosp. Reports* 7 (1899): 223.
———. "Clinical and Pathological Differential Diagnosis of the Female Breast." *Am. J. Med. Sci.* 135 (1908): 157.
Clark, J. G. "A More Radical Method of Performing Hysterectomy for Cancer of the Uterus." *Johns Hopkins Hosp. Bull.* 6 (1895): 120.
Crowe, S. J. "Recollection of William Stewart Halsted." *Bull. Johns Hopkins Hosp.* 84 (1949): 15.
———. *Halsted of Johns Hopkins: The Man and His Men.* Springfield, Ill.: Charles C Thomas, 1957.
Cullen, T. S. *Cancer of the Uterus.* New York: Appleton, 1900.
Finney, J. M. T. "A Personal Appreciation of Dr. Halsted." *Bull. Johns Hopkins Hosp.* 36 (1925): 28.
Galvin, G. A.; Jones, H. W., Jr.; and TeLinde, R. W. "Clinical Relationship of Carcinoma-in-Situ and Invasive Carcinoma of the Cervix." *J.A.M.A.* 149 (1952): 744.
Haagensen, C. D., and Lloyd, W. E. B. *A Hundred Years of Medicine.* New York: Sheridan House, 1943.
Halsted, W. S. "Intestinal anastomosis." *Bull. Johns Hopkins Hosp.* 2 (1891): 1.
———. "Operation for Carcinoma of the Breast." *Johns Hopkins Hosp. Reports* 2 (1891): 277.
———. "The Results of Operations for the Cure of Cancer of the Breast from June, 1889 to January, 1894." *Johns Hopkins Hosp. Reports* 4 (1895): 297. (Also *Annals of Surgery* 20 [1894]: 497.)
———. "Ligature and Suture Material. The Employment of Fine Silk in Preference to Cat Gut and the Advantages of Transfixation of Tissues and Vessels in Control of Hemorrhage. Also an Account of the Introduction of Gloves, Gutta Percha Tissue and Silver Foil." *J.A.M.A.* 40 (1913): 1119.
———. *Surgical Papers.* 2 vols. Baltimore: The Johns Hopkins University Press, 1924.
Heuer, G. J. "Dr. Halsted." *Bull. Johns Hopkins Hosp.* 90 (1952): 1.
Matas, R. "In Memoriam—William Stewart Halsted. An Appreciation." *Bull. Johns Hopkins Hosp.* 36 (1925): 2.
Park, Roswell. "An Epitome of the History of Carcinoma." *Johns Hopkins Hosp. Bull.* 14 (1903): 289.
Robb, H. *Aseptic Surgical Technique.* Philadelphia: J. B. Lippincott Co., 1894.
TeLinde, R. W., and Galvin, G. A. "The Minimum Histological Changes in Biopsies to Justify a Diagnosis of Cervical Cancer." *Am. J. Obst. Gyn.* 48 (1944): 774.
TeLinde, R. W., and Mattingly, R. F. *Operative Gynecology.* 4th Ed. Philadelphia and Toronto: J. B. Lippincott Co., 1970.
Welch, W. H. "In Memoriam—William Stewart Halsted. Address." *Bull. Johns Hopkins Hosp.* 36 (1925): 34.
Wertheim, E. *"Zur frage der radical operatus bein uterus krebs." Arch. Gynak.* 61 (1900): 627.
Wesson, Miley B. "Hugh Hampton Young." *J. Urol.* 57 (1947): 203.
Young, Hugh H. *A Surgeon's Autobiography.* New York: Harcourt, Brace & Co., 1940.

9. FOUNTAINHEAD OF AMERICAN PHYSIOLOGY:

H. NEWELL MARTIN AND HIS PUPIL WILLIAM HENRY HOWELL

Erlanger, J. "William Henry Howell, 1860–1945." *Biographical Memoirs, National Academy of Sciences* 26 (1951): 153.
Foster, M. "Henry Newell Martin." *Proc. R. Soc.* (Lond.), Series A, 60 (1896–1897): xx.

French, J. C. *A History of the University Founded by Johns Hopkins.* Baltimore: Johns Hopkins University Press, 1946.

Howell, W. H. "Vagus Inhibition of the Heart and Its Relation to the Inorganic Salts of the Blood." *Am. J. Physiol.* 15 (1906): 280.

———. "The Nature and Action of the Thromboplastic [Zymoplastic] Substances of the Tissues." *Am. J. Physiol.* 31 (1912): 1.

———. "The Coagulation of the Blood." *Harvey Lecture Series* 12 (1916): 272.

———. "The Purification of Heparin and its Chemical and Physiological Reactions." *Bull. Johns Hopkins Hosp.* 42 (1928): 119.

———. "Recent Advances in the Problem of Blood Coagulation Applicable to Medicine." *J.A.M.A.* 117 (1941): 1059.

———. "Celebration of the 60th Anniversary of William H. Howell's Graduation from the Johns Hopkins University." *Bull. Johns Hopkins Hosp.* 68 (1941): 291.

Howell, W. H., and Holt, E. "Two New Factors in Blood Coagulation—Heparin and Pro-antithrombin." *Am. J. Physiol.* 47 (1918–1919): 328.

Martin, H. N. "Study and Teaching of Biology. An Introductory Lecture Delivered at The Johns Hopkins University, October 23, 1876." *Popular Sci. Monthly* vol. 10, January 1877.

———. "The Direct Influence of Gradual Variations of Temperature upon the Rate of Beat of the Dog's Heart. (Croonian Lecture)." *Philos. Trans. R. Soc.* (Lond.) 174 (1883): 663.

———. "Modern Physiological Laboratories—What They Are and Why They Are." *Johns Hopkins Univ. Circular* vol. 3 (30), April 1884.

———. *Memoirs from the Biological Laboratory of the Johns Hopkins University. The Physiological Papers by H. Newell Martin.* Vol. 3. Baltimore: Johns Hopkins University Press, 1895.

Martin, H. N., and Sedgwick, W. T. "Observations on the Mean Pressure and the Character of the Pulse Wave in the Coronary Arteries of the Heart. *Studies from the Biological Laboratory of the Johns Hopkins University,* vol. 2, 1882.

McLean, J. "The Thromboplastic Action of Cephalin." *Am. J. Physiol.* 41 (1916): 250.

McLean, J. "The Relation between the Thromboplastic Action of Cephalin and Its Degree of Unsaturation." *Am. J. Physiol.* 43 (1917): 586.

10. A NEW SCHOOL OF ANATOMY: THE STORY OF FRANKLIN P. MALL,
FLORENCE R. SABIN, AND JOHN B. MAC CALLUM

Halsted, W. S. "Circular Suture of the Intestine—An Experimental Study." *Am. J. Med. Sci.* 94 (1887): 436.

———. "An Experimental Study of the Thyroid Gland of Dogs, with Especial Consideration of Hypertrophy of This Gland." *Johns Hopkins Hosp. Reports* 1 (1896): 373.

———. "An End-to-End Anastomosis of the Large Intestine by Abutting Closed Ends and Puncturing the Double Diaphragm with an Instrument Introduced Per Rectum." *Bull. Johns Hopkins Hosp.* 32 (1921): 98.

Heidelberger, M., and McMaster, P. "Florence R. Sabin." In *Biographical Memoirs of the National Academy of Sciences.* New York: Columbia University Press, 34 (1960): 272.

MacCallum, J. B. "On the Histology and Histogenesis of the Heart Muscle Cell." *Anat. Anz.* (Jena), 13 (1897): 609.

———. "On the Pathology of Fragmentatio Myocardii and Myocarditis Fibrosa." *Bull. Johns Hopkins Hosp.* 9 (1898): 208.

———. "On the Histogenesis of the Striated Muscle Fiber and the Growth of the Human Sartorius Muscle." *Bull. Johns Hopkins Hosp.* 9 (1898): 208.

———. "A Contribution to the Knowledge of the Pathology of Fragmentation, Segmentation and Fibrosis of the Myocardium. *J. Exp. Med.* 4 (1899): 409.

———. "On the Muscular Architecture of the Ventricles of the Human Heart." *Am. J. Anat.* 11 (1910): 211.

Mall, F. P. "The Contraction of the Vena Portae and its Influence Upon the Circulation." *Johns Hopkins Hosp. Reports* 1 (1896): 111.

———. "The Architecture and Blood Vessels of the Dog's Spleen." *Z. Morphol. Anthropol.* 2 (1900): 1.

———. "On the Circulation Through the Pulp of the Dog's Spleen." *Am. J. Anat.* 2 (1902–03): 315.

———. "A Study of the Structural Unit of the Liver." *Am. J. Anat.* 5 (1906): 227.

Malloch, Archibald. *Short Years: The Life and Letters of John Bruce MacCallum, 1876–1906.* Chicago: Normandie House, 1938.

Sabin, F. R. "A Model of the Medulla Oblongata, Pores and Midbrain of a Newborn Babe." *Johns Hopkins Hosp. Reports* 9 (1900): 925.

———. "On the Origin of the Lymphatic System from the Veins and the Development of the Lymph Hearts and Thoracic Duct in the Pig." *Am. J. Anat.* 1 (1901): 367.

———. "The Lymphatic System in Human Embryos with a Consideration of the Morphology of the System as a Whole." *Am. J. Anat.* 9 (1909): 43.

———. "The Origin and Development of the Lymphatic System." *Johns Hopkins Hosp. Reports* 17 (1916): 347.

———. "The Method of Growth of the Lymphatic System." *The Harvey Lecture Series* 11 (1915–16): 124.

———. "On the Origin of the Cells of the Blood." *Physiol. Rev.* 2 (1922): 38.

———. "Studies of Living Human Blood Cells." *Johns Hopkins Hosp. Bull.* 34 (1923): 277.

———. *Franklin Paine Mall, The Story of a Mind.* Baltimore: Johns Hopkins University Press, 1934.

II. JOHNS HOPKINS—THE BIRTHPLACE OF TISSUE CULTURE:

THE STORY OF ROSS G. HARRISON, WARREN H. LEWIS, AND GEORGE O. GEY

Carver, G. W. "Warren H. Lewis." In *Biographical Memoirs of the National Academy of Sciences.* New York: Columbia University Press, 39 (1967): 323.

Gey, G. O. "An Improved Technic for Massive Tissue Culture." *Am. J. Cancer* 17 (1933): 752.

———. "Some Aspects of the Constitution and Behavior of Normal and Malignant Cells in Continuous Culture." The Harvey Lectures, Series L, 1954–1955. New York: Academic Press, 1955.

———. "Cellular Responses to Viruses in Relation to Cancer." *Proceedings of the 3rd National Cancer Conference, 1957,* p. 453.

Gey, G. O., and Bang, F. B. "Cell Structure—A Comparative Study of the Cytological Characteristics of Normal and Malignant Cells with Phase and Electron Microscopy." *Anat. Rec.* 33 (1952): 98.

Gey, G. O.; Coffman, W. D.; Kubicek, M. T. "Tissue Culture Studies of the Proliferative Capacity of Cervical Carcinoma and Normal Epithelium." *Cancer Res.* 12 (1952): 264.

Gey, G. O., and Gey. M. K. "The Maintenance of Human Normal Cells and Tumor Cells in Continuous Culture." I. Preliminary Report: Cultivation of Mesoblastic Tumors and Normal Tissue and Notes on Methods of Cultivation." *Am. J. Cancer* 27 (1936): 45.

Gey, G. O.; Seegar, G. E.; and Hellman, L. M. "The Production of a Gonadotrophic Substance [Prolan] by Placental Cells in Tissue Culture." *Science* 88 (1938): 306.

Gey, G. O.; Svotelis, M.; Foard, M.; and Bang, F. B. "Long-Term Growth of Chicken Fibroblasts on a Collagen Substrate." *Exp. Cell. Res.* 84 (1974): 63.

Harrison, R. G. "Observations on the Living Developing Nerve Fiber." *Proc. Soc. Exp. Biol. Med.* 4 (1907): 140.

Harrison, R. G. "Regeneration of Peripheral Nerves." *Anat. Rec.* 1 (1908): 209.

———. "Embryonic Transplantation and Development of the Nervous System." *Anat. Rec.* 2 (1908): 385.

———. "The Outgrowth of the Nerve Fiber in a Mode of Protoplasmic Movement." *J. Exp. Zool.* 9 (1910): 787.

———. "The Cultivation of Tissues in Extraneous Media as a Method of Morphologic Study." *Anat. Rec.* 6 (1912): 181.

Harvey, A. McG. "Early Contributions to the Surgery of Cancer: William S. Halsted, Hugh H. Young and John G. Clark." *Johns Hopkins Med. J.* 135 (1974): 399.

Jones, H. W., Jr.; McKusick, V. A.; Harper, P. S.; and Wuu, K. D. "The HeLa Cell and a Reappraisal of Its Origin." *Obstet. Gynecol.* 38 (1971): 945.

Lewis, M. R., and Lewis, W. H. "The Cultivation of Tissue from Chick Embryos in Solutions of NaCl, CaCl$_2$, KCl, and NaHCO$_3$." *Anat. Rec.* 5 (1911): 277.

Lewis, M. R., and Lewis, W. H. "Mitochondria in Tissue Culture." *Science* 39 (1914): 330.

Lewis, W. H. "Pinocytosis." *Bull. Johns Hopkins Hosp.* 49 (1931): 17.

Lewis, W. H. "Locomotion of Lymphocytes." *Bull. Johns Hopkins Hosp.* 49 (1931): 29.

Lewis, W. H., and Gey, G. O. "Clasmatocytes and Tumor Cells in Cultures of Mouse Sarcoma." *Johns Hopkins Hosp. Bull.* 34 (1923): 369.

Lewis, W. H., and Lewis, M. R. "The Cultivation of Chick Tissues in Media of Known Chemical Constitution." *Anat. Rec.* 6 (1912): 207.

Nicholas, J. S. "Ross G. Harrison." In *Biographical Memoirs of the National Academy of Sciences.* New York: Columbia University Press, 35 (1961): 132.

Pattello, R. A., and Gey, G. O. "The Establishment of a Cell Line of Human Hormone-Synthesizing Trophoblastic Cells *in Vitro.*" *Cancer Res.* 28 (1968): 1231.

Russell, K. "Tissue Culture, a Brief Historical Review." *Clio. Med.* 4 (1969): 109.

Scherer, W. F.; Syverton, J. T.; and Gey, G. O. "Studies on the Propagation in Vitro of Poliomyelitis Viruses. IV. Viral Multiplication in a Stable Strain of Human Malignant Cells [Strain HeLa] Derived from an Epidermoid Carcinoma of the Cervix. *J. Exp. Med.* 97 (1953): 695.

12. CREATORS OF CLINICAL MEDICINE'S SCIENTIFIC BASE:
FRANKLIN PAINE MALL, LEWELLYS FRANKLIN BARKER, AND RUFUS COLE

Austrian, C. R. "Lewellys Franklin Barker." *Bull. Johns Hopkins Hosp.* 73 (1943): 401.

Barker, L. F. "The Laboratories of the Medical Clinic." *Johns Hopkins Hosp. Bull.* 18 (1907): 193.

———. "On Some of the Methods of Investigating Cardiovascular Conditions. The Jerome Cochran Lecture, Alabama State Medical Association, 1909." *Johns Hopkins Hosp. Bull.* 20 (1909): 297.

Barker, L. F.; Hirschfelder, A. D.; and Bond, G. S. "The Electrocardiogram in Clinical Diagnosis." *J.A.M.A.* 55 (1910): 1350.

"Carl Voegtlin, 1879–1960, First Director of Cancer Research of the Public Health Service and first chief of the National Cancer Institute." *J. Natl. Cancer Inst.* 25 (4) (1960): iii.

Chesney, A. M. *The Johns Hopkins Hospital and The Johns Hopkins University School of Medicine.* Vol. 3. Baltimore: The Johns Hopkins University Press, 1963.

Cole, R. "Lewellys Franklin Barker, 1867–1943." *Trans. Assoc. Am. Physicians* 58 (1944): 13.

Corner, G. *A History of the Rockefeller Institute (1901–1953).* New York: Rockefeller Institute Press, 1964.

Harvey, A. McG. "Medical Students on the March: Brown, MacCallum and Opie." *Johns Hopkins Med. J.* 134 (1974): 330.

Hirschfelder, A. D. "Some Observations upon Blood Pressure and Pulse Form." *Johns Hopkins Hosp. Bull.* 18 (1907): 262.

———. "Some Variations in the Form of the Venous Pulse." *Johns Hopkins Hosp. Bull.* 18 (1907): 265.

———. "The Rapid Formation of Endocarditic 'Vegetation.'" *Johns Hopkins Hosp. Bull.* 18 (1907): 267.

———. *Diseases of the Heart and Aorta.* 2nd ed. Philadelphia: J. B. Lippincott, 1913.

Kohlstaedt, K. Personal communication.

Sabin, F. R. *Franklin Paine Mall, The Story of a Mind.* Baltimore: The Johns Hopkins University Press, 1934.

Tillett, W. S. "Rufus Cole." *Trans. Assoc. Am. Physicians* 80 (1967): 9.

13. COMPLEAT CLINICIAN AND RENAISSANCE PATHOLOGIST:
LOUIS HAMMAN AND ARNOLD R. RICH

Cole, G. A.; Gilden, D. H.; Monjan, A. A.; and Nathanson, N. "Lymphocytic Choriomeningitis Virus: Pathogenesis of Acute Central Nervous System Disease." *Fed. Proc.* 30 (1971): 1831.

Dixon, F. J. "The Role of Antigen-Antibody Complexes in Disease." *Harvey Lecture Series* 58 (1963): 21.

Germuth, F. G., Jr., and McKinnon, G. E. "Studies on the Biological Properties of Antigen-Antibody Complexes: I. Anaphylactic Shock Induced by Soluble Complexes in Unsensitized Normal Guinea Pigs." *Bull. Johns Hopkins Hosp.* 101 (1957): 13.

Harvey, J. C. "The Writings of Louis Hamman." *Bull. Johns Hopkins Hosp.* 95 (1954): 178. (Contains the complete bibliography of Dr. Hamman.)

Holt, E. L., Jr. "Presentation of the George M. Kober Medal to Arnold Rice Rich." *Trans. Assoc. Am. Physicians* 71 (1958): 40.

Rich, A. R. "The Pathogenesis of the Forms of Jaundice." *Bull. Johns Hopkins Hosp.* 37 (1930): 338.

———. "The Pathology of Nineteen Cases of a Peculiar and Specific Form of Nephritis Associated with Acquired Syphilis." *Bull. Johns Hopkins Hosp.* 50 (1932): 357.

———. "The Role of Hypersensitivity in Periarteritis Nodosa as Indicated by Seven Cases Developing During Serum Sickness and Sulfonamide Therapy." *Bull. Johns Hopkins Hosp.* 71 (1942): 123.

———. "Additional Evidence of the Role of Hypersensitivity in the Etiology of Periarteritis Nodosa. Another Case Associated with a Sulfonamide Reaction." *Bull. Johns Hopkins Hosp.* 71 (1942): 375.

———. "A Peculiar Type of Adrenal Cortical Damage Associated with Acute Infections, and Its Possible Relation to Circulatory Collapse." *Bull. Johns Hopkins Hosp.* 74 (1944): 1.

———. "The Gordon Wilson Lecture. Visceral Hazards of Hypersensitivity to Drugs." *Trans. Am. Clin. Climat. Assoc.* 72 (1960): 46.

Rich, A. R., and McCordock, H. A. "The Pathogenesis of Tuberculous Meningitis." *Bull. Johns Hopkins Hosp.* 52 (1933): 5.

Rich, A. R., and Gregory, E. "The Experimental Demonstration That Periarteritis is a Manifestation of Hypersensitivity." *Bull. Johns Hopkins Hosp.* 72 (1943): 65.

Romano, J. "On Those From Whom We Learn." *Calif. Med.* 117 (1972): 72.

Rowe, W. T. "Protective Effect of Pre-irradiation on Infection in Mice." *Proc. Soc. Exp. Biol. Med.*, 92 (1956): 194.

Wainwright, C. W. "Dr. Hamman as I Knew Him." *Bull. Johns Hopkins Hosp.* 96 (1955): 29.

14. CLASSICAL DESCRIPTIONS OF DISEASE

Bernstein, A. "Antibody Responses in Infectious Mononucleosis." *J. Clin. Invest.* 13 (1934): 419.

Bernstein, A. "Infectious Mononucleosis." *Medicine* 19 (1940): 85.

Cushing, H. *The Life of Sir William Osler.* London: Clarendon Press, 1925.

Dewhurst, K. *Dr. Thomas Sydenham (1624–1689). His Life and Original Writings.* London: Wellcome Historical Medical Library, 1966.

Felty, A. R. "Chronic Arthritis in the Adult, Associated with Splenomegaly and Leukopenia." *Bull. Johns Hopkins Hosp.* 35 (1973): 122.

Harvey, A. McG. "Our Medical Heritage: Some Examples of Creative Scholarship." *Pharos* 36 (1973): 122.

Ireland, R. A.; Baetjer, W.; and Rührah, J. "A Case of Lymphatic Leukemia with Apparent Cure." *J.A.M.A.* 65 (1915): 948.

Keefer, C. S. "Report of a Case of Malta Fever Originating in Baltimore, Maryland." *Bull. Johns Hopkins Hosp.* 35 (1924): 6.

Longcope, W. T. "Infectious Mononucleosis [Glandular Form], with a Report of 10 Cases." *Am. J. Med. Sci.* 164 (1922): 781.

———. "The Generalized Form of Boeck's Sarcoid." *Trans. Assoc. Am. Physicians* 51 (1936): 94.

———. "Bronchopneumonia of Unknown Etiology [Variety X]. A Report of 32 Cases with Two Deaths." *Bull. Johns Hopkins Hosp.* 67 (1940): 268.

———. "Acceptance of the Kober Medal Award." *Trans. Assoc. Am. Physicians* 61 (1948): 25.

Longcope, W. T., and Freiman, D. G. "A Study of Sarcoidosis Based on a Combined Investigation of 160 Cases Including 30 Autopsies from the Johns Hopkins Hospital and the Massachusetts General Hospital." *Medicine* 31 (1952): 1.

Longcope, W. T., and Pierson, J. W. "Boeck's Sarcoid [sarcoidosis]." *Bull. Johns Hopkins Hosp.* 60 (1937): 223.

Longcope, W. T., and Winkenwerder, W. L. "Clinical Features of the Contracted Kidney Due to Pyelonephritis." *Bull. Johns Hopkins Hosp.* 53 (1933): 255.

MacLachlan, W. W. G. "Frank Alexander Evans (1889–1956)." *Trans. Assoc. Am. Physicians* 70 (1957): 13.

Osler, W. "The Chronic Intermittent Fever of Endocarditis." *Practitioner* (Lond.) 1 (1893): 181.

———. "Six Cases of Addison's Disease, with the Report of a Case Greatly Benefited by the Use of Suprarenal Extract." *Intern. Med. Magazine* 5 (1896): 3.

———. "On a Family Form of Recurring Epistaxis, Associated with Multiple Telangiectasis of the Skin and Mucous Membranes." *Johns Hopkins Hosp. Bull.* 12 (1901): 333.

———. "On the Educational Value of the Medical Society." *Boston Med. Surg. J.* 148 (1903): 275.

———. "Chronic Cyanosis with Polycythemia and Enlarged Spleen; A New Clinical Entity." *Am. J. Med. Sci.* 126 (1903): 187. (Also *Trans. Assoc. Am. Physicians* 18 (1903): 299).

———. "Chronic Cyanotic Polycythemia with Enlarged Spleen." *Br. Med. J.* 1 (1904): 121.

———. "Chronic Infectious Endocarditis." *Q. J. Med.* 2 (1908–1909): 219.

———. "Chronic Infectious Endocarditis, with an Early History Like Splenic Anemia." *Interstate Med. J.* 19 (1912): 103.

Sabin, F. R. "Studies of Living Human Blood-Cells." *Johns Hopkins Hosp. Bull.* 34 (1923): 277.

Sprunt, T. P., and Evans, F. A. "Mononuclear Leucocytosis in Reaction to Acute Infections ["Infectious Mononucleosis"]. *Johns Hopkins Hosp. Bull.* 31 (1920): 410.

Vaquez, H., and Quiserne: "De la polyglobulic progressive comme signe prognotic dans les cyanosis congenitales." *C.R. Soc. Biol.* 54 (1902): 915.

Wainwright, C. W. "Chester Scott Keefer, M.D." *Trans. Am. Clin. Climat. Assoc.* 84 (1972): xxxiii.

———. Personal communication.

Wilkins, R. W. "Chester Scott Keefer (1897–1972)." *Trans. Assoc. Am. Physicians* 85 (1972): 24.

Wintrobe, M. "Osler's Chronic Cyanotic Polycythemia with Splenomegaly." *Bull. Johns Hopkins Hosp.* 85 (1949): 75.

15. THE SECOND PROFESSOR OF GYNECOLOGY AND THE DEPARTMENT
OF ART AS APPLIED TO MEDICINE

Broedel, M. "The Origin, Growth and Future of Medical Illustration at The Johns Hopkins Hospital and Medical School. *Johns Hopkins Hosp. Bull.* 26 (1915): 185.

———. "Medical Illustration." *J.A.M.A.* 117 (1941): 668.

Cullen, T. S. "A Rapid Method of Making Permanent Specimens from Frozen Sections by the Use of Formalin." *Johns Hopkins Hosp. Bull.* 6 (1895): 67.

———. "Adenomyoma of the Round Ligament." *Johns Hopkins Hosp. Bull.* 7 (1896): 112.

———. *Adenomyoma of the Uterus.* Philadelphia: W. B. Saunders, 1908.

———. *Embryology, Anatomy, and Diseases of the Umbilicus Together with Diseases of the Urachus.* Philadelphia: W. B. Saunders, 1916.

———. "Bluish Discoloration of the Umbilicus as a Diagnostic Sign Where Ruptured Extrauterine Pregnancy Exists." In *Contributions to Medical and Biological Research,* Dedicated to Sir William Osler in Honor of his 70th Birthday, July 12, 1919, by His Pupils and Coworkers, p. 420. New York: P. B. Hoeber, 1919.

———. "Max Broedel, 1870–1941. Director of the First Department of Art as Applied to Medicine." *Bull. Med. Libr. Assoc.* 33 (1945): 5.

———. "John Albertson Sampson, 1873–1946." *Trans. Am. Gynecol. Soc.* 70 (1947): 273.

Ridley, J. H., and Edwards, J. K. "Experimental Endometriosis in the Human." *Am. J. Obstet. Gynecol.* 76 (1959): 783.

Robison, J. *Tom Cullen of Baltimore.* London: Oxford University Press, 1949.

Russell, W. W. "Aberrant Portions of the Müllerian Duct Found in an Ovary." *Johns Hopkins Hosp. Bull.* 10 (1899): 8.

Sampson, J. A. "Perforating Hemorrhagic [chocolate] Cysts of the Ovary. Their Importance and Especially Their Relation to Pelvic Adenomas of Endometrial Type ['Adenomyoma of the Uterus, Rectovaginal Septum, Sigmoid, etc.]." *Arch. Surg.* 3 (1921): 245.

Sampson, J. A. "The Development of the Implantation Theory for the Origin of Peritoneal Endometriosis." *Am. J. Obstet. Gynecol.* 40 (1940): 549.

Scott, R. B.; TeLinde, R. W.; and Wharton, L. R., Jr. "Further Studies on Experimental Endometriosis. *Am. J. Obstet. Gynecol.* 66 (1953): 1082.

TeLinde, R. W., and Scott, R. B. "Experimental Endometriosis." *Am. J. Obstet. Gynecol.* 60 (1950): 1147.

16. JOHN WHITRIDGE WILLIAMS—HIS CONTRIBUTIONS TO OBSTETRICS

Berkeley, C. "In Memoriam, John Whitridge Williams, 1866–1931." *J. Obstet. Gynaecol. Br. Commonw.* 39 (1932): 7.

Eastman, N. J. "The Contributions of John Whitridge Williams to Obstetrics. Presidential Address." *Am. J. Obstet. Gynecol.* 87 (1964): 1.

Guttmacher, A. F. "Reminiscences of John Whitridge Williams." *Johns Hopkins Alumni Mag.* 23 (1935): 233.

Kelly, H. A. "John Whitridge Williams (1866–1931)." *Am. J. Surg.* 15 (1932): 169.

Stander, H. J. "In Memoriam, Dr. John Whitridge Williams, 1866–1931." *Am. J. Obstet. Gynecol.* 22 (1931): 661.

Williams, J. W. "Deciduoma Malignum." *Johns Hopkins Hosp. Reports* 51 (1895): 461.

———. "Frequency of Contracted Pelvis in the First One Thousand Women Delivered in the Obstetrical Department of The Johns Hopkins Hospital." *Obstetrics* 1 (1899): 5, 6.

———. "A Case of Spondylolisthesis, with Description of the Pelvis." *Am. J. Obstet. Gynecol.* 41 (1899): 145.

———. "The Frequency and Significance of Infarcts of the Placenta." *Am. J. Obstet. Gynecol.* 41 (1900): 775.

———. "Subperitoneal Hematoma following Labor, Not Associated with Lesions of the Uterus." *Trans. Am. Gynecol. Soc.* 29 (1904): 186.

———. "The Clinical Significance of Glycosuria in Pregnant Women." *Am. J. Med. Sci.* 137 (1909): 1.

———. "Frequency of Aetiology and Practical Significance of Contraction of the Pelvic Outlet." *Surg. Gynecol. Obstet.* 8 (1909): 619.

———. "The Funnel Pelvis." *Am. J. Obstet. Gynecol.* 64 (1911): 106.

———. "The Limitations and Possibilities of Prenatal Care." *J.A.M.A.* 64 (1915): 96.

———. "Premature Separation of the Normally Implanted Placenta." *Surg. Gynecol. Obstet.* 21 (1915): 541.

———. "A Critical Analysis of 21 Years Experience with Caesarean Section." *Johns Hopkins Hosp. Bull.* 32 (1921): 173.

———. "The Problems of Effecting Sterilization in Association with Various Obstetrical Procedures." *Am. J. Obstet. Gynecol.* 1 (1921): 783.

———. "Spontaneous Labor Occurring Through an Obliquely Contracted, Kyphotic, Funnel Pelvis." *Johns Hopkins Hosp. Bull.* 33 (1922): 190.

———. "Note on Placentation in Quadruplet and Triplet Pregnancy." *Bull. Johns Hopkins Hosp.* 39 (1926): 271.

———. "Placenta Circumvalleta." *Am. J. Obstet. Gynecol.* 13 (1927): 1.

———. "Indications for Therapeutic Sterilization in Obstetrics." *J.A.M.A.* 91 (1928): 1237.

———. "A Clinical and Anatomical Description of the Naegale Pelvis." *Am. J. Obstet. Gynecol.* 18 (1929): 504.

Williams, J. W., and Sun, K. "A Statistical Study of the Incidence and Treatment of Labor Complicated by Contracted Pelvis in the Obstetric Service of The Johns Hopkins Hospital from 1896 to 1924." *Am. J. Obstet. Gynecol.* 11 (1926): 735.

17. THE FIRST FULL-TIME ACADEMIC DEPARTMENT OF PEDIATRICS:
THE STORY OF THE HARRIET LANE HOME

Asper, S. P., Jr. "Lawson Wilkins (1894–1963)." *Trans. Assoc. Am. Physicians* 76 (1964): 33.

Blackfan, K. D., and Maxcy, K. F. "Intraperitoneal Injection of Saline Solution." *Am. J. Dis. Child.* 15 (1918): 19.

Bongiovanni, A. M. "Introduction of Lawson Wilkins for the John Howland Award." *J. Pediatr.* 63 (1963): 803.

Bongiovanni, A. M. "Lawson Wilkins: Memorial (1894–1963)." *J. Clin. Endocrinol. Metab.* 24 (1964): 1.

Butler, A. M. "Presentation of the John Howland Medal and Award of the American Pediatric Society to Dr. James L. Gamble." *Am. J. Dis. Child.* 90 (1955): 483.

———. "James Lawder Gamble (1883–1959)." *Trans. Assoc. Am. Physicians* 73 (1960): 13.

Chesney, A. M. *The Johns Hopkins Hospital and The Johns Hopkins University School of Medicine.* Vols. 1 and 2. Baltimore: The Johns Hopkins University Press, 1943, 1958.

Davidson, W. C. "Pediatric Profiles, John Howland (1873–1926)." *J. Pediatr.* 46 (1955): 473.

Diamond, L. K. "Reflections on Pediatric Care." *Pharos* 37 (1974): 5.

Faber, H. K., and McIntosh, R. *History of the American Pediatric Society, 1887–1965.* New York: Blakeston Division, McGraw Hill Book Co., 1966.

Gamble, J. L. "The Metabolism of Fixed Base During Fasting." *J. Biol. Chem.* 57 (1923): 633.

———. "Presentation of the Kober Medal to Dr. Edwards A. Park." *Trans. Assoc. Am. Physicians* 63 (1950): 21.

———. "Acceptance of the Kober Medal Award." *Trans. Assoc. Am. Physicians* 64 (1951): 36.

————. "The Early History of Fluid Replacement Therapy." *Pediatrics* 11 (1953): 554.

Gamble, J. L.; Ross, S. G.; and Tisdall, F. F. "A Study of Acidosis Due to Kitone Acids." *Trans. Am. Pediatr. Soc.* 34 (1922): 289.

Grob, D. Personal communication.

Harrison, H. Personal communication.

Harrison, H. E., Edwards, A. Park. "An Appreciation of the Man." *Johns Hopkins Med. J.* 132 (1973): 361.

Howard, J. E. "Edwards A. Park (1877–1969)." *Trans. Assoc. Am. Physicians* 83 (1970): 28.

Howland, J., and Marriott, W. McK. "A Study of the Acidosis Occurring in the Nutritional Diseases of Infancy." *Trans. Assoc. Am. Physicians* 30 (1915): 330.

————. "Acidosis Occurring with Diarrhea." *Am. J. Dis. Child.* 11 (1916): 309.

————. "A Discussion of Acidosis with Special Reference to That Occurring in Diseases of Children." *Johns Hopkins Hosp. Bull.* 27 (1916): 63.

————. "Observations upon the Calcium Content of the Blood in Infantile Tetany and upon the Effect of Treatment by Calcium." *Q. J. Med.* 11 (1918): 289.

Howland, J., and Kramer, B. "Calcium and Phosphorus in the Serum in Relation to Rickets." *Am. J. Dis. Child.* 22 (1921): 105.

Howland, J., and Kramer, B. "Factors Concerned in the Calcification of Bone." *Trans. Am. Pediatr. Soc.* 34 (1922): 204.

Jospehs, H. Personal communication.

————. "Clinical Aspects of Sickle Cell Anemia." *Johns Hopkins Hosp. Bull.* 43 (1928): 397.

————. "Treatment of Anemia of Infancy with Iron and Copper. *Johns Hopkins Hosp. Bull.* 49 (1931): 246.

Kramer, B., and Howland, J. "Factors Which Determine the Concentration of Calcium and of Inorganic Phosphorus in the Blood Serum of Rats." *Johns Hopkins Hosp. Bull.* 33 (1922): 313.

Loeb, R. F. "Presentation of the Kober Medal to James L. Gamble." *Trans. Assoc. Am. Physicians* 64 (1951): 29.

Marriott, W. McK. "Some Phases of Pathology of Nutrition in Infancy." *Harvey Lecture Series* 15 (1919–20): 121.

Marriott, W. McK., and Howland J. "A Micro Method for the Determination of Calcium and Magnesium in Blood Serum." *J. Biol. Chem.* 32 (1917): 233.

Martzloff, K. H. "Thomas Stephen Cullen. Presidential Address." *Am. J. Obstet. Gynecol.* 80 (1960): 833.

McCollum, E. V.; Simmonds, N.; Parsons, H. T.; Shipley, P. G.; and Park, E. A. "Studies on Experimental Rickets. I. The Production of Rachitis and Similar Diseases in the Rat by Deficient Diets." *J. Biol. Chem.* 45 (1921): 333.

McCollum, E. V.; Simmonds, N.; Shipley, P. G.; and Park, E. A. "Studies on Experimental Rickets. IV. Cod Liver Oil as Contrasted with Butter Fat in the Protection against the Effects of Insufficient Calcium in the Diet." *Proc. Soc. Exp. Biol. Med.* 18 (1921): 275.

————. "Studies on Experimental Rickets. VIII. The Production of Rickets by Diets Low in Phosphorus and Fat-Soluble A." *J. Biol. Chem.* 47 (1921): 507.

————. "Studies on Experimental Rickets. VIII. The Production of Rickets by Diets Low in ficient in Calcium." *Am. J. Hygiene* 1 (1921): 492.

————. "Studies on Experimental Rickets. XII. Is There a Substance Other Than Fat-Soluble A Associated with Certain Fats Which Plays an Important Role in Bone Development?" *J. Biol. Chem.* 50 (1922): 5.

————. "Studies on Experimental Rickets. XVL. A Delicate Biological Test for Calcium-Depositing Substances." *J. Biol. Chem.* 51 (1922): 41.

————. "Studies on Experimental Rickets. XV. The Effect of Starvation on the Healing of Rickets." *Johns Hopkins Hosp. Bull.* 33 (1922): 31.

————. "Studies on Experimental Rickets. XXII. Conditions Which Must be Fulfilled in Preparing Animals for Testing the Anti-rachitic Effect of Individual Foodstuffs." *Johns Hopkins Hosp. Bull.* 33 (1922): 296.

McIntosh, R. "Reminiscences of the Harriet Lane Home Outpatient Department." *Johns Hopkins Med. J.* 132 (1973): 367.

Migeon, C. Personal communication.

Money, J. "Preface." In *The Diagnosis and Treatment of Endocrine Disorders in Childhood and Adolescence.* 3rd ed. Ed. by L. Wilkins. Springfield, Ill.: Charles C Thomas Co., 1965.

Park, E. A. "John Howland." *Science* 64 (1926): 80.

————. "Kenneth D. Blackfan (1883–1941)." *Trans. Assoc. Am. Physicians* 57 (1942): 7.

————. "Acceptance of the Kober Medal Award." *Trans. Assoc. Am. Physicians* 63 (1950): 26.

————. "Lawson Wilkins." *J. Pediatr.* 57 (1960): 317.

Powers, G. F.; Park, E. A.; Shipley, P. G.; McCollum, E. V.; and Simmonds, N. "The Prevention of Rickets in the Rat by Means of Radiation with the Mercury Vapor Quartz Lamp." *Proc. Soc. Exp. Biol. Med.* 19 (1921): 120.

Powers, G. F.; Park, E. A.; Shipley, P. G.; McCollum, E. V.; and Simmonds, N. "Studies on Experimental Rickets. XIX. The Prevention of Rickets in the Rat by Means of Radiation with the Mercury Vapor Quartz Lamp." *Johns Hopkins Hosp. Bull.* 33 (1922): 125.

Ross, S. G., and Josephs, H. "Observations on the Metabolism of Recurrent Vomiting." *Am. J. Dis. Child.* 28 (1924): 447.

Rowntree, L. G.; Marriott, W. McK.; and Levy, R. L. "A Simple Method for Determining Variation in Hydrogen-Ion Concentration of the Blood." *Trans. Assoc. Am. Physicians* 30 (1915): 227.

Schaffer, A. J. "Lawson Wilkins, 1894–1963." *Pediatrics* 33 (1964): 1.

Shipley, P. G.; Park, E. A.; McCollum, E. V.; Simmonds, N.; and Parsons, H. T. "Studies on Experimental Rickets. II. The Effect of Cod Liver Oil Administered to Rats with Experimental Rickets." *J. Biol. Chem.* 45 (1921): 343.

————. "Studies on Experimental Rickets. III. A Pathological Condition Bearing Fundamental Resemblances to Rickets of the Human Being Resulting from Diets Low in Phosphorus and Fat-Soluble A: The Phosphate Ion in Its Prevention." *Johns Hopkins Hosp. Bull.* 32 (1921): 160.

————. "Studies on Experimental Rickets. V. The Production of Rickets by Means of a Diet Faulty in Only Two Respects." *Proc. Soc. Exp. Biol. Med.* 18 (1921): 277.

Taussig, H. B. "Dr. Edwards A. Park: Physician, Teacher, Investigator, Friend." *Johns Hopkins Med. J.* 132 (1973): 370.

Veeder, B. "Pediatric Profiles: William McKim Marriott (1885–1936)." *J. Pediatr.* 47 (1955): 791.

Wilkins, L. "Modern Materia Medica." *Am. J. Dis. Child.* 104 (1962): 449.

18. JOHNS HOPKINS—ITS ROLE IN MEDICAL EDUCATION FOR WOMEN

Anderson, W. A., Ed. Chapter 31, "Hematopoietic System: Reticulo Endothelium, Spleen, Lymph Nodes, Blood and Bone Marrow, p. 1344. In John B. Miale, *Pathology*. St. Louis: C. V. Mosby Company, 1971.

Archibald, R. B., and Frenster, J. H. "Quantitative Ultrastructural Analysis of In Vivo Lymphocyte Reed-Sternberg Cell Interaction in Hodgkin's Disease." *Natl. Cancer Inst. Monogr.* 36 (1973): 239.

Austin, M. "Early Period. History of Women in Medicine—A Symposium." *Bull. Med. Libr. Assoc.* 44 (1956): 12.

Avery, M. E. Personal communication.

————. "The Alveolar Lining Area. A Review of Studies on Its Role in Pulmonary Mechanisms and in the Pathogenesis of Atelectasis." *Pediatrics* 30 (1962): 324.

————. "The Pulmonary Surfactant in Foetal and Neonatal Lungs." In *Bancroft Symposium*. Cambridge: Cambridge University Press, 1973.

Avery, M. E., and Mead, J. "Surface Properties in Relation to Atelectasis and Hyaline Membrane Disease." *Am. J. Dis. Child.* 97 (1959): 517.

Avery, M. E., and Said, S. "Surface Phenomena in Lungs in Health and Disease." *Medicine* 44 (1965): 503.

Belpomme, D.; Joseph, R.; Lavaros, L.; et al. "T-lymphocytes and Reed-Sternberg Cells in Spleen of Hodgkin's Disease." *Lancet* 291 (1974): 1417.

Blalock, A., and Taussig, H. B. "The Surgical Treatment of Malformations of the Heart in Which There is Pulmonary Stenosis or Atresia." *J.A.M.A.* 128 (1945): 189.

Chesney, A. M. *The Johns Hopkins Hospital and the Johns Hopkins University School of Medicine—A Chronicle.* Vol. 1. Baltimore: Johns Hopkins University Press, 1943.

Corea, G. "Lost Women: Dorothy Reed Mendenhall: Childbirth Is Not a Disease." *Ms.* 2 (1974): 98.

DeLemos, R. A.; Shermeta, D. W.; Knelson, J. H.; Kotas, R.; and Avery, M. E. "Acceleration of Appearance of Pulmonary Surfactant in the Fetal Lamb by Administration of Corticosteroids." *Am. Rev. Resp. Dis.* 102 (1970): 459.

Epstein, M. A.; Achong, B. G.; and Barr, Y. M. "Virus Particles in Cultured Lymphoblasts from Burkitt's Lymphoma." *Lancet* 1 (1964): 702.

Froslid, C. K. "Helen Taussig." *Science Year*, p. 389. Chicago: The World Book Science Annals, Field Enterprises, Educational Corp., 1967.

Garrison, F. H. *An Introduction to the History of Medicine*, 4th ed. Philadelphia: W. B. Saunders, 1929, p. 769.

Greenfield, W. S. "Specimens Illustrative of Pathology of Lymphadenoma and Leucocythemia." *Trans. R. Path. Soc.* (Lond.), 29 (1878): 272.

Henle, A.; Henle, W.; and Diehl, V. "Relation of Burkitt's Tumor Associated Herpes-Type Virus to Infectious Mononucleosis." *Proc. Nat. Acad. Sci.* 59 (1968): 94.

Jackson, H., Jr., and Parker, F., Jr. *Hodgkin's Disease and Allied Disorders*. New York: Oxford University Press, 1947.

Kaplan, H. S. *Hodgkin's Disease*. Cambridge, Mass.: Harvard University Press, 1972.

Leech, J. "Immunoglobulin Positive Reed-Sternberg Cells in Hodgkin's Disease." *Lancet* 1 (1973) 265.

Lukes, R. J; Trindle, B. H.; and Parker, J. W. "Reed-Sternberg-Like Cells in Infectious Mononucleosis." *Lancet* 2 (1969): 1003.

Luy, M. L. M. "Neonatal care—an investment for life [An Interview with Mary Ellen Avery]." *Modern Medicine* April 15, 1974, p. 14.

McGrew, E. "The Present. History of Women in Medicine—A Symposium." *Bull. Med. Libr. Assoc.* 44 (1956): 23.

Order, S. E., and Helman, S. "Pathogenesis of Hodgkin's Disease." *Lancet* 1 (1972): 571.

Ravitch, M. M., ed. *The Papers of Alfred Blalock*, p. xxxvi. 2 vols. Baltimore: Johns Hopkins University Press, 1966.

Reed, D. M. "On the Pathological Changes in Hodgkin's Disease with Special Reference to Its Relation to Tuberculosis." *Johns Hopkins Hosp. Reports* 10 (1902): 133.

Sternberg, C. "Über eine Eigenartige unter dem Bilde der Pseudoleukamie verlaufende tuberculose des lymphatischen Apparatus." *Zeitschrift F. Heilk.* 19 (1898): 21.

Taussig, H. Personal communication.

———. "Phocomelia and Thalidomide." *Am. J. Obstet. Gynecol.* 84 (1962): 979.

———. "A Lady's Hand Guides Fight on Heart Disease." *Business Week*, November 20, 1965, p. 130.

———. "History of the Blalock-Taussig Operation and Some of the Long Term Results on Patients with a Tetralogy of Fallot [The First James Bordley III Lecture]." Occasional Papers, Mary Imogene Bassett Hospital, Cooperstown, New York. Feb. 27, 1970.

———. "Medicine's Living History. Dr. Taussig Remembers the First Blue Baby Operation." *Medical World News*, January 28, 1972, p. 38.

Taylor, C. R. "The Nature of Reed-Sternberg Cells and Other Malignant 'Reticulum' Cells." *Lancet* 2 (1974): 802.

Thomas, C. B. Personal communication.

———. "The Prophylactic Treatment of Rheumatic Fever by Sulfanilamide." *Bull. N.Y. Acad. Sci.* 18 (1942): 508.

Thomas, C. B., and France, R. "A Preliminary Report of the Prophylactic Use of Sulfanilamide in Patients Susceptible to Rheumatic Fever." *Johns Hopkins Hosp. Bull.* 64 (1939): 67.

Wiernik, P. H. "Hodgkin's Disease in 1974." *Johns Hopkins Med. J.* 135 (1974): 25.

Wilson, E. *Upstate: Records and Recollections of Northern New York*. New York: Farrar, Strauss and Geroux, 1971.

Wright, D. H. "Reed-Sternberg-like Cells in Recurrent Burkitt Lymphomas." *Lancet* 1 (1970): 1052.

Wright, K. "19th Century or Transition Period. History of Women in Medicine—A Symposium." *Bull. Med. Libr. Assoc.* 44 (1956): 16.

19. CONTRIBUTIONS OF THE PART-TIME STAFF OF THE JOHNS HOPKINS HOSPITAL: MOORE, KING, AND GAY

Acquarone, P., and Gay, L. N. "A Survey of the Pollen Flora in Baltimore During 1929." *J. Allerg.* 11 (1931): 336.

Carliner, P. E.; Nadman, H. M.; and Gay, L. N. "Treatment of Nausea and Vomiting of Pregnancy with Dramamine—Preliminary Report." *Science* 110 (1949): 215.

Chesney, A. M. "Joseph Earle Moore, 1892–1957." *Trans. Assoc. Am. Physicians* 71 (1958): 31.

Gay, L. N. "The Treatment of Hay Fever and Pollen Asthma by Air Conditioned Atmosphere." *J.A.M.A.* 100 (1933): 1382.

Gay, L. N., and Carliner, P. E. "The Prevention and Treatment of Motion Sickness." *Bull. Johns Hopkins Hosp.* 84 (1949): 470.

Gay, L. N., and Herman, N. B. "The Treatment of 100 Cases of Asthma with Ephedrine." *Bull. Johns Hopkins Hosp.* 43 (1928): 185.

Hahn, R. Personal communication.

Hampton, A. O.; Prandoni, A. G.; and King, J. T. "Pulmonary Embolism from Obscure Sources." *Bull. Johns Hopkins Hosp.* 76 (1945): 245.

Harvey, A. McG., and Shulman, L. E. "Systemic Lupus Erythematosus and the Chronic Biologic False-Positive Test for Syphilis." In *Lupus Eryethematosus*, ed. E. L. Dubois. 2nd ed. Los Angeles: University of Southern California Press, 1974.

Keeney, E. L.; Pierce, J. A.; and Gay, L. N. "Epinephrine-in-Oil. A New Slowly Absorbed Epinephrine Preparation." *Arch. Intern. Med.* 63 (1939): 119.

King, J. T. "Determination of the Basal Metabolism from the CO_2 Elimination." *Johns Hopkins Hosp. Bull.* 34 (1923): 304.

———. "Stenosis of the Isthmus [Coarctation] of the Aorta." *Arch. Intern. Med.* 38 (1926): 69.

———. "The Chemical Recognition and Physical Signs of Bundle Branch Block." *Am. Heart J.* 3 (1928): 505.

———. "Bundle Branch Block. A Case Analysis with Especial Reference to Incidence and Prognosis." *Am. J. Med. Sci.* 187 (1934): 149.

———. Personal communication.

King, J. T., and Bramwell, J. C. *Principles and Practice of Cardiology.* London: Oxford University Press, 1942.

Moore, J. E., and Keidel, A. "The Treatment of Early Syphilis. I. A Plan of Treatment for Routine Use." *Bull. Johns Hopkins Hosp.* 39 (1929): 1.

Moore, J. E., and Lutz, W. B. "The Natural History of Systemic Lupus Erythematosus: An Approach to Its Study Through Chronic Biologic False Positive Reactors." *J. Chronic Dis.* 1 (1955): 297.

Moore, J. E., and Mohr, C. F. "Biologically False Positive Serologic Test for Syphilis. Type, Incidence, Cause." *J.A.M.A.* 150 (1952): 467.

Moore, J. E.; Shulman, L. E.; and Scott, J. T. "The Natural History of Systemic Lupus Erythematosus: An Approach to Its Study Through Chronic Biologic False Positive Reactors. *J. Chronic Dis.* 5 (1957): 282.

Nelson, R. A., Jr., and Mayer, M. M. "Immobilization of Treponema Pallidum in Vitro by Antibody Produced in Syphilitic Infection." *J. Exp. Med.* 89 (1949): 369.

Shulman, L. E., and Harvey, A. McG. "Hashimoto's Thyroiditis in False-Positive Reactors to the Tests for Syphilis." *Am. J. Med.* 36 (1964): 174.

Turner, T. B. "Protective Antibodies in the Serum of Syphilitic Rabbits." *J. Exp. Med.* 69 (1939): 857.

———. *Heritage of Excellence. The Johns Hopkins Medical Institutions, 1914–1947.* Baltimore: Johns Hopkins University Press, 1974.

20. CARDIOVASCULAR RESEARCH AT JOHNS HOPKINS

Andrus, E. C. "Alterations in the Activity of the Terrapin's Heart Relative to Slight Changes in the pH Value of the Perfusate." *Am. J. Physiol.* 48 (1919): 221.

———. Personal communication.

Andrus, E. C., and Carter, E. P. "Q-T Interval in Human Electrocardiogram in Absence of Cardiac Disease." *Trans. Soc. Clin. Invest., J.A.M.A.* 78 (1921, 1922).

———. "The Genesis of Normal and Abnormal Cardiac Rhythm." *Science* 58 (1923): 376.

———. "The Development and Propagation of the Excitatory Process in the Perfused Heart." *Heart* 11 (1924): 94.

———. "The Mechanism of the Action of the Hydrogen Ion upon the Cardiac Rhythm." *J. Clin. Invest.* 3 (1927): 555.

Andrus, E. C., and Drury, A. N. "The Influence of Hydrogen-Ion Concentration upon Conduction in the Auricle of the Perfused Mammalian Heart." *Heart* 11 (1924): 389.

Andrus, E. C., and Hill, W. H. P. "The Cardiac Factor in the 'Pressor' Effects of Renin and Angiotonin." *J. Exp. Med.* 74 (1941): 91.

Andrus, E. C.; McEachern, D.; Perlzweig, W. A.; and Herman, S. "Comparative Sensitivity to Oxygen-Want and Sodium Lactate of the Hearts of Normal and Thyroxinized Animals (with Notes on Chemical Analysis of Muscle)." *J. Clin Invest.* 9 (1930): 16.

Andrus, E. C., and Wilcox, H. B., Jr. "Anaphylaxis in the Isolated Heart." *J. Exp. Med.* 67 (1938): 169.

Barker, L. F.; Hirschfelder, A. D.; and Bond, G. M. "Personal Experience in Electrocardiographic Work with the Use of the Edelmann String Galvanometer (Smaller Model)." *Trans. Assoc. Am. Physicians* 25 (1910): 648.

Blalock, A. "Surgical Procedures Employed and Anatomical Variations Encountered in the Treatment of Congenital Pulmonic Stenosis." *Surg. Gynecol. Obstet.* 87 (1948): 385.

Blalock, A., and Taussig, H. N. "The Surgical Treatment of Malformations of the Heart in Which There is Pulmonary Stenosis or Pulmonary Atresia." *J.A.M.A.* 128 (1945): 189.

Burch, G. E., and DePasquale, N. P. *A History of Electrocardiography.* Chicago: Yearbook Medical Publishers, 1964.

Carter, E. P. "William Sydney Thayer (June 23, 1864–December 10, 1932)." *Bull. Johns Hopkins Hosp.* 52 (1933): 1.

Carter, E. P.; Richter, C. P.; and Greene, C. H. "A Graphic Application of the Principles of the Equilateral Triangle for Determining the Direction of the Electrical Axes." *Johns Hopkins Hosp. Bull.* 30 (1919): 162.

Craib, W. H. "A Study of the Electrical Field Surrounding Active Heart Muscle." *Heart* 14 (1927): 71.

Erlanger, J. "The Physiology of Heart Block in Mammals with Special Reference to Stokes Adams Disease." *J. Exp. Med.* 7 (1905): 676.

———. "A New Instrument for Determining Systolic and Diastolic Pressure in Man." *Am. J. Physiol.* 6 (1901): 22.

———. "A Physiologist Reminisces." *An. Rev. Physiol.* 26 (1964): 1.

Erlanger, J., and Hewlett, A. W. "A Study of the Metabolism in Dogs with Shortened Small Intestines." *Am. J. Physiol.* 6 (1901): 1.

Erlanger, J., and Hirschfelder, A. D. "Further Studies in the Heart-Block in Mammals." *Am. J. Physiol.* 15 (1906): 153.

Erlanger, J., and Hooker, D. R. "An Experimental Study of Blood Pressure and Pulse Pressure in Man." *Johns Hopkins Hosp. Rep.* 12 (1904): 145.

Eyster, J. A. E., and Hooker, D. R. "Instrument for Determination of Venous Pressure in Man." *Johns Hopkins Hosp. Bull.* 19 (1908): 274.

Harlan, H. D., et al. "The Thayer Memorial Exercises Held in the Hurd Memorial Amphitheatre, Feb. 24th, 1934." *Johns Hopkins Hosp. Bull.* 55 (1934): 201.

Hooker, D. R.; Kouwenhoven, W. B.; and Langworthy, O. R. "Effect of Alternating Electrical Currents on the Heart." *Am. J. Physiol.* 103 (1933): 444.

Howell, W. H. "Vagus Inhibition of the Heart in Its Relation to the Inorganic Salts of the Blood." *Am. J. Physiol.* 15 (1906): 280.

Howell, W. H., and Duke, W. W. "Experiments on the Isolated Mammalian Heart to Show the Relation of the Inorganic Salts to the Action of the Accelerator and Inhibitory Nerves." *J. Physiol.* 35 (1906): 131.

———. "The Effect of Vagus Stimulation on the Output of Potassium from the Heart." *Am. J. Physiol.* 21 (1908): 51.

Janeway, E. G. "Important Contributions to Clinical Medicine During the Past 30 Years from the Study of Human Blood Pressure." *Trans. Assoc. Am. Physicians* 30 (1915): 27.

Keefer, C. S., and Resnik, W. H. "Angina Pectoris: A Syndrome Caused by Anoxia of the Myocardium." *Arch. Intern. Med.* 41 (1928): 769.

Kouwenhoven, W. B.; Jude, J. R.; and Knickerbocker, G. G. "Closed Chest Cardiac Massage." *J.A.M.A.* 173 (1960): 1064.

Kouwenhoven, W. B., and Langworthy, O. R. "Cardiopulmonary Resuscitation: An Account of Forty-five Years of Research." *Johns Hopkins Med. J.* 132 (1973): 186.

Kouwenhoven, W. B.; Milnor, W. R.; Knickerbocker, G. G.; and Chesnut, W. R. "Closed Chest Defibrillation of the Heart." *Surgery* 42 (1957): 550.

"Lasker Awards Citations." *J.A.M.A.* 226 (1973): 876.

Lewis, J. K. "Stokes-Adams Disease. An Account of Important Historical Discoveries." *Arch. Intern. Med.* 101 (1958): 130.

Marshall, E. K., Jr. "Cardiac Output in Man." *Medicine* 9 (1930): 175.

McKusick, V. A. *Cardiovascular Sound in Health and Disease*, p. 23. Baltimore: Williams and Wilkins Co., 1958.

"Presentation of the Thayer Lectureship." *Bull. Johns Hopkins Hosp.* 41 (1927): 1.

Reid, E. G. *The Life and Convictions of William Sydney Thayer—Physician.* London: Oxford University Press, 1936.

Ross, R. S. "Presentation of American Heart Association Research Achievement Award to R. S. Bing, November 18, 1974."

Thayer, W. S. *Lectures on Malarial Fevers.* New York: D. Appleton and Co., 1897.

———. "On the Early Diastolic Heart Sound [the So-Called Third Heart Sound]." *Boston Med. Surg. J.* 158 (1908): 713. (Also *Trans. Assoc. Am. Physicians* 23 [1908]: 326.)

———. "Further Observations on the Third Heart Sound." *Arch. Intern. Med.* 4 (1909): 297. (Also *Trans. Assoc. Am. Physicians* 24 [1909]: 81.)

Thayer, W. S., and Blumer, G. "Ulcerative Endocarditis Due to Gonococcus, Gonorrheal Septicemia." *Johns Hopkins Hosp. Bull.* 3 (1896): 57.

Thayer, W. S., and Hewetson, J. *The Malarial Fevers of Baltimore.* Baltimore: The Johns Hopkins University Press, 1895.

21. HEMATOLOGICAL FIRSTS AT JOHNS HOPKINS

Auer, J. "Some Hitherto Undescribed Structures Found in the Large Lymphocytes of a Case of Acute Leukemia." *Am. J. Med. Sci.* 131 (1906): 1002.

Auer, J., and Lewis, P. A. "Acute Anaphylactic Death in Guinea Pigs: Its Cause and Possible Prevention; A Preliminary Note." *J.A.M.A.* 53 (1909): 458.

———. "Demonstration of the Cause of Acute Anaphylactic Death in Guinea Pigs." *Proc. Soc. Exp. Biol. Med.* 7 (1909): 103.

———. "Physiology of the Immediate Reaction of Anaphylaxis." *J. Exp. Med.* 12 (1910): 151.

Auer J., and Meltzer, S. J. "Anesthesia Produced by Magnesium Salts." *Proc. Soc. Exp. Biol. Med.* 2 (1904): 41.

Auer, J., and Meltzer, S. J. "Effects of Intraspinal Injection of Magnesium Salts upon Tetanus." *J. Exp. Med.* 8 (1906): 692.

Auer, J., and Meltzer, S. J. "Respiration by Continuous Intrapulmonary Pressure Without the Aid of Muscular Action." *Proc. Soc. Exp. Biol. Med.* 6 (1908): 106.

Brain, M. C. "Microangiopathic Hemolytic Anemia." *N. Engl. J. Med.* 281 (1969): 833.

Brem, T. H. "Verne Rheem Mason, 1889–1965." *Trans. Assoc. Am. Physicians* 79 (1966): 62.

Castle, W. B. "From man to molecule and back to mankind." In *Proceedings of the First National Symposium on Sickle Cell Disease, Washington, D.C., June 27–29, 1974.* Edited by J. I. Hercules, A. N. Schecter, W. A. Eaton, and R. E. Jackson. DHEW Publ. No. (NIH) 75–723, Bethesda, Md., 1974.

Castle, W. B. Personal communication.

Childs, B.; Zinkham, W.; Brown, E. A.; Kimbro, E. L.; and Torbert, J. W. "A Genetic Study of a Defect in Glutathione Metabolism of the Erythrocyte." *Bull. Johns Hopkins Hosp.* 102 (1958): 21.

Clough, M. C., and Richter, I. M. "A Study of an Autoagglutinin Occurring in a Human Serum." *Johns Hopkins Hosp. Bull.* 29 (1918): 86.

Dacie, J. V. *The Haemolytic Anemias; Congenital and Acquired.* Part II, *The Autoimmune Haemolytic Anemias.* 2nd ed. New York: Grune and Stratton, 1963.

Dacie, J. V. *The Haemolytic Anemias; Congenital and Acquired.* Part IV, *Drug-Induced Haemolytic Anemias.* 2nd ed. New York: Grune and Stratton, 1967.

Freiman, J. A. "Origin of Auer Bodies." *Blood* 27 (1966): 499.

Harvey, A. McG., and Janeway, C. A. "The Development of Acute Hemolytic Anemia During the Administration of Sulfanilamide." *J.A.M.A.* 109 (1937): 12.

Howell, W. H. "The Life-History of the Formed Elements of the Blood, Especially the Red Corpuscles." *J. Morphol.* 4 (1890): 57.

Huck, J. G. "Sickle Cell Anemia." *Johns Hopkins Hosp. Bull.* 34 (1923): 335.

Kinsella, R. "John Auer (1875–1948)." *Trans. Assoc. Am. Physicians* 61 (1948): 6.

Lerner, A. B., and Watson, C. J. "Studies of Cryoglobulins: Unusual Purpura Associated with Presence of High Concentrations of Cryoglobulin [Cold Perceptible Serum Globulin]." *Am. J. Med. Sci.* 214 (1947): 410.

Marsh, G. W., and Lewis, S. M. "Cardiac Hemolytic Anemia." *Semin. Hematol.* 6 (1969): 133.

Mason, V. R. "Sickle Cell Anemia." *J.A.M.A.* 79 (1922): 1318.

Meltzer, S. J., and Welch, W. H. "The Behavior of Red Blood Corpuscles When Shaken with Indifferent Substances." *J. Physiol.* (Lond.) 5 (1884–85): 255.

Monroe, W. M., and Strauss, A. F. "Intravascular Hemolysis—A Morphologic Study of Schizocytes in Thrombotic Purpura and Other Diseases." *South. Med. J.* 46 (1953): 837.

Moss, W. L. "Studies on Iso-agglutinins and Isohemolysins." *Trans. Assoc. Am. Physicians* 24 (1909): 419.

Moss, W. L. "Paroxysmal Hemoglobinuria—Blood Studies in Three Cases." *Johns Hopkins Hosp. Bull.* 22 (1911): 278.

Moss, W. L. "A Simple Method for the Indirect Transfusion of Blood." *Am. J. Med. Sci.* 147 (1914): 698.

Moss, W. L. "A Simplified Method for Determining the Isoagglutinin Group in the Selection of Donors for Blood Transfusion." *J.A.M.A.* 68 (1917): 1905.

Osler, W. "An Account of Certain Organisms Occurring in the Liquor Sanguinis [Communicated by Prof. J. Burdon Sanderson, Received May 6, 1874]." *Proc. R. Soc. Lond.* 22 (1873–74): 391. Also, *Month. Micr. J.* 12 (1874): 141.

———. "The Third Corpuscle of the Blood." *Med. News,* December 29, 1883, p. 3.

Pauling, L.; Itano, H. A.; Surger, S. J.; and Wills, I. C. "Sickle Cell Anemia, a Molecular Disease." *Science* 110 (1949): 543.

Rieder, R. F.; Zinkham, W. H.; and Holtzman, W. H. "Hemoglobin Zurich." *Am. J. Med.* 39 (1965): 4.

Sherman, I. J. "The Sickling Phenomenon with Special Reference to the Differentiation of Sickle Cell Anemia from the Sickle Cell Trait." *Bull. Johns Hopkins Hosp.* 67 (1940): 309.

Thayer, W. S. "Splenic Myelogenous Leukemia—Exhibition of a Patient." *Johns Hopkins Hosp. Bull.* 2 (1891): 84.

Toulmin, H. E. "Two Cases of Leukemia; Presented Before the Johns Hopkins Medical Society, March 2, 1891." *Johns Hopkins Hosp. Bull.* 2 (1891): 84.

Watson, C. J. "Presentation of the George M. Kober Medal to Maxwell M. Wintrobe." *Trans. Assoc. Am. Physicians* 87 (1974): 45.

———. Personal communication.

Weistock, R. Personal communication.

Wintrobe, M. M. *Clinical Hematology.* 6th ed. Philadelphia: Lea and Febiger, 1968, p. 1018.

———. "Classification of the Anemias on the Basis of Differences in the Size and Hemoglobin Content of the Red Corpuscles." *Proc. Soc. Exp. Biol. Med.* 27 (1930): 1071.

———. "The Erythrocyte in Man." *Medicine* 9 (1930): 195.

———. "A Hematological Odyssey, 1926–66." *Johns Hopkins Med. J* 120 (1967): 287.

———. "Anemia, Serendipity and Science." *J.A.M.A.* 210 (1969): 318.

———. Personal communication.

———. "Acceptance of the Kober Medal for 1974." *Trans. Assoc. Am. Physicians* 87 (1974): 58.

Wintrobe, M. M., and Buell, M. V. "Hyperproteinemia Associated with Multiple Myeloma. With a Report of a Case in Which an Extraordinary Hyperproteinemia Was Associated with Thrombosis of the Retinal Veins and Symptoms Suggesting Raynaud's Disease." *Bull. Johns Hopkins Hosp.* 52 (1933): 156.

Wintrobe, M. M.; Matthews, E.; Pollack, R.; and Dobyns, B. M. "A Familial Hemopoietic Disorder in Italian Adolescents and Adults." *J.A.M.A.* 114 (1940): 1550.

Wintrobe, M. M., and Shumacker, H. S., Jr. "The Occurrence of Macrocytic Anemia in Association with Disorder of the Liver." *Bull. Johns Hopkins Hosp.* 52 (1933): 387.

22. RESEARCH AT JOHNS HOPKINS ON THE THYROID GLAND AND ITS DISEASES

Astwood, E. B. "Chemotherapy of Hyperthyroidism." *Harvey Lecture Series,* 40 (1944–45): 195.

———. Personal communication.

———. "Treatment of Hyperthyroidism with Thiourea and Thiouracil." *J.A.M.A.* 122 (1943): 78.

———. "Thiouracil Treatment in Hyperthyroidism." *J. Clin. Endocrinol.* 4 (1944): 229.

———. "The Chemical Nature of Compounds Which Inhibit the Function of the Thyroid Gland." *J. Pharm. Exp. Therap.* 78 (1943): 79.

Astwood, E. B., and Bissell, A. "Effect of Thiouracil in the Iodine Content of the Thyroid Gland." *Endocrinology* 34 (1944): 282.

Chesney, A. M.; Clawson, T. A.; and Webster, B. "Endocrine Goiter in Rabbits. I. Incidence and Characteristics." *Bull. Johns Hopkins Hosp.* 43 (1928): 261.

Follis, R. H., Jr. "Presentation of the Kober Medal for 1960 to David Marine." *Trans. Assoc. Am. Physicians* 73 (1960): 51.

Halsted, W. S. "The Operative Story of Goitre." *Johns Hopkins Hosp. Reports* 19 (1920): 71.

Howard, J. E. "Treatment of Thyrotoxicosis." *J.A.M.A.* 202 (1967): 146.

———. Personal communication.

Lewis, P.; Lee, F. C.; and Astwood, E. B. "Some Observations on Intermedin." *Bull. Johns Hopkins Hosp.* 61 (1938): 198.

MacCallum, W. G. "The Pathology of Exophthalmic Goiter." *J.A.M.A.* 49 (1907): 1158.

Mackenzie, C. G. Personal communication.

———. "Differentiation of the Antithyroid Action of Thiouracil, Thiourea and PABA from Sulfonamides by Iodine Administration." *Endocrinology* 40 (1947): 137.

Mackenzie, C. G., and Mackenzie, J. B.: "Effect of Sulfonamides and Thioureas on Thyroid Gland and Basal Metabolism." *Endocrinology* 32 (1943): 185.

Mackenzie, J. B.; Mackenzie, C. G.; and McCollum, E. V. "Effect of Sulfanilyl Guanidine on Thyroid of Rat." *Science* 94 (1941), 518.

Mackenzie, J., and Mackenzie, C. G. "Effect of Prolonged and Intermittent Sulfonamide Feeding on the Basal Metabolic Rate, Thyroid and Pituitary." *Bull. Johns Hopkins Hosp.* 74 (1944): 85.

Marine, D. "On the Occurrence and Physiological Nature of Glandular Hyperplasia of the Thyroid [Dog and Sheep], Together with Remarks on Important Clinical [human] Problems. *Johns Hopkins Hosp. Bull.* 18 (1907): 359.

Marine, D.; Baumann, E. J.; Webster, B.; and Cipra, A. "Effect of Drying in Air on the Goiter-Producing Substance in Cabbage." *Proc. Soc. Exp. Biol. Med.* 27 (1930): 1025.

Nissen, R., and Wilson, R. H. L. *History of Chest Surgery*, p. 47. Springfield, Ill.: Charles C Thomas, 1960.

Richter, C. P., and Clisby, K. H. "Toxic Effects of Bittertasting Phenylthiocarbamide." *Arch. Path.* 33 (1942): 46.

Rienhoff, W. F., Jr. Personal communication.

———. "Gross and Microscopic Structure of the Thyroid Gland in Man." *Arch. Surg.* 19 (1929): 986.

———. "A New Conception of Some Morbid Changes in Diseases of the Thyroid Based on Experimental Studies of the Normal Gland and the Thyroid Gland in Exophthalmic Goiter." *West. J. Surg. Obst. Gyn.*, June 1931, p. 421.

———. "Pneumonectomy—A Preliminary Report of the Operative Technique in Two Successful Cases." *Bull. Johns Hopkins Hosp.* 53 (1933): 590.

———. "The Histological Changes Brought About in Cases of Exophthalmic Goiter by the Administration of Iodine." *Bull. Johns Hopkins Hosp.* 37 (1925): 285.

Turner, T. B. "Alan Mason Chesney (1888–1964)." *Trans. Assoc. Am. Physicians* 78 (1965): 17.

Webster, B. Personal communication.

Webster, B., and Chesney, A. M. "Studies in the Etiology of Simple Goiter." *Am. J. Path.* 6 (1930): 275.

Webster, B.; Marine, D.; and Cipra, A. "The Occurrence of Variations in the Goiter of Rabbits Produced by Feeding Cabbage." *J. Exp. Med.* 53 (1931): 81.

Webster, B.; Clawson, T. A.; and Chesney, A. M. "Endemic Goitre in Rabbits. II. Heat Production in Goitrous and Non-goitrous Animals." *Bull. Johns Hopkins Hosp.* 43 (1928): 278.

Webster, B., and Chesney, A. M. "Endemic Goiter in Rabbits. III. Effect of Administration of Iodine." *Bull. Johns Hopkins Hosp.* 43 (1928): 291.

Wilkins, L. "The Thyroid Gland." *Sci. Amer.*, March 1960, p. 119.

Williams, R. H., and Bissell, G. W. "Thiouracil in the Treatment of Thyrotoxicosis." *N. Engl. J. Med.* 229 (1943): 97.

23. MORE BRIGHT STARS IN THE JOHNS HOPKINS GALAXY

Asper, S. P. "Dr. Howard at Seventy." *Johns Hopkins Med. J.* 131 (1972): 79.

Berlin, R. D. [by invitation], and Wood, W. B., Jr. "Molecular Mechanisms Involved in the Release of Pyrogen from Polymorphonuclear Leucocytes." *Trans. Assoc. Am. Physicians* 75 (1962): 190.

Berlin, R. D., and Wood, W. B., Jr. "Studies on the Pathogenesis of Fever. XII. Electrolytic Factors Influencing the Release of Endogenous Pyrogen from Polymorphonuclear Leucocytes." *J. Exp. Med.* 119 (1964): 697.

Bigham, R. S., Jr.; Mason, R. E.; and Howard, J. E. "Total Intravenous Alimentation: Its Technics and Therapeutic Indicators." *South. Med. J.* 40 (1947): 238.

Bordley, J. E.; Hardy, W. G.; and Richter, C. P. "Audiometry with the Use of the Galvanic Skin Resistance Response." *Bull. Johns Hopkins Hosp.* 82 (1948): 569.

Collin, R. D., and Wood, W. B., Jr. "Studies on the Pathogenesis of Fever. VI. The Interaction of Leucocytes and Endotoxin in Vitro." *J. Exp. Med.* 110 (1959): 1005.

Conner, T. B., et al. "Unilateral Renal Disease as a Cause of Hypertension: Its Detection by Ureteral Catheterization Studies." *Ann. Intern. Med.* 52 (1960): 544.

Duncan, L. E., Jr.; Mirick, G. S.; and Howard, J. E. "Total Intravenous Alimentation; Its Effect on Mineral and Bacterial Content of Feces." *Bull. Johns Hopkins Hosp.* 82 (1948): 515.

Duncan, L. E., Jr.; Semans, J. H.; and Howard, J. E. "Adrenal Medullary Tumor [Pheochromocytoma] and Diabetes Mellitus: Disappearance of Diabetes After Removal of the Tumor." *Ann. Intern. Med.* 20 (1944): 815.

Edwards, H. T., and Wood, W. B., Jr. "A Study of Leukocytosis in Exercise." *Arbeitsphysiologie* 6 (1932): 73.

Frankfurter, F. "Personal Recollections of Jonas S. Friedenwald." *Johns Hopkins Hosp. Bull.* 99 (1956): 29.

Friedenwald, J. S. "A New Approach to Some Problems of Retinal Vascular Disease." *Am. Acad. Ophth. Otolaryng.*, November–December 1948, p. 73.

———. "The Formation of Intraocular Fluid." *Am. J. Ophthalmol.* 32 (1949): 9.

———. "Carbonic Anhydrase Inhibition and Aqueous Flow." *Am. J. Ophthalmol.* 39 (1955): 59.

———. "Current Studies on Acetazolamide [Diamox] and Aqueous Humor." *Am. J. Ophthalmol.* 40 (1955): 139.

Hahn, H. H.; Char, D. C.; Postel, W. B.; and Wood, W. B., Jr. "Studies on the Pathogenesis of Fever. XV. The Production of Endogenous Pyrogen by Peritoneal Macrophages." *J. Exp. Med.* 126 (1967): 385.

Harrop, G. A., and Thorn, G. W. "The Effect of Suprarenal Cortical Hormone upon the Electrolyte Excretion of the Intact Normal Dog. A Proposed Method of Comparative Assay." *J. Exp. Med.* 65 (1937): 757.

Howard, J. E. "Adventures in Clinical Research on Bones and Stones." *J. Clin. Endocrinol. Metab.* 21 (1961): 1254.

———. "Treatment of Thyrotoxicosis." *J.A.M.A.* 202 (1967): 706.

———. "Serendipity in Clinical Investigation. [On the Occasion of the Presentation of the Passano Award, June 17, 1965]." *J.A.M.A.* 207 (1969): 38.

———. "Hypertension Due to Ischemia of One Kidney: A Survey of 20 Years Experience." *Yale J. Biol. Med.* 41 (1969): 363.

———. Personal communication.

Howard, J. E., and Barker, W. H. "Paroxysmal Hypertension and Other Clinical Manifestations Associated with Benign Chromaffin Cell Tumors [pheochromocytomas]." *Bull. Johns Hopkins Hosp.* 61 (1937): 371.

Howard, J. E., and Cary, R. A. "Potassium as a Therapeutic Agent." *Trans. Am. Clin. Climatol. Assoc.* 60 (1948): 145.

Howard, J. E.; Duncan, L. E., Jr.; and Meyer, R. J. "Cellular Needs and Capability During Various Types of Starvation." *Transactions of Conference on Metabolic Aspects of Convalescence, 17th Meeting, sponsored by Josiah Macy, Jr., Foundation.* New York, March 29–30, 1948.

Howard, J. E., et al. "Relief of Hypertension by Nephrectomy in Four Patients with Unilateral Renal Vascular Disease." *Trans. Assoc. Am. Physicians* 66 (1953): 164.

———. "A Urinary Peptide with Extraordinary Inhibitory Powers Against Biological 'Calcification' [Deposition of Hydroxyapatite Crystals]." *Trans. Assoc. Am. Physicians* 79 (1966): 137.

———. "The Recognition and Isolation from Urine and Serum of a Peptide Inhibitor to Calcification." *Johns Hopkins Med. J.* 120 (1967): 119.

King, M. K., and Wood, W. B., Jr. "Studies on the Pathogenesis of Fever. III. The Leucocytic Origin of Endogenous Pyrogen in Acute Inflammatory Exudates." *J. Exp. Med.* 107 (1958): 279.

King, M. K., and Wood, W. B., Jr. "Studies on the Pathogenesis of Fever. IV. The Site of Action of Leucocytic and Circulating Endogenous Pyrogen." *J. Exp. Med.* 107 (1958): 291.

Kozak, M. S.; Hahn, H.; Lennarz, W. J.; and Wood, W. B., Jr. "Studies on the Pathogenesis of Fever. XVI. Purification and Further Chemical Characterization of Granulocytic Pyrogen." *J. Exp. Med.* 127 (1958): 341.

Maren, T. "Bicarbonate Formation in Aqueous Humor: Mechanism and Relation to Treatment of Glaucoma." *Invest. Ophthalmol.* 13 (1974): 479.

Moore, C. V. "William Barry Wood, Jr., 1910–1971." *Trans. Assoc. Am. Physicians* 84 (1971): 45.

———. "Presentation of the Kober Medal for 1971 to W. Barry Wood, Jr." *Trans. Assoc. Am. Physicians* 84 (1971): 47.

Moore, D. M.; Murphy, P. A.; Chesney, P. J.; and Wood, W. B., Jr. "Synthesis of Endogenous Pyrogen by Rabbit Leukocytes." *J. Exp. Med.* 137 (1973): 1263.

Richter, C. P. "A Behavioristic Study of the Activity of the Rat." *Comp. Psychol. Mongr.* 1 (1922): 1.

———. "Animal Behavior and Internal Drives." *Q. Rev. Biol.* 2 (1927): 307.

———. "The Electrical Skin Resistance." *Arch. Neurol. Psychiat.* 19 (1928): 488.

———. "Pathologic Sleep and Similar Conditions Studied by the Electrical Skin Resistance Method." *Arch. Neurol. Psychiat.* 21 (1929): 363.

———. "The Grasp Reflex of the Newborn Infant." *Am. J. Dis. Child.* 48 (1934): 327.

———. "Increase in Salt Appetite in Adrenalectomized Rats." *Am. J. Physiol.* 115 (1936): 155.

———. "The Pituitary Gland in Relation to Water Exchange." *Res. Publ. Assoc. Res. Nerv. Ment. Dis.* 17 (1936): 392.

———. "Two Day Cycles of Alternating Good and Bad Behavior in Psychotic Patients." *Arch. Neurol. Psychiat.* 39 (1938): 587.

———. "Total Self Regulatory Functions in Animals and Human Beings." *Harvey Lecture Series* 38 (1942): 63.

———. "The Development and Use of Alpha-naphthyl Thiourea [ANTU] as a Rat Poison." *J.A.M.A.* 129 (1945): 927.

———. "Domestication of the Norway Rat and Its Implication for the Problem of Stress." *Res. Publ. Assoc. Res. Nerv. Ment. Dis.* 29 (1949): 19.

———. "Phenomenon of Sudden Death in Animals and Man." *Psychosom. Med.* 19 (1957): 191.

———. "Hormones and Rhythms in Man and Animals." In *Recent Progress in Hormone Research*. Vol. 13, ed. Gregory Pincus. New York: Academic Press, 1957, pp. 105–159.

———. "Rats, Man and the Welfare State." *Am. Psychol.* 14 (1959): 18.

———. "Sleep and Inactivity: Their Relation to the 24-Hour Clock." *Res. Publ. Assoc. Res. Nerv. Ment. Dis.* 45 (1967): 8.

———. "Experiences of a Reluctant Rat-Catcher. The Common Norway Rat—Friend or Enemy." *Proc. Am. Phil. Soc.* 112 (1968): 6.

———. Personal communication.

Richter, C. P., and Clisby, K. H. "Phenylthiocarbamide Taste Thresholds of Rats and Human Beings." *Am. J. Physiol.* 134 (1941): 157.

Richter, C. P., and Ford, F. R. "Electromyographic Studies on Different Types of Neuromuscular Disturbances." *Arch. Neurol. Psychiat.* 19 (1928): 660.

Richter, C. P., and Hawkes, C. D. "Increased Spontaneous Activity and Food Intake Produced in Rats by Removal of the Frontal Poles of the Brain." *J. Neurol. Psychiat.* 2 (1939): 231.

Richter, C. P., and Hines, M. "Experimental Production of the Grasp Reflex in Adult Monkeys by Lesions of the Frontal Lobes." *Am. J. Physiol.* 101 (1932): 87.

———. "Increased Spontaneous Activity Produced in Monkeys by Brain Lesions." *Brain* 61 (1938) 1.

Richter, C. P., and Woodruff, B. G. "Lumbar Sympathetic Dermatomes in Man Determined by the Electrical Skin Resistance Method." *J. Neurophysiol.* 8 (1945): 323.

Shin, H. S.; Smith, M. R.; and Wood, W. B., Jr. "Heat Labile Opsonins to Pneumococcus. II. Involvement of C_3 and C_5." *J. Exp. Med.* 84 (1946): 387.

Smith, M. R.; Shin, H. S.; and Wood, W. B., Jr. "Natural Immunity to Bacterial Infections: The Relation of Complement to Heat Labile Opsonins." *Proc. Natl. Acad. Sci., U.S.A.* 63 (1969): 1151.

Smith, M. R., and Wood, W. B., Jr. "Heat Labile Opsonins to Pneumococcus. I. Participation of Complement." *J. Exp. Med.* 130 (1969): 1209.

Thomas, W. C., Jr., and Howard, J. E. "Studies on the Mineralizing Propensity of Urine from Patients With and Without Renal Calculi." *Trans. Assoc. Am. Physicians* 72 (1959): 181.

Thorn, G. W. "The Adrenal Cortex. I. Historical Aspects." *Johns Hopkins Med. J.* 123 (1968): 49.

Thorn, G. W., and Eisenberg, H. "Studies of Desoxycorticosterone." *Endocrinology* 25 (1939): 39.

Thorn, G. W.; Engel, L. L.; and Eisenberg, H. "The Effect of Corticosterone and Related Compounds on the Renal Excretion Electrolytes." *J. Exp. Med.* 68 (1938): 161.

Thorn, G. W.; Engel, L. L.; and Eisenberg, H. "Treatment of Adrenal Insufficiency by Means of Subcutaneous Implants of Pellets of Desoxycorticosterone Acetate [a Synthetic Adrenal Cortical Hormone]." *Bull. Johns Hopkins Hosp.* 64 (1939): 155.

Thorn, G. W., and Firor, W. M. "Deoxycorticosterone Acetate Therapy in Addison's Disease. Clinical Considerations." *J.A.M.A.* 231 (1940): 76.

Thorn, G. W.; Howard, R. P.; Emerson, K.; and Firor, W. M. "Treatment of Addison's Disease with Pellets of Crystalline Adrenal Cortical Hormone [Synthetic Desoxycorticosterone Acetate], Implanted Subcutaneously." *Bull. Johns Hopkins Hosp.* 64 (1939): 339.

Thorn, G. W.; Koepf, G. F.; and Clinton, M. "Renal Failure Simulating Adrenocortical Insufficiency." *N. Engl. J. Med.* 231 (1944): 76.

Thorn, G. W.; Koepf, G. F.; Lewis, R. A.; and Olsen, E. F. "Carbohydrate Metabolism in Addison's Disease." *J. Clin. Invest.* 19 (1940): 813.

Walsh, F. B., and Howard, J. E. "Conjunctival and Corneal Lesions in Hypercalcemia." *J. Clin. Endocrinol.* 7 (1947): 644.

Wolman, A. "Jonas S. Friedenwald—His Contribution to Medical Education in Israel." *Bull. Johns Hopkins Hosp.* 99 (1956): 37.

Wilkins, L., and Richter, C. P. "A Great Craving for Salt by a Child with Cortico-adrenal Insufficiency." *J.A.M.A.* 114 (1940): 866.

Wood, W. B., Jr. "The Action of Type-Specific Antibody upon the Pulmonary Lesion of Experimental Pneumococcal Pneumonia." *Science* 92 (1940): 15.

———. "Studies on the Mechanism of Recovery in Pneumococcal Pneumonia. I. The Action of Type-Specific Antibody upon the Pulmonary Lesion of Experimental Pneumonia." *J. Exp. Med.* 73 (1941): 201.

———. "The Mechanism of Recovery in Acute Bacterial Pneumonia." *Science* 104 (1946): 28.

———. "Studies on the Cellular Immunology of Acute Bacterial Infections." *Harvey Lecture Series* 47 (1951): 72.

———. "Studies on the Cause of Fever [Shattuck Lecture]." *N. Engl. J. Med.* 258 (1958): 1023.

———. "Phagocytosis, with Particular Reference to Encapsulated Bacteria." *Bacteriol. Rev.* 24 (1959): 41.

———. "The Pathogenesis of Fever." In *Infectious Agents and Host Reactions*, ed. S. Mudd. Philadelphia: W. B. Saunders Co., 1970.

Wood, W. B., Jr.; Smith, M. R.; and Watson, B. "Surface Phagocytosis—Its Relation to the Mechanism of Recovery in Pneumococcal Pneumonia." *Science* 104 (1946): 28.

———. "Natural Immunity to Bacterial Infections: The Relation of Complement to Heat Labile Opsonins." *J. Exp. Med.* 84 (1947): 387.

Woods, A. C. "Jonas S. Friedenwald: In Memoriam." *Bull. Johns Hopkins Hosp.* 99 (1956): 23.

24. JOHNS HOPKINS AND BIOMEDICAL COMMUNICATION

Ackerknecht, E. H. "Introduction." In *A Bibliography of the Writings of Henry E. Sigerist.* Ed. Genevieve Miller. Montreal: McGill University Press, 1966.

Billings, J. S. "The Plans and Purposes of The Johns Hopkins Hospital." In *Johns Hopkins Hospital. Addresses at the Opening of the Hospital.* Baltimore: Privately printed, 1889.

Burr, C. B. "Tribute to Henry Mills Hurd." *Am. J. Insanity* 46 (1899): 303.

Chesney, A. M. *The Johns Hopkins Hospital and The Johns Hopkins University School of Medicine—A Chronicle.* Vol. 2. Baltimore: Johns Hopkins University Press, 1958.

"Contributions to Embryology of the Carnegie Institution, Volume IX." Book Review. *Nature* 106 (1920): 170.

Cullen, T. S. "Henry Mills Hurd. The First Superintendent of The Johns Hopkins Hospital." *Johns Hopkins Hosp. Bull.* 30 (1919): 341.

Cushing, H. "The Binding Influence of a Library on a Subdividing Profession." *Bull. Johns Hopkins Hosp.* 46 (1930): 29.

Flexner, S., and Flexner, J. T. *William Henry Welch and the Heroic Age of American Medicine.* New York: Viking Press, 1941.

Fulton, J. F., et al. "A Farewell Dinner for Dr. and Mrs. Henry E. Sigerist." *Bull. Hist. Med.* 22 (1948): 5.

Richards, A. N. "*Journal of Biological Chemistry*. Recollection of Its Early Years and Its Founders." *Fed. Proc.* 15 (1956): 803.

Sabin, F. R. *Franklin Paine Mall. The Story of a Mind*. Baltimore: Johns Hopkins University Press, 1934.

Sigerist, H. E. "Preface." *Bull. Hist. Med.* 7 (1939): 1.

Temkin, O., et al. "In Memory of Henry E. Sigerist." *Bull. Hist. Med.* 31 (1957): 295.

Turner, T. B. *Heritage of Excellence. The Johns Hopkins Medical Institutions, 1914–1947*. Baltimore: Johns Hopkins University Press, 1974.

Voegtlin, C. "John Jacob Abel (1857–1938)." *J. Pharmacol. Exp. Ther.* 67 (1939): 373.

Weed, L. H. "Notes on Ceremonies Held in Connection with the Dedication of the William H. Welch Medical Library of The Johns Hopkins University." *Bull. Johns Hopkins Hosp.* 46 (1930): 3.

Welch, W. H. "In Memoriam: Dr. Christian A. Herter." *Johns Hopkins Hosp. Bull.* 22 (1911): 161.

Young, H. H. *A Surgeon's Autobiography*. New York: Harcourt, Brace & Co., 1940.

25. THE STORY OF CHEMOTHERAPY AT JOHNS HOPKINS:

PERRIN H. LONG, ELEANOR A. BLISS, AND E. KENNERLY MARSHALL, JR.

Bliss, E. A. Personal communication.

Dudley, Sir Sheldon R. *Our National Health Service; An Essay on the Preservation of Health*. London: Watts and Co., 1953.

Galdston, I. *Behind the Sulfa Drugs: A Short History of Chemotherapy*. New York: Appleton-Century-Crofts, 1943.

Long, P. H., and Bliss, E. A. "Observations on the Mode of Action of Sulfanilamide." *J.A.M.A.* 109 (1937): 1524.

———. "Para-amino Benzene Sulfonamide and Its Derivatives. Clinical Observations on their Use in the Treatment of Infections Due to Beta Hemolytic Streptococci." *Arch. Surg.* 34 (1937): 351.

Marin, T. H. "Eli Kennerly Marshall, Jr. (1889–1966)." *Bull. Johns Hopkins Hosp.* 119 (1966): 247.

Marshall, E. K., Jr. "A New Method for the Determination of Urea in Urine." *J. Biol. Chem.* 14 (1913): 283.

———. "A New Method for the Determination of Urea in Blood." *J. Biol. Chem.* 15 (1913): 487.

———. "The Comparative Physiology of the Kidney in Relation to Theories of Renal Secretion." *Physiol. Reviews* 14 (1934): 133.

———. "Scientific Principles, Methods and Results of Chemotherapy, 1946." *Medicine* 26 (1947): 155.

Marshall, E. K., Jr., and Vickers, J. L. "The Mechanism of the Elimination of Phenolsulfonephthalein by the Kidney—a Proof of Secretion by the Convoluted Tubules." *Johns Hopkins Hosp. Bull.* 34 (1923): 1.

Talalay, P. "Eli Kennerly Marshall, Jr. (1889–1966)." Minutes of the Advisory Board of the Medical Faculty, The Johns Hopkins University School of Medicine, January 31, 1966.

Tillett, W. S. "Perrin H. Long (1899–1965)." *Trans. Assoc. Am. Physicians* 79 (1966): 59.

26. DISCOVERIES AT JOHNS HOPKINS RELATED TO THE

NERVOUS SYSTEM AND ITS DISEASES

Blalock, A.; Harvey, A. McG.; Ford, F. R.; and Lilienthal, J. L., Jr. "The Treatment of Myasthenia Gravis by Removal of the Thymus Gland—Preliminary Report." *J.A.M.A.* 117 (1941): 1529.

Bard, P. "A Diencephalic Mechanism for the Expression of Rage with Special Reference to the Sympathetic Nervous System." *Am. J. Physiol.* 84 (1928): 490.

———. "Studies on the Cortical Representation of Somatic Sensibility." *Harvey Lecture Series* 33 (1937): 143. (Also, *Bull. N.Y. Acad. Med.* 14 [1938]: 585.)

———. "Central Nervous Mechanisms for Emotional Behavior Patterns in Animals." *Res. Publ. Assoc. Res. Nerv. Ment. Dis.* 19 (1939): 190.

———. "The Ontogenesis of One Physiologist." *Ann. Rev. Physiol.* 35 (1973): 1.

Bard, P., and Macht, M. B. "The Behavior of Chronically Decerebrate Cats." In *Ciba Founda-*

tion Symposium on the Neurological Basis of Behavior, pp. 55–75. Ed. J. London and A. Churchill. Boston: Little, Brown and Co., 1958.

Bard, P., and Mountcastle, V. B. "Some Forebrain Mechanisms Involved in Expression of Rage with Special Reference to Suppression of Angry Behavior." *Res. Publ. Assoc. Res. Nerv. Ment. Dis.* 27 (1947): 362.

Bard, P., and Rioch, D. "A Study of Four Cats Deprived of Neocortex and Additional Portions of the Forebrain." *Bull. Johns Hopkins Hosp.* 60 (1937): 73.

Bodian, D. "The Virus, the Nerve Cell, and Paralysis. A Study of Experimental Poliomyelitis in the Spinal Cord." *Bull. Johns Hopkins Hosp.* 83 (1948): 1.

———. "Experimental Studies on Passive Immunization Against Poliomyelitis. I. Protection with Human Gamma Globulin Against Intramuscular Inoculation, and Combined Passive and Active Immunization." *Am. J. Hyg.* 54 (1951): 132.

———. "A Reconsideration of the Pathogenesis of Poliomyelitis." *Am. J. Hyg.* 55 (1952): 414.

———. "Experimental Studies on Passive Immunization Against Poliomyelitis. III. Passive-Active Immunization and Pathogenesis After Virus Feeding in Chimpanzees." *Am. J. Hyg.* 58 (1953): 81.

———. "Emerging Concept of Poliomyelitis Infection." *Science* 122 (1955): 105.

Bodian, D., and Howe, H. A. "An Experimental Study of the Role of Neurones in the Dissemination of Poliomyelitis Virus in the Nervous System." *Brain* 63 (1940): 135.

———. "Experimental Studies on Intraneural Spread of Poliomyelitis Virus." *Bull. Johns Hopkins Hosp.* 68 (1941): 248.

———. "Non-paralytic Poliomyelitis in the Chimpanzee." *J. Exp. Med.* 81 (1945): 255.

Bodian, D.; Morgan, I. M.; and Howe, H. A. "Differentiation of Types of Poliomyelitis Viruses. III. The Grouping of Fourteen Strains into Three Basic Immunological Types." *Am. J. Hyg.* 49 (1949): 234.

Eccles, J. C., and Kuffler, S. W. "Initiation of Muscle Impulses at the Neuromuscular Junction." *J. Neurophysiol.* 4 (1941): 402.

Ford, F. R. *Diseases of the Nervous System in Infancy, Childhood and Adolescence.* 6th ed. Springfield, Ill.: Charles C Thomas, 1973.

Ford, F. R., and Woodhall, B. "Phenomena Due to Misdirection of Regenerating Fibers of Cranial, Spinal and Autonomic Nerves—Clinical Observations." *Arch. Surg.* 36 (1938): 480.

Harvey, A. McG. "The Actions of Quinine on Skeletal Muscle." *J. Physiol.* 95 (1939): 45.

———. "The Mechanism of Action of Quinine in Myotonia and Myasthenia." *J.A.M.A.* 112 (1939): 1562.

———. "Joseph Leo Lilienthal, Jr. (1911–1955)." *Trans. Assoc. Am. Physicians* 69 (1956): 19.

Harvey, A. McG., and Kuffler, S. W. "Motor Nerve Function with Lesions of the Peripheral Nerves. A Quantitative Study." *Arch. Neurol. Psychiat.* 52 (1944): 495.

Harvey, A. McG., and Lilienthal, J. L., Jr. "Observations on the Nature of Myasthenia Gravis. The Intra-arterial Injection of Acetylcholine, Prostigmine and Adrenaline." *Bull. Johns Hopkins Hosp.* 69 (1941): 566.

Harvey, A. McG.; Lilienthal, J. L., Jr.; and Talbot, S. A. "On the Effects of the Intra-arterial Injection of Acetylcholine and Prostigmine in Normal Man." *Bull. Johns Hopkins Hosp.* 69 (1941): 529.

———. "Observations on the Nature of Myasthenia Gravis." *Bull. Johns Hopkins Hosp.* 69 (1941): 547.

———. "Observations on the Nature of Myasthenia Gravis. The Effect of Thymectomy on Neuromuscular Transmission." *J. Clin. Invest.* 21 (1942): 579.

Harvey, A. McG., and Masland, R. L. "A Method for the Study of Neuromuscular Transmission in Human Subjects." *Bull. Johns Hopkins Hosp.* 68 (1941): 81.

———. "The Electromyogram in Myasthenia Gravis." *Bull. Johns Hopkins Hosp.* 69 (1941): 1.

Harvey, A. McG., and Whitehill, M. R. "Prostigmine as an Aid in the Diagnosis of Myasthenia Gravis." *J.A.M.A.* 108 (1937): 1329.

Howe, H. A., and Bodian, D. "Some Factors Involved in the Invasion of the Body by the Virus of Infantile Paralysis." *Sci. Monthly* 49 (1939): 391.

———. *Neural Mechanisms in Poliomyelitis.* New York: Commonwealth Fund, 1942.

———. "The Efficiency of Intranasal Inoculation as a Means of Recovering Poliomyelitis Virus from Stools." *Am. J. Hyg.* 40 (1944): 224.

———. "Passive Immunity to Poliomyelitis in the Chimpanzee." *J. Exp. Med.* 81 (1945): 247.

Howe, H. A.; Bodian, D.; and Morgan, I. M. "Subclinical Poliomyelitis in the Chimpanzee and Its Relation to Alimentary Reinfection." *Am. J. Hyg.* 51 (1950): 85.

King, A. B. "Dr. Ford as Seen by Former Students and House Officers." *Johns Hopkins Med. J.* 138 (1971): 103.

Kuffler, S. W. "Electric Potential Changes at an Isolated Nerve-Muscle Junction." *J. Neurophysiol.* 5 (1942): 18.

———. "Specific Excitability of the Endplate Region in Normal and Denervated Muscle." *J. Neurophysiol.* 6 (1943): 99.

———. "A Second Motor Nerve System to Frog Skeletal Muscle." *Proc. Soc. Exp. Biol. Med.* 63 (1946): 21.

———. "Discharge Patterns and the Functional Organization of the Mammalian Retina." *J. Neurophysiol.* 16 (1953): 37.

———. "The Two Skeletal Nerve-Muscle Systems in the Frog." *Arch. Exp. Pathol. U. Pharmakol.* 220 (1953): 116.

———. "Excitation and Inhibition in Single Nerve Cells." *Harvey Lecture Series* 54 (1958–59): 176.

Kuffler, S. W., and Hunt, C. C. "The Mammalian Small-Nerve Fibers: A System for Efferent Nervous Regulation of Muscle Spindle Discharge. *Res. Publ. Assoc. Res. Nerv. Ment. Dis.* 30 (1950): 24.

Marshall, W. H.; Woolsey, C. N.; and Bard, P. "Observations on Cortical Somatic Sensory Mechanisms of Cat and Monkey." *J. Neurophysiol.* 4 (1941): 1.

Martin, L. "Recollections of School Days with Frank Ford." *Johns Hopkins Med. J.* 128 (1971): 101.

McKhann, G. M. "Speaking of Dr. Ford for the Field of Neurology." *Johns Hopkins Med. J.* 128 (1971): 108.

Morgan, I. M. "The Role of Antibody in Experimental Poliomyelitis. III. Distribution of Antibody In and Out of the Central Nervous System in Paralyzed Monkeys." *Am. J. Hyg.* 45 (1947): 390.

———. "Immunization of Monkeys with Formalin-Inactivated Poliomyelitis Viruses." *Am. J. Hyg.* 48 (1948): 394.

———. "Distribution of Antibody to Poliomyelitis in Vaccinated and Paralytic Monkeys." *Fed. Proc.* 8 (1949): 618.

———. "Level of Serum Antibody Associated with Intracerebral Immunity in Monkeys Vaccinated with Lansing Poliomyelitis Virus." *J. Immunol.* 62 (1949): 301.

———. "Differentiation of Types of Poliomyelitis Viruses. II. By Reciprocal Vaccination-Immunity Experiments." *Am. J. Hyg.* 49 (1949): 225, 233.

———. "Persistence of Neutralizing Antibody for a Year Following Vaccination of Monkeys with Lansing Poliomyelitis Virus." *Proc. Soc. Exp. Biol. Med.* 75 (1950): 305.

Morgan, I. M.; Howe, H. A.; and Bodian, D. "The Role of Antibody in Experimental Poliomyelitis. II. Production of Intracerebral Immunity in Monkeys by Vaccination." *Am. J. Hyg.* 45 (1947): 379.

Mountcastle, V. M. "Philip Bard." *Physiologist* 18 (1975): 1.

Sperry, R. "The Growth of Nerve Circuits." *Sci. Am.* 201 (1959): 68.

Talbot, S. A., and Kuffler, S. W. "A Multibeam Ophthalmoscope for the Study of Retinal Physiology." *J. Opt. Soc. Am.* 42 (1952): 931.

Walsh, F. B. "Dr. Ford as He Appeared to His Colleagues." *Johns Hopkins Med. J.* 128 (1971): 105.

Woods, J. W.; Bard, P.; and Bleier, R. "Functional Capacity of the Deafferentiated Hypothalamus: Water Balance and Response to Osmotic Stimuli in the Decerebrate Cat and Rat." *J. Neurophysiol.* 29 (1966): 751.

Woolsey, C. N.; Marshall, W. H.; and Bard, P. "Representation of Cutaneous Tactile Sensibility in the Cerebral Cortex of the Monkey as Indicated by Evoked Potentials." *Bull. Johns Hopkins Hosp.* 70 (1942): 399.

Name Index

Abbott, Alexander C., 39, 266
Abel, John J., 6, 20, 22, 49–59, 92, 264, 343, 350, 367, 370–73, 396–98, 400, 407
Ackerknecht, Erwin H., 387
Albright, Fuller, 358
Amoss, Harold L., 395
Andres, Reuben, 291
Andrus, E. Cowles, 274, 275, 277–82
Ashford, Bailey, 21, 22
Astwood, Edwin B., 320, 325–27, 331
Auer, John, 51, 295, 296
Avery, Mary Ellen, 244–47
Avery, Oswald T., 136, 137, 318, 361

Baetjer, Frederick H., 60
Baetjer, Walter, 165
Bagley, Charles, 346
Bahnson, Henry T., 287
Baker, Benjamin M., 141, 142, 241
Bard, Philip, 260, 405–8, 416
Bardeen, Charles R., 22, 108, 119, 227, 373, 376
Barker, Halsey, 355, 356
Barker, Lewellys F., 40, 110, 125–29, 133–35, 166, 179, 221, 262, 266, 373, 375
Baumgartner, A., 71
Bean, Robert, 376
Becker, Bernard, 337
Becker, Hermann, 16, 179, 180, 182
Benjamin, John, 346
Bernstein, Alan, 166
Berthrong, Morgan, 337, 356
Billings, John S., 1, 4, 5, 43, 364, 367, 378, 380, 382, 384
Bills, Charles, 220
Bing, Richard, 283, 284
Blackfan, Kenneth, 60, 64, 68, 200, 206, 207, 244
Blalock, Alfred, 232, 236–38, 282–85, 422, 423
Bliss, Eleanor A., 392–96
Bloodgood, Joseph C., 71, 73–75, 180
Bloomfield, Arthur, 124, 172
Blumer, George, 220, 269
Bodian, David, 408, 410, 411, 414, 415
Boggs, Thomas R., 126, 127, 166
Bolton, B. Meade, 39
Bond, George S., 128, 129, 271

Booker, William D., 39, 195–98, 248
Bordley, James, 140
Bordley, John, 344
Bosler, Robert, 416
Bowditch, Henry P., 92, 367, 368
Bowman, Isaiah, 313, 389
Bridgman, Evelyth, 258
Broedel, Max, 16, 17, 68, 73, 173, 175, 178–80, 182, 183, 285, 316, 346, 373
Bronk, Detlev, 416
Brooks, Chandler, 407
Brown, James R., 8–10, 14, 22, 80, 248
Brown, Thomas R., 10, 18–22, 200, 294
Buell, Mary E., 309, 354

Carliner, Paul E., 260
Carrel, Alexis, 119–21, 283
Carroll, James, 40, 155
Carter, Edward P., 142, 241, 254, 255, 272–75, 277, 280, 281
Castle, William B., 169, 304, 308, 360
Chesney, Alan M., 22, 40, 196, 240, 251, 312, 317–22, 389, 399
Childs, Barton, 306
Clark, E. L., 101, 376
Clark, E. R., 101, 376
Clark, John G., 14, 16, 80–83, 179
Clark, William M., 120, 303, 360, 396
Clements, John A., 245
Clisby, Katherine, 323, 326
Clough, Mildred C., 164, 298, 302
Clough, Paul W., 257, 302
Cobb, Stanley, 343
Coburn, Alvin, 241, 242
Coffman, Ward, 122
Coghill, Robert D., 118
Cole, Gerald A., 146
Cole, Rufus, 126, 132–37, 240, 318
Colston, J. A. C., 378
Conley, C. Lockard, 291
Corner, George, 136, 376
Councilman, W., 266, 269, 367
Craib, William H., 272–77
Crawford, A. C., 51, 264
Crowe, Samuel J., 61, 68, 179
Cullen, Thomas S., 16, 40, 82, 83, 173–77, 179, 180, 182, 183, 186
Cushing, Harvey, 64, 68, 72, 179, 261, 338

Dandy, Walter E., 60–68, 179, 206, 304, 308, 402, 403
Dandy, Walter E., Jr., 66
Day, Robert, 337
Delfs, Eleanor, 326
Dieuaide, Francis, 272
Dobyns, B. M., 309
Douglas, Robert Gordon, 194
Duke, W. W., 265

Eastman, Nicholas, 326
Ecke, Robert, 408
Edsall, David, 159, 206
Ehrlich, Paul, 18, 23, 43, 170, 251, 266, 269, 291–94, 312, 372, 373, 390, 391, 394
Eisenberg, Harry, 350
Ellsworth, Reed, 350, 358
Emerson, Kendall, 354
Erlanger, Joseph, 261–64, 280
Evans, Frank A., 152, 165–68
Evans, Herbert M., 101, 316
Everett, Houston S., 15
Eyzaguirre, Carlos, 417, 418

Feinstone, W. Harry, 392
Felton, Lloyd D., 120
Felty, Augustus Rio, 152, 171, 172
Finney, John M. T., 36, 37, 40, 79, 248, 329, 331, 355
Firor, Warfield M., 64, 65, 351
Fisher, A. Murray, 310
Fitz, Reginald, 256, 268, 367
Fleischman, Walter, 223
Flexner, Simon, 37, 40–42, 106, 110, 125, 159, 198, 228, 266, 270, 370, 377, 394
Flint, Joseph H., 113, 262
Follis, Richard, 73
Ford, Frank R., 342, 343, 346, 401–5, 422
Ford, William W., 383
France, Richard, 241
Francis, W. W., 17
French, John C., 84
Friedenwald, Harry, 39, 333
Friedenwald, Jonas S., 333–39
Frontz, William A., 378

Gaither, Bradley, 10
Galvin, Gerald A., 82, 83
Gamble, James L., 202, 203, 206–10
Gamble, Thomas O., 194
Garrett, Mary E., 103, 225, 226
Gavin, Frank D., 39
Gay, Leslie N., 248, 257–60
Gemmill, Chalmers L., 407
Geraghty, John T., 53, 59, 377
Germuth, Frederick G., Jr., 147
Geschickter, Charles, 325
Gey, George O., 121–23

Gey, Margaret Koudelka, 123
Gilchrist, T. Caspar, 32–36
Gilden, Donald H., 146
Gilman, Daniel C., 5, 14, 22, 43, 51, 84, 85, 90–92, 150, 226, 365, 367, 375
Goldsborough, Francis C., 194
Goodell, Constantine, 12, 15
Goodnow, F., 382
Goodpasture, E., 318
Goodwin, Mary Stewart, 252
Gregg, Alan, 5, 313, 386, 387
Gregory, John E., 146
Grollman, A., 350, 351
Grumbach, M. M., 222
Guthrie, C. G., 167
Guttmacher, Alan Frank, 192

Hahn, Richard D., 252, 304
Halsted, William S., 5, 6, 8, 9, 16, 18, 22, 39, 60, 62, 65, 68, 69–74, 76, 78–80, 99, 100, 148, 159, 178–80, 195, 226, 248, 262, 266, 314–16, 327, 329, 331, 371, 380
Hamman, Louis, 67, 139–43, 149, 150, 221, 330
Harris, John W., 194
Harrison, Ross G., 101, 106, 114–19, 123, 373
Harrop, George, 317, 350, 351, 353
Hartman, Carl, 342, 350
Harvey, A. McGehee, 140, 150, 251, 305, 306, 399
Harvey, J. C., 139, 140
Henneman, Elwood, 407
Herman, Nathan, 258
Herter, Christian A., 39, 51, 368–72
Hewetson, W., 269
Hill, Philip, 282
Hines, Marion, 342, 346
Hirschfelder, Arthur, 126–29, 132, 264, 269
Holt, Emmett, 198–200, 203, 370
Holt, Emmett, Jr., 95, 148, 151, 344
Hood, Bowman J., 252
Hooker, Donald R., 263, 277, 280, 286, 374
Hopkins, H. Hanfield, 252
Horn, August, 16, 180, 182
Howard, Evelyn, 407
Howard, John E., 320, 331, 332, 354, 355–60
Howard, John Tilden, 20
Howard, Palmer, 354
Howe, Howard A., 408, 411, 415
Howell, William H., 6, 20, 85, 90–96, 147, 159, 262, 264, 265, 274, 277, 286, 288, 292, 342, 367, 396, 397, 400, 405, 406, 410, 411, 423
Howland, John, 199, 200, 202–11, 213–16, 220, 224, 233, 244, 409
Hubel, David, 417
Huck, John, 303
Hunner, Guy L., 15, 38
Hunt, Carlton C., 416, 417

Hunt, Reid, 40, 371, 373
Hurd, Henry M., 8, 9, 174, 229, 230, 365, 366, 369, 379
Hurst, A., 20
Huxley, Thomas, 1, 2, 85

Ingraham, Clarence D., 194

Janeway, Charles A., 244, 305, 306, 308, 326
Janeway, Edward G., 308
Janeway, Theodore C., 59, 199, 200, 215, 256, 264, 265, 306
Jennings, Herbert Spencer, 342
Jewitt, Hugh, 378
Johnson, J. M., 133
Johnson, Robert W., 39
Jones, Georgeanna Seegar, 326
Jones, Howard W., Jr., 82, 83, 122, 123
Jones, Walter, 50, 372, 396
Josephs, Hugh W., 214, 215
Joy, James, 211
Jude, James, 287

Keefer, Charles S., 118, 152, 167–70, 172, 308, 360
Keeney, Edmund L., 259
Keidel, Albert, 251
Kelly, Howard A., 5, 8–18, 38, 80, 81, 159, 175, 178–80, 182, 188, 189, 226, 248, 379
King, Arthur B., 403
King, Elizabeth, 225
King, John T., Jr., 248, 254–57, 260
Knox, J. Mason, 173
Koelle, George B., 336
Koepf, George, 354
Kouwenhoven, William B., 285–87
Kramer, Benjamin, 202, 209, 210, 213, 214, 216, 220
Krumrein, Louis, 310
Kuffler, Stephen W., 415–18
Kuttner, Ann, 240, 241

Langworthy, Orthello R., 286, 342, 346
Leutscher, John, 351
Lewis, Dean, 66, 67, 330
Lewis, Margaret R., 118–21, 376
Lewis, Warren H., 118–21, 376, 399
Lilienthal, Joseph L., 419
Lilienthal, Joseph L., Jr., 422–24
Lister, Joseph, 22, 24, 69, 70, 72, 78, 153
Loeb, Jacques, 27, 113, 119, 208, 350, 359, 371, 372
Loevenhart, Arthur, 133
Long, Perrin H., 241, 242, 325, 353, 390, 392–96
Longcope, Warfield T., 142, 152, 158–61, 164, 165, 241, 242, 258, 273, 317, 331, 351, 353, 354, 361, 383
Lord, Jere Williams, 33

Ludwig, Karl, 42, 43, 50, 98–100, 102, 126, 178, 180
Lynch, Frank W., 194

MacCallum, George A., 24, 108
MacCallum, John B., 24, 27, 84, 101, 107–13, 119
MacCallum, William G., 18, 20, 22–31, 84, 107, 108, 133, 148, 166, 204, 236, 262, 269, 316, 333, 342, 383
McCarty, Maclyn, 137
McCollum, Elmer V., 211, 213, 216, 220, 320, 323, 342, 371, 383
MacEachern, Donald, 142
McKelvey, John L., 194
Mackenzie, Cosmo G., 320–26
Mackenzie, John N., 248
Mackenzie, Julia B., 320–26
McKhann, Guy, 405
McLean, Jay, 94, 95, 359
Mall, Franklin P., 6, 39, 72, 75, 92, 97–103, 106–9, 112, 113, 118–20, 125, 126, 135, 159, 178–80, 212, 228, 262, 264, 266, 327, 328, 365, 367, 368, 373–76
Malloch, Archibald E., 26, 107–10
Marchetti, Andrew A., 194
Maren, Thomas, 335
Marine, David, 316–18, 322
Marriott, McKim, 202, 204–7, 210, 213
Marshall, Eli K., Jr., 320, 354, 383, 392, 394, 396–99, 405, 407
Marshall, Wade, 53, 407
Martin, Henry N., 2, 50, 84–91, 96, 118, 195, 262, 365, 405
Martin, Lay, 20
Mason, Verne Rheem, 302
Matthews, E., 309
Maxcy, Kenneth, 409, 410
Mayer, Manfred, 250
Meltzer, Samuel J., 290, 292, 296
Mencken, Henry, 182
Mendenhall, Dorothy Reed, 226–32, 295
Merritt, Houston H., 304
Meyer, Adolph, 341–43, 402
Meyer, William, 17, 70
Migeon, Claude, 223
Milnor, William, 286
Minot, C. S., 373–76
Minot, George, 40, 48, 167, 169, 256, 308, 311
Mohr, Charles F., 250, 252
Monjan, Andrew A., 146
Moore, Joseph Earle, 248–54, 260
Morgan, Isabel, 410, 411, 414
Morgan, Thomas H., 118, 119, 410
Morison, Robert Brown, 33, 248
Morrow, Glenn, 285
Morse, Arthur H., 194
Morton, Daniel G., 194
Mosenthal, Herman O., 377

Moss, William Lorenzo, 296, 297, 298
Mountcastle, Vernon, 407
Müller, Friedrich, 19, 125, 153
Murray, Anthony S., 16, 179

Nathanson, Neal, 146
Nelson, Robert, 250
Nichols, J. L., 29, 108
Nuttall, George H. F., 41, 266

Olsen, Betty, 354
Opie, Eugene L., 18, 22–31, 262, 370
Oppenheimer, Ella, 246, 342
Osler, William, 5, 6, 9, 12, 15, 17–19, 23, 24,
    26, 29, 40, 46, 50, 57, 80, 111, 113, 124,
    125, 133–35, 139, 140, 152–60, 166, 171,
    173, 195–98, 220, 226, 227, 229, 230, 248,
    263, 266, 268, 269, 288, 289, 294, 295, 347,
    350, 365, 367, 371, 379, 380

Padget, Paul, 252, 282
Park, Edwards A., 65, 199, 200, 202, 203,
    205, 209, 211, 213, 215–17, 221, 222, 231,
    233, 236–38, 342, 359
Parsons, Helen T., 211
Paul, John R., 166
Paulson, Moses, 20
Pearl, Raymond, 312, 342, 344
Peele, Talmadge, 408
Permutt, Solbert, 246
Pincoff, Maurice C., 166, 318, 355
Pirquet, Clemens von, 146, 196, 200, 223
Plass, Everett D., 194
Pleasants, J. Hall, 189
Pollack, R., 309
Powers, Grover P., 106, 200, 216
Pratt, Joseph, 257

Randolph, R. L., 248
Ravitch, Mark, 237, 238
Reed, Dorothy, 226–32, 295
Reed, Walter, 40, 155, 258
Reid, Mont, 318
Remsen, Ira, 22, 52, 53, 85, 182, 188
Resnick, William, 168
Retzer, Robert, 264
Rich, Arnold R., 95, 140, 144, 147–51, 322,
    323, 337, 361
Richardson, Edward H., 17
Richter, Curt P., 320, 323, 326, 340–47
Richter, Ina M., 164, 272, 298, 302
Ridley, J., 187
Rienhoff, William F., Jr., 141, 320, 327–31
Riley, Richard, 246
Rioch, David, 407
Rivers, Thomas, 409, 414
Robb, Hunter, 12, 14, 15, 40, 74, 248
Robinson, Canby, 258, 318, 319, 369
Robinson, Harry M., 251
Rous, P., 29
Rowe, Wallace P., 146

Rowland, Henry A., 85
Rowntree, Leonard G., 52–59
Rührah, John, 165
Russell, Frederick F., 132, 133, 377
Russell, William Wood, 38, 175, 179, 183,
    186

Sabin, Florence R., 97, 99, 101, 103–7, 119,
    121, 167, 170, 228, 229, 231, 373, 374, 376
Sampson, Albertson, 16, 81, 186, 187
Schaffer, Alexander, 246
Schenck, Benjamin R., 32, 36–38
Schlossberg, Leon, 285
Schwentker, Francis, 217, 222
Scott, Roger, 187
Scott, William W., 357
Sedgwick, William T., 86, 91
Sewall, Henry, 50, 91, 92, 98
Shepard, T. H., II, 222
Sherman, Irving J., 303, 304
Shipley, Paul G., 211, 212, 214, 216
Shryock, Richard H., 386
Shulman, Lawrence E., 250, 251
Sigerist, Henry E., 383–89
Simmonds, N., 211, 216
Slemons, J. Morris, 189, 194
Smith, M. Brewster, 347
Smith, Mary Ruth, 361
Smith, Richard M., 308
Smith, Winford H., 68, 354
Snowdon, Roy R., 256
Snyder, Charles D., 277, 407
Spencer, Frank, 284
Spencer, Madeline, 211
Sprunt, Thomas P., 152, 165–67
Stander, Henricus J., 194
Starling, E. H., 20, 262
Sternberg, George M., 39, 230
Stewart, H. A., 128
Srauss, A. F., 291
Streeter, George L., 101, 120, 376
Strong, Richard P., 20, 22
Sturgis, Cyrus, 257

Talbot, Samuel W., 286, 287, 416
Tappan, Vivian, 233
Taussig, Helen B., 232, 233, 236–39, 257, 282,
    283, 354
TeLinde, Richard W., 82, 83, 122, 187
Temkin Owsei, 385, 386
Thayer, William S., 18, 22, 23, 40, 139, 142,
    143, 150, 157, 256, 265–70, 293, 294, 330,
    355
Theobald, Samuel, 159, 248
Thomas, Caroline B., 240–44
Thomas, Henry M., 39, 248
Thomas, Henry M., Jr., 308, 309
Thomas, M. Carey, 103, 225
Thomas, Vivian, 238, 284, 285
Thomas, William C., Jr., 357
Thoms, Herbert, 194

Thorn, George W., 157, 350–54
Tillet, W. S., 159
Tisdall, Frederick, 202, 208
Toulmin, Henry, 292
Tower, Sarah, 342
Traut, Herbert F., 194
Trescher, John, 350, 402
Turner, B. B., 54
Turner, Thomas B., 249, 250, 252

Van Wyck, J. J., 222
Vaughan, Victor C., 49, 50, 98, 197, 377
Virchow, Rudolph, 12, 43, 153, 158, 268
Voegtlin, Carl, 27, 53, 126, 133, 204, 373

Wainwright, Charles, 143, 167
Walker, George, 251
Walsh, Frank B., 403
Walters, Henry, 182
Washington, John, 236
Watson, John B., 341, 342, 346
Webster, Bruce P., 317, 318
Weed, Lewis H., 318, 319, 376, 387, 410
Weistock, Regina, 310
Welch, William H., 5, 6, 18, 22, 26, 29, 30,
    36, 39–46, 51, 70, 72, 73, 79, 80, 99, 124,
    125, 158, 159, 174, 178, 189, 195, 199, 225–
    27, 229, 230, 262, 266, 288, 290, 315, 327,
    365, 367–71, 375–77, 380, 382–84

Whipple, George Hoyt, 40, 46–48
White, J. William, 74
Whitehill, Richard, 419
Wiesel, Torsten, 417
Wilkins, Lawson, 217, 220–24, 344, 354
Williams, John Whitridge, 16, 17, 40, 188–
    94, 376, 383
Williams, Miles Vaughan, 417, 418
Williams, Tiffany J., 194
Wilmer, William H., 240, 333
Wilson, Karl M., 194, 228
Winkenwerder, Walter A., 161
Wintrobe, Maxwell M., 155, 303, 309–13
Wislocki, George, 336, 337, 342, 407
Wolman, Abel, 339
Wood, W. Barry, Jr., 360–63
Woodhall, Barnes, 401, 402
Woods, Alan, 333–35, 416
Woolsey, Clinton, 407
Wright, J. H., 40

Yendt, Edmund, 357
Young, Hugh H., 10, 52, 53, 74–80, 222,
    251, 331, 358, 369, 377–79

Zierler, Kenneth, 291, 424
Zimmerman, E. L., 251
Zinkham, William, 306

Subject Index

Ablation, surgical, in study of cortical function, 407

Addison's disease: carbohydrate metabolism in, 352, 353; treatment of, 156, 350, 352

Adrenal cortex, tubular degeneration of, 149

Adrenal gland, extract of, 350; assay for, 351

Adrenogenital syndrome, 222

Allergy Clinic, development of, 258

American Journal of Anatomy, founding of, 373–75

American Journal of Hygiene, founding of, 376

American Pediatric Society, organization of, 196

Amino acids, isolation from blood, 54

Anaphylactic death, 296

Anatomical Record, 375

Anemia: microangiopathic hemolytic, 291; "secondary," treatment with copper and iron, 214; sulfonamide, 305. *See also* Sickle cell anemia

Aneurysm, infection of, 141

Angina pectoris, pathogenesis of, 168

Aorta, coarctation of, 257

Art as Applied to Medicine, Department of, 16, 175

Asthma, treatment of, 258

Auer bodies, 294

Axon, demonstration of nerve cell origin of, 114

Baltimore City Hospitals, 40; reorganization of, 189

Basal metabolism, 257

"Battle of Tin Horns," 109

Biologic clocks, 341

Biology, Department of, 90, 91

Birds, malarial infections of, 23, 24

Blalock-Taussig operation, 282

Blastomycosis, 32, 33

Blood: coagulation, 93; culture, 132; donors, 298; platelets, 288; staining technique, 268, 292

Blood pressure: measurement of, 127, 261, 263; study of, in man, 264

Bone, growth arrest lines in, 216

Bronchopneumonia, variety X, 164

Bulletin of the Johns Hopkins Hospital, founding of, 364

Bundle branch block: clinical diagnosis of, 254; electrocardiographic changes of, 272

Calcium: homeostasis, 359; metabolism, 28

Calculi, urinary, 357

Calorimeter, 202

Cancer: of breast, 70–72; early history of, 69; of prostate, 76; of uterus, 80

Carbohydrates, intolerance to, 214

Carbohydrate tolerance, 140

Cardiac catheterization, as a diagnostic tool, 284

Cardiac clinic: adult, organization of, 241; Harriet Lane Home, organization of, 233

Cardiac rhythm, mechanism of, 280

Cell, comprehensive description of components of, 120

Cervix, carcinoma-in-situ, 82

Chemical-biological course, 91

Chemotherapy, history of, 390–91

Child and maternal welfare, 231

Cholesterol, synthesis of, 207

Chorio-epithelioma, 189

Choriomeningitis, lymphocytic, viral, 146

Circulating anticoagulants, development of concept of, 95

Cirrhosis, hepatic, due to dietary deficiency, 149

Clinical-pathological conference, 140

Clinical scientists, training of, 134–35

Coarctation of aorta, operation for, 237

Cocaine, studies by Halsted, 72

Cold autoantibody, in mycoplasma infection, 298

Cooley's anemia, 310

Congenital heart disease, study of, 233–38

Coronary heart disease, factors in development of, 244

Coronary occlusion, symptomatology of, 140

Cryoglobulinemia, 308

Cullen's sign, 173

Cystoscope: air, technique of, 8, 14; Brown modification of, 8

Defibrillation of the heart, 286

Dehydration: circulatory failure in, 206; replacement therapy of, 206

Department L, organization of, 251
Dermatology: research in, 36; subdepartment of, 33
Desoxycorticosterone, 351
Diabetes mellitus, 30–31
Diarrhea, infantile, 198, 204
Ductus arteriosus, artificial construction of, 236
Dystocia, 189

Edelmann heart station, 129
Electrocardiography: contributions to, 272; doublet theory of, 274–76; introduction into Johns Hopkins Hospital, 128
Embryological studies, 101
Emphysema, 141
Encephalomyelitis, allergic, 217
Endocarditic vegetations, experimental production of, 128
Endocarditis: bacterial, due to gonococcus, 269; infectious, Osler's contributions to, 154
Endocrinology, graphic charts in study of, 223
Endometriosis: clinical and pathological types, 183; pathogenesis of, 187
Endothelial cell, 101
Eosinophilia, 18–21
Epilepsy, treatment of: with ketogenic diet, 221; by starvation, 208
Epinephrine: isolation of, 51; long-acting, 259
Erythrocytes, mechanical destruction of, 290
Eye, wound healing in, 336

Family clinic (Medicine I), organization of, 252
Felty's syndrome, 171
Fever, studies on mechanism of, 361, 362
Fluid, intraocular, formation of, 334, 335

"Gamblegrams," 209
Gamma-amino butyric acid, 417
Gammaglobulin, antibodies against poliomyelitis in, 411
Gas bacillus, 40, 41
Gastric contents, in diagnosis of tuberculosis, 197
Gastroenterology division, organization of, 20
Glaucoma, pathogenesis of, 334
Glomerular nephritis, relation of streptococcus to, 160
Goiter: due to dietary cabbage, 317, 318; endemic in rabbits, 317; experimental, due to iodine lack, 316; operative story of, 316; simple, thyroid administration for, 327
Gynecological pathology, first laboratory of, 174

Gynecology: Department of, 17; residency training program in, 15, 16

Hamman-Rich syndrome, 141, 142
Harriet Lane Home for Invalid Children, 196, 198, 200, 203–4, 209, 210, 214, 220, 221, 233, 237, 244
Heart: architecture of muscle of, 112; electrical axis, fixation of, 273; mammalian, method of study in isolation, 86, 87; muscle, fibrosis of, 110; muscle cell, histology and histogenesis of, 109
Heart block, experimental, 263
Heart failure, causes of, 139
Heart sound, third, 269
HeLa cell culture, 122
Heparin, discovery of, 94
Heritage of excellence, definition of, 5–7
Histochemistry, use in ophthalmic pathology, 336
History of medicine, early interest in, 380. See also Institute of the History of Medicine
Howell-Jolly bodies, 292
Hydrocephalus, 61, 62, 206
Hypertension, renal, 356
Hyperthyroidism, propylthiouracil and thyroid hormone in management of, 332
Hypoglycemia, spontaneous, 214
Hypophosphatemia, in rickets, 210
Hypothalamus, study of function of, 406
Hypothyroidism, in children, 221, 222

Institute of the History of Medicine, 382 ff.
Insulin, crystallization of, 51
Intensive Care Unit, organization of, 65
International Medical Congress of 1881, 153
Intervertebral disc, herniation of, 62, 64, 65
Intestinal contraction, 100
Iodine, changes produced in thyroid gland by, 329
Ions: inorganic, effect on heart, 93; inorganic, micro-measurement of, 210
Islets of Langerhans, discovery of relation to diabetes, 30, 31
Isoagglutinins, classification of, 297
Isuprel, value and dangers of, 259

Jaundice, classification of, 148
Johns Hopkins Hospital: address at opening of, 4; plans for and purposes of, 4
Johns Hopkins Hospital Reports, 365
Johns Hopkins School of Hygiene and Public Health, founding of, 46
Johns Hopkins University: address at opening of, 1; faculty selection, 84; plans for, 2
Johns Hopkins University School of Medicine, first class of, 18
Journal of Biological Chemistry, founding of, 370–72

Journal of Experimental Medicine, 41; founding of, 51, 367–70
Journal of Pharmacology and Experimental Therapeutics, 51; founding of, 373
Journal of Urology, founding of, 377

"Kensington Colt," 12
Kidney: artificial, 53, 54; blood supply of, 180; study of comparative physiology of, 397; study of function of, with phenol-sulphonphthalein, 52
Kidney stones, oxylate, prevention by phosphate, 357

Lead poisoning, bone x-rays in, 216
Leukemia: Auer bodies in, 294; study by Ehrlich's color analysis, 293;
Leukocytes, 360
Library: early facilities, 378–80; William H. Welch, 383
Liver, structural unit of, 102
Lung surfactant: effect of adrenal steroids in production of, 245; hyaline membrane disease due to deficiency of, 244; source of, 245
Lymphatic system, origin and development of, 101, 104

Magnesium salts, anesthetic properties of, 296
Malaria: aestivo autumnal type, 23; experimental, 398; studies of, 269
Malignant cell: cytological features of, 121; techniques of study of, 122, 123
Malta fever, porcine variety, 167, 168
Mammalian cells, culture of, *in vitro*, 119
Marine cycle, 317
Medical clinic, research laboratories in, 124
Medical education, improvements in, 97, 98
Medical genetics clinic, 254
Medical Society, educational value of, 153
Medicine and the Universities, 125
Medulla and midbrain, atlas of, 103
Metallic poisoning, treatment of, 160
Monocytes, studies in Malta fever by supravital staining of, 170
Mononuclear cells, origin and types, 170
Mononucleosis, infectious, 165
Morphine, administration of, to cyanotic child, 238
Motion sickness, 259
Muscles: limbs and trunk, development of, 119; voluntary, study of, 110
Muscle spindles, study of, 416
Myasthenia gravis, pathogenesis of, 421, 422
Myocardial blood flow, 284

Nephritis: experimental, production of, 160; salt-losing, resemblance to adrenal insufficiency, 351

Nerve impulses, chemical transmission of, 265
Nerves, regeneration of, 401
Nerve system: diseases of, in infancy and childhood, 404; embryonic transplantation and development of, 115; histogenesis of, 100; plasticity of, 401; small, in the frog, 417
Neurology, developmental, clinical aspects of, 404
Neuromuscular transmission: study of, in animals, 415; study of, in man, 421
Nitrogen balance, following injury, 359

Organs, study of structure and function of, 99, 101
Osler V, clinical research facility, 353
Osler's nodes, 155
Outpatient Center for Clinical Investigation, 254
Outpatient Department, organization of, 248
Ovarian agenesis, sexual infantilism with, 222
Ovary, "chocolate" cyst of, 186

Pancreatitis, hemorrhagic, 149
Para-amino-benzoic acid, goitrogenic activity, 322, 323
Paralysis, hypokalemic, 351
Parathyroid glands: anatomical studies of, 316; experiments in transplantation of, 315; research on function of, 26–28
Parathyroid hormone, action of, 358
Pathology, Department of, 39
Pelvis, contracted, 189
Periarteritis: due to drug hypersensitivity, 144; experimental, 146; role of hypersensitivity in, 144
Pharmacology: early development of, 49, first department of, 50; laboratory course in, 50
Pheochromocytoma, clinical recognition of, 355
Phonocardiography, technique for, 129
Pick's syndrome, early description of, 198
Pinocytosis, 121
Pithotomy Club, founding of, 29
Pituitary gland, posterior lobe, function of, 93
Placenta, infarction of, 190
Placing and hopping reactions, control of, 407
Plasmaphoresis, experiments on, 54, 55
Pneumonia: contribution to knowledge of, 135; mechanism of recovery from, 362
Poliomyelitis: experimental, immunization against, 410, 411; immunological types of virus, 411; neural mechanism in, 409; portal-of-entry of virus, 414; research

center for study of, 410; study of, 409; vaccine for, 414

Pollens, atmospheric, surveys of, 258

Polycythemia vera, 155

Postural reaction, cortical control of, 407

Potassium metabolism, 359

Practicing physicians, contributions of, 260

Prostate cancer: monograph on, 78; radical operation of Young, 76, 77

Prostatectomy: perineal method of Young, 75; suprapubic, 75

Pseudohermaphroditic-adrenocortical syndrome, 222

Psychohormonal research unit, 223

Pulmonary stenosis, experimental production of, 237

Pyelonephritis, chronic, contracted kidney due to, 161

Pyrogen, leucocyte, 361

Rat: activity cycles in, 341; dietary behavior in, 344; sudden death reaction in, 345; wild, behavior of, 345

Rat poisons, development of, 345

Reed-Sternberg cells, description of, 230

Reflex: grasp, 346; psychogalvanic, 343

Research Club (School of Medicine), 150

Research divisions, Department of Medicine, 126

Respiration, artificial, by continuous intrapulmonary pressure, 296

Resuscitation, cardiac, by external massage, 287

Retinitis, diabetic, 337

Rheumatic fever: study of, 233; sulfonamide prophylaxis in, 242

Rickets: blood calcium in, 204; curative effect of sunlight, 212; experimental, 211; pathogenesis of, 212–214; treatment with irradiated milk, 214

Rockefeller Institute, Hospital of the, organization of, 134

Rubber gloves, introduction of, in surgery, 73, 74

Sabin Building for Research, dedication of, 106

Sarcoidosis, of Boeck, 161

Scurvy, radiographic changes in, 216

Secretion, by kidney tubules, 397

Serum sickness, experimental, due to immune complexes, 147

Sickle cell anemia: abnormal hemoglobin in, 303; hereditary nature of, 302, 303; naming of, 302; splenic lesions in, 149; studies of, 214

Sickle cells, birefringence of, in polarized light, 303

Skin resistance, electrical, 343

Sleeping sickness, 57

Solubility product, calcium and phosphorus, 213

Somatic sensibility, cortical, mapping of, 407

Specialism, remarks on, by Osler, 197

Spleen, circulation of, 102

Spondylolisthesis, 189

Sporotrichosis, identification of, 36, 37

Sulfaguanidine, 398; goitrogenic activity of, 320–22

Sulfanilamide: method for determination of, 394; treatment of infections with, 392

Surgical technique, improvement of, by Halsted, 73

Syphilis: biological false positive test for, 249; congenital, clinic for, 220; experimental, immunity in, 319; latent, experimental, infectivity of organs in, 319; penicillin in treatment of, 252; renal lesion in, 149; research in, 251, 252

Taste, mechanism of, 345

Telangiectasia, hereditary, 156

Tetany: blood calcium in, 204; experimental study of, 27, 28; treatment of, by hydrochloric acid, 209

Thalassemia minor, 309

Thalidomide, phocomelia due to, 239

Thiourea: goitrogenic activity of, 323; in management of hyperthyroidism, 325–27; mode of action, 323, 324

Thoracic surgery, contributions to, 330

Thymectomy, in treatment of myasthenia gravis, 422, 423

Thymus, embryology of, 98

Thyroid: benign tumors of, in hyperthyroidism, 330; extirpation and transplantation in dogs, 315; reconstruction of, using wax model, 328

Thyroiditis, autoimmune, 251

Thyrotoxicosis, spontaneous remission in, 331

Tick bite fever, in Maryland, 212

Time lapse photography, 121

Tissue culture: in artificial medium, 120; method of, 115

Tissue diagnosis, frozen-section method of Cullen, 16

Tonometers, standardization of, 338

Transforming factor, pneumococcal, 137

Transfusion, indirect method of, 298

Treponema pallidum, demonstration of: in blood; in spinal and joint fluid, 319

Tuberculin, in diagnosis and treatment, 139

Tuberculosis: hypersensitivity and immunity in, 148; pulmonary, diagnosis of, in children, 197

Typhoid fever: high caloric diet in treatment of, 133; vaccination against, 133

Urea, method for determination of, 396

Ureter: female, catheterization of, 8, 10, 14; male, first catheterization of, 8

Uterus: adenomyoma of, 183; radical operation for cancer of, 80, 81

Venereal disease, control, course in, 252. *See also* Syphilis

Venous pulse, variations in form of, 127

Ventriculography, air, 60, 61

Vestibular reflexes, importance of, 402

Viremia, in poliomyelitis, 414

Visual system, function of, 417

Vital staining, study of living cells by, 106

Vitamin D, discovery of, 212, 213

Vitamins, role of, in blood formation, 312, 313

Vividiffusion, method of, 53, 54

Whipple's disease, 46–48

William H. Welch Medical Library, 383

Woman's Fund Committee, organization of, 226

About the Author ❧ A. McGehee Harvey
and Scientific Clinical Medicine
by Richard J. Johns, M.D.

COMMENT has been made in this series on the role of Mall, Barker, and Cole in the initiation of a scientific base for clinical medicine (Chapeter 12). It was A. McGehee Harvey, the author of this book, who brought this scientific approach to its full fruition. Dr. Harvey's highly visible implementation of scientific medicine came about through a fortuitous combination of circumstances, which included his personal attributes and interests, the influential position of the Department of Medicine at Johns Hopkins under his twenty-seven-year tenure as its director, and the concurrent national emphasis on scientific research during the post-World War II era.

Dr. Harvey's personal contributions to clinical research took the form of bringing techniques and discoveries in the basic biomedical or biophysical sciences to bear upon unsolved clinical problems. Not only was this fresh approach successful in Dr. Harvey's hands, but it also served as a model for his younger colleagues, and was woven into the structure of the Department of Medicine as it developed. Moreover, Dr. Harvey fostered the traditional approach to clinical investigation, that is, the careful analysis of aggregations of patients from which new insights were gained. This was done with equal scientific rigor, and was achieved both by personal precept and by embedding it into the regular departmental activities.

In addition to implementing a broad and varied program of scientific clinical *research*, he also brought the elements of the scientific method (scientific problem solving) to bear in an organized way upon clinical *practice* (clinical problem solving). The scientific approach to clinical practice was implemented so gradually, and it is now so widely accepted, that Dr. Harvey's key role in this remarkable change is scarcely perceived.

Dr. Harvey entered medical school at Hopkins from Washington and Lee University, with the firm intention of returning to Little Rock, Arkansas, as a general practitioner. Nevertheless, he soon became engaged in basic scientific research which had clear clinical relevance. In his first year he came under the influence of E. Kennerly Marshall, Jr., who was then the head of physiology. Dr. Harvey's interest in physiologic mechanisms led to studies with Marshall and W. W. Burgess on the site of action of antidiuretic hormone. Their comparative studies showed that the effect was seen only in species with a loop of Henle, leading to the conclusion that the observed effect was a stimulation of water reabsorption at that site. He first began his application of new techniques to the study of human disease when, as an assistant resident assigned to the heart station, he used the newly developed esophageal electrocardio-graphic lead to study the origin of paroxysmal tachycardias.

It was the advent of the drug Prostigmin, however, which kindled enduring in-terests in the physiological mechanisms of disease and led Dr. Harvey into an academic career. Prostigmin had been introduced in the treatment of myasthenia gravis, but the diagnostic specificity of the drug was undetermined. Dr. Harvey and Dr. M. R. White-hill demonstrated its diagnostic specificity in a controlled clinical trial in which they ad-ministered Prostigmin to a group of myasthenic patients and to a group of patients with a variety of other neuromuscular disorders.

This clinical study led Dr. Harvey to seek further fundamental knowledge of neuromuscular transmission, with a view to using that knowledge to investigate human disease. This approach of taking a clinical problem to the experimental laboratory and then bringing the new results and the new investigative techniques back to clinical studies is common now, but it was unusual in 1937. Dr. Harvey obtained one of the first American College of Physicians research fellowships, and was invited to work for two years in the laboratories of Sir Henry Dale at the National Institute of Medical Re-search in London. There, often in collaboration with another young scientist, G. L. Brown (the late Sir Lindor Brown), he engaged in a broad spectrum of basic studies of neuromuscular transmission, including the effects of curare, quinine, procaine, calcium, and tetanus toxin. They also studied the fundamental aspects of neuromuscular trans-mission in the fowl, in the extrinsic muscles of the mammalian eye, and in goats with congenital myotonia. In these studies he became proficient in quantitative electro-physiology and in the technique of the intra-arterial injection of substances close to their site of action.

At the completion of his fellowship, Dr. Harvey took the unusual step of working for a year at the Johnson Foundation of Biophysics at the University of Pennsylvania. He elected to do this in order to develop further the techniques he had used in England into methods suitable for the detailed study of neuromuscular function in man. These techniques revealed for the first time the nature of the block in neuromuscular trans-mission in myasthenia gravis and its similarity to partial curarization in man. In addi-tion to their intrinsic value, these studies opened up the entire field of neuromuscular investigation in human disease through the new techniques that Dr. Harvey developed.

When Dr. Harvey, at Dr. Longcope's invitation, returned to Hopkins as chief resident, he met Dr. Joseph L. Lilienthal, Jr., who shared Dr. Harvey's enthusiasm for quantitative physiologic studies of diseases in man. The fruits of this productive collab-oration are detailed in Chapter 26.

Assuming the directorship of the Department of Medicine in 1946, Dr. Harvey's personal interest in the use of basic scientific studies and techniques in the investigation of human disease found departmental expression in the formation of various divisional activities which were well ahead of their time: biomedical engineering (1946), clinical pharmacology (1955), cardiac catheterization laboratory (1955), medical genetics (1957), and clinical immunology (1963), to name but a few.

Dr. Harvey's use of the other, more traditional approach to clinical investigation—the scholarly inquiry into unusual clinical observations—also began early in his career. During the period of residency training each intern in medicine spent six weeks in the biological laboratory, during which he did all the bacteriology for the medical service. In this setting Dr. Harvey isolated an unusual organism, a *Salmonella suispestifer*, from a patient's blood stream. He then gathered twenty-one instances of this unusual infection and described for the first time its clinical features in adults. During his house staff days he engaged in similar studies of tuberculous pericarditis, Friedlander's pneumonia, amoebic hepatitis, and interatrial septal defect.

Under Dr. Harvey's leadership as physician-in-chief, this aspect of medical scholarship, one which is not limited to academicians but is open to all physicians, was made a regular part of the clinical clerkship. Each student prepared a "grand rounds paper" in which he investigated a clinical problem identified or an observation made while assigned to the in-patient service. The investigation usually involved a literature survey as well as an analysis of similar cases drawn from the hospital records. These reports were presented orally to Dr. Harvey, the visiting physician, the house staff, and fellow students at the end of each quarter. Many were of high quality and some were subsequently published. The quantitative impact of this exercise can be appreciated only when one recognizes that over two thousand medical students participated in this introduction to clinical scholarship under Dr. Harvey's personal tutelage. His own scholarship in this area served as a constant example through his and his colleagues' classic clinical studies of systemic lupus erythematosus, and other auto-immune diseases.

An entirely different contribution to clinical science also began with Dr. Harvey's appointment as director of the Department of Medicine. At age thirty-four, Dr. Harvey was a mature and well-trained internist, but despite his retentive memory for patients, he could not be regarded as having the wealth of clinical experience of some of his senior colleagues on the faculty. Characteristically, Dr. Harvey did not withdraw into clinical investigation and become a research professor, he immersed himself in clinical work. He consulted with the chief resident on a daily basis concerning problem patients; he made ward rounds three mornings a week; and he conducted that highly visible test of diagnostic acumen and judgment, the weekly clinical-pathological conference (Chapter 13). Rather than drawing upon a broad background of anecdotal experience, Dr. Harvey relied heavily upon his clinical skills in eliciting clinical information, followed by an organized, systematic, rational analysis of this information. This impressive application of the scientific method to clinical problem-solving won the respect of students, house staff, and faculty alike. Soon he was called into consultation on all manner of vexing diagnostic problems, both locally and internationally.

In addition to promulgating this systematic, scientific approach at Hopkins, Dr. Harvey reached a much larger audience with the publication, with Dr. James Bordley III, of their book, *Differential Diagnosis*. The approach was later extended in scope as the central theme of a new kind of medical textbook, *The Principles and Practice of Medicine*, of which Dr. Harvey is the chief editor. Thus, by precept and publication Dr. Harvey showed the way to scientific analysis of clinical problems, both diagnostic and therapeutic.

The national impact of the promulgation of these scientific principles by a single individual can be understood only by realizing the scope of Dr. Harvey's personal contact. As has been mentioned, more than two thousand medical students and eight hundred house officers have been taught these principles by him at the bedside. Furthermore, there is a multiplicative effect on this teaching of scientific principles in that there are presently sixteen departmental chairmen and eight medical school deans who received clinical training with Dr. Harvey. It was in this fashion that a new scientific approach was introduced into clinical medicine, a charge that was so gradual and disseminated so widely that it was scarcely perceived.

Dr. Harvey has said that ". . . the basic tools and concepts that we use in the pursuit of scientifically oriented practice stand out more vividly for us when cloaked in the robes of their historical origins." His own career in creative scholarship has contributed to this scientific practice, as well as to our insights into their historical origins.

References

Austrian, C. R., and Harvey, A. McG. "Friedlander's Pneumonia." *Internatl. Cl.* 3 (1937): 1.

Burgess, W. W.; Harvey, A. McG.; and Marshall, E. K., Jr. "The Site of the Antidiuretic Action of Pituitary Extract." *J. Pharmacol. Exp. Ther.* 49 (1933): 237.

Futcher, T. B., and Harvey, A. McG. "Amoebic Hepatitis." *Internatl. Cl.* 3 (1937): 1.

Harvey, A. McG. "The Origin of Paroxysmal Tachycardia as Determined by the Esophageal Electrogram." *Ann. Intern. Med.* 11 (1937): 57.

————. "Salmonella Suipestifer Infection in Human Beings." *Arch. Intern. Med.* 59 (1937): 118.

————. "Our Medical Heritage: Some Examples of Creative Scholarship." *Pharos* 36 (1973): 122.

Harvey, A. McG. et al., eds. *The Principles and Practice of Medicine.* 17th ed. New York: Appleton-Century-Crofts, 1968.

Harvey, A. McG., and Bordley, J., III. *Differential Diagnosis: The Interpretation of Clinical Evidence.* Philadelphia: W. B. Saunders, 1955.

Harvey, A. McG., and Masland, R. L. "A Method for the Study of Neuromuscular Transmission in Human Subjects." *Bull. Johns Hopkins Hosp.* 68 (1941): 81.

————. "The Electromyogram in Myasthenia Gravis." *Bull. Johns Hopkins Hosp.* 69 (1941): 1.

————. "Actions of Curarizing Preparations in the Human." *J. Pharmacol. Exp. Ther.* 73 (1941): 302.

Harvey, A. McG., and Whitehill, M. R. "Prostigmin as an Aid in the Diagnosis of Myasthenia Gravis." *J.A.M.A.* 108 (1937): 1329.

————. "Tuberculous Pericarditis." *Medicine* 16 (1937): 45.

Taussig, H. B.; Harvey, A. McG.; and Follis, R. H., Jr. "The Clinical and Pathological Findings in Interauricular Septal Defects." *Bull. Johns Hopkins Hosp.* 63 (1938): 51.